W9-CPF-182

Neuropsychiatry is a rapidly expanding field, linking the traditional areas of neurology and psychiatry, which has benefited greatly from recognition of the role of genetic and environmental determinants of psychiatric disorder particularly in childhood and adolescence. Based on 20 years of clinical experience and 18 years of research, Professor Gillberg has utilized his unique and detailed interdisciplinary knowledge of neurobiology, pharmacology, epidemiology and neuropsychiatry to compile this comprehensive reference to clinical assessment and treatment of the many neuropsychiatric disorders of childhood which, at a conservative estimate, affect 5 in every 100 children.

This is a unique and valuable reference resource that is sure to be welcomed by a wide range of professionals and researchers including child neurologists, psychiatrists, psychologists, speech therapists and special education teachers.

Clinical child neuropsychiatry

Clinical child neuropsychiatry

Christopher Gillberg

Annedals Clinics, Gothenburg, Sweden

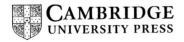

CAMBRIDGE
UNIVERSITY PRESS

PUBLISHED BY THE PRESS SYNDICATE OF THE UNIVERSITY OF CAMBRIDGE
The Pitt Building, Trumpington Street, Cambridge, United Kingdom

CAMBRIDGE UNIVERSITY PRESS
The Edinburgh Building, Cambridge CB2 2RU, UK
40 West 20th Street, New York NY 10011–4211, USA
477 Williamstown Road, Port Melbourne, VIC 3207, Australia
Ruiz de Alarcón 13, 28014 Madrid, Spain
Dock House, The Waterfront, Cape Town 8001, South Africa

http://www.cambridge.org

© Cambridge University Press 1995

This book is in copyright. Subject to statutory exception
and to the provisions of relevant collective licensing agreements,
no reproduction of any part may take place without
the written permission of Cambridge University Press.

First published 1995
Reprinted 1999
First paperback edition 2003

A catalogue record for this book is available from the British Library

Library of Congress cataloguing in publication data
Gillberg, Christopher, 1950–
Clinical child neuropsychiatry / Christopher Gillberg
         p.   cm.
Includes index.
ISBN 0 521 43388 6 (hardback)
1. Pediatric neuropsychiatry.   I. Title
[DNLM: 1. Mental Disorders–therapy.   2. Mental Disorders–in
infancy and childhood.   3. Neuropsychiatry–in infancy and childhood.
4.   Child Development Disorders–therapy.   WS 350.2 G475t 1995]
RJ 486.5.G54   1955
618.92´89–dc20
DNLM/DLC
for Library of Congress   94-33060 CIP

ISBN 0 521 43388 6 hardback
ISBN 0 521 54335 5 paperback

CONTENTS

PREFACE

This book is the result of stubbornness and 20 years of clinical experience with young patients. It is also the pressing by-product of 18 years of systematic research in the field of child neuropsychiatry.

When, in 1972, at the age of 22, I was first drawn to paediatrics and child psychiatry, two fields particularly attracted my attention: perinatal medicine and children with chronic disabling conditions. In perinatal medicine, my craving for drama and action was stilled. My longing for practical things was reciprocated by the infants who could not speak but who demanded to be handled with the utmost precision. In work with mentally and physically handicapped children and adolescents, my more reflective and analytical streaks prevailed. The interest in these divergent areas demanded a link, and I soon became obsessed with finding out the origins (first perinatal, later genetic) of chronic disability, and the pathways from infancy to childhood and later to adolescence and adulthood.

I owe a considerable debt to Bengt Hagberg, whom I met for the first time in 1972 and who introduced me to the 'neuroaspects' of children. It was also he who put me on to the tracks of research in 1975, and who taught me child neurology from 1977 and onwards. Bengt's need to associate all the diverse neurological and physical symptoms under various syndromal 'hats' served as an example for me in child psychiatry, whence I had erred already in 1974 and where I settled in 1978.

But, it was not Bengt who taught me child psychiatry. I had to learn that all by myself,

with just that little bit of necessary help from Gunilla Carlström. In the late 1970s, it was she who opened my eyes to the inner world of children, as we spent so many hundreds of hours together during the first epidemiological studies of children with attentional, motor and perceptual problems. And, it was not Bengt who taught me to be critical. My mother always told me I was born that way. But Olle Hansson, my tutor in scientific matters in the 1970s, helped me to combine criticism and analytical thinking (the little of it that I have) into something for which I am now often criticized; scepticism.

I believe that, had it not been for my encounter with young children with autism (and their parents) back in 1974, I would never have stayed so stubbornly and obsessively in child psychiatry. My need to find out what was at the root of the puzzling conditions, referred to as autism, has haunted me for almost 20 years now.

Meeting Iris Murdoch (Dame Iris) in 1980 changed many of my concepts: it was through her that I realized that the human condition will, most likely, never be captured in human frames. However, good may come from trying to analyse the contents held by the net weaved by human thinking and conceptions.

My encounter with Mary Coleman in Paris in 1983 led to the production of several books on autism with, and without, her stimulating collaboration. Writing these books made me realize that the neuroaspects of autism were stronger than generally acknowledged in the literature. Mary has remained the most exceptional friend in what was at first an uncertain field and now perhaps the most flourishing branch of the whole of psychiatry, i.e. child neuropsychiatry.

I also believe that, had I not met Lorna Wing and Uta Frith, I might never have become obsessed with Asperger syndrome. The realization that this syndrome overlaps with autism, and with some dominant traits in certain people I know, inspired new hope that child psychiatry (and child neuropsychiatry in particular) might hold more keys to a better understanding of humans and their brains than any other discipline in medicine. Again, the Aspergers in Dame Iris's fiction have made me think again about the bounds of this disorder.

Had I not spent time with all my friends and colleagues at the NYU Medical Center (Magda Campbell, Richard Perry, Judy Shay, Nilda Gonzales, Laura Sanchez, Kay Spencer, Jeanette Cueva and Jorge Armenteros, in particular), I would not have been in a position to have a personal clinical point of view in the field of child and adolescent psychopharmacology. I am also grateful to Ed Kollodny, Ruth Nass and Rene Guttmann at NYU, whose inspiring discussions have coloured the section on disintegrative disorder, Asperger syndrome and Landau–Kleffner syndrome.

The development in the last couple of years in the field of the new genetics (and, for that matter, in the field of the old genetics) has made it impossible not to regard child neuropsychiatry as one of the most fascinating scientific fields of all. The concept of the behavioural phenotype is among the most challenging and astounding that has emerged in the latter half of this century. A considerable portion of this book is devoted to all the named neuropsychiatric syndromes that now compete for space within that frame.

In the end, it was David Taylor, who, I suspect quite unwittingly, set me on the track to writing a textbook on child neuropsychiatry. His inspiring, unconventional, indeed, according to some contemporaries, idiosyncratic, general approach to clinical medicine (and, in particular, to neuropsychiatry) made me realize that the gap between research and clinical work needs to be constantly spanned by new bridges, and that in child psychiatry the gap is wider than in most other disciplines.

As with any clinical textbook, the people behind the syndromes constitute the real backbone. The young patients and their parents have been my most reliable source of inspiration and information. If it had not been for them, and for Carina, my wife and fellow child psychiatrist, the constant discussant with the soundest clinical judgement, this book would not have been conceived at all.

The book is intended for a wide readership, including child (and adult) psychiatrists and psychologists, paediatricians and child neurologists, speech therapists and special education teachers. I hope to be able to strike a tone which will appeal to other potential readers as well, including the families of children affected by neuropsychiatric disorders.

Christopher Gillberg, October 1994

ACKNOWLEDGEMENTS

I am grateful to Carina Löf for all her unselfish support in the production of this book.

Jan Wahlström provided helpful comments on the section of 'Genetic factors'. Sonya Heyerdahl took time out to help me with the section on hypothyroidism.

Marit Korkman wrote the brief section on the NEPSY test, and I am indebted to her for allowing me to include her text.

The Sunnerdahl and Wilhelm and Martina Lundgren foundations funded part of my six months at NYU Medical Center, New York, and this contributed to better informed sections on the psychopharmacological sections of this book.

Part I:
General methodological concerns

1 Introduction to clinical child neuropsychiatry

Over the last 20 years, child and adolescent psychiatry has managed to establish itself as a flourishing branch of medicine. Several major textbooks appeared (e.g. Rutter & Hersov, 1977; Rutter & Hersov, 1985; Noshpitz *et al.*, 1987; Lewis, 1991; Rutler, Taylor & Hersov, 1994) and thousands of empirically based studies were published. The clinical and research areas covered by child and adolescent psychiatry are enormous ranging from infant psychiatry to adolescent problems and from family relationship problems and sexual abuse to autism and anorexia nervosa.

The need for subspecialization gradually emerged, and volumes relating specifically to 'developmental psychiatry' (Rutter, 1980) and 'developmental neuropsychiatry' (Rutter, 1984) were published. These were fine pioneering works which contributed to the gradual, albeit usually implicit, delineation of 'child neuropsychiatry'. However, most of the work published to date has been in the format of individual scientific papers or classical research reviews. Clinical aspects have been summarily dealt with, if at all.

A textbook specifically on 'clinical child neuropsychiatry' has been needed for some time. To the best of my knowledge, this is the first such book to be published. It aims to cover those *infancy, childhood or adolescent onset disorders in which mental, emotional and behavioural problems predominate at one or other stage of development and for which biological factors have been shown to play a major pathogenetic/contributory role.* The emphasis, as the title implies, is on clinical aspects, but reference will be made throughout to empirical studies and results which underpin the clinical conclu-

sions. The scope of the clinical field surveyed is perhaps most clearly evident in the Contents, but Chapter 2 (on epidemiology) also contains summary information, and I shall therefore not dwell further on it in this context.

There are many instances in which the empirical basis for clinical recommendations is limited or lacking altogether. Obviously, in such circumstances, the views expressed, to a considerable extent mirror my own clinical approach. Wherever possible I have tried to indicate which conclusions represent my own personal opinion (and that of colleagues) rather than scientific fact.

References

Lewis, M. (Ed.) (1991). *Child and Adolescent Psychiatry. A Comprehensive Textbook.* Baltimore, Maryland: Williams & Wilkins.

Noshpitz, J.D., Call, J.D., Cohen, R.L. *et al.* (Eds.) (1987). *Basic Handbook of Child Psychiatry.* New York: Basic Books.

Rutter, M. (1980). *Scientific Foundations of Developmental Psychiatry.* London: Heinemann Medical.

Rutter, M. (Ed.) (1984). *Developmental Neuropsychiatry.* Edinburgh: Churchill Livingstone.

Rutter, M., Hersov, L. (Eds.) (1977). *Child Psychiatry. Modern Approaches.* Oxford: Blackwell Scientific.

Rutter, M., Hersov, L. (Eds.) (1985). *Child and Adolescent Psychiatry. Modern Approaches.* Oxford: Blackwell Scientific.

Rutter, M., Taylor, E., Hersov, L. (Eds.) (1994). *Child and Adolescent Psychiatry. Modern Approaches.* Oxford: Blackwell Scinentific.

2 Epidemiological overview

There are at least two ways to provide an epidemiological framework for child neuropsychiatry. The first is to find some reasonable overall boundary for child neuropsychiatry and establish what proportion of all child psychiatric disorders or of all children and adolescents have a neuropsychiatric component. The other is to review the various epidemiological studies which have tried to establish prevalence figures for specific syndromes.

In this overview, I shall attempt both approaches, even though I shall rely on the second one in trying to establish the boundaries of child neuropsychiatry within the broader field of child and adolescent psychiatry.

In defining child neuropsychiatry in Chapter 1, I included the following criteria.

1. Problem onset in infancy, childhood or adolescence.
2. Major mental, emotional or behavioural impairment is the most important clinical problem during at least one phase of development.
3. Important biological contributory factors are present in the genesis of the disorder or the shaping of symptomatology.

In deciding which disorders belong to this field, some, at the present stage, appear to be uncontended candidates, whereas others are likely to cause some dispute. In the first of these categories, mental retardation and other severe learning disorders, autism and the syndromes contained in the behavioural phenotype category, are the most obvious examples. Obsessive compulsive disorders, paranoid disorders and, in particular, anorexia nervosa, on the other hand, make borderline candidates. Some researchers and clinicians would certainly jump at the suggestion of including them among the child neuropsychiatric conditions. I shall not try to affront those who consider anorexia nervosa an example of a purely psychogenic class of disorders, but will try to make a case for the future inclusion of a subgroup with this condition among the neuropsychiatric disorders of childhood and adolescence.

In the present context, without deciding on the exact boundaries of child neuropsychiatry, I aim to present prevalence figures for conditions currently established, believed or proposed to belong among the neuropsychiatric disorders of childhood.

Table 2.1 details epidemiological data for child neuropsychiatric disorders according to age and sex (for conditions in which sex ratios have been published). Almost all the relevant data pertain to urban populations. In those few instances where data from urban and rural areas have been compared, no clear trend for a particular bias has emerged (e.g. Steffenburg & Gillberg 1986; Ahlsén *et al.*, 1994). This is unlike the situation in general child psychiatry where a number of studies have established that the rate of psychiatric disorder is consistently higher in urban than in rural populations (Rutter, 1973; Lavik, 1977, Gillberg, 1991).

Overall, at the very least, 5% of all children in the general population show clear signs of a neuropsychiatric disorder before adult age.

Table 2.1. *Epidemiological overview of child ne*

Disorder/syndrome	Prevalence n/1000 (boy:girl ratio)	Age g		
Autism (infantile autism, autistic disorder)	0.4–1.6 (2.6–6:1)	prepu		1979
			Sweden	Gillberg et al., 1991
			Canada	Bryson, Clark & Smith, 1988
			Japan	Sugiyama & Abe, 1989
Asperger syndrome	3.6–7.1 (3:1)	prepubertal	Sweden	Ehlers & Gillberg, 1993
Mental retardation with major psychiatric problems (autism not included)	3.7 (2:1)	adolescents	Sweden	Gillberg et al., 1986a
DAMP:				
severe	12	7 year-olds	Sweden	Gillberg et al., 1982
mild	30–59	7 year-olds	Sweden	Gillberg et al., 1982
ADHD	46 (3–9:1)	5 year-olds	Canada	Offord et al., 1989
Dyslexia	c. 50	prepubertal		Rutter, 1978a; true rate difficult to assess
Tourette syndrome	5.9 (8:1)	prepubertal	USA	Comings et al., 1990
Teenage psychosis	5.4 (1:1)	13–19 year-olds	Sweden	Gillberg et al., 1986b
Major neurological disorder (e.g. epilepsy, cerebral palsy) with major psychiatric problems (autism or mental retardation not included)	2.0 (3:1)	children and adolescents	Sweden	pooled results from several Swedish studies
Anorexia nervosa	6.0 (1:9)	under 18 year-olds	Sweden	Råstam et al., 1989
Total	50–90 (2.5–3:1)	0–19 year-olds	Sweden	pooled data from several Swedish population-based studies:overlap between groups (e.g. DAMP and Tourette) taken into account

Depending on exactly which defining criteria are used, as many as 9% of the general population may be considered to suffer from a child neuropsychiatric disorder.

There is, inevitably, some overlap across diagnostic boundaries in the field. For instance, the DAMP categories are not exclusive: most children with DAMP (deficits in attention, motor control and perception) develop dyslexia (Gillberg & Gillberg, 1989), and possibly the majority of all children with dyslexia have shown signs of DAMP when younger. All children with DAMP also meet criteria for ADD (attention deficit disorder with or without hyperactivity). However, not all children with ADD (or ADHD/attention deficit hyperactivity disorder/) meet DAMP criteria. DAMP is often an antecedent of psychosis with teenage onset (Hellgren, Gillberg & Enerskog, 1987), Tourette syndrome is often associated with ADHD. Severe DAMP often shows 'autistic traits', and the majority diagnosed as suffering from Asperger syndrome meet criteria for DAMP (Gillberg & Gillberg, 1989). Anorexia nervosa can occasionally be preceded by Asperger syndrome or some other autistic-like condition (Råstam, 1992).

Autism

Infantile autism (Rutter, 1978b; APA, 1980) is commonly regarded as a very rare disorder. The first population-based study yielded a prevalence figure as low as 2 per 10000 among 8–10 year-olds (Lotter, 1966). Later studies have reported considerably higher rates. Virtually all studies from the late 1980s have found prevalence rates close to or above 10 per 10000. Some have argued that this could be the result of gradually looser autism concepts, including that of 'autistic disorder' (APA, 1987). This does not seem to be an adequate explanation (Gillberg, Schaumann & Steffenburg, 1991). Better screening, refined diagnostic measures, and a real increase of autism among the offspring of immigrants who have arrived from far-away cultures, plus the increasing awareness that typical autism may well appear in

populations of neurologically handicapped children, are some of the important factors contributing to a rate of autism several times higher than that traditionally reported.

The clinical implication, of course, is that child psychiatrists and pediatricians need to be better informed about autism and be prepared to diagnose this condition more often than they have done in the past, so that parents and children may have access to the best possible help available for the problems specifically related to autism.

Boy:girl ratios in autism are in the range of 2–6:1 (Wing, 1993; Gillberg, 1994). The more recent population-based studies tend to show the lowest male:female ratios.

Asperger syndrome and other autistic-like conditions

Asperger syndrome (Wing, 1981) is now often conceptualized as a form of high-functioning autism. Whether it is truly on a continuum with autism or represents a special variant of social impairment syndromes (or 'disorders of empathy') remains to be seen, but it is already clear that, in certain families, there is considerable overlap with some individuals showing Asperger syndrome and others classical autism (Gillberg & Coleman, 1992).

No clearly population-based studies had been published before 1993. A Swedish estimate of at least 0.26% among school-age children was the only published figure before that date (Gillberg & Gillberg, 1989). A new population-based study from Göteborg reported that 'typical' Asperger syndrome occurs in at least 0.36% of the 8–16 year-old population (Ehlers & Gillberg, 1993). If Asperger syndrome is conceptualized as a variant of a broader class of empathy disorders, the prevalence for the broader class is higher than 1% of the general population of children (Gillberg, 1992).

By 'tradition', Asperger syndrome is regarded as an almost exclusively male condition, with boy:girl ratios at least in the 5–15:1 range. In recent years, some authors have challenged this view (see Chapter 5), suggesting that the Asperger phenotype in females might be slightly different from that in males.

Other autistic-like conditions include childhood disintegrative disorder (WHO, 1992), an extremely rare condition with autistic symptomatology appearing at the age of 30–50 months in children with previously normal, or almost normal, development (Volkmar, 1992).

Mental retardation with marked psychiatric problems

0.7–1.0% of all children in the 8–13 year-old age range are clearly classifiable as mentally retarded, i.e. they have a tested IQ under 70 (Hagberg et al., 1981; Gillberg et al., 1983). Of these, half to two-thirds show major psychiatric problems, at least during the teenage period (Gillberg et al., 1986a). Some of these have autism, but even if autism is excluded, the rate of severe psychiatric problems in teenage individuals with mental retardation is very high. At least 0.37% of the general population of teenagers have the combination of mental retardation and psychiatric disorder. There is a slightly moderately increased boy to girl ratio in mental retardation as compared with the general population. Among children with mental retardation and psychiatric problems the boy:girl ratio is further increased (c. 2:1).

Behavioural phenotype syndromes

Within the group of mental retardation plus psychiatric problems, there are quite a few individuals who suffer from specific named syndromes, such as Williams and Prader–Willi syndrome (see Chapter 10). These syndromes, with a known biological (often genetic) basis, very often show typifying behavioural features which are at least as specific as some of the physical identifying traits. The total prevalence for such syndromes clearly exceeds 2 per 1000 children born. For some of these syndromes, epidemiological data are only now beginning to appear. Thus, for instance, the rate of Prader–Willi syndrome in a rural population in Sweden

was 0.013% of all people under age 25 years (Åkefeldt, Gillberg & Larsson, 1991). However, not all individuals with these named syndromes are mentally retarded: the vast majority have severe learning problems, but a substantial proportion score above IQ 70 on formal testing.

DAMP (deficits in attention, motor control and perception)

The estimates of prevalence for attention deficits or attention deficit hyperactivity disorders (ADHD) which have been published so far have not been acceptable from an epidemiological perspective, except in a very few cases. Also, the diagnostic criteria used have been widely discrepant, even across the few clearly population-based studies that exist. Attention deficits exist in 2–14% of the general population of school-age children, depending on the type of criteria used (Gillberg & Gillberg, 1990; Sergeant & Steinhausen, 1992). In Sweden, 1.2% of 7 year-olds have been reported to suffer from the combination of severe cross-situational ADD (attention deficit disorder) and a multitude of motor control/perceptual dysfunctions (MPD) (including speech and language problems) (Gillberg et al., 1982). This combination of deficits has been labelled DAMP (deficits in attention, motor control and perception) (Gillberg, Gillberg & Groth, 1989). A further 5.9% have milder variants of DAMP including ADD and MPD, but with less pervasive problems in the MPD field. There is important overlap between severe DAMP and so-called Asperger syndrome and 'autistic traits'. DAMP (and ADD/ADHD without MPD) is 3–4 times more common in boys than in girls.

Dyslexia/dysgraphia/dyscalculia

–DAMP is often followed by obvious signs of reading–spelling, writing and maths problems. Reading–spelling problems are often referred to as dyslexia, writing difficulties as dysgraphia, and maths problems as dyscalculia. Depending on the exact definition of what constitutes dyslexia, dysgraphia and dyscalculia, such conditions occur, singly or in various combinations, in at least 5% of all children around the age of 10–11 years (Rutter, 1978a).

Tourette syndrome

Motor *or* vocal tics are very common, occurring in many per cent of all school-age children (and showing considerable overlap with DAMP and Asperger syndrome). Multiple motor *and* vocal tics (= Tourette syndrome) are considerably less common, but might nevertheless occur in 0.1–1.0% of all school-age boys (Comings, 1990; Robertson *et al.*, 1993). There is a striking excess of boys in this group as well. Unfortunately, there have been no clearly population-based studies of Tourette syndrome. Almost all of the studies cited in relation to Tourette syndrome epidemiology have been based on clinical materials. It is only the study of Comings, Himes & Comings. (1990) and a study of Israeli conscripts (Apter *et al.*, 1993) that come close to true population studies. In those studies the range was substantial: 1.05% of all school-age boys had definite Tourette syndrome in the USA. The corresponding figure in girls was 0.13%. In Israeli 16–17 year-olds the rate was reported at 0.04%. Although the latter is likely to be an underestimate, it is hard to account for the enormous discrepancy between these two studies.

Anorexia nervosa

The inclusion of anorexia nervosa among child neuropsychiatric disorders will almost definitely irritate some authors who believe this condition to be a clear-cut example of a psychosocially determined disorder. Nevertheless, the data suggesting a genetic background in some cases (Holland, Sicotte & Treasure, 1988), the follow-up data implicating a relatively restricted outcome even in cases with high IQ and good social background (Steinhausen, Rauss-Mason & Seidel, 1991), the clear evidence that starvation in anorexia *leads to* severe neuro-

muscular problems (Alloway *et al.*, 1985), and the recent suggestion that, in certain cases, there might be overlap between anorexia nervosa, on the one hand, and autism/autistic-like conditions/Asperger syndrome on the other (Råstam & Gillberg, 1992) all indicate that, at least a subgroup with anorexia nervosa has several roots in child neuropsychiatry.

The only clearly population-based study including a reasonable number of cases with this condition found a prevalence in girls under 18 years of 1.1%. The corresponding prevalence in boys was 0.1% (Råstam, Gillberg & Garton, 1989; Råstam, 1992).

Adolescent onset psychosis

The appearance of severe hallucinations, delusions, thought disorder, confusion or mania in teenage has been collectively referred to as 'teenage psychosis'. Over the whole teenage period, from 13–19 years of age, 0.5% of all people develop teenage psychosis requiring treatment in hospital. This is almost certainly an underestimate of the true population prevalence, even though it has been argued that severe cases of this kind are likely to attract medical attention and require hospital treatment (Gillberg *et al.*, 1986b). Girls and boys seem to be equally prone to develop psychosis in teenage, but boys more often receive a diagnosis of schizophrenia or schizophreniform disorder, and girls more often receive a diagnosis of depression.

Major neurological disorders with major psychiatric problems

It has been clearly demonstrated that major neurological disorders involving brain problems carry an increased risk of being accompanied by major psychiatric problems (Rutter, Graham & Yule, 1970). Thus, for instance, in childhood epilepsy, the rate of psychiatric disorder is increased almost ten times above the base rate in the general population. In 'uncomplicated' cerebral palsy, the rate is at least double that in the general population of children. In infantile, shunt-operated, hydrocephalus, the prevalence of major behaviour problems is high, but is strongly linked with concomitant mental retardation (Fernell, Gillberg & von Wendt, 1991*a*, *b*).

Summary and conclusion

At least 5, possibly 9 to 10% of the general population of school-age children demonstrate some kind of major neuropsychiatric problem. Many of the various disorders in this field need to be worked up and diagnosed by doctors specifically trained in the field of clinical child neuropsychiatry. Neuropsychiatric problems make up 25–50% of all consultations in child and adolescent psychiatry in Sweden (Gillberg, I.C. 1987), and it is unlikely that the figure is lower in other countries. Considering that all the disorders referred to here are severe, and with far-reaching consequences for psychosocial adaptation, they will not go unrecognized in countries with child psychiatric services, at least not in any large proportion of the cases.

References

Ahlsén, G., Gillberg, I.C., Lindblom, R., Gillberg, C. (1994). Tuberous sclerosis in Western Sweden. A population study of cases with early childhood onset. *Archives of Neurology*, **51**, 76–81.

Åkefeldt, A., Gillberg, C., Larsson, C. (1991). Prader–Willi syndrome in a Swedish rural county: epidemiological aspects. *Developmental Medicine and Child Neurology*, **33**, 715–21.

Alloway, R., Reynolds, E.H., Spargo, E., Russell, G.F. (1985). Neuropathy and myopathy in two patients with anorexia and bulimia nervosa. *Journal of Neurology, Neurosurgery and Psychiatry*, **48**, 1015–20.

American Psychiatric Association. (1980). *Diagnostic and Statistical Manual of Mental Disorders*. Washington, DC: APA.

American Psychiatric Assocation. (1987). *Diagnostic and Statistical Manual of Mental Disorders*. Third Edition, Revised. Washington, DC: APA.

Apter, A., Pauls, D.L., Bleich, A., Zohar, A.H.,

Kron, S., Ratzoni, G., Dycian, A., Kotler, M., Weizman, A., Gadot, N., Cohen, D.J. (1993). An epidemiologic study of Gilles de la Tourette's syndrome in Israel. *Archives of General Psychiatry*, **50**, 734–8.

Bryson, S.E., Clark, B.S., Smith, I.M. (1988). First report of a Canadian epidemiological study of autistic syndromes. *Journal of Child Psychology and Psychiatry*, **29**, 433–45.

Comings, D. (1990). *Tourette Syndrome and Human Behavior*. Duarte, CA: Hope Press.

Comings, D.E., Himes, J., Comings, B.G. (1990). An epidemiological study of Tourette syndrome in a school district. *Journal of Clinical Psychiatry*, **51**, 463–9.

Ehlers, S., Gillberg, C. (1993). The epidemiology of Asperger syndrome. A total population study. *Journal of Child Psychology and Psychiatry*, **34**, 1327–50.

Fernell, E., Gillberg, C., von Wendt, L. (1991*a*) Behavioural problems in children with infantile hydrocephalus. *Developmental Medicine and Child Neurology*, **33**, 388–95.

Fernell, E., Gillberg, C., von Wendt, L. (1991*b*). Autistic symptoms in children with infantile hydrocephalus. *Acta Paediatrica Scandinavica*, **80**, 451–7.

Gillberg, C. (1991). Outcome in autism and autistic-like conditions. *Journal of the American Academy of Child and Adolescent Psychiatry*, **30**, 375–82.

Gillberg, C. (1992). The Emanuel Miller Memorial Lecture 1991: Autism and autistic-like conditions: subclasses among disorders of empathy. *Journal of Child Psychology and Psychiatry*, **33**, 813–42.

Gillberg, C. (1994). The prevalence of autism and autism spectrum disorders. *In* Verhulst, F.C.,Koot, H.M. (Eds.) *The Epidemiology of Child and Adolescent Psychopathology*. Oxford: Oxford University Press.

Gillberg, C., Coleman, M. (1992). *The Biology of the Autistic Syndromes*. 2nd edition. London, New York: MacKeith Press, Cambridge University Press.

Gillberg, C., Gillberg, I.C. (1989). Six-year-old children with perceptual, motor and attentional deficits: outcome in the six-year perspective. *In* Sagvolden, T.,Archer, T. (Eds.) *Attention Deficit Disorder Clinical and Basic Research*. Hillsdale, NJ.: Erlbaum Associates.

Gillberg, C., Rasmussen, P., Carlström, G., Svenson, B., Waldenström, E. (1982). Perceptual, motor and attentional deficits in six-year-old children. Epidemiological aspects. *Journal of*

Child Psychology and Psychiatry, **23**, 131–44.

Gillberg, C., Svenson, B., Carlström, G., Waldenström, E., Rasmussen, P. (1983). Mental retardation in Swedish urban children: some epidemiological considerations. *Applied Research in Mental Retardation*, **4**, 207–18.

Gillberg, C., Persson, E., Grufman , M., Themnér, U. (1986*a*). Psychiatric disorders in mildly and severely mentally retarded urban children and adolescents: epidemiological aspects. *British Journal of Psychiatry*, **149**, 68–74.

Gillberg, C., Wahlström, J., Forsman, A., Hellgren, L., Gillberg, I.C. (1986*b*). Teenage psychoses--epidemiology, classification and reduced optimality in the pre-, peri- and neonatal periods. *Journal of Child Psychology and Psychiatry*, **27**, 87–98.

Gillberg, C., Schaumann, H., Steffenburg, S. (1991). Is autism more common now than 10 years ago? *British Journal of Psychiatry*, **158**, 403–9.

Gillberg, I.C. (1987). *Deficits in Attention, Motor Control and Perception: Follow-up from Pre-School to Early Teens*. MD Thesis. Uppsala: University of Uppsala.

Gillberg, I.C., Gillberg, C. (1989). Asperger syndrome – some epidemiological considerations: a research note. *Journal of Child Psychology and Psychiatry*, **30**, 631–8.

Gillberg, I.C., Gillberg, C. (1990). Hyperactivity and attention deficit. *Current Opinion in Pediatrics*, 694–99.

Gillberg, I.C., Gillberg, C., Groth, J. (1989). Children with preschool minor neurodevelopmental disorders. V: Neurodevelopmental profiles at age 13. *Developmental Medicine and Child Neurology*, **31**, 14–24.

Hagberg, B., Hagberg, G., Lewerth, A., Lindberg, U. (1981). Mild mental retardation in Swedish school children. I. Prevalence. *Acta Paediatrica Scandinavia*, **70**, 441–4.

Hellgren, L., Gillberg, C., Enerskog, I. (1987). Antecedents of adolescent psychoses: a population-based study of school health problems in children who develop psychosis in adolescence. *Journal of the American Academy of Child and Adolescent Psychiatry*, **26**, 351–5.

Holland, A.J., Sicotte, N., Treasure, J. (1988) Anorexia nervosa: evidence for a genetic basis. *Journal of Psychosomatic Research*, **32**, 561–71.

Lavik, N. (1977). Urban–rural differences in rates of disorder. *In* Graham, P. (Ed.) *Epidemiological Approaches to Child Psychiatry*. London: Academic Press.

Lotter, V. (1966). Epidemiology of autistic conditions in young children. I. Prevalence. *Social Psychiatry*, **1**, 124–37.

Offord, D.R., Boyle, M.H., Fleming, J.E., Blum, H.M., Grant, N.I. (1989). Ontario Child Health Study. Summary of selected result. *Canadian Journal of Psychiatry*, **34**, 483–91.

Råstam, M. (1992). Anorexia nervosa in 51 Swedish adolescents. Premorbid problems and comorbidity. *Journal of the American Academy of Child and Adolescent Psychiatry*, **31**, 819–29.

Råstam, M., Gillberg, C. (1992). Background factors in anorexia nervosa. A controlled study of 51 teenage cases including a population sample. *European Child & Adolescent Psychiatry*, **1**, 54–65.

Råstam, M., Gillberg, C., Garton, M. (1989). Anorexia nervosa in a Swedish urban region. A population-based study. *British Journal of Psychiatry*, **155**, 642–6.

Robertson, M.M., Channon, S., Baker, J., Flynn, D. (1993). The psychopathology of Gilles de la Tourette's syndrome. A controlled study. *British Journal of Psychiatry*, **162**, 114–17.

Rutter, M. (1973). Why are London children so disturbed? *Proceedings of the Royal Society of Medicine*, **66**, 1221–5.

Rutter, M. (1978*a*). Prevalence and types of dyslexia. *In* Benton, A.L.,Pearl, D. (Eds.) *Dyslexia*. New York: Oxford University Press.

Rutter, M. (1978*b*). Diagnosis and definition of childhood autism. *Journal of Autism and Childhood Schizophrenia*, **8**, 139–61.

Rutter, M., Graham, P., Yule, W. (1970). *A Neuropsychiatric Study in Childhood*. London: S.I.M.P./William Heinemann Medical Books Ltd.

Sergeant, J., Steinhausen, H.-C. (1992). European perspectives on hyperkinetic disorder. *European Child & Adolescent Psychiatry*, **1**, 34–41.

Steffenburg, S., Gillberg, C. (1986). Autism and autistic-like conditions in Swedish rural and urban areas: a population study. *British Journal of Psychiatry*, **149**, 81–7.

Steinhausen, H.-C., Rauss-Mason, C., Seidel, R. (1991). Follow-up studies of anorexia nervosa: a review of four decades of outcome research. *Psychological Medicine*, **21**, 447–54.

Sugiyama, T., Abe, T. (1989). The prevalence of autism in Nagoya, Japan: A total population study. *Journal of Autism and Developmental Disorders*, **19**, 87–96.

Volkmar, F.R. (1992). Childhood disintegrative disorder: Issues for DSM-IV. *Journal of Autism and Developmental Disorders*, **22**, 625–42.

WHO (1992). *The ICD-10 Classification of Mental and Behavioural Disorders. Clinical descriptions and guidelines.* Geneva: Author.

Wing, L. (1981). Asperger's syndrome: a clinical account. *Psychological Medicine*, **11**, 115–29.

Wing, L. (1993) The definition and prevalence of autism: a review. *European Child & Adolescent Psychiatry*, **2**, 1–14.

Wing, L., Gould, J. (1979). Severe impairments of social interaction and associated abnormalities in children: epidemiology and classification. *Journal of Autism and Developmental Disorders*, **9**, 11–29.

3   Background factors

Most child and adolescent psychiatric problems are multifactorially determined. This means that, whenever discussing aetiology, both biological, social and psychological factors have to be taken into account.

It goes without saying that, with a definition of child neuropsychiatry such as the one given in Chapter 1, biological factors are of crucial importance in all cases falling within this sub-branch of child psychiatry. Even so, social and psychological factors are often of major importance, too.

This chapter deals briefly with some of the major issues in the field of aetiological and pathogenetic factors in child neuropsychiatry. It is divided into five different sections: (1) genetic factors, (2) reduced optimality in the pre- and perinatal periods, (3) major environmentally determined brain damage, (4) sociocultural influences and (5) psychological factors.

Genetic factors

The influence of genetic factors on the child's intellectual, emotional and behavioural development is widespread and very important (Plomin, 1994). However, for many years, and especially during the 1960s, 1970s and early 1980s, the contribution of genes to the psychiatric disorders of childhood was grossly underestimated in many clinical settings. With the advent of appropriate twin, adoption and family studies, and, in particular, following the development in the new genetics (with more and

more sophisticated methods for studying genes at the DNA level), the under-emphasis of genetic factors has, almost too drastically, been turned into a strong emphasis. Sometimes, one has almost sensed an over-reliance on genetic factors when trying to account for various mental and behavioural phenomena.

This section deals with some of the various types of studies which have been used in order to demonstrate the contribution of genetic factors in the causation chain of events in child psychiatry, in general. Specific examples of studies from the narrower field of child neuropsychiatry are selected for illustration purposes.

The longitudinal study of temperament

There is a widely accepted folk meaning of temperament, involving some notion of stable behavioural dispositions (Bates 1989a). Temperament (or temperamental style) is discernible early in life and persists over time and across situations. For instance, it allows other people to have a sense of knowing what a person is likely to do in a given situation (Prior, 1992). In spite of this general acceptance of the term 'temperament', researchers have been unable to agree on a definition; indeed, most authors agree that a satisfactory definition does not exist (Bates, 1989b).

The reports by Thomas and Chess in New York (from the so-called New York Longitudinal Study (NYLS)) on the long-term follow-up of temperamental characteristics in children, have provided the best evidence to date that early observable childhood temperamental factors (not equivalent with personality factors according to Chess (1993)) play an important role in the shaping of personality, psychiatric disorder and life events (Thomas, Chess & Birch, 1968; Thomas & Chess, 1977). These authors propose a biosocial or transactional model in which temperament, whilst biological in origin, exerts its effects in transactional dynamics with the environment. This model implies several things: (1) the 'goodness of fit' between the individual's temperament and his/her environment will influence the psychosocial adjustment of the individual, (2) continuity and stability of temperament over time will be less striking, and (3) the longitudinal study of temperament is extremely complex.

Nine factors were intuitively derived by Thomas and Chess (1977) in modelling the temperament of children. These factors have since been shown repeatedly to cluster in a clinically (and statistically) meaningful way. The stability of some of these factors over time and their stronger concordance in monozygotic as compared with dizygotic pairs can be taken as supportive of a considerable genetic contribution to their expression. The nine factors are: (1) activity level, (2) approach–withdrawal, (3) adaptability, (4) mood, (5) intensity, (6) threshold to respond, (7) distractibility, (8) persistence and (9) rhythmicity. In addition, cluster factors labelled 'easy child', 'difficult child', comprising (a) low rhythmicity, (b) high intensity, (c) withdrawal tendency, (d) negative mood and (e) poor adaptability, and 'slow to warm up child' have been proposed. The easy–difficult temperament score (calculated by adding the five scores outlined in connection with the difficult child and dividing the sum by 5) at age 3 years in the NYLS sample was found to be related to the same construct of the early adult life period (Chess & Thomas, 1984). The clinical relevance of the 'difficult child' concept has been demonstrated in a Swedish sample (Persson-Blennow & McNeil, 1982).

Buss and Plomin (1984) have argued for a more constitutional/heritable theory of temperament. They propose three general temperament factors: (1) sociability, (2) emotionality and (3) activity. Heritability estimates have been found to be greatest for these three factors (and, possibly, for a fourth factor, i.e. shyness). It is obvious that several of the factors suggested by Thomas and Chess can be subsumed under the more general categories proposed by Plomin and his colleagues (Plomin & Dunn, 1986).

There is some debate as to whether 'temperament' and 'personality' should be regarded as separate, identical or overlapping constructs. Some researchers (e.g. Plomin, 1989) do not appear to differentiate between them. There is empirical data confirming their overlap (Prior et al., 1986). Nevertheless, other influential authors in the field (notably Chess, 1993), regard temperament as clearly separate from personality. Rutter (1987) seems to regard temperament as a non-premeditated style of responding, independent of cognition. In this sense, it would appear to be a useful construct only in infants and very young children who are minimally influenced in their behavioural responses by cognitive processes.

It is clear that there are links between 'difficult temperament' and psychiatric disorder (Thomas, Chess & Birch, 1968). It also appears that strong temperamental traits, whether considered difficult or not, may render a child vulnerable to particular types of psychiatric disorder. This seems to be the case for girls with high 'emotionality' who tend, more often than others, to develop major depression (Goodyear et al., 1993).

An excellent review of childhood temperament has been published by Prior (1992), and the interested reader is referred to this reference for more in-depth information.

Twin studies

For many years, twin studies were regarded as the superior way of studying genetic factors in medicine generally, and in psychiatry in particular. Significantly higher concordance rates in identical (monozygotic) twin pairs than in nonidentical (dizygotic) pairs were taken as strong evidence for genetic influences. This was based on the assumption of a generally rather similar environment for twins, and the notion of mono-zygotic twins sharing all their genes (which is not true in all cases), and dizygotic twins shar-ing on average 50% of theirs. If there is no unique contribution of twin environments, dizygotic twins should be no more similar than singleton birth siblings. If a particular trait or disorder is determined purely by a fully pene-trant autosomal dominant gene, the concor-dance rate for dizygotic twins should be 0.50 compared to 1.0 for monozygotic twins. If a trait or disorder is determined purely by the presence of a mutant autosomal recessive gene, the expected concordance for dizygotic twins would be 0.25. When the inheritance is more complex, concordance rates for monozygotic and dizygotic twins are not expected to approxi-mate these Mendelian segregation ratios. Under these circumstances, a significantly greater concordance for monozygotic twins is usually taken as evidence for the contribution of genetic factors to the trait or disorder being studied. Penrose (1953) suggested a useful rule in evaluating the data from twin studies: if the monozygotic twins show a rate of concordance more than four times that of the dizygotic twins, then multiple gene determination is more likely than any simple major single gene inheritance. Thus, for instance, the findings of 36–89% concordance for autism in monozygotic twins and 0% concordance in dizygotic same-sexed pairs (Gillberg, 1992) suggest that some expla-nation other than a single major gene locus is called for in this disorder. Penrose (1953) further pointed out that it is important to take account of variability of phenotype and the possible influence of environmental factors. Thus, for instance, in twin studies of autism, it would probably be inappropriate to focus only on the most narrowly defined autism pheno-type: Asperger syndrome and other 'disorders of empathy' (and yet other extensions of the core phenotype) need to be monitored as well.

One of the major advantages of twin studies is that they allow the study of the two indivi-duals in the twin pairs at approximately the same point of life development. Most other genetic studies require assessments at different developmental ages of the individuals in a family. This entails considerable problems relating to reliability and validity aspects: which are the adult phenotypes of childhood dis-orders, and how does one make appropriate retrospective diagnoses of childhood con-ditions in adulthood?

However, there are a number of caveats pertaining to twin studies. First of all, there may be concern that identical twins experience a psychosocially more homogeneous environ-ment than do non-identical twins. However, the available evidence does not unequivocally sup-port such a notion, and there is, in fact, some evidence that monozygotic twins may be con-sciously treated more 'individually' than frater-nal twins by their parents. Also, there have been a number of studies of twins reared apart from infancy, which have shown that, at least with regard to IQ and certain personality traits, differences between mono- and dizygotic pairs remain, suggesting a major genetic influence (e.g. Pedersen et al., 1984). Even though studies of twins reared apart are conceptually superior to those of twins reared together, several problems make most of them less than adequate. For rare disorders (and even for disorders which are not extremely common) it is almost impossible to obtain a large enough number of twin pairs, and there is usually some doubt as to whether there might be bias in the selection procedure. Therefore, studies of twins reared together have provided the broadest data base in the field. Nevertheless, there must be some caution in accepting a purely genetic interpretation of data from twin studies of certain disorders, in particular if the disorder has its onset only after several years of life. The first twin study of anorexia nervosa (Holland et al., 1984) showed monozygotic twins to be concordant for anorexia nervosa in more than half the pairs, but dizygotic twins only in one pair. This has been interpreted as showing a very important genetic contribution to the development of eating disorders comprising severe restriction of food intake (Holland, Sicotte & Treasure, 1988). However, anorexia nervosa has long been regarded as, at least partly, a cultural phenomenon. Imitating a twin who looks almost exactly like yourself (monozygotic) might be more common than imitation of a twin who looks clearly different from yourself (dizygotic).

Secondly, the confounding effects of pre-, peri- and neonatal problems are not easily dealt with. Twins experience more perinatal problems than singletons, and it is difficult, regardless of whether prospectively or with hindsight, to attribute a differential effect of intrauterine and perinatal adversities, which may well exist within a pair, to one particular twin.

Thirdly, it is very rare for a published twin study to be based on a population sample of twins. In most instances, a population basis for a twin study would be required for the results to be generalizable.

Fourthly, the establishment of zygosity needs to be done with great care (DNA fingerprinting is certain, but blood grouping on many variables is also acceptable in most instances).

Also, one point rarely considered in reviews of twin studies is the possibility that twins may be atypical of the general population and, hence, that results obtained on the genetics within twin samples, may not necessarily pertain to other groups. Thus, for instance, twinning per se could, conceivably, predispose to certain genetic disorders or be associated with a disease for other reasons. For instance, twinning has been shown to be a possibly associated background factor in developmental language disorder (Robinson, 1991) and autism (Gillberg et al., 1990). Monozygotic twins could be more liable than dizygotic twins to develop a particular problem.

The conclusion to be drawn from this is that, even though twin studies may provide strong evidence for a genetic component, such as in the case of autism (Folstein & Rutter 1977; Steffenburg et al., 1989), the results may not be informative with respect to the degree to which autism in the general population can be regarded as 'purely hereditary' (Gillberg, 1991). In other words: even though a perfect twin study can provide strong support for the notion of a particular trait or disorder being inherited in some cases, it will not necessarily provide an indication as to how much of the total variance of the disorder in the general population is attributable to genetic factors.

Adoption studies

Adoption studies in child neuropsychiatry provide perhaps the most powerful instrument for separating out the effects of biological and social background (Bohman, 1981). There are a number of different strategies which may be used, all of which have some advantages. There are also a number of limitations, such as (1) the risk for selective placement (adoption agencies tending to match adoptive and biological parents), (2) the risk that biological parentage could reflect obstetric rather than (or as well as) genetic factors (even though controls could be introduced to overcome this problem), (3) the lack of adequate data in most studies on the biological father (and hence an over-reliance on data pertaining to the biological mother, who, at least theoretically, may be the least important biological background factor), (4) the increased risk that mothers and fathers who give up their children for adoption may have mental disorders and the correspondingly increased likelihood that the adopting parents will be relatively free of such disorder, (5) the environmental risks associated with the atypicality of the adoptee studies, and (6) the great difficulty encountered when trying to collect reliable diagnostic assessments of the biological parents.

The various types of adoption studies are briefly described in the following.

Adoptees' study

In adoptees' studies, the biological parent is taken as the starting point in order to examine the rate of disorder in the offspring adopted away in early childhood and reared in a non-related household.

Adoptees' family design

The adoptees' family studies use some specific disorder as their starting point, and examine the segregation of this among biological and adoptive family members, or compare the biological relatives of adoptees with the specified disorder with those of control adoptees.

Cross-fostering design

In the cross-fostering studies, individuals born to normal parents, but reared by adoptive parents, one of whom developed a specific disorder, are compared with individuals born to parents, one of whom had that disorder, but reared by normal parents.

Adopted sibling design

In adopted sibling studies, the concordance between genetically related pairs of adult adoptees reared apart and that of genetically unrelated pairs of adoptees who have been reared together, are compared.

Parent–offspring adoption design

In parent–offspring adoption studies, parent–offspring correlations for a disorder or trait in adoptive and non-adoptive families are compared.

Family genetic studies

The study of the segregation of a disorder in an extended family has long been one of the tools for examining the heritability of pathology and also for establishing the mode of transmission (autosomal dominant, autosomal recessive and sex-linked (usually sex-linked recessive) to mention but a few of the better known) genetic disorders. Recently, the emergence of tools for examining genes at the DNA level has led to the refinement of genetic linkage studies. Linkage studies are meticulous examinations of several generations of a family with regard to the distribution of a particular gene; when disorder in an individual is coupled with linkage with a particular DNA probe and non-disorder is uncoupled with that probe, linkage is taken as evidence of the influence of a gene corresponding to the DNA probe in the causation of the disorder. In order to understand the assets and drawbacks of linkage studies better, a brief review of the current status of molecular genetics is appropriate (see the next section).

The study of sib pairs concordant for a particular disorder provides a reasonable tool for the evaluation of genetic factors in childhood and adolescence. The advantage of this type of study over many other types of family study is that it does not require any assumption about the mode of inheritance. In a disorder with genetic loading, it is usually easier to accumulate a large number of concordant sib-pairs than it is to collect, for instance, a large number of concordant twin-pairs. Also the separate effects of pre- and perinatal events is considerably easier to disentangle in the case of sib-pairs as compared with twin-pairs.

A particular case of sib-pair is the dizygotic twin pair. In rare disorders (like Rett syndrome), a single concordant dizygotic twin pair may provide a better basis for studying a 'candidate' gene than a set of multiple concordant monozygotic twins (see below).

Molecular genetics

Molecular neurobiology is an area of great potential promise for clinicians and scientists concerned with developmental and neuropsychiatric disorders of childhood. Molecular genetics have changed the whole prospect of child neuropsychiatry dramatically in the past few years. The discovery of the gene for the fragile X syndrome, as well as of the genetics of Angelman and Prader–Willi syndromes, have enormous theoretical (and clinical) implications. The fact that the clustering of a set of complex behavioural characteristics (such as turning away on greeting, gaze avoidance and cluttering of speech in the fragile X syndrome or overeating, stubbornness, skin-picking and outbursts of rage in Prader–Willi syndrome) can be aetiologically linked to a particular genetic problem (the pathological enlargment of a specific DNA-base-pair repeat (CGG) on the X chromosome in the fragile X syndrome and the absence of normal paternal DNA at the q11–13 location of chromosome 15 in Prader–Willi syndrome) casts some doubt on the notion that, for all complex human behaviour, there has to be a very complex explanation involving a long chain of transactional and interactional events. The realization that many of the so-called behavioural phenotype syndromes may be caused by (relatively) simple genetic defects has sparked renewed interest in the field of learning disorders (in which many of the behavioural phenotype syndromes cluster). The advent of much more refined molecular genetics methods has opened the possibility that, even in child psychiatry, many previously unexplained phenomena could turn out to have a much more specific genetic basis than previously believed.

Since about 1960, methods have been developed that allow the study of direct and indirect associations between point mutations in one or several genes, on the one hand, and medical/psychiatric disorder on the other.

Restriction enzymes are used to 'digest' the DNA-molecule at specific sites. EcoRI is an example of such an enzyme 'cutting' the DNA-molecule every time the base sequence of cytosine–adenine–adenine–thymine–thymine–cytosine appears on one of the two DNA-strings (and hence guanine–thymine–thymine–adenine–adenine–guanine on the other). The length of the DNA fragment that is recognized by any one particular restriction enzyme varies from 1 to several dozen basepairs. When a restriction enzyme is added to a preparation of DNA, the 'digestive process' results in several different DNA fragments of varying lengths. The higher the number of basepairs recognized by the restriction enzyme, the fewer and longer the resulting DNA fragments.

A so-called *probe* consists of a well-defined DNA fragment, whose sequence (usually) is known and whose location on a chromosome has been mapped. The probe can be part of a gene (or the actual gene) but, more often, it represents anonymous DNA fragments without a known gene function.

Cloning refers to the process by which an identified fragment of DNA (for instance, from humans) is multiplied. With the help of enzymes, the identified DNA fragment can be inserted in the DNA from a bacteriophage (a virus usually present in the intestinal bacterium *E.coli*). Through division within the bacterium, the bacteriophage produces many copies of the DNA fragment. Further copies are produced when the bacteria themselves divide. In this manner a particular probe or gene can be multiplied. For instance, the gene for growth hormone production can be operated into a bacteriophage and large quantities of the gene are then produced.

Several methods for studying human DNA exist. One of the better known of these is the so-called *'Southern's blot'*. A blood sample is drawn from the patient, and DNA is prepared from the cells (usually lymphocytes). Appropriate restriction enzymes are added (which cut the DNA strands at specific 'restriction' sites that range from four to eight bases in length) and the result is a preparation with DNA fragments of varying length. This preparation is then placed on an agarose-gel-plate and subjected to electrophoresis. Depending on the length of the fragments, they will move at different speeds in the electrical field. Through special treatment, the bindings of the double-stranded DNA are broken up, resulting in single-stranded DNA in which the bases stick out. A probe containing radioactive phosphorus is then added. If, and when, the DNA of the probe completely corresponds to that of the single-stranded DNA of the patient, *hybridisation* occurs (i.e. the two single strands of DNA, one from the patient, the other from the probe, combine). The patient DNA corresponding to the probe can then be visualized by exposing the radiation (from the radioactive phosphorus) on a film (autoradiography).

The Southern blot technique can be used in various ways to decide whether an individual suffers from a particular genetic disorder. The simplest way is to identify the exact mutation. So far, this is possible in a relatively small number of conditions in child neuropsychiatry (e.g. the fragile X syndrome, neurofibromatosis type 1). In *linkage analysis*, an indirect approach is used instead. The concordance of two separate abnormalities in a large family tree is examined. The first of these is usually the particular disorder being studied and the other is the variation, or the 'restriction fragment length polymorphism' (*RFLP*) of individual bases of the proband's two chromosomes (that can be measured using Southern blot techniques). The distance from the actual site of the gene and the RFLP is measured in centimorgans, and the statistical accuracy with which linkage occurs is presented as a '*lod score*'. A lod score of more than 3 indicates that the chance that linkage does not occur is less than one in a thousand. This level of accuracy is currently accepted as sufficient for use in clinical diagnosis. The higher the lod score, the stronger the probability of a true concordance between disorder and the base variation (i.e. the RFLP).

Northern blots constitute a chromatographic method for the analysis of RNA and is similar to Southern blot technique.

PCRs (polymerase chain reactions) are a series of reactions comprising the use of oligonucleotide primers and DNA polymerase employed in order to amplify a particularly interesting sequence of DNA, e.g. a mutant gene.

Cytogenetics

Chromosomal analysis continues to be one of the most important aids in genetic diagnosis, in spite of the ever-growing number of new techniques and applications of molecular genetics. In clinical practice and in clinical research, chromosomal examination (after chromosomal culture) will help reveal aneuploidies (abnormalities involving the number of chromosomes), the fragile X syndrome (although molecular genetic techniques are taking over in this field) and other structural chromosomal aberrations (deletions, inversions, duplications and translocations). In research, chromosomal analysis can also help identify minute deletions, the location of which may then help guide gene research into a particular area on a particular chromosome. Further improvements in karyotype analyses over the course of the next several years hold promise of greater clinical application and specificity of findings as well as decreased expenditure of manpower and money.

Application of molecular biology in child neuropsychiatry

In research, RFLPs are already being used in linkage studies of familial autistic disorder and Tourette syndrome. It should be kept in mind that RFLPs do not usually represent the actual genes themselves but may be located thousands (even millions) of bases away from the site of the crucial aberrant gene. Additionally, even if a mutant gene is present, it may not always be detected by RFLP analysis. Nevertheless, linkage analysis using RFLP (or PCRs) has become the standard first step in identifying candidate loci for genetic diseases. The limitations of the method diminish or disappear once the mutant gene is discovered and chemically identified.

Some genetic disorders with particular interest for the child neuropsychiatrist can now be diagnosed at the molecular level. At the time of going to press with this book, this is true of the fragile X syndrome, Prader–Willi syndrome, Angelman syndrome, neurofibromatosis type 1, carbohydrate-deficient glucoprotein (CDG) syndrome, Huntington disease, and Duchenne muscular dystrophia. It is possible that Williams syndrome too should be included in this list, but the evidence is yet too limited to make a firm conclusion.

Reduced optimality in pre-, peri-, neo- and postnatal periods

General overview

It is currently believed that pre- and perinatal risks play a relatively small role in the panorama of pathogenetic factors in child neuropsychiatry. However, this may be due both to a relative dearth of acceptable studies in the field and a possible current over-emphasis on genetic factors (Rutter *et al.*, 1990*a*, *b*; Bayley, 1993), which, in turn, could be seen as a reaction against the previous over-emphasis of psychosocial and brain damage factors in the aetiology of child psychiatric disorder, generally.

It is clear that pre- and perinatally acquired brain damage may have far-reaching consequences for the later psychological development of the child (Rutter, 1981, 1982). Intrauterine rubella infection, thalidomide embryopathy and perinatally acquired hydrocephalus have all been shown to be associated with a relatively strong risk of later psychiatric or intellectual disorder or both. However, it seems equally certain that major brain damage, which, in all probability, was acquired in the pre- or perinatal periods, in some cases, may contribute little, if anything, to later psychiatric disorder (Lorber, 1981). For instance, in one study, a trained nurse in a psychiatric hospital was shown to have very little left of her frontal, parietal and occipital lobes (according to MRI scan), but yet was able to function adequately. Such cases beg the question: 'Is your brain really necessary?'

– Some neuropsychiatric disorders with childhood onset are associated with reduced optimality in the pre- and perinatal periods (Gillberg & Gillberg, 1991). Optimality in this context is a concept developed by Heinz Prechtl's group in Groningen (Prechtl, 1980). It refers to states, for instance, during pregnancy, that have been shown, through operationalized criteria, to be 'optimal', in the sense that no harmful effects (according to the definitions used) have occurred. It was originally applied in the prospective studies of pregnancies and of newborn infants in order to be able to define single or sets of risk factors for abnormal neurological development. It has later been used mostly as a basis for defining varying degrees of 'reduced' optimality (Kyllerman & Hagberg, 1983) in cerebral palsy, autism (Gillberg & Gillberg, 1983; Piven et al., 1993), DAMP (Gillberg & Rasmussen, 1982), adolescent onset psychosis (Gillberg et al., 1986) and mental retardation (Gillberg et al., 1991). In all of these studies, neurological and neuropsychiatric disorders have been shown to have higher scores for reduced optimality (i.e. deviations from the optimality state) than carefully matched controls. This could be taken to mean that negative influences in the pre- and perinatal periods could have affected brain development/ structure adversely, and that the incurred damage/dysfunction is the cause or in other ways directly associated with the neuropsychiatric symptoms. However, careful analysis of the patterns of reduced optimality has revealed that most of the reductions have occurred in the prenatal period. The perinatal period is hardly

implicated at all (but the neonatal period is). This could be taken as indirect evidence of genetic factors being important: a genetically impaired foetus might trigger a series of negative intrauterine events which, in themselves, may have nothing to do with the later development of neuropsychiatric disorder. Transactional effects are, of course, also a possibility: the genetically deviant foetus triggers the reductions of optimality which, in turn, affect the brain negatively. Clinical evidence suggests that this may be an important chain of events in Down syndrome: the genetically determined hypotonia and immunological problems predispose to poor breathing and severe infections in the newborn period, which, in turn, may lead to structural brain damage. This could be the reason why some children with Down syndrome, usually with 'non-Down-syndrome-associated signs of brain damage', rather than showing a sociable phenotype, exhibit irritability, autistic symptoms and, indeed, occasionally full-blown autistic disorder (Howlin, Wing & Gould, 1994).

Also, it is clear that one negative factor is often associated with the development of more negative factors. Thus, in epidemiological studies of neuropsychiatric disorders it is rare for single factors to surface. There is strong evidence that severe and widespread brain damage sustained in utero can be followed by completely normal psychological development (see above). However, accumulations of, sometimes seemingly rather minor, negative events are relatively common. One interpretation of this is that it may be worse for the brain to constantly have a slight reduction of optimality (meaning that the brain never gets a chance to develop optimally) than to be affected by single major blows (providing that the brain does not die).

Intra-uterine reductions of optimality are often associated with relative deprivation of supply to the foetus and lightness/smallness for gestational age. Statistical levels of –2 standard deviations below the norm for weight/height relative to gestational age may not be surpassed, but, clinically, it is clear that the child has not been adequately nourished. In such cases, calories may not be freely available (from liver or subcutaneous tissues) immediately after birth. The imposed starvation faced (and managed) by most infants could, in these extreme instances, lead to hypoglycaemia, neuroglycopoenia and brain damage. This would be a plausible chain of events in cases with severely reduced prenatal optimality and newborn status consistent with the picture of 'clinical dysmaturity' (i.e. birthweight clearly under normal relative to gestational age, height and parental weight/height in combination with a large, possibly scaling, skin costume). Potentially, early feeding of such newborn infants could reduce the rate of brain problems that might later lead to neuropsychiatric problems.

The effect of alcohol, toxins and other drugs on the developing brain

It is clear that intra-uterine exposure of the foetus to massive amounts of alcohol can produce severe brain damage with long-term clinical sequelae for the growing child. It is also clear that intra-uterine exposure to certain drugs (such as thalidomide and phenytoin) may have devastating effects on the development (including the evolution of neural structures) of the foetus. It is much less certain what the consequences of intra-uterine exposure to a number of other drugs (such as the neuroleptics and the benzodiazepines) might be (van Baar 1990; Strömland & Miller 1993). This is a fast-growing area of research, which, unfortunately, so far, has been hampered by a whole host of methodological problems.

Alcohol

The foetal alcohol syndrome (see section on specific syndromes, Chapter 10) in a severe form is ample evidence of the harmful effects of intra-uterine exposure to large quantities of alcohol (Clarren & Smith, 1978). However, there is still considerable controversy regarding the 'dose–response' relationship in this field (Streissguth, Barr & Sampson, 1990). It seems that long-term exposure to alcohol in foetal life can result in brain dysfunction which may present with symptoms in early childhood on a spectrum from hyperactivity and mild learning

disabilities to severe mental retardation. The range of associated physical anomalies have been reported to be lacking or minor in the former case and minor–major in the latter.

Lead

There is an association between lower IQ and body lead measured by levels in blood or tooth dentine (Rutter, 1980; Fergusson et al., 1988; Taylor 1991). This finding is consistent but small, particularly when compared with major determinants of IQ such as parental IQ and family circumstances. No study has yet provided a good guideline as to what might be considered 'dangerously high normal' blood lead levels. It has been known for a long time that 'above normal levels' (blood levels exceeding 40 μg/dl) cause severe neuropathy. The majority of studies over the last ten years have examined the effects of chronic exposure to 'high normal' levels of lead in the environment. In the studies comparing 'high' and 'low' normal blood lead results, mean IQ has been 4–6 points lower in the 'high' group.

The possible association of chronic low-grade lead exposure and psychiatric problems (other than low IQ) is more controversial. Many studies show a negative effect on measures of psychopathology, but it has proved more difficult than in the case of IQ to determine the mechanisms underlying this possible effect (Taylor, 1991).

Cadmium

In one study (Norén, Hulthe & Gillberg, 1987) there was a suggestion of an association between high levels of dentine cadmium and attention deficits in the child. However, since, to the author's knowledge, no replication studies have been published, no conclusions can be drawn in this area.

Anti-epileptic drugs

Several of the anti-epileptic drugs (diphenylhydantoin, ethosuximide) have been shown to have teratogenic properties (Trimble, 1988). Some of these (like diphenylhydantoin) are rarely used in the treatment of epilepsy nowadays. Others (such as ethosuximide) are still in use for the treatment of very rare variants of epilepsy. The type of teratogenic effects is only partly known (Nakane *et al.*, 1980). This is due, to some extent, to the fact that many patients with severe epilepsy are treated with several different drugs, making it difficult to tease out the effect of any one individual substance. Also, —severe epilepsy in the mother can produce brain abnormality in the foetus through asphyxiation of the foetal brain during extended maternal seizure activity. Nevertheless, it seems that facial skeletal and skin defects (such as in cleft palate syndrome) and mental retardation may be particularly common features of the difenyl-hydantoin teratogenic syndrome (Hanson & Smith, 1975).

Neuroleptics

The effects of maternal neuroleptic medication on the developing foetal brain are poorly under-stood in spite of the fact that such drugs have been in clinical use for more than 40 years. The administration of large doses of neuroleptics to the mother during the third term is often followed by prolonged neurological upset in the newborn baby.

Antidepressants

No clear permanent harmful effects on the offspring have been documented after maternal medication with clomipramine or imipramine. However, withdrawal symptoms with tremor and seizures have been noted in newborns whose mothers were on such medication during the final weeks of gestation.

Cocaine and other central stimulants

In the late 1980s, a number of reports raised the possibility that maternal cocaine and 'crack'-abuse might lead to brain dysfunction in the foetus with subsequent development of autistic symptoms in the baby (Gillberg & Coleman, 1992). Subsequent studies have indicated that haptic defensiveness and a wide variety of social abnormalities may be more salient features of so-called 'crack babies' and that autism and typical autistic symptoms may be just one of the outcomes, albeit in a small proportion of the cases (Davis & Fennoy, 1991). Major and minor neurological anomalies without a typical syndrome have also been noted by several auth-ors (Burkett, Yasin & Palow, 1990; Hoyme *et al.*, 1990; Good *et al.*, 1992). Visual recognition memory (but not visual evoked potential) was impaired in infants prenatally exposed to cocaine and amphetamines. One study indi-cated that 6 weeks after birth the only remain-ing problem in infants exposed to cocaine in utero was one of automatic instability (Black, Schuler & Nair, 1993).

Lithium

There is no doubt that lithium carries the risk of teratogenesis if ingested during pregnancy. Cardiac abnormalities rather than central ner-vous system dysfunction appear to be the most common type of outcome. Lithium should be avoided altogether in pregnancy. ⨯

Benzodiazepines

There is still considerable controversy regard-ing the possible teratogenic properties of the benzodiazepines. Nevertheless, it seems clear that, at least in some cases, very severe malfor-mations of the foetal brain and other parts of the body may occur when the mother has been treated with benzodiazepines in pregnancy (Laegreid *et al.*, 1989; Laegreid, Hagberg & Lundberg, 1992). It is sometimes difficult, or indeed impossible, to separate the effects of alcohol, smoking, illicit drug taking and benzo-diazepines in certain cases which may have been exposed to any combination of these different agents.

Thalidomide

Thalidomide causes well-known abnormalities of limb development (phocomelia, etc.), deaf-ness, ophthalmological problems (including unusual disturbances of ocular motility) and facial skeletal abnormalities (Strömland & Miller, 1993). Just recently, a report appeared in which at least 4 out of 100 individuals with well-documented thalidomide embryopathy had autistic disorder (Strömland *et al.*, 1994). The possibility was raised that, since thalido-mide caused damage to the foetus during day 20–36 post-conceptionally, autism, in certain cases, may be caused by abnormal brain development occurring during this period.

Other drugs

A considerable number of drugs are known to affect brain and other nervous tissue development. These include several drugs classified as antibiotics (sulphonamides, chloramphenicol). The clinician working up a child with an unaccounted-for-neuropsychiatric disorder whose mother was on any kind of medication in pregnancy should consult a textbook of teratology or a major review chapter (such as Strömland, Miller & Cook, 1993) in order to analyse the various possibilities.

Brain damage

The distinction between structural and metabolic normal and abnormal development becomes less and less tenable. Structural and metabolic disorders are both the expression of an underlying disorder in genetic programming (Casaer, 1993). Even in the normal brain, cell death occurs. For instance, during the course of development, in animals, there is a 10–50% reduction of synaptic connections (and of cells providing these synaptic connections).

Factors other than those outlined in the section on reduced optimality, including alcohol and drugs, can cause brain damage and neuropsychiatric disorder. Brain damage increases the risk that the child will develop psychiatric disorder quite considerably, but there is no consistent pattern of symptoms associated with such damage (Rutter, 1981; Rutter, 1982). The Isle of Wight study, the only population-study ever which looked specifically at the association of measures of brain damage with psychiatric disorder in children, found that, in 10–11 year-old rural children, the rate of psychiatric disorder increased if there was a physical handicap and that if this handicap was due to a brain problem, the rate was even higher (Rutter, Graham & Yule, 1970). The highest rate of psychiatric disorder was found in children who had the combination of epilepsy and other brain disorders (such as cerebral palsy). The general conclusions were that (a) brain damage increases the risk for psychiatric disorder over and above the level explained by the presence of a physical disorder as such and (b) abnormal brain function rather than loss of brain function is associated with the highest rate of disorder. It is quite surprising that this landmark study has never been replicated. It is now more than 25 years old and there is a need for replication both in a rural and an urban setting. We cannot continue to quote forever *one* (albeit excellent) study as clear-cut evidence of the associations just outlined.

Even though there appears to be little, if any, correlation between crude measures of brain damage and particular syndromes (Rutter, 1982), this does not mean that brain damage cannot lead to very specific psychiatric problems in the child. Indeed there are many leads indicating that specific brain dysfunction can lead to specific neuropsychiatric behavioural profiles. The Prader–Willi syndrome and the fragile-X syndrome, to mention but two, are associated with specific genetic abnormalities, and, in all likelihood, with specific patterns of brain dysfunction. These syndromes are also associated with fairly specific behavioural phenotypes (see Chapter 10). What is strikingly clear, however, is that an overall measure of brain dysfunction, such as widespread EEG-abnormality, cannot be taken as an indication of specific neuropsychiatric problems, such as hyperactivity or attention deficits.

The relationship of so-called brain damage factors to reduced optimality in the pre-, peri- and neonatal periods has already been highlighted in the previous section. It may merit reiterating that transactional effects are likely to be important in the aetiology of many child neuropsychiatric disorders. Genetic factors may cause the foetus to be prone to various kinds of brain damage. These could result for instance (1) from immunological deficiencies increasing the propensity for being permanently brain damaged by incidents which might have been better sustained in the absence of the genetic factor or (2) on the basis of hypotonia which increases the risk that the child will not sustain the trauma of the birth process as readily as would a normotonic child or (3) as a consequence of genetically derived postnatal hypotonia leading to breathing dysfunction increasing the risk of having a common infection turning into pneumonia which, in turn. may end in septicaemia, meningitis, encephalitis and brain damage. In clinical practice, it is common to encounter a combination of factors which *might* indicate brain damage, but it is often impossible with hindsight to separate out whether these factors should be viewed as reflecting brain damage, genetic problems or a combination of both. One factor which has relatively high predictive validity for later neuropsychiatric problems is premature birth. Being born much prior to term, and in particular, having a very low birthweight, carries a high risk of school failure and social interaction problems. Hack *et al.* (1994) found that children with birthweights under 750 g had lower IQ. more motor–perceptual dysfunction. attention deficits and social interaction abnormalities than children with normal birthweight. Children in the 750–1500 g bithweight range had problem rates in-between the other two groups. The risk of intracranial haemorrhage is considerable in very premature children and this might be the link between low birthweight and later neuropsychiatric problems.

It is clinically difficult, not to say impossible, to determine the extent to which reduced optimality or 'brain damaging factors', *potentially* harmful to brain development, has indeed *caused harm* to the individual child. Markers for brain dysfunction, whether reflected as neurochemical abnormalities, neurological signs in the newborn period, autopsy findings on neonates and older children, CAT-scan abnormalities or deviations on ultrasound scans, and their relationship both to each other, and to measures of reduced optimality, and long-term follow-up results will provide indications of the contribution of pre-, and perinatal risk factors to the neuropsychiatric outcome of children and adolescents. The studies that have been performed to date have shown that (a) very low birth weight infants, because of respiratory stress syndrome (associated with acidosis and hypercarbia) and immaturity factors (delivery factors appear not to be very important), often suffer intraventricular haemorrhage which may cause death, but usually survive. The bleeds most often occur at the head of the caudate and extend from there into the ventricles or other areas of the brain (Caesar & de Vries, cited in Taylor, 1991); (b) children with evidence of haemorrhage have a high risk of developmental delay, a risk that tends to increase with age (as more types of dysfunction can be detected) (Costello *et al.*, 1988); (c) leukomalacia (appearing as cystic lesions round the ventricles and in subcortical white matter, or showing as transient areas of increased density to echo) compromises the newborn neurological state and is followed by floppy infant syndrome and often, at least in the case of extensive lesions, by cerebral palsy. Frontoparietal cysts are reported to lead to better outcomes but may produce hyperactivity (around age 2 years) (Casaer & deVries, 1991); (d) moderate hypoglycaemia shows a strong dose–response relationship with developmental delay (Hack *et al.*, 1994) and hypoglycaemia diagnosed on five or more separate days predicts a three-fold increase in neurodevelopmental impairment at 18 months (Lucas, Morley & Cole, 1988); and (e) intrapartal and neonatal asphyxia in isolation constitute a minor risk factor and should not be taken as an index that the brain has been damaged (Hall, 1989).

In summary, many of the old 'truths' (such as neonatal hypoxia being an important cause of later psychiatric disorder) need to be re-examined in the light of new knowledge emerging as a result of ever more refined instruments being applied in the study of brain damage sustained in the pre- and perinatal periods.

Child neuropsychiatric disorders resulting from brain damage due to particular acquired agents (viruses, bacteria and trauma) are described in detail in Chapters 10 and 12.

Sociocultural influences

A whole spectrum of sociocultural influences, not specifically associated with the 'family network', affect the development of normal and abnormal children. [Age-peers, friends of the family, day nursery staff and settings, school (both as an academic stress and as regards relationships with teachers and other school staff), general psychosocial circumstances (housing, urban–rural settings, economy, etc.) and the (often accidental) effects of major life events (including road accidents, being part of major disasters and physical and sexual abuse (see below also under Family Discord)) all contribute to the enormous complexity of children's lives.] However, even though psychosocial circumstances generally have far-reaching effects on the psychological well-being of children (Rutter, 1975), it is much less clear how the various factors in isolation affect the child's development. Incidentally, it would be reasonable to assume that, just as with reduced optimality in the intrapartal period, sociocultural factors would be more likely to have an impact if acting together rather than in isolation. With regard to neuropsychiatric disorders specifically, very little is known about the meaning of psychosocial influences. Furthermore, many of the psychosocial influences which are known, or suspected, to adversely affect child development are also those that have been established to carry a high risk of harmful genetic or brain effects (e.g. alcoholism or cocaine abuse in the parents, psychiatric disorder or mental retardation in the mother, etc.). This makes it even more difficult to disentangle the effects of nature and nurture. What is known about the very harmful effects of a 'negative psychosocial milieu' pertains mostly to child psychiatric broad band disorders, such as 'conduct disorder'. It is not immediately clear that what has been learnt about psychosocial effects in such disorders can be translated to the area of specific neuropsychiatric disorder. Nevertheless, some of the major observations in the field of psychosocial influences in general child and adolescent psychiatry will be briefly summarized here to serve as a background for the understanding of health and development in child neurospsychiatric disorders.

Sociocultural influences, in the broadest sense of the word, also comprise factors directly associated with differences in ethnic and cultural origin. Such factors are clearly of import in the shaping of symptoms related to child neuropsychiatric disorders (e.g. grandiose delusions in schizophrenia would be more likely to involve being a king in a monarchy like Sweden than in a republic like the US, where, perhaps delusions about being president would be expected). Also, symptoms of a disorder, while not necessarily shaped by the sociocultural factors, may be more difficult to cope with in a particular social setting (e.g. DAMP is more commonly encountered in the lower social classes in western societies, and this could, at least in part, be due to poorer parental coping skills and possibilities in a subgroup among those in the lower social classes (Gillberg et al., 1983; Taylor et al., 1991), whereas in other societies, higher social status might mean stricter norms and less tolerance and hence seemingly higher rates of DAMP in upper social classes; Asperger syndrome, depending on the particular interest pattern of the individual affected, may be easy to cope with in a highly intellectual setting or in a rural area, but may be more difficult to accommodate in a different setting). Sociocultural factors may also contribute in different ways to the aetiology of the disorder (such as in the case of anorexia nervosa, which appears to be very rare in cultures in which starvation is a common problem, but common in settings where there is an abundancy of food; [DAMP and mental retardation, in some cases, may be caused by less than optimal intra-uterine environments leading to brain dysfunction and the reduced optimality, in turn, may be caused by sociocultural factors such as drug or alcohol abuse). Sociocultural factors may also influence the epidemiology of neuropsychiatric disorders in ways which are only indirectly connected with underlying aetiology (e.g. autism is possibly more common in the first generation offspring of parents who have migrated; adopted children may have higher rates of some neuropsychiatric disorders).

The influence of sociocultural factors on neuropsychiatric disorders (and vice versa) will be discussed in more detail in connection with the description of the individual syndromes.

It may need stressing here that many child

neuropsychiatric disorders are surprisingly similar in their symptomatology regardless of the sociocultural setting. Judging from the author's own experience, core symptoms of autism are the same in the US, the UK, Uganda, Zimbabwe, France, India, Jordan, Israel, Iran, Japan, the republic of China, Australia, Chile and Sweden. This, according to the published reports, is also true of most of the so-called behavioural phenotype syndromes.

Familial factors

Very sophisticated research methodology would be required in order to tease out the specific aetiological/pathogenetic contribution of family factors to symptoms encountered in clinical child neuropsychiatry. By and large, studies performed to date have not been able to clearly disentangle such effects from those primarily associated with the child's disorder, from familial genetic influences or from general psychosocial factors.

Nevertheless, some studies have implicated important family factors in *the production of symptoms* in certain child neuropsychiatric disorders (e.g. in attention disorders). Other studies in the fields of child health and general child psychiatry contribute to our understanding of family influences in child development and adjustment/maladjustment. Evidence from these studies will be reviewed here as it pertains to the understanding of the neuropsychiatrically disordered child or adolescent. Some of the evidence will be reviewed in a little more detail in sections on specific disorders.

Before we move on, however, it is important to make note of the fact that environmental influence is not necessarily shared by children growing up in the same family. Salient environmental influences, factors which may well be of pathogenetic importance in an individual case, may be specific to each child, not general to an entire family (Plomin, 1994).

Parental death

The death of one or both of one's parents is bound to occur in the lives of most people, and it is usually a psychological trauma regardless of when in life it happens. There has been a lot of theoretical work on the meaning of parental loss for children but the actual empirical data is quite scanty.

As with many types of psychological trauma, the impact of parental death on infants and children depends to a large extent on the situation before (type of attachment/bonding, amount of care given/experienced and the presence/absence of other important caregivers) and after the loss (presence/absence of other important caregivers, such as the presence of one parent still alive, grandparents, siblings, general psychosocial situation, economical circumstances etc.). Nevertheless, there is probably no disputing the fact that losing one or both parents before adult age is among the most serious life events that can affect an individual.

There are few prospective studies of children and adolescents relating to the impact of parental death (Goodyer, 1993). However, retrospective controlled studies of cross-sectional samples with particular disorders can tell us something about the contribution of parental death in the causation of psychiatric abnormality even though they are not necessarily informative with regard to the impact of parental death in the general population. In teenage onset psychosis and anorexia nervosa there are some indications that parental death may be an important antecedent of disorder in certain cases (Hellgren, Gillberg & Enerskog, 1987; Gillberg & Råstam, 1992).

Adoption

This is not the place to review the literature on adoption. For recent overviews, the interested reader is referred to Bohman (1981).

Before the 1960s, adoption in western societies often concerned children born in the same area (or at least country) as the adopting parents. Genetic risks and poor social circumstances singly or in combination were often part of the picture. In recent years, in western societies, this pattern has changed completely, and the majority of adopted children now have been born in other countries, often far away from the culture in which they are subsequently raised.

To the genetic risks and early psychosocial disadvantage are now added cultural risk factors. Also, it seems likely, although not proven, that intra-uterine starvation, perinatal problems and neonatal hazards may be more common in children adopted to western societies from developing countries.

It is only very recently that it has been realized that the psychiatric risks associated with being an adopted child from a far-away country may be considerable (Verhulst, Althaus & Versluis-Den Bieman, 1990a, b).

Autism is clearly over-represented in the offspring of mothers who have migrated (Wing, 1993). It now seems that adopted children from far-away countries may also run an increased risk of developing autism (Gillberg & Gillberg, in press).

Fostering

Fostering is sometimes used as a means of positive intervention for children whose lives with their biological parents are in turmoil or for whom, for other reasons, there is a need to be raised and supported by 'foster-parents'. It should go without saying that, from the point of view of the child's mental health, the effects of fostering may be anything from very beneficial to detrimental. In western cultures it is becoming increasingly recognized that, to achieve successful fostering of a child, at least after the first few years of life, great efforts need to be made to assure the best possible 'quality' of the foster-parents (a very important task for the local social authorities), the best possible 'fit' of foster-parents and child (including extensive information about the nature of the child's problems and/or background situation) and thoughtful follow-up (including paying attention to the child's needs, not least as regards relationships with the biological family, the foster-parents' needs, not least emotional and financial, and the needs of the biological parents).

Many neuropsychiatrically disordered children are being cared for in foster-homes. Sometimes, as in the case of autism and Tourette syndrome, the foster-parents may have been given the false impression (perhaps by the social authorities) that the severe behavioural problems exhibited by the child will automatically subside or even disappear altogether once the child adapts in the foster-home. The neuropsychiatrist, in such cases, has an important, and often difficult, task trying to set 'treatment' or 'intervention' goals at a realistic level.

Divorce

As late as in the 1970s, many textbooks proposed that divorce be considered one of the major causes of child turmoil and disorder. This was at a time when, in western societies, divorce was still considered very abnormal. Even now, when divorce in some countries is more common than unbroken marriages, divorce is likely to play a major role in causing emotional upset in children and teenagers (Wallerstein, 1991). However, the long-term effects of divorce are not well understood and may, at best, be considered complicated. As is often the case in child psychiatry, transactional (Rutter, 1985) and interactive effects are likely to be of utmost importance. Thus, for instance, the reasons for divorce and the situation, support and social/emotional 'network' following it, are possibly more important factors than the divorce as such (Rutter, 1985). Nevertheless, Wallerstein's studies from the US have indicated that divorce in itself carries enormous emotional impact, and that even five years after, the sadness and upset experienced by the child at the time are recalled in astonishing detail, showing that it has probably been 'near the surface' in all the intervening time. Girls, on average, may cope better than boys with divorce in the long term (Wallerstein & Kelly, 1980; Hetherington, Cox & Cox, 1978; Hetherington, 1985). Boys of divorce (one–six years after the event) score lower on achievement tests, show a narrower range of effect and have fewer social relationships than do girls of divorce of the same age.

Whether or not divorce has particular effects in neuropsychiatrically disordered children has not been extensively studied. There have been some earlier indications that parents of children with cerebral palsy, epilepsy and DAMP tended to divorce at a higher rate than parents of children in the general population (Anderson, Clarke & Spain, 1982; Ward & Bower, 1978; Gillberg & Rasmussen, 1982), but it is unclear whether this still holds.

The notion that parents of patients with anorexia nervosa tend to stick together more often than other parents was not borne out by a population study of anorexia nervosa (Råstam & Gillberg, 1991). If anything, there was a slight tendency (though not statistically significant) in the opposite direction. The old conclusion may have been caused by referral bias leading to only a selected group of anorexia patients and their families' consulting services. This latter conclusion was indirectly supported by the population study in which only about a third of all anorexia nervosa cases had consulted specialists (psychiatrists or other doctors particularly knowledgeable in the field of eating disorders).

One-parent families

In older studies in child psychiatry, one-parent families and broken homes (sometimes, but by no means always, equivalent) were often cited as the factors most often associated with disorder in the child (Jonsson & Kälvesten, 1964; Rutter, 1977, 1985). It is clear that, on average, single-parent families are often characterized by female heads of household, poverty and the presence of young children (Luthar & Zigler, 1991; Zigler & Finn-Stevenson, 1991). Poverty, at least, is known to be associated with increased risk of mental disorder. Single-parent families are more isolated than two-parent families. The lack of social support may be indirectly important in producing emotional and behavioural problems in children (and perhaps particularly in neuropsychiatrically disordered children): it has been well established that the availability of a social support system often mediates the negative consequences of stress (Garmezy & Rutter, 1985).

There can be little doubt that single parents face more difficulty raising children than do parents who have the support of a spouse, other relative or friend. Also, most single parents have more financial problems (see above). Nevertheless, it is equally clear that many single parents do very well, and raise children who are emotionally stable and well adjusted.

In recent years, the number of single-parent families has increased dramatically as divorce rates have increased. In the late 1980s, more than 55% of all new Swedish marriages ended in divorce within a ten-year period (see also above). This means that the number of single parents has increased. Consequently, cultural norms have changed (just as the changed norms have themselves contributed to the increased divorce rate). The connotations of being raised by a single parent are no longer the same as 20–30 years ago (when many of the studies suggesting an effect of single parentship were performed). In fact, the 'norm' (if by norm is meant that which is most 'normal'/frequent) as this book is written, is *not* being raised in an 'unbroken home'. Therefore the study of the effects, if any, of being raised by a single parent is no longer as straightforward as it appeared to be when a broken home was (at least from the statistical point of view) something out of the ordinary.

Homosexual parents

There is a dearth of studies of children raised by homosexual parents. One of the few systematic investigations in the field described the emotional and psychosocial development of children raised by lesbian mothers. No significant differences could be established between school-age children with a lesbian parent background and those with a heterosexual 'single parent' background (Golombok, Spencer & Rutter, 1983).

Family discord

Family discord is a common associated feature in all sorts of child psychiatric disorders, be they neuropsychiatric or not (Rutter, 1975).

It seems clear that, sometimes, such discord in itself *causes* the child's problems (Rutter & Hersov, 1985). This may be particularly true of child disorders for which there is 'diffuse' rather than 'specific' symptomatology, i.e. unspecified conduct and emotional disorder. Also, it stands to reason that family discord may aggravate problems in a family already burdened by the presence of disability and handicap in one or several children.

However, in other instances, it is quite possible that the child's primary (neuropsychiatric) disorder may contribute to the development of family discord or that disorder and discord may exist as independent variables.

In attention deficit hyperactivity disorder (ADHD) and deficits in attention, motor control and perception (DAMP), several different lines of evidence suggest the contribution of the disorder as such to the development of discord. The stimulant–placebo-controlled double blind studies of ADHD show convincingly that, when attention problems are specifically treated with stimulants, family discord decreases, parental interference reduces and child peer interaction improves (Barkley et al., 1985; Barkley, 1988; Barkley et al., 1990). Also, mothers of children with DAMP have a psychiatric consultation rate which increases from child age 3 to 4 years significantly more than does the corresponding rate in mothers of children who do not have DAMP (Gillberg, 1983).

An interesting study by Breslau and Prabucki (1987) suggested that, in certain instances, family discord may exist independently of disorder in the child or that disorder may protect against the negative effects of discord. Family discord produced significantly fewer negative effects (depression in particular) in hyperactive (brain dysfunctional?) children than in children judged to be psychiatrically normal.

Deviant family interaction and sexual abuse

Family interactions are important in all families, regardless of whether or not they contain deviant children (Oberfield & Gabriel, 1991). To what extent family interaction styles can cause, contribute to, or modify, child psychiatric symptoms is, by and large, unknown, in spite of many ill-founded claims that there may be even aetiological links. Sometimes, a child psychiatric disorder can cause family interac-

tion to change, at least in negative, perhaps also in positive ways.

Disorders such as anorexia and bulimia nervosa (and other so-called psychosomatic disorders) have been partly or completely attributed to unusual/deviant styles of family interaction (e.g. Minuchin et al., 1975; Ekberg & Gillberg, 1977). However, even though there are indications that family problems are more common in such disorders than in the general population without eating disorders (Råstam & Gillberg, 1991), there is no empirical evidence to support the notion of a particular family interaction style in such families.

Sexual abuse has also been implicated as a pathogenetic factor in eating disorders. Intrafamilial sexual abuse is often not distinguished from sexual abuse involving extrafamilial perpetrators. The patchy evidence that exists in the field (Folsom et al., 1993) suggests that childhood sexual abuse may be a frequent background factor in bulimia nervosa, but that, in anorexia nervosa, it may be less prevalent than in other psychiatric disorders. In fact, in one community-based study of anorexia nervosa, the rate of reported childhood sexual abuse (whether familial or not) was lower than in a comparison group of non-eating disordered individuals from the general population. Reported childhood sexual abuse in a community sample of adult women was associated with higher prevalence of reported eating disorder symptoms (Anderson et al., 1993), but the overlap of possible consequences of the sexual abuse and the consequences of the matrix of disadvantage from which it so often emerges are so considerable 'as to raise doubts about how often, in practice, it operates as an independent causal element' (Anderson et al., 1993).

Whether or not there is a specific correlation of child neuropsychiatric disorder and sexual abuse, familial or extra-familial, remains an open issue at this stage. Clinical reports suggest that disorders involving cognitive and/or social dysfunction might predispose the individual to sexual abuse (Witt-Engerström & Forslund, 1992; Haracopos, 1988). For instance, a severely mentally retarded person might be abused because the perpetrator may judge that she/he will not be able to tell. A young man with Asperger syndrome may be more likely than normal males to be 'taken advantage of', because he may be socially extremely naïve. Incidentally, he may also, unwittingly, himself contribute to suspicion of having been homo- sexually abused, when, in fact, he himself selected homosexual contacts because of his social dysfunction, restricting his interaction with females.

Children with severe attention deficits appear to be more resilient than normal children to the effects of family dysfunction (Breslau, 1990). This statement seems to be in superficial con- flict with the general observation that family problems are much more common in popula- tions of children with severe attention deficits than in control populations (Taylor *et al.*, 1991). However, attention deficits in the child may well contribute to family dysfunction (rather than the other way around) according to studies by Barkley (1988), and Taylor (1989), and, even though family problems might contri- bute to the development of attention deficits, once such symptoms occur, they may not be strongly influenced by the presence or not of family dysfunction. Interestingly, it has been repeatedly shown that central stimulants, which effectively reduce many of the clinical problems associated with attention deficits, quickly improves family function and parental (in addi- tion to peer) interaction with the affected child.

Sibling relationships

The influence of siblings on development and mental health of children and adolescents has received relatively little attention in child psy- chiatric research (Dunn & Kendrick, 1982; Lamb, 1991). In a number of conditions (such as autism, mental retardation (Down syndrome in particular) and neurological disorders (including cerebral palsy and hydrocephalus)), studies of siblings have been performed. The general conclusions from such studies are that siblings may have important positive effects on the abnormal child and that siblings themselves may be both positively and negatively affected by the presence of an abnormal child in the family (McHale, Sloan & Simeonsson, 1986; McHale & Gamble, 1989; Gath, 1990; Bågen- holm & Gillberg, 1991; Fernell, Gillberg & von Wendt, 1992; Dallas, Stevenson & McGurk, 1993*a, b*). At least in the case of Down syn- drome, there is a higher rate of behavioural problems in the older sisters, possibly caused by their carrying an undue burden of care (Gath, 1974).

Other relatives

If there is a relative lack of studies concerning the importance of sibling relationships in rela- tion to child psychiatric disorders, the absence of studies relating to the impact of relationships with other relatives is virtually complete. The emergence of more sophisticated studies of 'informal social networks' will hopefully remedy this shortcoming. Clinically, it is clear that relatives often play a major part in the lives of young children and adolescents.

Psychological factors

Psychological factors are always of utmost importance in the analysis of problems in indi- vidual children or adolescents, almost regard- less of the particular kind of neuropsychiatric diagnosis being considered. The way a young person's situation is perceived by him/herself, for obvious reasons, will be among the most important factors to take into account when making a decision as to the current level of functioning and when opting for interventions.

It is often the case that psychological factors are taken into consideration when discussing problems occurring in the adolescent popula- tion. A teenager often has excellent ability to communicate experiential problems. However, this may not be true in cases of schizophrenia, autism, depression or mental retardation. In younger children, individual psychological factors are often overlooked in an unacceptable way. This may be true even when, superficially, a lot of effort may appear to have been invested in the examination of the child's psyche, such as when unvalidated projective tests, rather than direct interview, are cited as evidence in favour of this or the other opinion.

In child neuropsychiatry it is mandatory always to consider the problems being assessed from the point of view of the child or adolescent: 'what would it be like to suffer from this particular neuropsychiatric disorder?" For instance, in DAMP, there are attentional problems, motor clumsiness and automatization problems already in the first few years of life. Even though the very young child will not be able to understand that there are problems (because he/she does not know what it would be like *not* to have those problems), it will not be long before other people (siblings, age-peers and parents) will make him/her aware that he cannot live up to the same expectations that most other children do. Self-image is likely to suffer in the process (Barkley, 1990), even though there are probably those whose attentional problems are so pervasive that they might be less aware than age-peers of the critical attitudes of others and so may have less negative *personal experiences* of scolding and less-than-positive interactions with others (Breslau & Prabucki, 1987). In an interesting British study, three year-olds in a community sample were subdivided into those who performed best and worst on neuromotor screening examination. It was clear already at that young age that the children who fared worst on the motor test were also those who appeared to have the lowest level of self-esteem.

Children with a mental age of at least seven years can usually be relied upon to provide a reliable account of mood and anxiety problems (Gillberg, 1983). It appears that parents may be less accurate in this respect. Specifically, parents suffering from depression may under-report depression in their own children. Even parents who do not suffer from depression tend to under-report depression and anxiety disorders in their children. This may be particularly true in the case of adolescent daughters, but children of all age groups appear to be affected by parental underreporting of emotional problems (Weissman *et al.*, 1987).

As regards behaviour and developmental problems, mothers are usually very reliable informants. Unless there are highly atypical circumstances, a thorough interview with young children's mothers remains the best single source of information for the clinician required to make an assessment of the child with a possible neuropsychiatric disorder. However, in most instances, the child should also be interviewed, separately, whenever required.

References

Abel, E.L., Sokol, R.J. (1986). Fetal alcohol syndrome is now leading cause of mental retardation. *Lancet*, **ii**, 1222.

Anderson, E.M., Clarke, L., Spain, B. (1982). *Disability in Adolescence*. London: Methuen.

Anderson, J., Martin, J., Mullen, P., Romans, S., Herbison, P. (1993). Prevalence of childhood sexual abuse in a community sample of women. *Journal of the American Academy of Child and Adolescent Psychiatry*, **32**, 911–19.

Bågenholm, A., Gillberg, C. (1991). Psychosocial effects on siblings of children with autism and mental retardation; a population-based study. *Journal of Mental Deficiency Research*, **35**, 291–307.

Barkley, R.A. (1988). The effects of methylphenidate on the interactions of preschool ADHD children with their mothers. *Journal of the American Academy of Child and Adolescent Psychiatry*, **27**, 336–41.

Barkley, R.A. (1990). *Attention Deficit Hyperactivity Disorder*. New York: Guilford Press.

Barkley, R.A., Karlsson, J., Pollard, S., Murphy, J.V. (1985). Developmental changes in the mother–child interactions of hyperactive boys: effects of two dose levels of Ritalin. *Journal of Child Psychology and Psychiatry*, **26**, 705–15.

Barkley, R.A., Fischer, M., Edelbrock, C.S., Smallish, L. (1990). The adolescent outcome of hyperactive children diagnosed by research criteria. I. An 8 year prospective follow-up study. *Journal of the American Academy of Child and Adolescent Psychiatry*, **29**, 546–57.

Bates, J.E. (1989a). Application of temperament concepts. *In* Konstamm, G.A., Bates, J.E.,Rothbart, M.K. (eds.) *Temperament in Childhood*. Chichester: Wiley.

Bates, J.E. (1989b). Concepts and measures of temperament. *In* Konstamm, G.A., Bates,

J.E.,Rothbart, M.K. (eds.) *Temperament in Childhood*. Chichester: Wiley.

Bayley, A. (1993). The biology of autism – editorial. *Psychological Medicine*, **23**, 7–11.

Bohman, M. (1981). The interaction of heredity and childhood environment: some adoption studies. *Journal of Child Psychology and Psychiatry*, **22**, 195–200.

Black, M., Schuler, M., Nair, P. (1993). Prenatal drug exposure: neurodevelopmental outcome and parenting environment. *Journal of Pediatric Psychology*, **18**, 605–20.

Breslau, N. (1990). Does brain dysfunction increase children's vulnerability to environmental stress? *Archives of General Psychiatry*, **47**, 15–20.

Breslau, N., Prabucki, K. (1987). Siblings of disabled children. Effects of chronic stress in the family: published erratum appears in *Archives of General Psychiatry* 1988 Feb;45(2):196. *Archives of General Psychiatry*, **44**, 1040–6.

Burkett, G., Yasin, S., Palow, D. (1990). Perinatal implications of cocaine exposure. *Journal of Reproductive Medicine*, **35**, 35.

Buss, A.H., Plomin, R. (1984). *A Temperament Theory of Personality Development*. Wiley: New York.

Casaer, P. (1993). Old and new facts about perinatal brain development. *Journal of Child Psychology and Psychiatry*, **34**, 101–9.

Casaer, P., deVries, L. (1991). Pre- and peri-natal risk factors for psychosocial development. *In* Rutter, M.,Casaer, P. (Eds.) *Biological Risk Factors for Psychosocial Disorders*. Cambridge: Cambridge University Press.

Chess, S. (1993). Childhood Temperament. Paper given at Grand Rounds, New York University.

Chess, S., Thomas, A. (1984). *Origins and Evolution of Behavior Disorders*. New York: Brunner/Mazel.

Clarren, S.K., Smith, D.W. (1978). The fetal alcohol syndrome. *New England Journal of Medicine*, **298**, 1063–7.

Costello, A.M.d.L., Hamilton, P.A., Baudin, J., Townsend, J., Bradford, B.C., Stewart, A.L., Reynolds, E.O.R. (1988). Prediction of neurodevelopmental impairment at four years from brain ultrasound appearance of very preterm infants. *Developmental Medicine and Child Neurology*, **30**, 711–22.

Dallas, E., Stevenson, J., McGurk, H. (1993*a*). Cerebral-palsied children's interactions with siblings-I. Influence of severity of disability, age and birth order. *Journal of Child Psychology and Psychiatry*, **34**, 621–47.

Dallas, E., Stevenson, J., McGurk, H. (1993*b*). Cerebral-palsied children's interactions with siblings-II. Interactional structure. *Journal of Child Psychology and Psychiatry*, **34**, 649–71.

Davis, E., Fennoy, I. (1991). Growth and development in infants of cocaine abusing mothers. *Biological Psychiatry*, **31**, 194A.

Dunn, J., Kendrick, C. (1982). *Siblings: Love, Envy and Understanding*. Oxford, Cambridge MA: Blackwells, Harvard University Press.

Ekberg, M., Gillberg, C. (1977). Familjeterapi vid anorexia nervosa–ett behandlingsalternativ. Family therapy in anorexia nervosa–an alternative treatment. *Läkartidningen*, **74**, 647–50 (in Swedish).

Fergusson, D.M., Fergusson, J.E., Horwood, L.J., Kinzett, N.G. (1988). A longitudinal study of dental lead levels, intelligence, school performance and behaviour. *Journal of Child Psychology and Psychiatry*, **29**, 781–824.

Fernell, E., Gillberg, C., von Wendt, L. (1992). Self-esteem in children with infantile hydrocephalus and their siblings. Use of the Piers-Harris self-concept scale. *European Child & Adolescent Psychiatry*, **1**, 227–32.

Folsom, V., Krahn, D., Nairn, K., Gold, L., Demitrack, M.A., Silk, K.R. (1993). The impact of sexual and physical abuse on eating disordered and psychiatric symptoms: a comparison of eating disordered and psychiatric inpatients. *International Journal of Eating Disorders*, **13**, 249–57.

Folstein, S., Rutter, M. (1977). Infantile autism: a genetic study of 21 twin pairs. *Journal of Child Psychology and Psychiatry*, **18**, 297–321.

Garmezy, N., Rutter, M. (1985). Acute reactions to stress. *In* Rutter, M.,Hersov, L. (Eds.) *Child and Adolescent Psychiatry. Modern Approaches*. Oxford: Blackwell Scientific Publications.

Gath, A. (1974). Sibling reactions to mental handicap: a comparison of the brothers and sisters of mongol children. *Journal of Child Psychology and Psychiatry*, **15**, 187–98.

Gath, A. (1990). Down syndrome children and their families. *American Journal of Medical Genetics Suppl*, **7**, 314–16.

Gillberg, C. (1983). Perceptual, motor and attentional deficits in Swedish primary school children. Some child psychiatric aspects. *Journal of Child Psychology and Psychiatry*, **24**, 377–403.

Gillberg, C. (1991). Outcome in autism and autistic-like conditions. *Journal of the American Academy of Child and Adolescent Psychiatry*, **30**, 375–82.

Gillberg, C. (1992). The Emanuel Miller Memorial

Lecture 1991: Autism and autistic-like conditions: subclasses among disorders of empathy. *Journal of Child Psychology and Psychiatry*, **33**, 813–42.

Gillberg, C., Coleman, M. (1992). *The Biology of the Autistic Syndromes*. 2nd edition. London, New York: Mac Keith Press, Cambridge University Press.

Gillberg, C., Gillberg, I.C. (1983). Infantile autism: a total population study of reduced optimality in the pre-, peri-, and neonatal period. *Journal of Autism and Developmental Disorders*, **13**, 153–66.

Gillberg, C., Gillberg, I.C. (1991). Note on the relationship between population-based and clinical studies: the question of reduced optimality in autism: letter. *Journal of Autism and Developmental Disorders*, **21**, 251–3.

Gillberg, C., Rasmussen, P. (1982). Perceptual, motor and attentional deficits in seven-year-old children: background factors. *Developmental Medicine and Child Neurology*, **24**, 752–70.

Gillberg, C., Råstam, M. (1992). Do some cases of anorexia nervosa reflect underlying autistic-like conditions? *Behavioural Neurology*, **5**, 27–32.

Gillberg, C., Svenson, B., Carlström, G., Waldenström, E., Rasmussen, P. (1983). Mental retardation in Swedish urban children: some epidemiological considerations. *Applied Research in Mental Retardation*, **4**, 207–18.

Gillberg, C., Wahlström, J., Forsman, A., Hellgren, L., Gillberg, I.C. (1986). Teenage psychoses–epidemiology, classification and reduced optimality in the pre-, peri- and neonatal periods. *Journal of Child Psychology and Psychiatry*, **27**, 87–98.

Gillberg, C., Ehlers, S., Schaumann, H., Jakobsson, G., Dahlgren, S.O., Lindblom, R., Bågenholm, A., Tjuus, T., Blidner, E. (1990). Autism under age 3 years: a clinical study of 28 cases referred for autistic symptoms in infancy. *Journal of Child Psychology and Psychiatry*, **31**, 921–34.

Gillberg, C., Steffenburg, S., Wahlström, J., Gillberg, I.C., Sjöstedt, A., Martinsson, T., Liedgren, S., Eeg-Olofsson, O. (1991). Autism associated with marker chromosome. *Journal of the American Academy of Child and Adolescent Psychiatry*, **30**, 489–94.

Gillberg, I.C., Gillberg, C. (1994). Autism in immigrants. A population-based study from a Swedish rural and urban area. *Journal of Intellectual Disability Research*, (in press).

Golombok, S., Spencer, A., Rutter, M. (1983). Children in lesbian and single-parents households: psychosexual and psychiatric appraisal. *Journal of Child Psychology and Psychiatry*, **24**, 551–72.

Good, W.V., Ferreiro, D.M., Golabi, M., Kabori, J.A. (1992). Abnormalities of the visual system in infants exposed to cocaine. *Ophthalmology*, **99**, 341.

Goodyer, I.M. (1993). Recent stressful life events: their long term effects. *European Child & Adolescent Psychiatry*, **2**, 1–9.

Goodyear, I.M., Ashby, L., Altham, P.M.E., Vize, C., Cooper, P.J. (1993). Temperament and major depression in 11 to 16 year olds, *Journal of Child Psychology and Psychiatry*. **34**, 1409–23.

Hack, M., Taylor, H.G., Eiben, R., Schatschneider, C., Meruri-Minich, N. (1994). School-aged outcomes in children with birth weights under 750 g, *New England Journal of Medicine*, **31**, 802–3.

Hall, D. (1989). Birth asphyxia and cerebral palsy. *British Medical Journal*, **299**, 279–82.

Hanson, J.W., Smith, D.W. (1975). The fetal hydantoin syndrome. *Journal of Pediatrics*, **87**, 285.

Haracopos, D. (1988). *Hvad med mig?* Svendborg: Andonia. (In Danish.)

Hellgren, L., Gillberg, C., Enerskog, I. (1987). Antecedents of adolescent psychoses: a population-based study of school health problems in children who develop psychosis in adolescence. *Journal of the American Academy of Child and Adolescent Psychiatry*, **26**, 351–5.

Hetherington, E.M. (1985). Long-term effects of divorce and remarriage on the adjustment of children. *Journal of the American Academy of Child and Adolescent Psychiatry*, **24**, 518–30.

Hetherington, E.M., Cox, M., Cox, R. (1978). The aftermath of divorce. *In* Stevens, J.J.,Matthews, M. (Eds.) *Mother–child, father–child relations*. Washington, DC: National Association for the Education of Young Children.

Holland, A.J., Hall, A., Murray, R., Russell, G.F.M., Crisp, A.H. (1984). Anorexia nervosa: A study of 34 twin pairs and one set of triplets. *British Journal of Psychiatry*, **145**, 414–19.

Holland, A.J., Sicotte, N., Treasure, J. (1988). Anorexia nervosa: evidence for a genetic basis. *Journal of Psychosomatic Research*, **32**, 561–71.

Howlin, P., Wing, L., Gould, J. (1994). The recognition of autism in children with Down's Syndrome: implications for intervention. *Developmental Medicine and Child Neurology*, in press.

Hoyme, H.E., Jones, K.L., Dixon, S.D., Jerrett, T., Hanson, J.W., Robinson, L.K., Msall, M.E. & Allanson, F.E. (1990). Prenatal cocaine exposure and fetal vascular disruption. *Pediatrics*, **85**, 743.

Jonsson, G., Kälvesten, A.-L. (1964). *222 stockholmspojkar. En socialpsykiatrisk undersökning av pojkar i skolåldern (English summary)*. Stockholm: Almqvist & Wiksell. (In Swedish.)

Kyllerman, M., Hagberg, B. (1983). Reduced optimality in pre- and perinatal conditions in a Swedish newborn population. *Neuropediatrics*, **14**, 37–42.

Laegreid, L., Olegård, R., Wahlström, J., Conradi, N. (1989). Teratogenic effects of benzodiazepine use during pregancy. *Journal of Pediatrics*, **114**, 126.

Laegreid, L., Hagberg, G., Lundberg, A. (1992). The effect of benzodiazepines on the fetus and the newborn. *Neuropediatrics*, **23**, 18–23.

Lamb, M. (1991). Infancy. *In* Lewis, M. (Ed.) *Child and Adolescent Psychiatry. A Comprehensive Textbook*. Baltimore, Maryland: Williams & Wilkins.

Lorber, J. (1981). Is your brain really necessary? *Nursing Mirror*, **152**, 28–9.

Lucas, A., Morley, R., Cole, T.J. (1988). Adverse neurodevelopmental outcome of moderate neonatal hypoglycaemia. *British Medical Journal*, **297**, 1304–8.

Luthar, S.S., Zigler, E. (1991). Vulnerability and competence: a review of research on resilience in childhood. *American Journal of Orthopsychiatry*, **61**, 6–22.

McHale, S.M., Gamble, W.C. (1989). Siblings relationships of children with disabled and nondisabled brothers and sisters. *Developmental Psychology*, **25**, 421–9.

McHale, S.M., Sloan, J.L., Simeonsson, R.J. (1986). Sibling relationships of children with autistic, mentally retarded, and nonhandicapped brothers and sisters. *Journal of Autism and Developmental Disorders*, **16**, 399–413.

Minuchin, S., Baker, L., Rosman, B., Liebman, R., Milman, L., Todd, T. (1975). A conceptual model of psychosomatic illness in children. *Archives of General Psychiatry*, **32**, 1031–8.

Nakane, Y., Okuma, T., Takahashi, R. *et al.* (1980). Multi-institutional study on the teratogenicity and fetal toxicity of anti-epileptic drugs: a report of collaborative study group in Japan. *Epilepsia*, **21**, 663.

Norén, J., Hulthe, P., Gillberg, C. (1987). Analysis of lead and cadmium in deciduous teeth by means of potentiometric stripping analysis. *Swedish Dental Journal*, **11**, 45–52.

Oberfield, R., Gabriel, H.P. (1991). Prematurity, birth defects, and early death: Impact on the family. *In* Lewis, M. (Ed.) *Child and Adolescent Psychiatry. A Comprehensive Textbook*. Baltimore, Maryland: Williams & Wilkins.

Pedersen, N.L., Friberg, L., Floderus-Myrhed, B., G.E., Plomin, R. (1984). Swedish early separated twins: identification and characterization. *Acta Genetica Medicae et Gemellologiae*, **33**, 243–50.

Penrose, L.S. (1953). The genetic background of common diseases. *Acta Genetica et Statistica Medica*, **4**, 257–65.

Persson-Blennow, I., McNeil, T. (1982). Questionnaires for measurement of temperament in one- and two-year old children: development and standardization. *Journal of Child Psychology and Psychiatry*, **21**, 37–46.

Piven, J., Simon, J., Chase, G.A., Wzorek, M., Landa, R., Gayle, J., Folstein, S. (1993). The etiology of autism: pre-, peri-, and neonatal factors. *Journal of the American Academy of Child and Adolescent Psychiatry*, **6**, 1256–63.

Plomin, R. (1994). The Emanuel Miller Memorial Lecture 1993. Genetic research and identification of environmental influences. *Journal of Child Psychology and Psychiatry*, **35**, 817–34.

Plomin, R. (1989). Environment and genes. Determinants of behavior. *American Psychologist*, **44**, 105–11.

Plomin, R., Dunn, J. (Eds.) (1986). *The Study of Temperament: Changes, Continuities and Challenges*. Hillsdale, NJ: Lawrence Erlbaum.

Prechtl, H.F.R. (1980). The optimality concept. *Early Human Development*, **4**, 201–5.

Prior, M. (1992). Childhood temperament. *Journal of Child Psychology and Psychiatry*, **33**, 249–79.

Prior, M., Crook, G., Stripp, A., Power, M., Joseph, M. (1986). The relationship between temperament and personality: an exploratory study. *Personality and Individual Differences*, **7**, 875–81.

Råstam, M., Gillberg, C. (1991). The family background in anorexia nervosa: a population-based study. *Journal of the American Academy of Child and Adolescent Psychiatry*, **30**, 283–9.

Robinson, R.J. (1991). Causes and associations of severe and persistent specific speech and language disorders in children. *Developmental Medicine and Child Neurology*, **33**, 943–62.

Rutter, M. (1975). *Helping Troubled Children*. Harmondsworth: Penguin.

Rutter, M. (1977). Separation, loss and other family relationships. *In* Rutter, M.,Hersov, L. (Eds.) *Child Psychiatry: Modern Approaches*. Oxford: Blackwell Scientific.

Rutter, M. (1980). Raised lead levels and impaired cognitive/behavioural functioning: a review of the evidence. *Developmental Medicine and Child Neurology*, **Suppl. 42**, 1–36.

Rutter, M. (1981). Psychological sequelae of brain

damage in children. *American Journal of Psychiatry*, **138**, 1533–44.

Rutter, M. (1982). Syndromes attributed to minimal brain dysfunction in childhood. *American Journal of Psychiatry*, **139**, 21–33.

Rutter, M. (1985). Family and school influences on cognitive development. *Journal of Child Psychology and Psychiatry*, **26**, 683–704.

Rutter, M. (1987). Temperament, personality and personality disorder. *British Journal of Psychiatry*, **150**, 443–58.

Rutter, M., Hersov, L. (Eds.) (1985). *Child and Adolescent Psychiatry. Modern Approaches.* Oxford: Blackwell Scientific.

Rutter, M., Graham, P., Yule, W. (1970). *A Neuropsychiatric Study in Childhood.* London: S.I.M.P./William Heinemann Medical Books Ltd.

Rutter, M., Bolton, P., Herrington, R., Le Couteur, A., McDonald, H., Simonoff, E. (1990*a*). Genetic factors in child psychiatric disorders. Review of research strategies. *Journal of Child Psychology and Psychiatry*, **1**, 3–37.

Rutter, M., Mac Donald, H., Le Couteur, A., Harrington, R., Bolton, P., Bailey, A. (1990*b*). Genetic factors in child psychiatric disorders – II. Empirical findings. *Journal of Psychology and Psychiatry*, **31**, 39–83.

Steffenburg, S., Gillberg, C., Hellgren, L., Andersson, L., Gillberg, I.C., Jakobsson, G., Bohman, M. (1989). A twin study of autism in Denmark, Finland, Iceland, Norway and Sweden. *Journal of Child Psychology and Psychiatry*, **30**, 405–16.

Streissguth, A.P., Barr, H.M., Sampson, P.D. (1990). Moderate prenatal alcohol exposure: Effects on child IQ and learning problems at age 7 years. *Alcoholism, Clinical and Experimental Research*, **14**, 662.

Strömland, K., Miller, M. (1993). Thalidomide embryopathy: revisited 27 years later. *Acta Ophthalmologica*, **71**, 238–45.

Strömland, K., Miller, M., Cook, C. (1993). Ocular teratology. *Survey of Ophthalmology*, **35**, 429–46.

Strömland, K., Nordin, V., Miller, U., Akershöm, B., Gillberg, C. (1994). Autism in thalidomide embryopathy: a population study. *Developmental Medicine and Child Neurology*, **36**, 351–6.

Taylor, E. (1989). On the epidemiology of hyperactivity. *In* Sagvolden, T.,Archer, T. (Eds.) *Attention Deficit Disorder. Clinical and Basic Research.* Hillsdale, New Jersey: Lawrence Erlbaum Associated.

Taylor, E. (1991). Developmental neuropsychiatry.

Journal of Child Psychology and Psychiatry, **32**, 3–47.

Taylor, E., Sandberg, S., Thorley, G., Giles, S. (1991). *The Epidemiology of Childhood Hyperactivity.* London: Institute of Psychiatry.

Thomas, A., Chess, S. (1977). *Temperament and Development.* New York: Brunner/Mazel.

Thomas, A., Chess, S. (1984). Genesis and evolution of behavioral disorders: from infancy to early adult life. *American Journal of Psychiatry*, **141**, 1–9.

Thomas, A., Chess, S., Birch, H.G. (1968). *Temperament and Behavior Disorders in Children.* New York: New York University Press.

Trimble, M. (1988). *Biological Psychiatry.* Chichester: John Wiley and Sons.

van Baar, A. (1990). Development of infants of drug dependent mothers. *Journal of Child Psychology and Psychiatry*, **31**, 911–20.

Verhulst, F.C., Althaus, M., Versluis-Den Bieman, H.J.M. (1990*a*). Problem behavior in international adoptees: I. An epidemiological study. *Journal of the American Academy of Child and Adolescent Psychiatry*, **29**, 94–103.

Verhulst, F.C., Althaus, M., Versluis-Den Bieman, H.J.M. (1990*b*). Problem behavior in international adoptees: II. Age at placement. *Journal of the American Academy of Child and Adolescent Psychiatry*, **29**, 104–11.

Wallerstein, J.S. (1991). The long-term effects of divorce on children: a review. *Journal of the American Academy of Child and Adolescent Psychiatry*, **30**, 349–60.

Wallerstein, J.S., Kelly, J.B. (1980). *Surviving the Breakup.* New York: Basic Books.

Ward, F., Bower, B.D. (1978). A study of certain social aspects of epilepsy in childhood. *Developmental Medicine and Child Neurology*, **20**, Suppl no 39.

Weissman, M.M., Wickramaratne, P., Warner, V., John, K., Prusoff, B.A., Merikangas, K.R., Gammon, G.D. (1987). Assessing psychiatric disorders in children. *Archives of General Psychiatry*, **44**, 747–53.

Wing, L. (1993). The definition and prevalence of autism: A review. *European Child & Adolescent Psychiatry*, **2**, 1–14.

Witt-Engerström, I., Forslund, M. (1992). Mother and daughter with Rett syndrome. *Developmental Medicine and Child Neurology*, **34**, 1022–3.

Zigler, E.F., Finn-Stevenson, M. (1991). National policies for children, adolescents, and families. *In* Lewis, M. (Ed.) *Child and Adolescent Psychiatry.* Baltimore, Maryland: Williams & Wilkins.

4   A brief review of normal development

Normal development varies widely. The variation is partly accounted for by factors associated with IQ, sex, personality, intrafamilial/genetic characteristics and social influences, but much of the variance is poorly understood. This chapter does not aim to be a comprehensive survey of all aspects of normal development. It is intended as a background for a better understanding of the degree to which symptoms seen in abnormal states deviate qualitatively or quantitatively from the so-called norm. The reader wanting a more detailed description and fuller theoretical background of normal development is referred to specific textbooks on this topic (e.g. Illingworth, 1979; Lewis, 1982) or to comprehensive appraisals of the state-of-the-art as regards research findings (Rutter, 1980, 1984).

However, recent developments in social/cognitive psychology (e.g. Astington, Harris & Olson, 1988; Frith, 1989; Baron-Cohen, 1990; Duncan, 1986; Ozonoff, Pennington & Rogers, 1991), and in particular in the fields of 'shared attention', 'theory of mind', and 'executive function' have changed some of the conceptual framework for understanding normal social, communicative and cognitive development, and there are, as yet, no good comprehensive texts on normal development that adequately take these changes into account. Because of this dearth of good reviews, the current section will focus mostly on the recent expansion of knowledge in the fields of social interaction and communication.

Developmental milestones

Before discussing the important new insights gained with reference to the child's 'inner world', Table 4.1, outlining some of the outwardly obvious developmental milestones can serve as a crude point of reference.

The Table shows approximate dates at which certain selected developmental milestones are usually attained.

Normal variability

There can only be rough guidelines for normal child development. Normal inter-individual variation is wide for many variables. For instance, it is usually stated that unsupported walking is achieved at age 10–16 months, but in fact a child starting to walk at age 10 months may well be abnormal, perhaps belonging in a group of children with so-called attention deficit hyperactivity disorder (ADHD, see below), whereas another one, starting to walk at age 20 months may well turn out to be a highly intelligent child with familial late onset walking.

Sex differences

Girls are, on the whole, earlier in their development than boys (Rutter, 1980) and demonstrate a more rapid rate of maturation, even though for some measures, differences across sexes in the preschool years are relatively small (Prior *et al.*, 1993). This does not hold for certain gross motor skills (such as onset of walking) or visuospatial skills (boys are, for instance, earlier

Table 4.1. *Some developmental milestones*

Developmental milestone	Approximate age first noted
Gaze contact	1–2 hrs
Smile	0–4 wks
Vocalizing other than crying	2–8 wks
Social smile	2–3 mths
Begins to lift head in prone position	2–3 mths
Laughs aloud	2–4 mths
Bimanual (visually guided) coordination in reaching for objects	4–6 mths
Pulls self to stand holding on to furniture	5–10 mths
Sits steadily unsupported	7–10 mths
Responds to own name	7–10 mths
Sits self up on floor	8–10 mths
Pincer grip	9–12 mths
Waves bye-bye	9–12 mths
Holds out object to adult but will not release it	9–12 mths
One word with meaning	9–14 mths
Simple pretend play (e.g. peek-a-boo)	10–14 mths
Walks unsupported	10–16 mths
Holds out object to adult and will release it	11–14 mths
Shakes head for 'No"	12–16 mths
Walks up stairs, one hand held	16–20 mths
Complex pretend play (with toys)	18–24 mths
Goes up and down stairs alone, 2 feet per step	20–26 mths
Uses 'I', 'me', 'you'	2–2 1/2 yrs
Mutual play with other children	2–2 1/2 yrs
Five-word sentences comprehensible to strangers	2–3 yrs
Mainly dry by day	2–5 yrs
Mainly dry by night	2 1/2–6 yrs
Speech generally intelligible to strangers	2 1/2–5 yrs
(Imaginary companion)	(3–4 yrs)[a]
Skips on one foot	3 1/2–4 1/2 yrs
Tells 'stories'	3 1/2–4 1/2 yrs
Draws 'a man'	3 1/2–4 1/2 yrs
Emerging time concepts: distinguishes morning/evening	4 1/2–6 yrs

Note: [a] not a universal phenomenon.

and better than girls at jigsaws). Girls, as a group, seem to be particularly early in the development of some social and communication skills (Maccoby & Jacklin, 1980). Most girls have a 'peak' spurt of speech and language development around age 1.5–2 years. Some boys show a similar spurt even before this age, but most are later and have their corresponding spurt between the ages of 2 and 3 years. The normal range of variation in the development of speech and language skills appears to be considerably greater in boys than in girls. Limited evidence from studies of cerebrospinal fluid levels of homovanillic acid (the end-product of brain dopamine) indicates that girls may have significantly lower levels than boys (Gillberg, Svennerholm & Hamilton-Hellberg, 1983; Shaywitz *et al.*, 1984), a finding which could be taken to reflect a higher degree of maturation in CNS functioning, given the well-established negative correlation of homovanillic acid and age.

The systematic scientific study of sex differences in development is relatively scanty. Studies of development and developmental disability should always subdivide according to sex, but, so far, not enough attention has been paid to this need.

Shared attention and social referencing

Around age 9–14 months, normal children of both sexes begin to show clear signs that they want to share other people's attention, indicating joint points of reference (such as the lamp above the kitchen table). Not only do they indicate the objects as such; in doing this, they also look at people as if to check whether they too are interested and perhaps are looking at the same thing. It is possible that this drive for shared attention (Mundy & Sigman, 1989) is present in even younger infants, but, so far, clear examples of shared attention *behaviours* have not been documented before the end of the second half of the first year of life. It is also possible that a 'theory of mind' (see below) might be necessary for the appearance of signs of shared attention, and that shared attention is the first outward reflection of the presence of this mind theory. Baron-Cohen (1994) has postulated an 'eye direction detector, which develops in the infant period in normal children. He suggests that such a mechanism might be crucial for the development of awareness of other people as goal-directed beings capable of attending to objects.

Parallel to the appearance of shared attention behaviours, there is usually also the typical interest in peek-a-boo games and objects that disappear out of sight. This is not necessarily connected with shared attention, and the child may participate in peek-a-boo games in an imitative fashion without really sharing a joint external reference point with the other person.

Similar to the notion of shared attention is the concept of social referencing (Walden & Ogan 1988). Social referencing is s a process of emotional communication in which one's perception of other persons' interpretations is used to form one's own understanding of that event (Feinman, 1982). A four-level sequence of development leading to the ability to participate in social referencing has been proposed (Klinnert et al., 1983). First emerges the ability to discriminate among emotional expressions, for instance, on mother's or father's face. Then follows the gradual recognition of the meaning of these various expressions. After that comes emotional responsiveness. Finally, the ability to refer to another person and interactive regulation of behaviour appear. It is this final stage which is usually referred to as social referencing. The first links in this chain of development are observable already at age 6–9 months (Walden & Ogan, 1988).

More complex forms of social interaction and empathy: the emergence of 'theory of mind'

The normal infant is socially responsive and already ready to interact immediately after birth. New-borns have been demonstrated to fixate, give gaze contact and even to imitate slightly after intensive coaxing. This should not be taken to mean that the new-born baby has good social interaction skills typical of older children. It does imply that the old notion of a 'normal autistic phase' in early development was mistaken.

The necessary basic skills for developing a superficially acceptable 'social competence' are, in a sense, there from the beginning. Gaze contact, imitation and turn-taking are all necessary if there is ever going to be the kinds of behaviours associated with gossiping, interaction at cocktail- and tea-parties or small talk at the bus station. These behaviours are best termed 'superficial social competence skills'. It is likely that it is possible to strengthen such skills through training and practice. This would be evidenced by the observation that girls tend to be better at such things than boys (girls often get more training in these areas than boys when they are young). On the other hand, there could be qualitative biological differences between boys and girls in this respect already from infancy.

Possibly separate from superficial social competence skills, there appear towards the end of the child's first year obvious signs that he/she has developed a 'theory of mind', that is an ability to impute mental states such as knowing and believing to other people and to oneself. For instance, if a 12-month-old baby, turning the pages of a picture book, is stopped in this activity by another person firmly putting his/her hand over the child's, the child will look the other person in the eye rather than just try to get rid of the hand. It seems reasonable to assume that underlying *this* kind of gaze contact would be the presumption on the part of the child that the other person has an intention in doing what he/she is doing. In other words, the child has a theory of mind. As he/she grows older he will become aware that there are a variety of mental states in other people and that there is not necessarily a correspondence between superficial social competence skills and these states of mind. The child even begins to be able to think: 'He thinks she thinks'. He/she will then also be able to gradually develop a more sophisticated understanding of complex social cues and interactions and of other people's many-faceted feelings. A theory of mind would also be necessary for the development of a generally good 'human' intelligence. Without a theory of mind the child will not be able to ask meaningful questions of other people (either verbally or non-verbally), and his use of language and 'communication' will not be appropriate for acquiring new skills. Rote memory skills need not be affected at all, however, and some children who appear to lack a theory of mind may be thought of as 'idiots savants' (see Frith, 1989) and show remarkable skills in one or two areas.

A theory of mind is a prerequisite for developing empathy (the ability to reflect intuitively and correctly about other people's thoughts and feelings). Empathy, in turn, is necessary for the development of sympathy and compassion (terms often semantically confused with empathy). However, empathy is not all that is necessary to develop these 'talents'. For instance, sociopaths/psychopaths may have good empathic skills (necessary when deliberately trying to deceive people) and yet generally show little compassion or sympathy with anybody but themselves (Gillberg, 1993).

Many children show signs of compassion and sympathy before age 2 years, for instance, in approaching and wanting to hug, kiss and comfort somebody who has been hurt or is crying.

It is common knowledge that we are all different in our superficial social competence skills and in respect of empathy skills and compassion. Perhaps all these three variables are, to a considerable extent, biologically determined, discrete, or only partly overlapping, functions which are distributed in much the same way as IQ along a spectrum from superior skills to severe dysfunction. This line of reasoning is in keeping with the writings of Frith (e.g. Frith, 1991). Maybe, in the lowermost portion of each spectrum, there exists a small group affected by environmentally caused dysfunction or specific genetic disorders (such as in the case of brain damage in cases with very low IQ). If this were the case, there would be similar types of social dysfunction caused either by brain damage/dysfunction, genetic disorders or by simply being on the lowermost end of the normal distribution.

There is, as yet, very little empirical evidence to support the construct of three independent social variables along the lines suggested. Nevertheless, there is emerging evidence that, in principle, theory of mind skills may show the same type of developmental changes with age as do functional capacities associated with varying levels of cognitive endowment as reflected in different levels of IQ (Happé, 1991). Gillberg (1992) has suggested that empathy and theory of mind skills may be regarded as synonymous constructs, and that the concept of an 'empathy quotient' (EQ) might be useful when trying to develop new tests of skills trying to tap this type of underlying neuropsychological function.

Social dysfunction syndromes seen in the light of recent developments in normal social/cognitive psychology

Social dysfunctions and problems of various kinds are the hallmarks of many of the neuropsychiatric disorders of childhood. Autism and autism spectrum disorders, including so-called Asperger syndrome are now the best known of such conditions. Both seem to share severe problems of empathy. People with autism are generally deficient in superficial social competence skills, empathy and, to some extent, compassion. IQ is often low as well. People with Asperger syndrome are, invariably, deficient in empathy and, to some extent, compassion. IQ is often normal or high. Such people are likely to be diagnosed as Asperger syndrome if superficial social competence skills are also impaired. However, there could be Asperger cases with relatively well-developed superficial skills of this kind who would then be accepted as belonging in a normal group in spite of severe empathy deficits. Girls, in particular, might have relatively good social competence skills and yet be severely deficient in the development of empathy skills. A diagnosis of Asperger syndrome in such girls will probably not be thought of, much less made. Children with deficits in attention, motor control and perception (DAMP) often have slight dysfunctions in all three areas (and sometimes in overall intelligence as well). Psychopaths need only be deficient in compassion and must, almost by definition, have good empathy skills. It appears that an analysis in terms of superficial social competence skills, empathy and compassion (and IQ) in patients showing social dysfunction might be useful and have far-reaching practical implications. So far, most psychiatric/neuropsychiatric evaluations do not make use of this model for analysis. The following presentation of neuropsychiatric problems in childhood will also rely on a more conservative phenotypical structure, and various syndromes will be described mainly as they show in outward symptoms and signs. Nevertheless, an awareness of the briefly surveyed expansion of our knowledge as regards children's social and cognitive development, is likely to be helpful when trying to understand children affected with neuropsychiatric problems in more depth.

Intellectual development

Intellectual development and the development of intelligence are often considered synonymous. Intelligence is 'the broadest and most pervasive cognitive trait, and is conceived of as being involved in virtually every kind of cognitive skill' and 'it is a quintessentially high-level skill at the summit of a hierarchy of intellectual skills' (Butcher, 1970). Intelligence is also 'what intelligence tests measure, a sample of current intellectual performance' (Madge & Tizard, 1980). Tested IQ is a *relatively* stable variable: more than 87–90% of all children show less than 30 points IQ variation from age 2–18 years if several tests are performed during this period (Honzik, Macfarlane & Allen, 1948; Moffitt *et al.*, 1993) and more than 80% show less than 15 points variation if only one retest is undertaken (Vernon, 1976). Stability over time is further increased if the first IQ-test is undertaken after age 6 years. Before age 2 years, IQ-tests have strong predictive validity only in the case of severely and profoundly mentally retarded children.

Cognitive development is rapid during the first few years of life and continues at a fast rate throughout childhood to adolescence. Thereafter the rate is much slower and most people reach a point (perhaps in early adult life) beyond which they do not increase their intelligence capacities. In adult age, IQ is defined by tests which yield normally distributed results in the general population and have a mean of 100. In childhood, IQ can be conceptualized in similar terms, but also as the equivalent of a developmental quotient (DQ) in which mental age is divided by chronological age and multiplied by 100. When used in this way, a child with an IQ of 50 around age 8 years can be seen roughly as having 50% of normal development for chronological age and therefore performing similarly to a normal 4 year-old.

Spearman (1927) found that people who did well on one cognitive task usually also did well on most of the other cognitive tasks. He hypothesized that a 'general' (g) factor, or 'mental energy', was in operation. Children with emotional and behaviour problems, as we shall see, very often have cognitive profiles which are extremely uneven and which cannot be predicted by a specific g-factor level.

Both genes and environmental factors play a

part in determining individual differences in IQ, but their relative contribution is not clearly established. That there are strong genetic determinants for IQ is now widely accepted. The overall effects of environment on the development of intelligence in individuals falling within the normal range of intelligence are probably less pronounced, except in grossly abnormal situations, such as *extreme* psychosocial deprivation and long-term near starvation. The Dunedin study of IQ at ages 7, 9, 11 and 13 years showed a remarkable consistency over time in most cases (n = 794). However, a subgroup of 13% showed IQ changes that clearly exceeded what was expected from sources of measurement errors. However, even in this subgroup, long-term change tended to be small: most of the children whose IQs were depressed bounced back within a few years, and those whose IQs were increased fell back to previous levels. In the words of the authors, the data suggest the 'hopeful thought that children really are wonderfully resilient' (Moffitt *et al.*, 1993).

Development of handedness

There are clear relationships between handedness of parents and offspring but the patterns are not easily fitted to any Mendelian inheritance mode. Concordance for handedness is not very high in twins and the difference in rate between monozygotic and dizygotic twins is small. Annett (1975) proposed that what is inherited is not the direction of asymmetry, but whether or not there is symmetry ('the right shift theory'). Thus, handedness is not as straightforward a behaviour or trait as believed by many laymen and clinicians (Bishop, 1990). Abnormal factors commonly underlie handedness. This statement holds regardless of whether right- or lefthandedness is considered.

However, a considerably larger proportion of individuals who are left-handed than of those who are right-handed are so for pathological reasons (Bishop 1980; Gillberg, Waldenström & Rasmussen, 1984). Also, it appears that mixed handedness may be an indicator of various forms of brain dysfunction (Bishop, 1990).

Handedness (or rather hand preference) is usually established by age 6 years (Fennell, Bowers & Morris, 1983). Those who prefer the right hand at this stage show much greater stability of handedness over the next 5 years as compared with ambidextrous children. There is even some stronger stability as compared with left-handers. Consistent hand-preference is often present long before age 6 years. Cohen (1966) found that already at age 8 months, consistent hand preference was significantly related to advanced developmental status, and Kaufmann, Zalma & Kaufmann, (1978) and Tan (1985) confirmed that preschool 'unestablished' hand preference correlated with poor motor skills.

Some notes on differential diagnostic aspects in relation to motor skills development

Early childhood clumsiness is a marker for neurodevelopmental and neuropsychiatric problems in later childhood and adolescence (Shaffer *et al.*, 1985; Hellgren, Gillberg & Gillberg, 1994). Clumsiness is usually hard to define in terms of operationalized criteria and either constitutes a sum abnormality score for various kinds of neurodevelopmental assessment ratings or a subjective clinical 'gestalt' impression (Losse *et al.*, 1991). The most salient features of the clumsiness appear to be in coordination of movements, associated movements of other parts of the body when trying to perform, and a general lack of control over motor movements at times when the individual is not concentrating his/her full attention on the performance.

It is obvious that many of the best-known neuropsychiatric disorders of childhood are associated with motor clumsiness. This is certainly true of DAMP (Gillberg IC, Gillberg & Groth, 1989) and Asperger syndrome (Gillberg, 1991), which include motor clumsiness as a diagnostic criterion (at least according to some definitions). It may hold equally true in developmental language disorders (Robinson, 1991), Tourette syndrome (Comings, 1990), hyperkinetic disorders (Taylor *et al.*, 1991) and adolescent onset psychosis (Hellgren, Gillberg & Enerskog, 1987). The longitudinal studies of young children with motor clumsiness suggest that affective and anxiety disorders may, at least to some extent, be predicted by childhood 'minor neurological dysfunction' (clinically roughly equivalent to clumsiness) (Shaffer *et al.*, 1985, Hellgren *et al.*, 1994).

Clumsiness is one of several markers for neurodevelopmental delay and/or deviance. Its clinical implication has been under-rated in child psychiatry. Not only is the diagnosis of clumsiness a worthwhile tool in the overall neuropsychiatric evaluation of any child with psychiatric problems; it provides clues as to ways of understanding and helping troubled children. Many young individuals suffer from 'undiagnosed' clumsiness in connection with their more obvious emotional or behavioural problems. A better understanding of the effects of the clumsiness *per se* on the psychological well-being of the individual (as well as of its status as a marker for neurodevelopmental problems generally), will contribute to more rational intervention and to better psychological adjustment of the child (or adolescent).

References

Annett, M. (1975). Hand preference and the laterality of cerebral speech. *Cortex*, **11**, 305–28.

Astington, J., Harris, P., Olson, D. (1988). *Developing Theories of Mind.* Cambridge: Cambridge University Press.

Baron-Cohen, S. (1990). Autism: a specific cognitive disorder of 'mind-blindness'. *International Review of Psychiatry*, **2**, 81–90.

Baron-Cohen, S. (1994). Origins of a theory of mind: the eye-direction detector. *International Journal of Psychology* (in press).

Bishop, D.V.M. (1980). Handedness, clumsiness and cognitive ability. *Developmental Medicine and Child Neurology*, **22**, 569–79.

Bishop, D.V.M. (1990). *Handedness and Developmental Disorders. Clinics in Developmental Medicine. No. 110.* London: Mac Keith Press.

Butcher, H.J. (1970). *Human Intelligence: Its Nature and Assessment.* London: Methuen.

Cohen, A.I. (1966). Hand preference and developmental status of infants. *Journal of Genetic Psychology*, **108**, 225–37.

Comings, D. (1990). *Tourette Syndrome and Human Behavior.* Duarte, CA: Hope Press.

Duncan, J. (1986). Disorganization of behavior after frontal lobe damage. *Cognitive Neuropsychology*, **3**, 271–90.

Feinman, S. (1982). Social referencing in infancy. *Merril-Palmer Quarterly*, **29**, 83–7.

Fennell, E.B., Bowers, D., Morris, R. (1983). The development of handedness and dichotic listening asymmetries in relation to school achievement: a longitudinal study. *Journal of Experimental Child Psychology*, **35**, 248–62.

Frith, U. (1989). Autism and 'theory of mind'. *In* Gillberg, C. (Ed.) *Diagnosis and Treatment of Autism.* New York: Plenum Press.

Frith, U. (1991). Autistic psychopathy in childhood. Hans Asperger. Translated and annotated by Uta Frith. *In* Frith, U. (Ed.) *Autism and Asperger Syndrome.* Cambridge: Cambridge University Press.

Gillberg, C. (1991). Clinical and neurobiological aspects of Asperger syndrome in six family studies. *In* Frith, U. (Ed.) *Autism and Asperger Syndrome.* Cambridge: Cambridge University Press.

Gillberg, C. (1992). The Emanuel Miller Memorial Lecture 1991: autism and autistic-like conditions: subclasses among disorders of empathy. *Journal of Child Psychology and Psychiatry*, **33**, 813–42.

Gillberg, C. (1993). Empathy disorders: basic problems in several psychiatric handicap conditions. *Läkartidningen*, **90**, 467–70. (In Swedish).

Gillberg, C., Svennerholm, L., Hamilton-Hellberg, C. (1983). Childhood psychosis and monoamine metabolites in spinal fluid. *Journal of Autism and Developmental Disorders*, **13**, 383–396.

Gillberg, C., Waldenström, E., Rasmussen, P. (1984). Handedness in Swedish 10-year-olds. Some background and associated factors. *Journal of Child Psychology and Psychiatry*, **25**, 421–32.

Gillberg, I.C., Gillberg, C., Groth, J. (1989). Children with preschool minor neurodevelopmental disorders. V: Neurodevelopmental profiles at age 13. *Developmental Medicine and Child Neurology*, **31**, 14–24.

Happé, F. (1991). The autobiographical writings of three Asperger syndrome adults: problems of interpretation and implications for theory. *In* Frith, U. (Ed.) *Autism and Asperger Syndrome.* Cambridge: Cambridge University Press.

Hellgren, L., Gillberg, C., Enerskog, I. (1987).

Antecedents of adolescent psychoses: a population-based study of school health problems in children who develop psychosis in adolescence. *Journal of the American Academy of Child and Adolescent Psychiatry*, **26**, 351–5.

Hellgren, L., Gillberg, C., Gillberg, I.C. (1994). Children with deficits in attention, motor control and perception (DAMP) almost grown up: the contribution of various background factors to outcome at age 16 years. *European Child & Adolescent Psychiatry*, **3**, 1–15.

Honzik, M.P., Macfarlane, J.W., Allen, L. (1948). The stability of mental test performance between two and eighteen years. *Journal of Experimental Education*, 309–24.

Illingworth, R.S. (1979). *The Normal Child*. 7th Edn. Edinburgh: Churchill Livingstone.

Kaufmann, A.S., Zalma, R., Kaufmann, N.L. (1978). The relationship of hand dominance to the motor coordination, mental ability, and right–left awareness of young normal children. *Child Development*, **49**, 885–8.

Klinnert, M., Campos, J., Emde, R., Svedja, M. (1983). Social referencing: emotional expressions as behavior regulators. *In* Plutschik, R.,Kellerman, H. (Eds.) *Emotion: Theory, Research and Experience. Vol. 2. Emotions in Early Development*. Orlando, FL: Academic Press.

Lewis, M. (1982). *Clinical Aspects of Child Development*. Philadelphia: Lea & Febiger.

Losse, A., Henderson, S.E., Elliman, D., Hall, D., Knight, E., Jongmans, M. (1991). Clumsiness in children–do they grow out of it? A 10-year follow-up study. *Developmental Medicine and Child Neurology*, **33**, 55–68.

Maccoby, E.E., Jacklin, C.N. (1980). Sex differences in aggression: a rejoinder and reprise. *Child Development*, **51**, 964–80.

Madge, N., Tizard, J. (1980). Intelligence. *In* Rutter, M. (Ed.) *Developmental Psychiatry*. London: Heinemann Medical.

Moffitt, T.E., Caspi, A., Harkness, A.R., Silva, P.A. (1993). The natural history of change in intellectual performance: Who changes? How much? Is it meaningful? *Journal of Child Psychology and Psychiatry*, **34**, 455–506.

Mundy, P., Sigman, M. (1989). Specifying the nature of the social impairment in autism. *In* Dawson, G. (Ed.) *Autism: New Perspectives on Nature, Diagnosis and Treatment*. New York: Guilford.

Ozonoff, S., Pennington, B.F., Rogers, S.J. (1991). Executive function deficit in high-functioning autistic individuals: relationships to theory of mind. *Journal of Child Psychology and Psychiatry*, **32**, 1081–5.

Prior, M., Smart, D., Sanson, A., Oberklaid, F. (1993). Sex differences in psychological adjustment from infancy to 8 years. *Journal of the American Academy of Child and Adolescent Psychiatry*, **32**, 291–304 discussion 305.

Robinson, R.J. (1991). Causes and associations of severe and persistent specific speech and language disorders in children. *Developmental Medicine and Child Neurology*, **33**, 943–62.

Rutter, M. (1980). *Scientific Foundation of Developmental Psychiatry*. London: Heinemann Medical.

Rutter, M. (Ed.) (1984). *Developmental Neuropsychiatry*. Edinburgh: Churchill Livingstone.

Shaffer, D., Schonfeld, I., O'Connor, P., Stokman, C., Trautman, P., Shafer, S., Ng, S. (1985). Neurological soft signs. Their relationship to psychiatric disorder and intelligence in childhood and adolescence. *Archives of General Psychiatry*, **42**, 342–51.

Shaywitz, S.E., Shaywitz, B.A., Cohen, D.J., Young, J.G. (1984). Monoaminergic mechanisms in hyperactivity. *In* Rutter, M. (Ed.) *Developmental Neuropsychiatry*. London: Churchill Livingstone.

Spearman, C. (1927). The doctrine of two factors. Reprinted in: Wiseman, S. (1967). (Ed.) *Intelligence and Ability: Selected Readings*. Harmondsworth: Penguin.

Tan, L.E. (1985). Laterality and motor skills in four-year-olds. *Child Development*, **56**, 363–73.

Taylor, E., Sandberg, S., Thorley, G., Giles, S. (1991). *The Epidemiology of Childhood Hyperactivity*. London: Institute of Psychiatry.

Vernon, P.E. (1976). Development of intelligence. *In* Hamilton, V.,Vernon, M.D. (Eds.) *The Development of Cognitive Processes*. London and New York: Academic Press.

Walden, T.A., Ogan, T.A. (1988). The development of social referencing. *Child Development*, **59**, 1230–40.

Part II:
Clinical disorders

5 Mental retardation and other severe learning disorders: an overview

Mental retardation is not a disease or specific disability. It is an administrative cover-all blanket term for a variety of different genetic, social and specific medical conditions sharing the one common feature that individuals affected test (reliably) below IQ 70 (or 67–73) on specific IQ tests (see below). In certain countries, a diagnosis of mental retardation will not be made unless the affected individual is in need of the support of society for his daily life.

Mental retardation is subgrouped according to the level of tested IQ. Profound mental retardation is the term often used for cases with IQ under 20. If this category is used at all, then severe mental retardation is the term used for cases with IQ of 20–34/39 and moderate mental retardation for cases with IQ in the 35/40–49/54 range. Mild mental retardation is the category applied to cases with IQ in the 50/55–69/74 range.

It is becoming increasingly common to include only two levels, i.e. severe mental retardation (SMR) for cases with IQ < 50 and mild mental retardation (MMR) for IQ-levels in the 50–69 range. Borderline intellectual functioning is the term applied when IQ is in the 70–84 range. This subgrouping system is the one which will be used in this chapter.

The DSM-III-R (the Diagnostic and Statistical Manual of Mental Disorders. Third Edition Revised, 1987) includes four levels of severity of mental retardation. Mild mental retardation corresponds to IQ-levels of 50–55 to approximately 70. Moderate mental retardation is diagnosed in cases with an IQ of 35–40 to 50–55, severe mental retardation in cases with IQ 20–25 to 25–40 and profound mental retardation in cases with IQ below 20–25.

Prevalence

Mild mental retardation is more common than severe mental retardation, but claims that it is about seven times more common, such as in the DSM-III-R (APA 1987), seem to have no support in the modern literature.

Recent Swedish studies have suggested that unequivocal mental retardation occurs in less than 1% of all school-age children. Hagberg et al. (1981) found that 0.7% of all 10–13 year-olds in one Swedish urban area had tested IQ < 70–73 and were in need of extra educational or psychosocial support. Slightly less than half of the children had severe mental retardation (i.e. they had an IQ < 50) and the remaining had mild mental retardation (IQ 50–70). Hagberg's group acknowledged that a number of borderline cases might have been missed, and that tested IQ in the Swedish population of children tended towards a higher mean than 100. On follow-up during the teenage period, almost 1% of the population was classified as mentally retarded. Mild mental retardation was about twice as common as severe mental retardation. Gillberg et al. (1983) found that 1% of the whole 7–8 year-old population in a Swedish urban area (Göteborg) had tested IQ < 73 and needed special education. They also found 1% of children in that age group who had tested IQ close to 73 (without clearly and constantly falling below this level) and who required special education.

These prevalence figures are considerably lower than reported in earlier studies. One possible explanation is that the IQ-tests used were standardized long ago and that they now yield a 'falsely high' IQ score. Another contributory factor could be the early stimulation in day-care centres and similar settings which could lead to a 'transiently higher' IQ score in early childhood. This would be supported by the findings of Hagberg *et al.* that 'new' mental retardation cases continued to be diagnosed even in adolescence, after the effects of early stimulation had subsided.

Severe mental retardation (IQ < 50) occurs at a rate of 0.3–0.4% already at age 3 years, because it is commonly diagnosed in the first few years of life. The rate is then relatively stable for several years, but will eventually begin to drop a little because of the increased mortality rate. The rate of severe mental retardation has been surprisingly stable over time and culture (Lewis, 1929; Kushlik, 1961; Åkesson, 1961; Wing, 1971; Bernsen, 1977; Hagberg & Kyllerman, 1983). Mild mental retardation (IQ 50–70) is diagnosed in only a very few cases during the first years of life, because, with milder degrees of retardation, it becomes progressively more difficult to recognize that the child is actually handicapped. Most cases of mild mental retardation are diagnosed from age 3–7 years, but, as has already been pointed out, prevalence will continue to increase throughout the school years, at least if no screening IQ-test is performed at a young age.

The rate of mental retardation will also depend on cultural factors, such as social deprivation, early stimulation programmes, the tolerance level in society (both in the positive and negative sense of that word) and access to and provision of special education services.

Boys are affected by mental retardation more often than girls. The boy:girl ratio is in the range of 1.3–1.9:1. Some mental retardation conditions are much more common in boys than in girls (e.g. the fragile X syndrome and autism), but very rarely the reverse is true (e.g. the Rett syndrome).

Background factors

Having a low tested IQ can depend on a wide variety of factors. Several hundred different medical conditions can cause mental retardation. Genetic and social factors can also contri-bute to cause mental retardation (Thompson & O'Quinn, 1979). The panorama of aetiologies varies with the degree of mental retardation and with a number of geographic/cultural factors and factors associated with ante- and perinatal care. A brief overview of the various causes of mental retardation will be provided according to a subdivision of cases into those with severe and those with mild mental retardation.

Background factors in moderate, severe and profound mental retardation (IQ < 50)

The aetiology of severe mental retardation can often be established with accuracy. A number of major chromosomal abnormalities are associated with severe mental retardation. Enzyme deficiencies due to single (or in some cases multiple) gene defects can sometimes be demonstrated. Certain disorders carrying a high risk of severe mental retardation are inherited in autosomal recessive fashion. In such disorders, carrier-status in clinically unaffected (or mildly affected) relatives can sometimes be identified. In yet other cases, physical or behavioural features cluster together in such a way that the diagnosis of a specific syndrome can be made even without the identification of a biological marker. However, in such syndromes, there are always 'borderline' variants for which a case can be made both for inclusion and exclusion. In several cases, aetiology cannot be established with certainty, but, inference suggests a plausible cause. This applies to many cases of perinatal asphyxia, infections and environmental toxins (such as intra-uterine alcohol poisoning), factors which have demonstrable brain damaging properties, but for which there is no proven cause–effect relationship in the individual case. Finally, there are cases of unknown aetiology, including some with a familial loading and some with great reductions of pre-, peri- and neonatal optimality (see below).

Hagberg and Kyllerman (1983) found a definite or highly probable cause of severe mental retardation in just over 80% of cases (Fig. 5.1). Two-thirds of these were of prenatal and about one-sixth each were of perinatal and postnatal origin. The prenatal factors were chromosomal

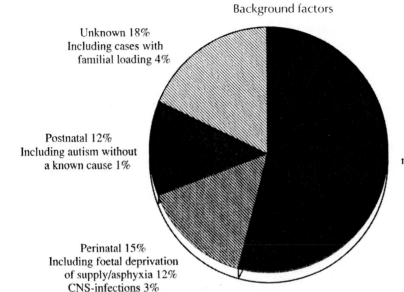

Unknown 18%
Including cases with
familial loading 4%

Postnatal 12%
Including autism without
a known cause 1%

Perinatal 15%
Including foetal deprivation
of supply/asphyxia 12%
CNS-infections 3%

Prenatal 55%. Including
chromosomal and other
genetic factors 34%
multiple congenital anomalies
and specific syndromes 10%
pregnancy factors including
infections 8%

Fig. 5.1.

in more than half the cases (trisomy 21 being much the most common type). In a further 20%, multiple anomalies were present in the absence of chromosomal abnormalities. Prenatal infections accounted for 13% of the prenatal factors. Clear genetic disorders without demonstrable chromosomal abnormality constituted less than 10% of the prenatal factors. The perinatal factors were fetal deprivation and asphyxia in most cases and perinatal CNS-infections in a minority. The postnatal factors were variable and could not be easily grouped. Of those 18% of severe mental retardation cases who had an unknown aetiology, slightly less than one in four had a familial clustering.

Background factors in mild mental retardation (IQ 50–70)

It is more difficult to arrive at a correct aetiological diagnosis in mild mental retardation. In the study by Hagberg and Kyllerman (1983) a definite or highly probable cause was found in just under 45% of the cases (Fig. 5.2). Psychosocial factors contribute considerably more to the aetiological variance in this group than in severe mental retardation.

More than half of the known or probable causes were of prenatal origin. However, the pattern was very different from that seen in severe mental retardation. Foetal alcohol exposure was the single most common factor, accounting for one-third of the prenatal cases. (Foetal alcohol syndrome is now believed to be the leading 'cause' of mental retardation in the western world (Abel & Sokol, 1986)). Identifiable chromosomal abnormalities were much less common than in the severely retarded group, but syndromes with multiple congenital anomalies were relatively common. Perinatal factors were relatively common and almost all of these were associated with foetal deprivation and asphyxia. Only 1 out of 91 cases of mild mental retardation appeared to have been caused by perinatal CNS-infection. Postnatal factors were a rare cause for mild mental retardation. Of those 55% of mild mental retardation cases without a known or probable cause, more than half showed familial clustering.

Background factors in borderline intellectual functioning (IQ 71–84)

It is usually very difficult to establish the cause of borderline intellectual functioning. A number of cases with IQs in the 71–84 range can be accounted for by their being on the lower portion of the normal distribution for intellec-

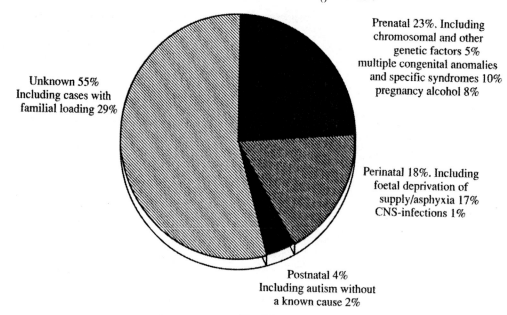

Unknown 55%
Including cases with
familial loading 29%

Prenatal 23%. Including
chromosomal and other
genetic factors 5%
multiple congenital anomalies
and specific syndromes 10%
pregnancy alcohol 8%

Perinatal 18%. Including
foetal deprivation of
supply/asphyxia 17%
CNS-infections 1%

Postnatal 4%
Including autism without
a known cause 2%

Fig. 5.2.

tual capacity, and the same probably applies to some of the mild mental retardation cases. Indirect evidence from studies of children with deficits in attention, motor control and perception (Gillberg & Rasmussen, 1982) suggests that pre-, peri- and postnatal brain damaging factors play a role in about one-third of the cases. It has been proposed that 'reduced optimality' in pregnancy and the peri- and postnatal periods might be more important than the occurrence of single major events. Reduced optimality is defined as any departure from the defined optimal state for any specified factor/ condition during the pre-, peri- and neonatal periods. A high reduced score would indicate a low level of optimality. The level of reduced optimality seems to be greater in borderline intellectual functioning than in severe mental retardation (Gillberg, Gillberg & Steffenburg, 1990; Gillberg & Gillberg, 1991). The reduced optimality could reflect both constitutional defects in the foetus and events which could lead to brain dysfunction. There might be important interactions between genetic factors and environmental factors associated with the reduced optimality . – Many studies also sug-

gest that psychosocial factors (including understimulation) are of considerable importance in this group (Craft, 1985).

Summary of background factors in mental retardation

Known genetic disorders (including Down syndrome) accounted for 47% of severe mental retardation cases, but only for 5% of mild mental retardation cases in the Hagberg and Kyllerman (1983) study. Intra-uterine infections were responsible for 10% of severe retardation, but were not encountered at all in the mildly retarded group. Foetal alchohol exposure was not a contributory factor in the severely retarded group, but accounted for 9% of the mild mental retardation cases. However, it is well known that intra-uterine exposure to alcohol may lead to severe mental retardation (Edwards, 1983; Strömland & Miller, 1993). The failure to document alcohol as a background factor in the Swedish study may be just a reflection of the relatively small number of cases involved rather than of alcohol being unimportant in the aetiological panorama of severe mental retardation. Foetal deprivation with or without asphyxia contributed about 20% of cases in both groups. The numbers that remained unexplained were 18% in the severely retarded and 55% in the mildly retarded group, but the tendency to familial clustering was much greater in the latter group, indicating the possible presence of one or several genetic factors. In the group with borderline intellectual functioning genetic factors, psychosocial factors and reduced optimality in the pre-, peri- and neonatal periods appear to interact in a complex pattern to cause mild (but clinically often very important) reductions of IQ.

A number of environmental factors, such as foetal exposure to drugs and postnatal exposure to lead and other toxins, could, theoretically contribute to cause mental retardation in certain individuals. There is ample evidence that lead can lower IQ (Needleman & Gatsonis, 1990), but the extent to which it may be involved in the causation of mental retardation has not been analysed. More research is warranted in this field.

It should be self-evident that, depending on the part of the world one is living in, the aetiological panorama of mental retardation will differ. For instance, if there is widespread starvation, intra-uterine malnourishment will be a major cause of mental retardation. Certain genetic conditions are more common in some countries than in others. These, and other factors, account for the wide variation both as regards prevalence and background factors in mental retardation.

The clinical picture in the mental retardation syndromes

Mental retardation is not *one* syndrome. This needs pointing out again and again, because many clinicians seem to regard mental retardation as some sort of syndromal diagnosis. Depending on underlying aetiology, the clinical picture varies very much from one underlying syndrome to another. Within syndromes, the clinical picture may vary as a consequence of such factors as personality ('temperament'),

associated disorders (such as epilepsy and motor impairment), degree of intellectual disability (which, of course, is very variable even within syndromes) and psychosocial environment.

Developments in the last 30 years have made it obvious that there is no clinical picture common to people with mental retardation. It is rare, even for the 'cognitive profile' to be smooth and even. It is the rule, rather than the exception, that there is some degree of 'irregularity' in the test profile. For example, if a person has an overall tested IQ of about 60, it would not be surprising if, in one area, he would receive a subscale IQ of 80 and in another area of 45. Unfortunately, even though this insight is acknowledged by most clinicians, in clinical practice it is still common to encounter the notion of 'simple' mental retardation or 'uncomplicated mental retardation', often with the implication that the person is a 'typical' example of a mental retardation case with generally (end evenly) low IQ. The term 'uncomplicated mental retardation' is also, usually inadvertently, used to infer that there is nothing else the matter except a generally low IQ level. Such 'uncomplicated' cases are extremely rare, if, indeed, they exist at all. Most people with so-called mental retardation have complications such as associated epilepsy, motor handicaps, other physical problems and/ or (in a majority of all cases) psychiatric disorder.

The fact that mental retardation is not a uniform syndrome has particular importance in much of the research literature on mental retardation and autism. Control groups of children and adults with mental retardation are often included for contrast in studies of background factors and outcome in autism. Rarely, if ever, is there a detailed description of the people with mental retardation other than to say that they were matched for IQ and sex and that they 'did not have autism'. Unfortunately, such information is not very informative if more detail is not provided. Some degree of autistic symptomatology is very often found even in people with mental retardation who do not meet all the diagnostic criteria for autism. Thus, unless the mental retardation group is examined specifically with a view to diagnosing autistic symptomatology, it cannot really be used to control for IQ only. This is not merely an academic dispute: it has far-reaching consequences in clinical practice. Because so much of the literature on autism makes use of mental retardation 'control' groups that have not been worked up in detail in respect of autistic symptoms, conclusions such as 'This is a case of pure autism' and 'This is definitely a case of mental retardation without autism' are apt to linger. In reality, the dividing line is nowhere near as clear as such statements would imply.

Finally, there are people with Down syndrome who have low normal or normal tested IQ levels. The same applies in Prader–Willi syndrome, Williams syndrome and other disorders originally conceptualized as invariably associated with mental retardation. In fact, mental retardation may not be the most typical 'symptom' in some of these syndromes. Prader–Willi syndrome, for instance, appears to be more clearly defined by the presence of a certain set of behaviour/psychiatric problems than by the degree of the learning disorder (even if the presence of a learning disorder seems to be universal). This implies that many of the syndromes thought of as 'mental retardation syndromes' are better grouped in an overall class of 'neuropsychiatric disorders', in which mental retardation is a common, but certainly not invariable, concomitant.

For these reasons, the clinical picture of mental retardation is not detailed here, but instead will be presented in connection with a number of named syndromes both in the chapter dealing with autism and autistic-like conditions, and in that describing 'other' neuropsychiatric syndromes.

Associated handicaps in mental retardation

The common association of mental retardation and other types of central nervous system afflictions is accounted for by the fact that mental retardation is often caused by widespread brain damage/dysfunction. Thus, cerebral palsy, epilepsy and visual and hearing impairments are much more common in mental retardation than in the general population.

Table 5.1 shows the prevalence of associated neurological and psychiatric handicaps in severe and mild mental retardation.

It is undisputed that severe mental retardation is more often associated with severe brain damage than is mild mental retardation. It is equally clear that, although both mild and severe mental retardation carry very high risks of associated handicaps, the association is stronger for severe retardation. The Isle of Wight study, (Rutter, Graham & Yule, 1970) demonstrated that the link between psychiatric disorder and neurological handicap was often mediated by brain damage. For instance, similar degrees of functional handicap resulted in higher rates of psychiatric disorder if the functional disability had resulted from brain damage. It is reasonable to assume that the major reason for severe mental retardation being so often associated with other handicapping conditions is the underlying brain damage. This is definitely true of epilepsy and motor neuron disorders.

Table 5.1. *Associated handicaps in mental retardation*

Associated handicap	SMR (%)	MMR (%)
Cerebral palsy	21	9
Epilepsy	37	12
Severe hearing impairment/deafness	8	7
Severe visual impairment/blindness	15	1
Hydrocephalus	5	2
One or more of above handicaps	40	24
Infantile autism	8	4
Other severe psychiatric abnormality	56	53

Note: Based on Hagberg & Kyllerman (1983) and Gillberg *et al.* (1986), cited in Rasmussen (1990).

Psychiatric/behavioural problems in mental retardation

Children with mental retardation show much higher rates of moderate and severe psychiatric abnormality than do children of normal intelligence (Rutter *et al.*, 1970; Corbett, 1979). A recent Swedish study revealed that more than half of school-age children with mild mental retardation, and almost two-thirds of those with severe mental retardation had major psychiatric/behavioural problems of some kind or other (Gillberg *et al.*, 1986).

Some behavioural problems are particularly common in the population of children with mental retardation. Autism and other severe social impairments appear to be more than 100 times more common in cases with mental retardation than in children of normal intelligence. Classical autism affects about 5% of all children with mental retardation but less than 0.05% of normally intelligent children. Autistic-like conditions, including Lorna Wing's triad (Wing & Gould, 1979, see below), are even more common. Every fourth to every third child with severe mental retardation is affected by such conditions (Gillberg *et al.*, 1986).

Motor stereotypies, regardless of associated autistic-like symptoms are also very common in mental retardation (Corbett, 1985).

Extremes of hyperactive behaviour are also much more common in mental retardation (see below in the section on deficits in attention, motor control and perception). Hypoactivity is less common, although not rare, in young children with mental retardation. In adolescence, many previously hyperactive children with autism become moderately or even severely hypoactive, spending long hours doing nothing. Obesity and concomitant reduction of activity level may or may not be a cause of, or associated with, hypoactivity.

Strange eating habits (or rather mouthing habits) are also very common in severe mental retardation. Pica is over-represented in mentally retarded populations. It consists of extremely odd mouthing behaviours such as putting flowers, newspapers, razor-blades, soil or sand in the mouth and then swallowing. Pica can lead to gastrointestinal obstruction, diarrhoea and stomachache, sometimes requiring immediate surgical intervention. There is also a high rate of other eating disorder behaviours, such as rumination and limitation in the range of foods preferred.

The symptoms mentioned so far are especially prevalent in the severely retarded population. In children with mild mental retardation, these problems are relatively common also, but, in general, the behavioural/psychiatric problems encountered in mildly retarded subjects, are more similar to those of children (particularly young children) with normal intelligence.

Medical work-up

An adequate medical work-up must include a meticulous history-taking concentrating on hereditary/familial and psychosocial circumstances, on the one hand, and on psychomotor development and associated handicaps on the other. The clinical examination of the child should always include a full paediatric and neuromotor assessment (including a thorough search for skin changes, to rule out neurocutaneous disorders, and examination of hand function, to rule out Rett syndrome and variants of that disorder), evaluation of the child's growth chart and assessment of minor physical anomalies and other signs which might help suggest a specific medical syndrome. A brief evaluation of neuropsychiatric/behavioural traits which might help in differential diagnosis should also be included. This should focus on symptoms suggestive of autism, Tourette syndrome and other specific neuropsychiatric syndromes, including those grouped with the behavioural phenotypes.

Hearing and vision must always be examined as comprehensively as possible. This may have to involve auditory brainstem response examination, visual evoked response examination and neuroophthalmological assessment under general anaesthesia in certain cases.

Laboratory investigations should always be considered only after some sort of preliminary diagnostic evaluation has been undertaken. However, chromosomal analysis is often indicated, particularly if there is a multitude of minor physical anomalies, congenital malformations or autism. The same holds for neuroradiological examinations (particularly if there is a suspicion of cerebral malformation), EEG (which is mandatory whenever there are symptoms suspected of having a convulsive character) and certain biochemical blood and urine screens (such as amino acids, organic acids and saccharides in urine).

The neuropsychological work-up

Mental retardation should never be diagnosed until at least two IQ-tests (or Vineland interviews or clinical assessments) have been performed. The IQ tests should be at least 3 months apart and both must indicate that the child's IQ is under 70.

One cannot expect to make accurate 'IQ diagnoses' in children under age 3 years, other than with regard to separating out those with severe and profound levels of mental retardation from the rest. From around age 7–8 years much more reliable IQ estimates can be made, using well-standardized tests such as the WISC-R.

Because of the difficulties associated with testing children with social and language impairments, some more details of various tests used with children are provided in the chapter on empathy disorders (Chapter 6).

Management, treatment and education

No cure is currently available for most mental retardation conditions. Nevertheless, some forms of mental retardation are preventable through immunization programmes (e.g. rubella embryopathy) and screening followed by diet (e.g. PKU) or substitution therapy (e.g. hypothyroidism).

Early diagnosis, education of the family and special education measures for the affected child are crucial elements in most treatment/ management programmes for children with mental retardation. In the section on autism, these and other aspects of treatment, as well as the need for special services, are illuminated in more detail. Many of the things that apply in autism are relevant in mental retardation generally, and, rather than being redundant on the matter, I refer the reader to this section. Also, in individual mental retardation syndromes, more or less specific interventions may be available. In such instances, these are referred to in the special section on 'Other neuropsychiatric disorders' under a specific syndrome.

Outcome

No general prognosis can be made for all children with mental retardation. Outcome is dependent on underlying aetiology. Children with progressive brain disorders have a poor psychosocial prognosis when compared with those with non-progressive brain damage. Even in disorders which have traditionally been regarded as 'non-progressive', empirical study has revealed that the picture is more complicated. For instance, Down syndrome is very often associated with Alzheimer-type dementia, and the type of familial mental retardation associated with the fragile X chromosome abnormality may show plateauing or even some deterioration at, or before, puberty. Bearing these reservations in mind, it is, however, possible to make the general statement that most children diagnosed in the pre-school period as having an IQ under 50 will still be mentally retarded in adult age. Those diagnosed as having an IQ under 70 in the early school years are likely to have a significant intellectual handicap also in adult age.

References

Abel, E.L., Sokol, R.J. (1986). Fetal alcohol syndrome is now leading cause of mental retardation. *Lancet*, **ii**, 1222.

Åkesson, H. (1961). *Epidemiology and Genetics of Mental Retardation in a Southern Swedish Population*. Uppsala: University of Uppsala Press.

American Psychiatric Association. (1987). *Diagnostic and Statistical Manual of Mental Disorders*. Third Edition – Revised. Washington, DC: APA.

Bernsen, A.H. (1977). Severe mental retardation among children in a Danish urban area. *In* Mittler, P. (Ed.) *Research to Pratice in Mental*

Retardation. Baltimore: University Park Press.

Corbett, J. (1985). Mental retardation: Psychiatric aspects. *In* Rutter, M.,Hersov, L. (Eds.) *Child and Adolescent Psychiatry: Modern Approaches*. Oxford: Blackwell Scientific.

Corbett, J.A. (1979). Psychiatric morbidity and mental retardation. *In* James, F.E.,Snaith, R.P. (Eds.) *Psychiatric Illness and Mental Retardation*. London: Gaskell Press.

Craft, M. (1985). Classification, criteria, epidemiology and causation. *In* Craft, M., Bicknell, J.,Hollins, S. (Eds.) *Mental Handicap*. London: Bailliere Tindall.

Edwards, G. (1983). Alcohol and advice to the pregnant woman. *British Medical Journal*, **286**, 247–8.

Gillberg, C., Gillberg, I.C. (1991). Note on the relationship between population-based and clinical studies: the question of reduced optimality in autism: letter. *Journal of Autism and Developmental Disorders*, **21**, 251–3.

Gillberg, C., Rasmussen, P. (1982). Perceptual, motor and attentional deficits in seven-year-old children: background factors. *Developmental Medicine and Child Neurology*, **24**, 752–70.

Gillberg, C., Svenson, B., Carlström, G., Waldenström, E., Rasmussen, P. (1983). Mental retardation in Swedish urban children: some epidemiological considerations. *Applied Research in Mental Retardation*, **4**, 207–18.

Gillberg, C., Persson, E., Grufman , M., Themnér, U. (1986). Psychiatric disorders in mildly and severely mentally retarded urban children and adolescents: epidemiological aspects. *British Journal of Psychiatry*, **149**, 68–74.

Gillberg, C., Gillberg, I.C., Steffenburg, S. (1990). Reduced optimality in the pre-, peri-, and neonatal periods is not equivalent to severe peri- or neonatal risk: a rejoinder to Goodman's technical note [comment]. Comment on: *Journal of Child Psychology and Psychiatry* 1990, Jul 31, 5, 809–12. *Journal of Child Psychology and Psychiatry*, **31**, 813–15.

Hagberg, B., Kyllerman, M. (1983). Epidemiology of mental retardation – a Swedish survey. *Brain and Development*, **5**, 441–9.

Hagberg, B., Hagberg, G., Lewerth, A., Lindberg, U. (1981). Mild mental retardation in Swedish school children. I. Prevalence. *Acta Paediatrica Scandinavia*, **70**, 441–4.

Kushlick, A. (1961). Subnormality in Salford. *In* Susser, M.W.,Kushlick, A. (Eds.) *A report on the Mental Health Services in the City of Salford for the year 1960*. Salford: Salford Health Department.

Lewis, E.D. (1929). *The Report on the Mental Deficiency Committee*. London: HMSO.

Needleman, H.L., Gatsonis, C.A. (1990). Low-level lead exposure and the IQ of children. A meta-analysis of modern studies. *JAMA*, **263**, 673–8.

Rasmussen, P. (1990). Psykisk utvecklingsstörning. *In* Gillberg, C.,Hellgren, L. (Eds.) *Barn- och ungdomspsykiatri*. Stockholm: Natur & Kultur. (In Swedish.)

Rutter, M., Graham, P., Yule, W. (1970). *A Neuropsychiatric Study in Childhood*. London: S.I.M.P./William Heinemann Medical Books Ltd.

Strömland, K., Miller, M. (1993). Thalidomide embryopathy: revisited 27 years later. *Acta Ophthalmologica*, **71**, 238–45.

Thompson, J.R.S., O'Quinn, A. (1979). *Developmental Disabilities*. New York: Oxford University Press.

Wing, L. (1971). Severely retarded children in a London area: prevalence and provision of services. *Journal of Psychological Medicine*, **1**, 405–15.

Wing, L., Gould, J. (1979). Severe impairments of social interaction and associated abnormalities in children: epidemiology and classification. *Journal of Autism and Developmental Disorders*, **9**, 11–29.

6 Disorders of empathy: autism and autism spectrum disorders (including childhood onset schizophrenia)

General review

The literature (e.g. Itard, 1801; Haslam, 1809; Frith, 1989a) contains descriptions of people living several hundred years ago, who, according to our present-day terminology, would have fulfilled criteria for infantile autism (Rutter, 1978; APA, 1980) or autistic disorder (APA, 1987; APA, 1994). Obviously, autistic syndromes are not 'new' conditions typical of urban and industrialized societies of the twentieth century (as has been proposed by Tinbergen & Tinbergen, 1983), even though current concepts and definitions are less than 50 years old. There is no strong indication that autism is more common in urban than in rural areas or that, in 'classical' form it is more common now than, say 10 or 20 years ago (Gillberg et al., 1991a; Gillberg, 1992a).

Autism

Previous definitions and concepts

The US child psychiatrist Leo Kanner (1943) (born in Austria) and the Austrian paediatrician Hans Asperger (1944) were the first to describe the type of empathy disorders encompassed in the 'autistic continuum' (Wing, 1989a), highlighting the specificity of the social interaction deficit which has, ever since, been regarded as the core symptom of autism. Kanner was working and publishing in the US, and his reports and his views were well known to most people working in child psychiatry already in the 1950s and 1960s. Asperger, on the other hand, who worked in Vienna and published in German, did not receive widespread recognition for his contribution until the 1980s (Wing, 1981a) and early 1990s (Frith, 1991). Whether to regard Kanner's 'early infantile autism' and Asperger's 'autistic psychopathy' as synonymous, different sections on an autism spectrum, partly biologically and psychologically overlapping disabilities or clearly different conditions, has been the subject of considerable debate. Here, the 'syndromes' will be described separately, even though, more likely than not, they can, at least regarding some key features, be conceptualized as existing on a continuum.

A number of labels and named syndromes, some of which can be regarded as synonymous and others which can be seen as partly overlapping entities, are shown in Table 6.1.

In the following, unless otherwise specified, 'autism' will be used throughout when referring to the syndrome of autism (outlined below). In other circumstances, the word autism can also be used in its original Bleulerian sense to describe the particular quality of naïve egocentric thinking encountered in schizophrenia (Bleuler, 1919).

Current definitions of autism

All currently accepted definitions of autism include three main criteria which have to be met for a diagnosis to be made. These are (1) disturbance of reciprocal social interaction, (2) disturbance of communication (including language comprehension and spoken language)

Table 6.1. *Synonyms and partly overlapping labels in the field of autism spectrum disorders*

Label	Reference
Infantile autism	Rutter, 1978; APA, 1980
Autistic disorder	APA, 1987
Early infantile autism	Kanner, 1943
Childhood autism	Wing, 1981*a*
Autistic syndrome	Coleman & Gillberg, 1985
Triad of social impairments	Wing & Gould, 1979
Pervasive developmental disorder	APA, 1980
Childhood schizophrenia	Bender, 1947
Autistic psychopathy	Asperger, 1944
Asperger syndrome	Wing, 1981*a*
Atypical child syndrome	Rank, 1949
Symbiotic psychosis	Mahler, 1952
Disorder of empathy	Gillberg, 1992*a*

and (3) restriction of normal variation in behaviour and imaginative activities leading to extreme restriction in the behavioural repertoire. The various specific symptoms associated with each criterion tend to be slightly differently emphasized in different manuals, but the basic symptom categories are the same throughout.

Some authors require onset before age 30–36 months to make the diagnosis of autism. This early age of onset criterion tends to be a prerequisite in particular when the prefix 'infantile' is used.

The criteria currently most used in the field are those of the DSM-III (APA, 1980) and the DSM-III-R (APA, 1987). The ICD–10 criteria (1993) and the criteria of the DSM-IV (1994) have just been published, and it is likely that, in the next decade, they will replace the old criteria and that, in turn, they will, at the end of this period, be replaced by new criteria. The different sets of criteria are outlined in Table 6.2. Some studies have suggested that the DSM-III-R criteria may diagnose more individuals with autism than the DSM-III (Volkmar *et al.*, 1988). Field trials of the DSM-IV criteria suggest that this new set may again diagnose fewer

cases with autism. The implicit assumption is that the DSM-IV would be more like the DSM-III when it comes to the diagnosis of autism. However, there have been no population studies comparing any of these manuals and therefore it is not appropriate to draw any conclusion regarding higher or lower specificity of any of the sets of diagnostic criteria as compared with the others. Because the few studies that have been published in the field have all referred to clinically referred samples (usually tertiary referrals), selection bias may have skewed the materials in ways which makes it impossible to decide whether or not it may be those factors rather than the 'true' syndrome of autism which contribute to the prevalence difference obtained when applying different sets of diagnostic criteria. From the 16 acceptable population-studies published in the field (Wing, 1993), there is no indication that variability in diagnostic criteria account for differences in prevalence obtained in different studies. However, none of the population studies has specifically examined the influence of changing from one set of criteria to another.

Lorna Wing (1989*a*) has argued that the specificity of infantile autism or 'Kanner autism' is in doubt. She has shown that a number of mentally handicapping conditions and brain damage syndromes show the same triad of social, communicative and behavioural impairments, and that a case for separating out a diagnosis of 'pure' Kanner autism sometimes cannot be made. Even when the phenomenology is clearly concordant with Kanner's descriptions, background factors and outcome tend to vary considerably (Wing & Gould, 1979; Gillberg & Steffenburg, 1987; Gillberg, Steffenburg & Jakobsson, 1987). Wing has shown that, in mentally handicapped individuals, the presence of one of the problems included in the triad dramatically increases the risk that one or both of the other two types of problems will be present as well. Gillberg and Coleman (1992) have advocated for a similar line of reasoning when referring to the 'autistic syndromes'. It has gradually become accepted that autism is a behavioural symptom constellation signalling underlying nervous system

Table 6.2. *Diagnostic criteria for autism*

Diagnostic label	Reference	Diagnostic criteria
Infantile autism	DSM-III (APA, 1980)	Pervasive lack of responsiveness to other people
		Gross deficits in language development, and, if speech is present, peculiar patterns such as echolalia, metaphorical language and pronominal reversal
		Bizarre responses to environment, for instance resistance to change, peculiar interests
		Absence of clear signs suggestive of schizophrenia
Autistic disorder	DSM-III-R (APA, 1987)	Qualitative impairment in reciprocal social interaction as manifested by at least two of the following five:
		1. marked lack of awareness of the existence or feelings of others
		2. no or abnormal seeking of comfort at times of distress
		3. no or impaired imitation
		4. no or abnormal social play
		5. gross impairment in ability to make peer friendships
		Qualitative impairment in verbal and non-verbal communication and in imaginative activity as manifested by at least one of the following six:
		6. no mode of communication
		7. markedly abnormal non-verbal communication
		8. absence of imaginative activity
		9. marked abnormalities in the production of speech
		10. marked abnormalities in the content of speech
		11. marked impairment in the ability to initiate or sustain a conversation with others, despite adequate speech
		Markedly restricted repertoire of activities and interests as manifested by at least one of the following five:
		12. stereotyped body movements
		13. persistent pre-occupation with parts of objects
		14. marked distress of changes in trivial aspects of environment
		15. unreasonable insistence on following routines in precise detail
		16. markedly restricted range of interests and a pre-occupation with one narrow interest
		Onset during infancy or childhood
		At least eight of the 16 specified items must be fulfilled
Childhood autism	ICD–10 (WHO, 1993)	Qualitative abnormalities in reciprocal social interaction, as manifested by at least two of the following four:

Table 6.2. (*cont.*)

Diagnostic label	Reference	Diagnostic criteria
		• failure adequately to use eye-to-eye gaze, facial expression, body posture and gesture to regulate social interaction
		• failure to develop peer relationships that involve a mutual sharing of interests, activities and emotions
		• rarely seeking and using other people for comfort and affection at times of stress or distress and/or offering comfort and affection to others when they are showing distress or unhappiness
		• lack of spontaneous seeking to share enjoyment, interests, or achievements with other people
		• lack of socio-emotional reciprocity as shown by an impaired or deviant response to other people's emotions; or lack of modulation of behaviour according to social context; or a weak integration of social emotional, and communicative behaviours
		Qualitative impairments in communication as manifested by at least one of the following
		• a delay in, or total lack of, development of spoken language that is *not* accompanied by an attempt to compensate through the use of gesture or mime as an alternative mode of communication (often preceded by a lack of communicative babbling)
		• lack of varied spontaneous make-believe or (when younger) social imitative play
		• relative failure to initiate or sustain conversational interchange
		• stereotyped and repetitive use of language or idiosyncratic use of words or phrases
		Restricted, repetitive and stereotyped patterns of behaviour, interests and activities, as manifested by at least one of the following four:
		• encompassing preoccupation with stereotyped and restricted patterns of interest
		• apparently compulsive adherence to specific, non-functional, routines or rituals
		• stereotyped and repetitive motor mannerisms
		• preoccupations with part-objects or non-functional elements of play material
		Developmental abnormalities must have been present in the first 3 years for the diagnosis to be made
Autistic disorder	DSM-IV (APA, 1994)	Qualitative impairment in social interaction, as manifested by at least two of the following four:
		• marked impairment in the use of multiple nonverbal behaviours such as eye-to-eye gaze, facial expression, body postures, and gestures to regulate social interaction

Table 6.2. (*cont.*)

Diagnostic label	Reference	Diagnostic criteria
		• failure to develop peer relationships appropriate to developmental level • a lack of spontaneous seeking to share enjoyment, interests, or achievements with other people (e.g. by a lack of showing, bringing, or pointing out objects of interest) • lack of social or emotional reciprocity
		Qualitative impairment in communication as manifested by at least one of the following four: • delay in, or total lack of, the development of spoken language (not accompanied by attempt to compensate through alternative modes of communication such as gesture or mime) • marked impairment in ability to initiate or sustain a conversation with others (if speech present) • stereotyped and repetitive use of language or idiosyncratic language • lack of varied spontaneous make-believe play or social imitative play appropriate to developmental level
		Restricted repetitive and stereotyped patterns of behaviour, interests and activities as manifested by at least one of the following four: • encompassing preoccupation with one or more stereotyped and restricted patterns of interest that is abnormal either in intensity or focus • apparently inflexible adherence to specific, non-functional routines or rituals • stereotyped and repetitive motor mannerisms • persistent preoccupation with parts of objects
		At least six of the above 12 items must be fulfilled
		Delay or abnormal functioning in at least one of following areas before age three: social interaction, language as used in social communication and symbolic or imaginative play
		Not better accounted for by Rett's disorder or childhood disintegrative disorder

dysfunction. The evidence for a specific 'nuclear autism' disease entity is largely lacking.

Many authors (starting with Gillberg, 1990) now use the term 'autism (or autistic) spectrum disorders'. Gillberg (1990) has used it to cover the range of triad disorders including 'Kanner' autism, Asperger syndrome and other autistic-like triad conditions (including 'autistic traits' encountered in DAMP and mental retardation). Szatmari (1992), on the other hand, has used it as a blanket term for the non-autism autistic-like conditions including Asperger syndrome.

Both the ICD–10 and the DSM use the term pervasive developmental disorders (PDD) to cover the triad syndromes, including childhood autism/autistic disorder. The DSM-III-R has two categories under PDD: autistic disorder and pervasive developmental disorder not otherwise specified (PDDNOS). Many authors disagree with this terminology, arguing that autism and autistic-like conditions (including Asperger syndrome) are not always pervasive (the highest functioning cases definitely are not pervasive), and that other pervasive disorders (such as profound mental retardation) would need to be subsumed under the PDD diagnosis (which they are not) for the label to make logical sense (Baird *et al.*, 1991; Gillberg, 1991*a*; Happé & Frith, 1991; Wing, 1992).

One additional problem of the PDD (in the ICD-10 and the DSM-IV-draft) is the inclusion of Rett syndrome as one of the specified variants of PDD. This is conceptually at odds with current understanding of autism and autistic-like conditions. Autism and autistic-like conditions are behaviourally defined syndromes. Rett syndrome is a neurological syndrome, just like tuberous sclerosis, which is defined on the basis of a number of symptoms and signs rather than on any kind of diagnostic marker (such as a blood or urine test). Rett syndrome, just like tuberous sclerosis, often has a course involving a protracted period of autistic and autistic-like symptoms. Rett syndrome, unlike tuberous sclerosis, often runs a course in which the autistic and autistic-like symptoms subside. Why then would one want to include Rett syndrome, *and not tuberous sclerosis*, with the autistic-like conditions or PDD? It seems that the only sensible thing in the current state of our knowledge would be to diagnose autism (or autistic-like condition depending on whether or not full criteria for autism are met) on one axis for psychiatric disorder, and Rett syndrome (or tuberous sclerosis) on another axis for associated medical condition.

In the following presentation, PDD will not be used as a diagnostic or generic term, unless specifically motivated in the text. Rett syndrome will not be treated as one specific variant of autistic-like conditions. Instead, the label 'autism spectrum disorders' will be used to cover the following: 'autism', 'Asperger syndrome', 'childhood disintegrative disorders' and 'other autistic-like conditions'. Rett syndrome can occur associated with any of these diagnoses (depending on diagnostic criteria for these disorders being met or not).

'Empathy disorder' will be used to cover a broader range of disorders showing some autistic traits and comprising 'autism spectrum disorders' as well as subgroups of other named syndromes (including some cases of elective mutism, DAMP, anorexia nervosa and obsessive compulsive personality disorder) (Fig. 6.1). Empathy disorder was recently proposed to be synonymous with clinical disorder of social interaction reflecting delay or deviance in the development of theory of mind (Gillberg, 1992*a*) (Fig. 6.2). It is not suggested that theory of mind deficits (Frith, 1991) are the only dysfunctions underlying this broader category of clinical disorder. Rather, empathy disorder is conceptualized as a blanket term, similar in some ways to PDD, but covering a broader spectrum of problems with no requirement of 'pervasiveness' or of appearance of first symptoms at a particularly early age in development.

The clinical picture in autism

Autism, like most syndromes, presents with a different clinical picture in each case, depending on factors such as sex, age at examination, IQ and personality style among other things. There is a stereotype, even in the minds of some laymen, that autism always comes in one shape, that all children with autism are copies of each other and that every single child needs exactly the same approach with respect to intervention. This notion is mistaken. It seems to have arisen as a result of all the studies of tertiary referral cases of autism. Inevitably, in such studies, it is likely that the most typical cases will be chosen for referral. The wide range of autistic-type problems encountered in community samples may be missed in such a highly specialized setting.

Early onset

Most clinicians and researchers agree that the behavioural disorder, or some major indication of abnormal development, has been apparent

Disorders of empathy

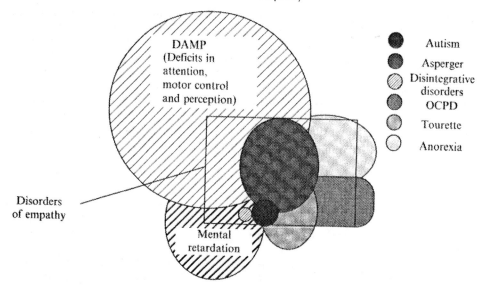

Fig. 6.1. Differential diagnosis in autism. Overlap with other clinical syndromes

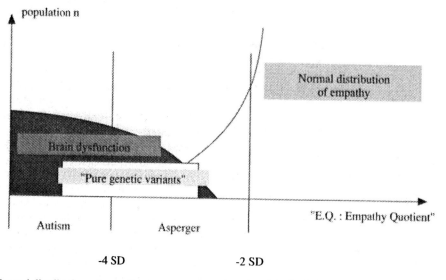

Fig. 6.2. Normal distribution of empathy, 'pure genetic variants' and brain dysfuncion in autism and Asperger syndrome.

before the age of 30 to 36 months (Rutter, 1978; APA, 1980; Coleman & Gillberg, 1985; WHO, 1993). However, some would require an even earlier age of onset, while others (Lotter, 1966, 1967; Wing & Gould, 1979) would allow the appearance of first symptoms to be delayed until the child's fifth birthday. Some authors have gone further still (Bohman *et al.*, 1983), and have accepted cases with onset up to the age of 7 years. Nevertheless, the age limit of 2½ to 3 years is widely accepted.

Evans-Jones and Rosenbloom (1978), while arguing that disintegrative psychosis (child-hood disintegrative disorder in the ICD-10) forms a separate diagnostic category from autism, maintain that sometimes the symptoms (which are often symptoms compatible with a diagnosis of autism) may begin before 2½ years of age, and yet not qualify the child for a diagnosis of autism but rather for disintegrative psychosis.

Even though the criterion of early onset rarely causes much dispute, the description of typical autistic syndromes beginning in pre-viously normal people between the age of 4 and 31 years in connection with herpes encephalitis (DeLong, Beau & Brown, 1981; Gillberg, 1986; Gillberg, I.C., 1991) shows clearly that the matter cannot be regarded as settled. As has already been noted, the DSM-III-R does not include early onset among the diagnostic criteria.

In the great majority of cases with autistic syndromes, however, onset is quite clearly during the first few years and often even in the first six months of life. Wing (1989a) has sug-gested that 'infantile autism' is congenital in approximately 80% of cases. In the remaining 20% there is either too scanty evidence from the medical history, or there are definite clues that the typical symptoms began sometime between the age of 6 and 20 months. Only rarely are there cases that commence around age 30 months or later. Cases with documented set-back after a period of clearly normal develop-ment are rare, but their relative frequency within the whole group is not known. In the author's experience, there is a subgroup of individuals with autism who develop within the

normal range up until about age 18 months and then plateau. They may have developed a few (or even many) single words. Once the plateau is reached, they often become mute for many months (indeed sometimes for many, many years), as though they have no grasp of the meaning of using the words for communica-tion. Parents and doctors may believe that the child has deteriorated, when, in fact, this has not occurred. The child's brain, in such cases, may have had enough capacity for normal motor and behavioural development until 18–24 months, whereafter the demands for much more complex development (particularly involving social interaction) can no longer be met. Such cases are sometimes distinguished from 'early infantile' autism on the one hand and 'childhood disintegrative disorder' on the other and referred to as 'late onset autism' (Volkmar & Cohen, 1989).

Many authors have assumed that the early onset of the disorder is one of the reasons for symptoms taking on such a stereotyped and primitive appearance. While this seems reason-able in a developmental-theoretical perspec-tive, the whole notion is contradicted by the clear documentation of Kanner-type autism with onset as late as 14 years of age.

Conversely, it should be made clear that symptom onset after, for instance, 18 months of age does not mean that the disorder may not be congenital.

Abnormality of social relatedness

The disturbance of social relatedness, as of all other symptoms, has to be out of proportion in comparison with the often concomitant mental retardation. The central features of this abnor-mality seem to be egocentricity, lack of recipro-city in social interaction with other humans, poorly developed empathy skills, and a failure to recognize the uniqueness of other human beings (Wing, 1980, 1989b, 1991; Rutter 1983; Gillberg 1992a, 1993).

Frith (1989b) has suggested that the basic failure in autism is the lack of early develop-ment of a 'theory of mind', such that a child with autism cannot conceive that other people think and feel and certainly cannot *intuit* what they think and feel. This 'underdeveloped' theory of mind will inevitably lead to extreme deficits in empathy, showing in all interactions with people. The empathy deficits, however, will not affect the ability to observe the world or to reason logically about visible and audible realities. Neither will basic emotions such as anger, fear or happiness necessarily be affected. The child will rely, more than other children, on the observable world and judge it by its physical characteristics only. Recording of physical events may be unimpaired, and memory skills for such events can sometimes be excellent. The child may be happy, fearful or angry during the course of such events, but he/she will not be able to share these effects in an emotionally appropriate reciprocal fashion.

Some children with autism already during the first three years of life (and to a lesser extent later also) display, in Kanner's words (1943), an 'extreme autistic aloneness'. Others are described as 'easy so long as they are left to themselves in their bed or in their room'. Still others are difficult, 'terrible', or scream at all hours and need little sleep. Imitation and imitation play are deficient or lacking (personal observations). Feeding and sucking difficulties are very common (Wing, 1980).

The 'typical' child with autism avoids eye contact, stares into thin air or is observed to have an abnormal gaze contact from before the end of the first year of life (Mirenda, Donnellan & Yoder, 1983). Many gaze out of the corner of the eye and only very briefly. Quite a number do not show anticipatory movements when about to picked up, may resist being held or touched, and will not 'adjust' to 'fit' in a hug or something similar. However, contrary to popular belief, many children with autism enjoy body contact, which may constitute their only mode of 'communication' with other people. Infants who later receive a diagnosis of autism have often seemed to lack initiative, and the interested curiosity and exploratory behaviour seen in normal babies is often completely lacking.

Frequent responses include: 'He was so happy if we left him all to himself, but started to scream as soon as someone picked him up'; 'She was stiff to hold'; or 'I don't know what it was, but he just wasn't "there".' Humans, animals and soft and hard objects may be treated alike. People are often treated by the child as if they were technical tools, there only for the benefit of the child to reach certain objects (exemplified by the child who leads their mother's hand, not only by the hand but by the wrist, to their spoon, and then directs the spoon via the mother's hand/wrist to their own mouth). The child does not usually come to parents, brothers or sisters, or anybody else for that matter, for help or comfort.

However, not all children with autism show these typical features and, to be sure, even in those who do, there is often a gradual decrease in the severity of symptoms.

Typical of all in the early preschool years is a failure to develop normal relationships with age-peers. This inability usually persists throughout childhood, adolescence and often into adult life.

As the child grows older, the abnormalities of social relatedness become less immediately obvious, particularly if the child is seen in familiar surroundings. The resistance to being touched and held often decreases with age, even though rough-and-tumble play is sometimes preferred to gentle stroking. The gaze avoidance behaviour may decrease. There is evidence (Rutter, 1978; Mirenda et al., 1983) to suggest that it is not the amount of gaze contact that is abnormal in autism, but rather that, at least after infancy, there is a qualitative difference, the gaze of people with autism being stiffer and lasting longer on an individual basis. It could be that an 'eye direction detector' function is missing or abnormal in autism (Baron-Cohen, 1994), i.e. the child fails to notice how other people visually attend to various objects and incidents. In some instances, e.g. autism associated with the fragile X chromosome abnormality, there is clear gaze avoidance (Hagerman, 1989, 1992), and it seems likely that, with the emergence of more and more aetiological subgroups, a multifaceted view of gaze abnormalities in autism will emerge. What is already quite clear at this stage is that gaze avoidance is definitely not a necessary feature of autism at any age.

Symptoms pertaining to the avoidance of visual or physical contact are often classified in the category of social abnormalities. However, several authors including Wing (1980) and the present author (Coleman & Gillberg, 1985; Gillberg *et al.*, 1990) would argue that these abnormalities are best dealt with in the context of abnormal sensory responses. Be that as it may, the result of the changes in the child in these respects is that the child becomes somewhat more co-operative and easy to relate to. Unfortunately, the inability to play reciprocally with age peers remains sadly unchanged throughout the years in most cases, although this characteristic may not be as conspicuously apparent in the school-age child with autism as it was in that same child during the preschool years.

In some cases, and at some stages of development, the abnormality of social relatedness takes on the form of a lack of selectivity and distance. However, even in children with autism who show seemingly attention-seeking, distance-lacking behaviour, the inability to reciprocate and the failure to treat humans as anything but objects are clearly evident. These hallmarks differentiate them from superficially similar behaviour seen in emotionally deprived children.

The highest functioning children with autism, including those with Asperger syndrome, may eventually develop primitive (and even elaborate) theory of mind (or empathy) skills (Gillberg & Coleman, 1992). However, perhaps because of the lack of such skills in early childhood, and hence the failure to foster reciprocal social interaction in a natural child interaction setting, the *automatic use of such skills in an intuitive fashion* may not occur even when the functional deficit is no longer present.

Abnormalities of communication development (including language)

Usually from a very early age, the child with autism shows major problems in the comprehension of human mime, gesture and speech, and, accordingly, shows little social use of communication skills. Social imitation is lacking or deficient, and common early imitation play such as waving bye-bye or doing pat-a-cake is not elicitable. Some, though by no means all, perhaps not even the majority (Gillberg *et al.*,

1990), do not babble, and some yield strange monotonous sounds instead of the varied babble patterns heard in normal children.

Abnormal babbling is often inferred to be a crucial symptom of abnormal language development in autism. Actually, there is little scientific evidence to uphold such a view, and some children with autism have indeed babbled in what appears to be a normal fashion. The few studies which have examined early language development (according to parental interview data) of children with autism do not suggest clear-cut abnormalities of babble (Dahlgren & Gillberg, 1989; Gillberg *et al.*, 1990). In fact, language and babbling may be more discrete functions and not as intrinsically interwoven as hitherto believed (Zetterström, 1983).

Almost without exception, children with autism are delayed in their development of spoken language. This delay runs parallel with an impairment in the understanding of spoken language, which may vary from an almost total lack of understanding to more subtle deviances leading to literal interpretation. An example of this kind of literal interpretation is provided by the 10 year-old girl with autism with a full-scale WISC IQ of 100 who appeared panic stricken when the nurse, about to do a simple blood test said: 'Give me your hand: it won't hurt.' The girl calmed down immediately when another person, who knew her well, said: 'Stretch out your index finger.' The girl had understood, at the first instruction, that she was required to cut off her hand and give it to the nurse. Comprehension is usually severely impaired even in such high-functioning persons with autism who may excel in the use of vocabulary.

Many children with autism learn to follow simple instructions if given in a particular social context, but appear to fail to grasp the meaning of these instructions when given out of that context. Quite unlike deaf children, children with autism make little, if any, use of mime or gesture. Very often they seem to misinterpret human facial expressions and begin to laugh when somebody cries, or become frightened at the sound of human laughter.

Approximately one in two children with autism fail to develop useful spoken language. The vast majority of these are also mentally retarded (usually severely or profoundly so). Of those who do develop speech, all show major abnormalities of speech development, such as sustained phases of seemingly non-communicative immediate and/or delayed echolalia (present only during short phases and integrated with the development of communicative speech in normal children), avoidance or confusion of personal pronouns (such as the substitution of 'you', 'he' or the child's first name for 'I', 'he' for 'she' and 'you' for 'we', thought to be a consequence of the echolalia), confusion of prepositions, and repetitive speech without talking with so much as to someone. The echolalia encountered in autism is often so well developed that the casual listener/observer will have difficulty in recognizing the severity of the abnormality of language. Some may parrot whole conversations and go on talking as if at a cocktail party or ask endless questions. Those who constantly ask questions often become very irritating for people around them. It is sometimes difficult to understand why they should want to ask all these questions when everybody knows that they know all the answers. If a theory of mind deficit underlies autism, it becomes easier to accept that, in autism, you can only ask questions that already have an answer which is well known to the person asking. If you cannot conceive that other people have mental states or, as it were 'inner worlds', how can you ask them about matters unknown to you?

Quite a number of people with autism eventually develop some communicative language, but, nevertheless, retain some of their echolalia in that they whisper in an echolalic fashion every question directed at them. This may be particularly common in autism associated with the fragile X chromosome abnormality (Gillberg, 1992b). The whispered (echoed) question may then be followed by a formally 'adequate' response.

A minority of people with autism not only parrot conversations in an echolalic fashion, but imitate one's every movement and gesture. This phenomenon is sometimes referred to as echopraxia.

Some talking children with autism have very good rote memory skills and can repeat whole conversations word by word. However, these same children may have great difficulty, or may not be at all able, to extract meaning from sentences based on the order and the meaning of the words (Hermelin & O'Connor, 1970).

Some non-speaking people with autism may be able to imitate and sing songs with baffling accuracy and some may even know the words of the song without being able to repeat them without singing.

In speaking children with autism, it has been commonly noted that they can relate a series of real events if allowed to do so according to their own rigid structure of telling about the events, but cannot do it if interrupted by questions or remarks. Especially in brighter children with autism, there may be quite a lot of spontaneous speech. Rarely, if ever, do they communicate to others about their feelings and needs, or do so in a fashion which does not take account of the social setting. They may hold lengthy and detailed disquisitions on the subject of a given, concrete experience, such as a dinner, or travelling on a bus, but will usually be unable to answer even simple questions about this same topic, in spite of having no difficulty at all 'recreating' the whole journey from start to finish in their own very concrete, descriptive words.

It is important to make note of the fact that comprehension of spoken language is always seriously compromised in autism. Even in high-functioning individuals who have well-developed expressive speech, there are usually severe comprehension problems. They may be able to understand most single words such as substantives and verbs (and even adjectives referring to visible or audible phenomena) and yet have enormous difficulty comprehending what these words mean if sequenced together and, particularly, if set in a social context. In other words, their pragmatic comprehension skills are very limited. Some high-functioning people with autism may have better skills with regard to language comprehension if they are allowed to read a text than if they hear the same text spoken by somebody. It appears that spoken language produces few if any 'mental states/ pictures' in people suffering from the syndrome of autism. Alternatively, it may be that their 'automatic' use of language may be severely impaired so that, in a naturalistic setting (such as in social encounters), they may not be able to pay attention to spoken language in an automatic fashion. Their attention may be overfocused on one or other particular aspect of the interacting person's communication, such as pitch, volume or inflection, rather than on the semantic contents.

There are often grammatical immaturities consistent with the overall developmental level of the child's speech (Bartak, Rutter & Cox, 1975).

Typically, there are peculiarities in respect to vocal volume and pitch, with a tendency to use staccato-like or scanning speech. Problems of pronunciation arise when using spontaneous, but no echo phrases (Wing, 1966; Howlin, 1982). Phrased differently, this sometimes implies that, when language spoken by people with autism sounds stiff or monotonous, it is more likely to be communicative than when it sounds 'perfect' or 'just as though it had been spoken by somebody else'.

Judging from the, so far limited, study of high-functioning people with autism, it appears that a flat prosody may be more characteristic than any other problems in the language domain.

Finally, it is important to note the non-verbal communication problems, such as standing too far off, too close up, looking at the mouths rather than the eyes of other people, prolonged eye closing during communication with others, stiff staring gaze, and other abnormalities of mime and gesture which usually prevail throughout the life of people on the autism spectrum. Little facial mimicry (including stiff and stereotyped smiles, on the one hand, and 'depressed' appearance on the other) and an extreme restriction/poverty, or indeed lack, of gestures are typical of almost all cases.

Restricted, repetitive and stereotyped behaviour, activities and interests

Children with autism often form bizarre attachments to certain objects or parts of objects, such as stones, curls of hair, pins, pieces of plastic toys or metals. They may also be fascinated by any object that glitters (glasses, earrings, necklaces, etc.). The objects are usually selected because of some particular quality (e.g. colour, surface texture) and are carried or followed around by the child, who becomes distressed or even frantic if anybody tries to remove them. Other children line up toys or household equipment for hours on end. Round and spinning objects, such as wheels of toy cars, coins, gramophone records and tape recorders often hold a distinct fascination for children with autism.

Many children, adolescents and adults with autism demand that certain routines be adhered to in a pathologically rigid fashion. One 6 year-old boy insisted that his mother had to put the frying pan on the stove and heat some butter in it before he would have his breakfast. This 'show', as it were, had to be put on every morning or he would scream for hours, refusing to eat altogether. Another boy of 7 would eat only if one of the legs of his father's chair was one inch away from one leg of the dinner table and his mother had one elbow on the table. A girl of 4 would scream in rage if her mother did not always walk on the same pavement on her way to the post office. A child of 1 year would scream for hours if his mother, when taking him out in his pram, did not always take him twice around the block going to the right (as she had done the very first time she took him out in the pram).

It is often impossible to predict what environmental change will cause the emotional outbursts. On the whole, it appears that minor changes tend to be more upsetting and to cause more severe temper tantrums than do major changes. For instance, a 5 year-old boy cried desperately for almost an hour until his mother realized that she had removed a book from one of the shelves of the bookcase. When she put it back, he stopped crying within seconds. This boy, who was considered by his parents and professionals as unable to cope with even the smallest kind of environmental change, accepted going abroad without any outward reaction at all.

The 'insistence on sameness' may also affect the verbal skills of the child, who may demand that only certain words or phrases be used or that things be talked about or repeated in exactly the same fashion. As noted above, standard questions with demands for standard answers are common.

Especially during the school years and after, some relatively brighter persons with autism show unusual preoccupations with, for example, weather reports, birthdays or train schedules.

Various other ritualistic and obsessive–compulsive phenomena are common. Some people with obsessive–compulsive disorders are very much aware that their rituals are unhelpful and limit their capacity for doing other things. People with autism are usually not as well aware of the handicapping nature of their own rituals, but their obsessive–compulsive behaviours may be very similar to those of people who are diagnosed as suffering from obsessive–compulsive disorder. Also among children with the latter diagnosis, there are many who are not aware that their rituals are 'negative'. It has been my experience that some children receive a diagnosis of obsessive–compulsive disorder when, in fact, they show all the hallmarks of autism. Conversely, many children with classical autism would also qualify for a diagnosis of obsessive–compulsive disorder.

Some authors include less complex stereotypic behaviour, such as simple stereotypies or toe-walking, among the elaborate repetitive routines. Even though some stereotypies, especially hand-flapping with flexion of the elbows and extremely 'high' tip-toeing, appear to be rather typical of autism, most authors do not include these kinds of stereotypic behaviours as necessary criteria for a diagnosis of autism. Nevertheless, in low-functioning individuals with autism, elaborate motor routines (stereotypies) may be the only way of 'expressing' the repetitive behaviour pattern considered essential for a diagnosis of autism to be made.

One way of looking at the 'behavioural criterion' of the autism diagnosis would be to say that the restricted pattern reflects the fact that you can only do what you know how to do. People with autism, because of their inability to communicate with the 'inner worlds' of other people, have to learn through copying what they see, hear or sense in other ways. This will

necessarily mean a severe restriction of the behavioural repertoire even in high-functioning cases. In low-functioning cases, repetitive motor patterns may be the only behaviours individuals with autism may know how to do, whereas in higher functioning cases, more elaborate patterns of behaviour may be possible.

Problems which are almost universal but not among the diagnostic criteria

Perhaps the most characteristic symptom of autism which is not currently included as a necessary diagnostic criterion is the abnormal response to sensory stimuli.

Of these symptoms, an abnormal response to sound may be thought of as the most characteristic of all. In my experience, all children with typical autism have shown abnormal responses to sensory stimuli when very young. The child who 'acts deaf' and does not react at all when an explosion is suddenly heard near by may moments later turn at the sound of a paper being removed from a chocolate. Many children with autism cover their ears to shut out even 'ordinary' noise levels. There may also be strange reactions, such as the covering of ears or eyes at a special sound. There is often an extreme variability in the reaction to sound and light from one second to another.

Reduced or otherwise abnormal sensitivity to pain, heat or cold is often encountered in autism. A typical example is that of a boy who seemingly derives pleasure by biting the back of his hand. Some children withdraw or squeal if touched or stroked lightly, but enjoy being handled roughly. Other kinds of tactile stimuli may give pleasure to a child who can stand for half-hours just feeling and scratching differently textured surfaces.

One boy of 7 years was 'helping' his mother by the stove. He put his hand down and did not remove it until the smell of burnt flesh attracted his interest. He had to undergo several operations after this, but his hand function was never totally recovered. He did not seem to experience pain or heat from the burn wound. Another boy of 9 years got up early on one extremely cold morning and went out, naked, to play in the snow for what must have been more than an hour without feeling the need for warm clothes (and, incidentally, without any untoward consequences).

Abnormal responses to visual stimuli are probably present in a large majority of young children with autism, who often give the impression of having difficulty recognizing the things they see. People may ask the parents if the child is blind; in fact, every now and then autism is mistaken for blindness. Some children with delayed visual maturation show many or all of the symptoms of autism (Goodman & Ashby, 1990). The peculiarities of gaze, reported in the section on abnormality of social relatedness, could also be taken as evidence of abnormal perceptual responses, as could the extreme fascination with contrasts of light (including that produced by shadows in the sunshine).

Children with autism often want to smell people and objects. This is a characteristic not usually encountered in normal development or in mental retardation without major autistic features.

Perceptions relating to auditory and tactile stimuli may be more impaired in autism than are perceptions of visual and, especially, olfactory stimuli. The two latter functions make their first intracranial nerve connections at a higher level in the nervous system than do the two former. A preference for proximal stimuli has also been experimentally evidenced in autism (Hermelin & O'Connor, 1970, 1990; O'Connor & Hermelin, 1990; Pring & Hermelin, 1993). Masterton and Biederman (1983) have argued that proprioceptive input dominates over visual input in children with autism. They see this dominance as the effect of an alternative strategy to compensate for a lack of visual control over fine motor performance. In this context, it is of some interest that certain children, who otherwise yield good gaze contact, can talk coherently only when avoiding gaze contact.

Although abnormal sensory responses in autism are regarded by many as 'primary' and, in their view, should therefore be included among the diagnostic criteria, the most influential diagnostic manuals do not do this. Neverth-

eless, most authorities agree that, for instance, 'undue sensitivity to sound' is an extremely common feature in autism and that it differentiates autism from, for instance, dysphasia (Rutter, 1978, 1983). In a prospective study of children with autism seen before their third birthday, 'abnormal responses to sensory stimuli' was the class of symptoms which most clearly distinguished autism from mental retardation (Gillberg et al., 1990). Similar findings were reported by Ornitz (1989).

Other common problems

Hyperactivity is a very common symptom, especially in young children with autism. Sleep problems are most often apparent in infancy, when the child may keep the whole family awake by crying, but may sometimes continue right through to adulthood. Many people with autism are awake for long periods each night. An almost total lack of initiative is a dominating problem in certain children with autism.

Food fads are the rule rather than the exception. Many children with autism have great problems chewing. Hard objects are sometimes orally preferred to soft ones. Anorexia nervosa has been described in autism and autistic-type features may be common in anorexia nervosa.

Self-injurious behaviour (head banging, wrist or knuckle biting, chin knocking, cheek smacking, eye poking, hair tearing, clawing, etc.) is seen in many children with autism. It has been proposed as being concomitant to the mental retardation, but in fact could not be, since such behaviour is often seen even in children with autism of normal intelligence.

Cognitive profile

Many children with autism are mentally retarded. However, it appears that there are certain characteristics in the cognitive patterns of a majority that differentiate them from children without autism regardless of whether they are mentally retarded or not.

First, it is well established (Shah & Frith, 1983), that some, though not all, show 'islets' of special abilities, particularly in the fields of rote memory (e.g. numerical skills), music, art and visuospatial skills (such as is sometimes demonstrated in a particular aptitude with jigsaw puzzles).

Secondly, many seem to have an impaired memory for recent events (Boucher, 1981). Specifically, their memory difficulties impair their ability to recall past activities in response to 'open' or 'uninformative' questions (Boucher & Lewis, 1989). Such problems would be compatible with underlying theory of mind problems. The memory difficulties might therefore not be 'true' memory deficits but depend on the way in which the 'memory imprint' is approached.

Thirdly, children with autism perform better than mental-age-matched retarded and normal children in respect to 'concrete' discrimination. However, tasks requiring 'formal' discrimination are more difficult for the child with autism (Maltz, 1981). Their concrete way of interpreting and solving problems is often evident throughout life, even in those few with relatively high intellectual functioning.

Fourthly, on the WISC, there is a particular test profile with peaks and troughs (Bartak *et al.*, 1975; Ohta, 1987; Rumsey & Hamburger, 1988) in certain areas. A recent study has shown a particular profile also on the Griffiths test (Sandberg *et al.*, 1993). Visuospatial skills (as reflected on the performance and gross motor subscales) show superior results, whereas language-associated (hearing and language subscale) and 'intuition/empathy' (practical reasoning)-associated tests yield extremely low results.

It is the unusual cognitive profile of children with autism that has given rise to the widespread speculation that they are indeed of superior intelligence, and just hiding their phenomenal capacity behind a shell of autism. Unfortunately, a large body of research is agreed that this view of autism is mistaken and that most children with autism, even those showing almost unbelievable splinter skills, are clearly mentally retarded. All have cognitive problems (Rutter, 1983).

Summary of diagnostic criteria

There are many children with one or two of the three major criteria proposed for diagnosing autism. What term do we apply to them? Are they autistic, autistic-like, children with autistic features or what? The matter can hardly be regarded as settled.

At the present stage, we would argue for an umbrella definition, namely that of 'the autistic syndromes' or, possibly, 'autism and autistic-like conditions', to cover the whole group of severe disorders on the autism spectrum. This term would clinically, be roughly equivalent to that of 'pervasive developmental disorders', but it would not be conceptually as confusing. based on the foregoing discussion, all autistic syndromes in our view share these characteristics:

1. severe abnormality of reciprocal social relatedness;
2. severe abnormality of development of communication, usually prominently noted in abnormalities of the production and, perhaps particularly, comprehension of spoken language;
3. rigid and restricted behavioural repertoire and imaginative skills as manifested in elaborate routines, insistence on sameness, restricted play patterns or interests and motor stereotypes.

All symptoms have to be out of phase with the overall intellectual level of the child. For a diagnosis of the 'complete autistic syndrome', 'childhood autism' or just 'autism', all three symptoms have to be present in severe and typical form.

In cases with all three symptoms represented in atypical form or with two of the symptoms in typical form, we suggest that 'partial autistic syndrome' or 'autistic-like condition' be diagnosed. This category would equate with 'pervasive developmental disorder not otherwise specified' (PDD NOS) in the DSM-III-R (APA, 1987).

In cases not meeting criteria for these two groups, but showing some autistic features, I suggest that 'autistic features' be diagnosed.

'Asperger syndrome' might be the diagnostic label selected for certain children falling in one of the above groups.

Prevalence

Recent studies suggest that autism prevalence (whether one defines autism according to Rutter, DSM-III or DSM-III-R-criteria) is at least in the range of 1–1.2 per 1000 (see Gillberg *et al.*, 1991*a*; Gillberg & Coleman, 1992; Wing, 1993; Gillberg, 1994 for recent overviews). Older studies suggested a lower prevalence rate (around 0.2–0.5 per 1000). It has been proposed that higher prevalence could be accounted for by more inclusive criteria in later diagnostic manuals, such as the DSM-III-R (Hertzig *et al.*, 1990). However, no good evidence from population studies has been put forward to support this notion. To the contrary, there is limited evidence that the reasons for the relatively high recent figures are an increasing awareness of the existence of autism generally and particularly in severely and profoundly mentally retarded people, and the fact that immigrants arriving in industrialized countries in recent years tend to bear children with autism more often (Akinsola & Fryers, 1986; Gillberg *et al.*, 1987, 1991*a*, Gillberg, 1992*b*; Wing, 1993). The figure of 1 per 1000 children born developing autism before age 10 years does not include Asperger syndrome cases. An average autism prevalence rate of 0.8 per 1000 children born was reported by Wing (1993) as she surveyed all the acceptable autism epidemiological studies that had been published from 1966 to 1992.

Sex ratios

In classic autism cases, boys tend to outnumber girls by at least 3 to 1 (Wing, 1981*b*). Among cases with severe and profound mental retardation, the ratio tends to be lower and in those with higher IQ it tends to be considerably higher.

It has been proposed that the same kind of underlying empathy disorder might be present in more girls than hitherto acknowledged (Kopp & Gillberg, 1992). Girls could have the same type of core deficit as boys with autism, but they would not receive a diagnosis of autism because they do not show all the symptoms of autism which are typically associated with the male prototype.

Perhaps the sex ratios for autism would be different if autism was conceptualized on the basis of some more basic construct than that of Kanner autism. Kanner autism was first described in boys, and it has been taken for granted too long that autism in girls must appear in exactly the same guise in girls. Girls in the general population appear to be more interested and participate more readily in two-way social interactions already at an early age. Their language development is earlier than that of boys. Their pattern of interests is definitely different in that they are not so exclusively devoted to mechanical aspects of objects and may not be equally insistent on routine. Thus, it would take more to meet the full clinical picture of autism if you are female than if you are male, even if a basic and characteristic autism empathy deficit were present to the same degree as in a male who would unreservedly be diagnosed as suffering from autism.

Interestingly, in recent reviews of the autism prevalence literature, Wing (1993) and Gillberg (1994) found that, in the European studies, the sex ratios were not as high as previously believed. In fact, a male:female ratio of 2:1 rather than 3–5:1 was the rule.

Associated handicaps

Mental retardation is present in 65–88% of autism cases, given the extension of today's autism concept. If Asperger syndrome is included, and if it becomes accepted that girls with social deficits and learning disorders may suffer from an 'autistic condition', the rate of clear mental retardation would drop considerably, perhaps even to below 20%. Nevertheless, it has been shown convincingly that all children with autism (and other autism spectrum disorders) have cognitive deficits.

Epilepsy occurs in 30–40% of all autism cases before 30 years of age (Gillberg, 1991*b*). About half this proportion represents various epilepsy types (including infantile spasms) with onset in early childhood. The other half is mostly adolescent onset epilepsy. Partial complex seizures and generalized tonic-clonic seizures are the most common types of epilepsy. However, all sorts of seizures can occur in conjunction with autism, and there is often a variety of different seizures types occurring within the same individual. It is not uncommon for a child with autism to have all of the following: juvenile myoclonic epilepsy, partial complex epilepsy and generalized tonic clonic epilepsy.

Hearing problems are relatively common. A hearing deficit of 25 dB or more is present in about 20% of all children with typical autism (Steffenburg, 1991). The hearing deficits in autism have mostly been described as neurogenic, but there is increasing evidence that a considerable fraction of all hearing deficits encountered in autism may be of the peripheral type (Gordon, 1993). Indeed, some of the abnormalities documented with the use of brainstem auditory evoked response examination may be attributable to peripheral lesions secondarily affecting brainstem pathways.

Visual problems are also common (but also difficult to diagnose). On the basis of results from one Swedish study, about half of all children with autism, who function at a level high enough to permit a comprehensive opthalmological assessment, have refraction errors or squints or both (Steffenburg, 1991).

A considerable proportion of people with autism have expressive dysphasia 'superimposed' on their autistic type speech and language abnormalities. No systematic epidemiological study has explored the possible interrelationships between autism and dysphasia. It has been the experience of the present author that about one in five of all classically autistic cases has a severe expressive speech and language problem in addition to autism.

Major motor control abnormalities are uncommon in classical autism in childhood. However, follow-up into adult age (von Knorring, 1991, von Knorring & Hägglöf, 1993; Gillberg et al., in preparation) reveals that many develop disturbances of gait, ataxic movements and overall motor clumsiness with increasing age. Furthermore, some children with autism show hypotonia and mild ataxia in early childhood (Coleman & Gillberg, 1985). Also, children with spastic tetraplegia exhibit social interaction and communication deficits in a relatively large proportion of the cases, even when the effects of concomitant severe mental retardations have been taken into account.

Associated specific medical conditions

A large number of specific medical conditions have been found to be associated with autism or autistic symptoms at a rate higher than that found in the general population. Conversely, in autism, one finds a high rate of associated medical conditions such as the fragile X syndrome, other chromosomal abnormalities, tuberous sclerosis, neurofibromatosis, hypomelanosis of Ito, Moebius syndrome and Rett syndrome. In a population-based study of autism in western Sweden, Steffenburg (1991) found that 37% had an associated medical condition of this type. The neurocutaneous disorders alone (tuberous sclerosis, neurofibromatosis and hypomelanosis of Ito) are likely to account for 10–15% of all autism cases (Gillberg & Forsell, 1984; Zappella, 1992; Hunt & Shepherd 1993; Gillberg et al., 1994) and the fragile X-syndrome for another 3–10% (Hagerman, 1989). In young girls with autism, Rett syndrome should always be considered the first option for differential diagnosis. If there is autism and epilepsy, the risk that the child may be suffering from tuberous sclerosis or Rett syndrome (in the case of girls) is very high.

Table 6.3 shows some of the correlations between autism and specific medical conditions which have been reported in the literature up to now.

The pathogenetic chain of events in autism

Reduced optimality in the pre-, peri- and neonatal periods has been found to be considerably more 'pathological' in autism than in a number of other developmental disorders such as mental retardation without autistic traits, syndromes associated with deficits in attention, motor control and perception and teenage psy-

Table 6.3. *Associated medical conditions in autism documented in at least two studies*

Medical condition	Important reference
Fragile X syndrome	Hagerman, 1989
Other sex chromosome anomalies	Hagerman, 1989
Marker chromosome syndrome (partial tetrasomy 15)	Gillberg *et al.*, 1991*b*
Other chromosome anomalies	Hagerman, 1989
Tuberous sclerosis	Hunt & Dennis, 1987
Neurofibromatosis	Gillberg & Forsell, 1984
Hypomelanosis of Ito	Åkefeldt & Gillberg, 1991
Rett syndrome	Coleman & Gillberg, 1985
Moebius syndrome	Ornitz, Guthrie & Farley, 1977
PKU	Friedman, 1969
Lactic acidosis	Coleman & Blass, 1985
Purine disorders	Gillberg & Coleman, 1992
Rubella embryopathy	Chess, Korn & Fernandez, 1971
Herpes encephalitis	Gillberg, 1986
CMV infection	Stubbs, 1978
Williams syndrome	Reiss *et al.*, 1985
Duchenne muscular dystrophy	Komoto *et al.*, 1984

chosis (Gillberg & Gillberg, 1991). These disorders in turn are associated with reductions of optimality greater than those which are to be expected in normal children. Bleedings in pregnancy, high maternal age, pre- and postmaturity, clinical dysmaturity and hyperbilirubinaemia are among the factors which contribute to high reduced optimality scores in autism (Gillberg & Gillberg, 1983; Bryson, Smith & Eastwood, 1989). The added negative effects of several factors which deviate from the optimal state in pregnancy and the newborn period could lead to a suboptimal environment for the developing nervous system which could cause brain dysfunction showing later as autistic symptomatology. However, the interpretation of reduced optimality is not straightforward. For instance, a study by Piven *et al.* (1993) using

the same method (but not the same type of populations or controls) as Gillberg and Gillberg (1989*a*) found the same high rate of reduced optimality in the pre- and perinatal periods, but after controlling for the effect of being first- or late-born in a sibship (both of which occurred more often in the autism group), differences were no longer significant.

Clear brain-damage risks (such as haemolytic anaemia caused by blood group incompatibility, severe and protracted asphyxia, etc.) are also associated with some cases of autism (e.g. Folstein & Rutter, 1977). Such findings imply that typical autism can arise on the basis of unspecific brain damage.

There is now increasing evidence that, at least in some cases, genetic factors are in operation in autism. Three well-designed twin studies have all shown a strong concordance for autism in monozygotic twins and no concordance in dizygotic twins (Folstein & Rutter, 1977; Steffenburg *et al.*, 1989, Bolton & Rutter, 1990; Bailey *et al.*, 1993). Family studies of population-based series of autism cases have demonstrated a 50–100-fold autism risk increase for siblings of children with autism as compared with children in the general population. Family studies (e.g., Bowman, 1988) show that, in certain families, Asperger syndrome, autistic-like conditions and autism cluster in such a way as to suggest the presence of a strong heritability for some kind of autism-associated trait. Rutter's group has suggested that it is not autism as such which is inherited but rather that some kind of cognitive disorder is transmitted which will in certain cases turn into autism if environmental insults of some kind are added (Folstein & Rutter, 1977). Other authors (Gillberg, Gillberg & Steffenburg, 1992; Szatmari, Boyle & Offord, 1993) have argued that some kind of social or 'social cognitive' deficit factor might be at the root of the hereditary component which is obviously present in some families with children with autism. The family case studies rather favours the notion of an 'Asperger trait' (or 'empathy disorder') running in some families (or that many members of some families fall in the lowermost portion of the normal distribution of empathy skills) (Gillberg, 1992*a*). If unassociated with brain damage this trait may breed 'true' as 'Asperger symptoms' or empathy disorder. If combined with brain damage, such as in the case of intrauterine rubella infection, this trait might produce autism (Gillberg, 1992*a*). Most of the family studies would support the notion of a cognitive deficit (dyslexia-language-associated) running in certain families, but a few studies have not been able to find evidence for this (e.g Steffenburg, 1990). A few studies have documented a high rate of affective disorders (including schizoaffective disorders in the first-degree relatives) (Steffenburg, 1991; Gillberg *et al.*, 1992; DeLong & Noria, 1993). A small fraction of this mood disorder heredity was accounted for by the fragile X syndrome. There could be several different hereditary factors which, in interaction with other factors, could produce the same end result. Thus, there might be Asperger-associated heredity in some families and dyslexia-associated heredity in others. Hereditary affective disorder might be a common trait in both these groups.

In a recent study by Steffenburg (1991) of a total population cohort of children with autism, 1 in 3 had a clear associated medical condition, less than 1 in 10 had a 'pure' hereditary form, and almost all of the remainder had major signs of brain dysfunction revealed by comprehensive neurobiological work-up. Less than half of the medical conditions would have been disclosed had not the neurobiological examination been comprehensive.

Several different theories regarding the aetiology of autism have been proposed over the last 20 years. It seems that autism can be the end result of quite a number of different aetiologies, ranging from tuberous sclerosis and the fragile X chromosome abnormality to well-defined metabolic disorders. Do these aetiologies share a common feature, i.e. that they impinge on the same brain structures or functional systems? In recent years, the brainstem and temporal lobes of the brain have been most often implicated in studies of neurophysiology/neuroradiology in autism. Also, some studies have drawn attention to the possible role of the prefrontal areas, the cerebellum and the basal ganglia. The target areas for the brain's dopaminergic nerve fibres

arising in the brainstem are the mesolimbic structures in the temporal lobes and prefrontal areas and in the basal ganglia. The dopamine system has been reported to be abnormal in autism (Gillberg & Svennerholm, 1987; Barthèlèmy *et al.*, 1989). One theory proposes that the diverse aetiologies all affect this functional dopamine system in the brain and that, when dopamine systems become dysfunctional, many of the typical autism symptoms ensue (Coleman & Gillberg, 1985). Support for this theory is also provided by recent preliminary observations that babies born to crack mothers show many of the characteristic features of autism from the first few months of life (Gillberg & Coleman, 1992). Crack affects the brain's dopamine systems. However, alternative theories, such as hyperserotonaemia problems, locus ceruleus dysfunction and endorphin imbalance have been advanced (Cook, 1990). The various theories need not be exclusive. At the present stage it does not seem likely that one pathogenetic chain of events will ever be discovered to account for all autism cases.

In summary, autism is best conceptualized as a behavioural disorder, not quite so specific as previously believed, with multiple aetiologies. Autism is a sign that there is something wrong in the nervous system. It is best regarded as belonging with the other major neurohandicapping conditions, such as mental retardation, cerebral palsy and epilepsy. It sometimes occurs in conjunction with other disorders and handicaps, and there should no longer be a need to discuss whether a child has, e.g. 'autism *or* a hearing deficit' in a case where it is clear that both diagnoses apply.

Medical work-up in autism

A medical work-up is required in all cases of autism (and in many instances of autistic-like conditions). Tables 6.4 and 6.5 list the essentials in any work-up of a child under age 10 years who receives a diagnosis of autism for the first time. In older children, those with normal IQ, and in children for which a clear aetiology is at once suspected, the work-up should perhaps be differently tailored.

Steffenburg's study (1990), among others,

Table 6.4. *Neuropsychiatric assessment in autism*

Assessment

1. History
- detailed structured assessment of autistic symptoms using standard questionnaire (such as the HBS, DISCO, ADI or CARS)
- review of optimality in pre-, peri- and neonatal periods (medical records *required*)
- review of postnatal, potentially brain-damaging events (medical records usually needed)
- review of previous medical illness, growth patterns, overall level of functioning in various developmental areas, development of handedness, etc.
- detailed psychiatric history:
    family factors and psychosocial milieu
    temperament and attention span of child
    heredity (especially autism, autistic-like conditions including detailed discussion of symptoms in near relatives suggestive of Asperger syndrome, 'schizoid personality', learning disorders, mental retardation, 'childhood psychosis', 'schizophrenia', 'paranoia' affective disorders, obsessive-compulsive disorders, psychiatric disorders generally including anorexia nervosa and elective mutism, tuberous sclerosis, neurofibromatosis, geniuses). Do not forget to enquire about kinship.

2. General physical examination
- measurement of cranial circumference, height, weight, auricle length and interpupillary distance
- assessment with respect to minor physical anomalies, meticulous physical examination (often needs repeating) including search for diagnostic skin changes (tuberous sclerosis, neurofibromatosis, hypomelanosis of Ito)
- inspection of external genitals in males (prepuce, penile and testicular size and volume)
- assessment of heart beat variation

3. Age-appropriate neurodevelopmental/neurological examination

4. Psychological evaluation
- should be performed by experienced clinical psychologist who knows how to do cognitive testing in children with autism and knows which test is appropriate according to child's age, developmental level, language and degree of cooperation; choice of test depends on availability, but for school age children and adults the Wechsler scales are those with the most comprehensive empirical basis

5. Laboratory examinations
- see Table 6.5.

has demonstrated that a comprehensive medical work-up is required in autism. She found a clear aetiology in more than one-third of the cases (and signs of major unspecific brain dysfunction in another 50%). More than half of the clear aetiologies would not have been disclosed without an exhaustive work-up of the kind suggested in Table 6.5.

Even in those many cases for which a clear aetiology cannot be established, the medical work-up is important for psychological reasons. The parents need to know that their doctor has done what is currently the best possible work-up in the field of autism. The fact that so many turn out to have demonstrable signs of brain dysfunction, even when no exact cause can be established, is often helpful rather than, as some seem to fear, contributing to pessimistic attitudes in parents and others working to help the affected child. The disorder becomes less mysterious, and some of the child's problems take on a less baffling, less threatening character.

Neuropsychological work-up

The notion that children with autism cannot be reliably tested, or indeed tested at all, with

Table 6.5. *Relevant laboratory analyses in all medium/low-functioning, and certain high-functioning, cases with autism and autistic-like condition*

Analysis	Finding	Reference
• Chromosomal (including in a folic-acid-depleted medium)	Fragile X q27.3	Hagerman, 1989
	XYY	Gillberg *et al.*, 1984
	Deletions, e.g. 15p	Kerbeshian *et al.*, 1990
	Partial tetrasomy 15	Gillberg *et al.*, 1991
	Other	Hagerman, 1989
• FMR-1-DNA gene analysis	Fragile X gene mutation	Verkerk *et al.*, 1991
• CAT-scan/MRI-scan	Tuberous sclerosis	Gillberg *et al.*, 1987
	Intrauterine infections	Chess *et al.*, 1971
	Neurofibromatosis	Gillberg & Forssell, 1984
	Hypomelanosis of Ito	Åkefeldt & Gillberg, 1990
	Migration disorders	Gillberg & Coleman, 1992
	Other	Tsai, 1989
• CSF-protein[a]	Progressive encephalopathy	Wing & Gould, 1979
• EEG	Tuberous sclerosis	Steffenburg, 1990
	Subclinical epilepsy	Gillberg & Schaumann, 1983
	Epileptogenic discharge	Gillberg & Schaumann, 1983
	Self-injurious behaviour	Coleman, 1989
	Other	Gillberg & Coleman, 1992
• Auditory brainstem response examination	Brainstem dysfunction	Coleman & Gillberg, 1985
• Ophthalmologist	Poor vision, fundus abnormalities	Steffenburg, 1991
• Oto-laryngologist (including hearing test)	Poor hearing, anatomy	Smith *et al.*, 1988
• Blood		
phenylalanine	high	Friedman, 1969
uric acid	high	Coleman & Gillberg, 1985
lactic acid	high	Coleman & Blass, 1985
pyruvic acid	high	Coleman & Gillberg, 1985
herpes titer	seroconversion	Gillberg, 1986
• 24-hour urine		
metabolic screen including muco-polysaccharidosis		Coleman & Gillberg, 1985
uric acid	high	Coleman & Gillberg, 1985
calcium	low	Coleman, 1989

Note: [a] if there is a nearby laboratory doing CSF amino acids (phenylalanine in particular), CSF monoamines CSF endorphins and CSF glial fibrillary acidic protein, these tests should be considered if the child is having a lumbar puncture anyway (to exclude progressive encephalitis/encephalopathy)

conventional psychometric cognitive measures has strongly restricted empirical study in the field. This has led to a situation in which the neuropsychology of autism has become a fairly small branch on the now rather healthy tree of autism research. However, recent years have witnessed an increasing interest in the basic psychology of autism, and some of the most interesting developments in all of autism research have emerged from neuropsychologically inclined studies of young children with autism and of adult high-functioning men with autism. During the 1980s, there were basically four seats of innovative research studies in the neuropsychological domain which have had a profound influence on the way we now think about autism. Uta Frith and her colleagues (Baron-Cohen, Leslie & Frith, 1985; Leslie & Frith, 1988; Baron-Cohen, 1989*a*) have studied the 'theory of mind' concept; Deborah Fein and Lynn Waterhouse have focused on the neuropsychological heterogeneity in groups of patients diagnosed as autistic or autistic-like (Waterhouse & Fein, 1989); Peter Hobson (1984, 1986*a,b*, 1987) has studied various aspects of egocentricity and perception along Piagetian lines; and Judith Rumsey and her co-workers (Rumsey *et al.*, 1988) have expanded the field of study of cognitive abilities in high-functioning adult males with autism. These studies, and a handful of other more 'isolated' attempts at finding core neuropsychological features in autism (Dawson & McKissick, 1984; Whitehouse & Harris, 1984), have considerably changed our whole conceptual framework in autism research. The pioneering work of Hermelin and O'Connor (1970) is still influential, and has inspired some of the most important recent studies by the Frith group, for instance. This chapter reviews selectively the work done to date in an attempt to summarize what is currently known concerning the neuropsychology of autism.

Cognition and cognitive strategies in autism

In spite of assertions to the contrary, it has been documented for decades that many children with autism are also mentally retarded (i.e. they test reliably below IQ 70 on conventional IQ tests), (Clark & Rutter, 1979). The proportion of children with autism who also show mental retardation has varied somewhat between studies, but most authors agree that the figure is somewhere in the range of 65 to 85% (Lotter, 1967; Wing & Gould, 1979; Bohman *et al.*, 1983; Gillberg, 1984; Gillberg & Steffenburg, 1987). Recent studies suggesting a much higher prevalence rate for Asperger syndrome (usually with IQ > 70) possibly equivalent with high functioning autism than for autism 'proper' (Gillberg & Gillberg, 1989*b*; Wing, personal communication) could imply that the rate of clear mental retardation in autism, although much higher than in the general population, might be in the 10 to 25% range instead. At any

rate, most authorities agree that even within the range of so-called normal intellectual functioning, children with autism (and Asperger syndrome) all show cognitive problems.

Defining features of autism (notably social, language and symbolic play deficits) make it clear that various cognitive functions associated with these deficits are likely to be particularly affected. The long-standing debate as to whether autism is either cognitive or social tends to miss the point. The issue really is not whether it is cognitive or social but rather how the social and cognitive deficits can be conceptualized as emerging from one common 'primary' dysfunction. However, with regard to neuropsychological views of autism, the semantic squabble over 'cognitive', on the one hand, and 'social' on the other, still has far-reaching consequences in that the former is being regarded as 'cortical' (new brain) and the latter 'subcortical' (old brain) dysfunction. The overall point in this connection is that there is danger that the way we use words ('cognitive', 'language', and 'social', for instance) might substantially influence the way in which we conceptualize autism as primarily this or the other, when in fact it may be neither. For example, much emphasis has been put on language (supposedly more 'cognitive' than 'social') as a 'primary' deficit in autism, even though there is now good evidence that people with autism can have excellent (at least formal expressive) language skills (Wing, 1980; Gillberg *et al.*, 1987; Rumsey *et al.*, 1988), and that language deficits often associated with autism (e.g. pronominal reversal) might be conceptualized as delay rather than deviance (Oshima-Takana & Benaroya, 1989). This emphasis has led to expectations that neuroimaging techniques aimed at visualizing cerebral cortical areas would show much promise in the disclosure of the common neurobiological denominator in autism. So far, such studies have by and large been disappointing.

Cognitive impairment is usually thought of as a global phenomenon: all cognitive functions in a child with cognitive impairment are expected to be affected. This is a gross oversimplification even in children who are mentally retarded but do not show autism (cf. Down syndrome and William syndrome, two mental retardation syndromes with clearly different cognitive profiles). In autism, it is essential that the cognitive impairment be recognized as showing in (sometimes extremely) uneven cognitive profiles (Frith, 1989a). Verbal abilities are usually poorer than performance skills, comprehension is quite often much more impaired than word production, fine motor skills may be better than gross motor skills, and a variety of measures reflecting rote memory skills demonstrate good or even superior results (Wing, 1980; Ohta, 1987). The typical profile on the WISC is one with relatively good results on Block Design and good results in Picture Assembly, but poor or very poor results on Comprehension and Picture Arrangement (Lockyer & Rutter, 1970; Ohta, 1987; Rumsey & Hamburger, 1988; Frith, 1989a). It has recently been suggested (Frith, 1989a) that a 'cognitive profile' of this kind might be diagnostic of autism or at least highly suggestive of autism or autism spectrum disorders. On the Block Design subtest, individuals with autism perform better than normals and mentally retarded subjects, particularly when presented with unsegmented designs. This suggests that they need less of the normally required effort to cement a gestalt, a 'whole', and this thus supports Frith's hypothesis (Frith, 1989a) of weak central coherence as a characteristic of information processing in autism (Shah & Frith, 1983). Some recent studies further suggest that with increasing age, the Similarities subtest of the Wecshler scales may tend to more abnormal results in autism (and other disorders of empathy). This may be because scoring on this subscale is done differently according to the child's age: in the younger age group, literal and concrete similarities are awarded scores, but with increasing age, only the more abstract similarities are accepted. For instance, the similarity of a dog to a cat may well be accepted to be 'both have fur' at age seven years, but only 'both are animals' will be awarded a full score at age 15 years. Young and old people with autism may well be able to notice the obvious (that is that both are furry animals), but will continue to miss the salient feature (that is that both are 'animals') even as they grow older. Equally, the result on the Object Assembly subtest may decline over the years. This may be because people with autism have problems disregarding detail and, with increasing age, the requirement for faster performance on this task puts more emphasis on the conception of the whole object for successful completion (Nydén, Ehlers, Gillberg, 1994; Gillberg I.C. et al., 1994).

In a number of children, adolescents and adults with autism there is, in addition, an 'islet of special ability' (Shah & Frith, 1983). Something like every 1:2 have an area of functioning which stands out as exceptionally good compared with other areas. In a very few cases (c.5% according to O'Connor & Hermelin 1989; fewer still according to the present authors) there may exist extraordinary 'savant skills' (Treffert, 1989), such as shown by Raymond (Dustin Hoffman) in the Barry Levison film, Rain Man. Such individuals ('idiots savants' or 'autistic savants') usually show extremely superior rote memory abilities, musical giftedness or mathematical skills. Similar, though not quite such striking giftedness (not so striking because of the overall better cognitive level), is also seen in cases with autism spectrum disorders (e.g. Asperger syndrome, Wing, 1981a).

It appears that many children with autism rely on visuospatial rather than temporal processing (Hermelin & O,Connor, 1970), and that meaningful information tends to be less often correctly identified (Aurnhammer-Frith, 1969). Many children with autism show excellent skills with jigsaw puzzles but cannot conceive on the notion of time. This is unlike normal children who tend to extract as many meaningful clues as possible in trying to solve problems. Also, whereas normal children will make use of several clues, children with autism will often depend on single piece of information when attending to a task.

Recent developments in the field of cognitive neuropsychology and autism

In the 1980s, the focus of neuropsychological studies in autism shifted gradually from language and other conservative measures of cognition to the description and delineation of social and pragmatic deficits. Two relatively distinct theories have emerged which have been subjected to systematic scientific study. For the purpose of brevity, they will be referred to here as the affective theory (Hobson, 1986a) and the meta representation theory (Baron-Cohen, 1988). Because both, particularly the latter, are currently influential in guiding research and in clinical concepts of autism, they will be described in this context. In the past few years, a partly competing theory of 'executive function' (i.e. frontal lobe) deficits in autism has evolved (Ozonoff, Pennington & Rogers, 1991; McEvoy, Roger & Pennington, 1993). It is mentioned only in passing since it has yet to assert its status as a theory which can account for the whole range of autistic symptomatology. The prediction that follows from this theory is that individuals with autism will be dysfunctional on tests tapping strategic, flexible plans of action and power to inhibit responses and/or defer them to a more appropriate time (Welsch, Pennington & Grossier, 1991). It seems clear from a number of studies (e.g. McEvoy et al., 1993) that relatively high-functioning young individuals with autism are, indeed, deficient in these domains. However, this is not to say that such deficits are primary or even basically involved in the pathogenetic chain of events in autism.

The affective theory goes back to Kanner's original assertions that children with autism have 'inborn disturbances of affective contact' (our quotes) and to the theories of Piaget. In the affective theory, autism is seen as stemming from an affective deficit which is primary and irreducible, and involves a dysfunction in the ability to perceive other people's mental states as reflected in their bodily expressions. This primary affective dysfunction underlines the social and communication problems. Support for the theory has been generated by a number of interesting experiments concerned with various aspects of emotion recognition in children with autism (see review by Hobson, Ouston & Lee, 1988). However, the studies by Marian Sigman and her group (Sigman & Ungerer, 1984; Sigman et al., 1986; Sigman & Mundy,

1989) have demonstrated convincingly that some attachment behaviours, eye contact and reaching after tickling are usually preserved in autism. Such behaviours can all be seen as primarily 'affective' variables. Also, most authorities agree that children with autism may have well developed primary emotions such as anger and gladness.

The meta representation theory, sometimes also referred to as the 'cognitive theory' (to distinguish it from the affective theory), argues rather differently that mental states with content (such as 'invisible' knowing and believing and not 'obvious' happiness and anger) are not directly observable but have to be inferred.

The ability to impute mental states with content to other people has been referred to as a 'theory of mind' (Premack & Woodruff, 1978). This 'theory' is present in normal children from at least 4 years of age (Hogrefe, Wimmer & Perner, 1986) but could be in operation much earlier, perhaps even before age 1 year (Leslie, 1987). The specific cognitive peaks and troughs encountered in autism (low scores on comprehension and picture arrangement and high on block design on the WISC; low scores on hearing and speech and practical reasoning and high on motor and performance on Griffiths) could be taken to indicate the lack of a core capacity for coherence in autism. Uta Frith (1989a, b) and her collaborators (Baron-Cohen et al., 1985; Baron-Cohen, 1990) have proposed a theory to account for the basic psychological features of autism. They hypothesize that underlying the behavioural symptoms of autism is a central disorder of empathy characterized by inability or decreased capacity to conceive of other people's mental states (such as knowing and believing). If a deficit of this kind exists, then it could explain the lack of coherence and need for coherence in autism. If you do not understand that behind people's actions are thought-out purposes and wilful planning, much of what people do will stand out as incomprehensible. What they say will be even more 'uncommunicative': not understanding that the spoken words are a 'message from the mind' makes spoken language something you may learn to imitate but not a tool for communication. Not having a well-developed theory of mind will lead to extreme deficits in reciprocal social interaction, in communication and 'creative' imagination. However, not having a theory of mind does not necessarily affect memory of visuospatial skills, areas in which many people with autism excel. Feats of rote memory and jigsaw puzzle solving are fairly common in autism. These are skills that are not dependent on having a theory of mind. Such skills are reflected in high scores on block design and performance. The theory predicts that only specific social capacities should be constantly restricted in autism (namely, those that require a concept of other people's wishes, beliefs and thoughts, e.g. reciprocal social interactions or 'empathy'), whereas other special capacities might be spared (i.e. those that require only perception of the observable world, e.g. face recognition). The theory further predicts that the pragmatics of existing language skills in a child with autism will be specifically impaired. A number of simple, yet-thought provoking experiments have been performed to test this theory (for a review see Baron-Cohen, 1990. In one of these, two dolls, Sally and Anne, were presented to normal children, children with Down syndrome and children with autism. In Sally's basket was a marble, but in Anne's box was nothing. Sally then 'left the room', meaning that she could no longer see what was going on. In the meantime, Anne moved the marble to her box. When Sally 'came back', the children participating in the study were asked: 'Where will Sally look for the marble?' Children with Down syndrome and normal children said she looked where it was when she left the room (a false but reasonable belief), whereas most of the children with autism said she would look in the box, where it actually is (a true but unreasonable belief). Children with autism under age 11 years and with a mental age under 6 years constantly fail this task according to Baron-Cohen (1990). One way to account for this finding, and similar findings from other experiments, would be the lack of a theory of mind; if the child cannot understand that Sally has a mind (a belief/thought about the marble being

where it once was), s/he will believe only what s/he sees or hears. There is now considerable support for its validity, not only from Frith's group, but also from past research (for review see by Baron-Cohen, 1988) and from independent experimenters (e.g. Dawson & Fernald, 1987, and indirectly from van Bourgondien & Mesibov, 1987).

Even though there have been experimental studies that have challenged the theory of mind theory of autism (Prior, Dahlstrom & Squires, 1990), the accumulating evidence is such that it is hard to dismiss. The theory provides a plausible account for the developmental changes in the clinical picture of autism across time and IQ levels. Impairments in 'first order belief attribution' (e.g. 'I think he thinks') may be typical of the most severely affected people with autism, whereas impairments of 'second order belief attribution' (e.g. 'I think he thinks she thinks') may typify high-functioning cases diagnosed as Asperger syndrome (see also Baron-Cohen, 1989b). A proposed deficient theory of mind in autism has the merit of making comprehensible to parents and professionals alike some of the mystifying features of autism. A theory of this kind has the great merit of being testable at several levels and also of providing a clinically relevant model for the development of autism.

The affective and meta representation theories are not necessarily mutually exclusive and there may be potential in trying to examine to what extent they can be reconciled. Both provide excellent possibilities for empirical study and have fuelled the previously speculation-loaded area of autism psychology with a number of interesting experiments which have already yielded important theoretical and clinical insights.

Another suggested primary deficit, possibly underlying the theory of mind (or 'mentalizing') deficit (although not necessarily clinically manifest before it), is 'weak central coherence' (Frith, 1989; Happé, 1994). In autism there is obviously an impairment in the normal cognitive process by which meaning is derived through the weaving together of otherwise piece-meal information. This lack of 'drive' for central coherence could explain both the typical autism impairments *and* the preserved (and even superior) skills.

Is psychological testing in autism useful?

It is often, though by no means always, problematic to test a young child with autism using conventional IQ tests. Problems are most likely to occur, of course, if the tester is not very well acquainted with the underlying deficits and clinical manifestations of autism. In order for it to be worthwhile testing a child with autism, testing and results on tests must have some meaning. So what are IQ tests and other tests in autism good for?

IQ tests in childhood have been shown to be the best available single instrument for roughly predicting outcome in autism (Rutter, 1983). A very low IQ (< 50) in childhood usually predicts a similar IQ and relatively poor social outcome in adult age. As has already been pointed out above, some IQ tests yield a typical 'profile' in autism. On the WISC (for school-age children), peaks in block design (and picture assembly) and troughs in word comprehension and picture arrangement are typical. In the Griffiths developmental scale (Griffiths, 1970), children with autism peak in motor and daily life activities but score very poorly on the hearing/language scales (Sandberg et al., 1993). For these, and other, reasons it is clear that IQ testing is essential in the work-up of any child and for predicting outcome in a reasonable way.

Results on specific tests of language performed in childhood can also help establish a fairly accurate prognosis. Useful speech at age 5 years is one of the best predictors of outcome (Gillberg, 1991c). In particular, it is helpful to try to pinpoint the receptive deficits (which, contrary to earlier assertions, are often even more pronounced than the expressive skill deficits) and to find out to what extent there might be added problems of 'pure' dysphasia over and above any language-communication deficits that could be accounted for by autism alone.

Finally, psychometric assessment is required

because children with autism are unique individuals: though they share some core deficits, they are quite different from each other. A detailed test of various functional capacities will help provide a fuller picture of assets and deficits, such that a better understanding of what will be the most useful coping strategies can be achieved.

All children with autism also need a comprehensive neuropsychological work-up. This must always include some kind of cognitive/intellectual testing or evaluation. No single measure in childhood will be able to predict outcome in autism better than an IQ-test: IQ under 50 around age 5–8 years almost invariably means a relatively poor outcome (see below) whereas IQ over 70 at this age predicts that outcome may quite often be relatively good (see below).

The kind of test one chooses will vary from one culture to another. Whatever the test, it should be performed by somebody knowledgeable in the field of autism, i.e. a psychologist both clinically and theoretically experienced with testing and evaluating children with autism.

Four different cognitive/developmental tests/scales seem to be very useful in autism, i.e. the WISC-R, the Leiter International Scale, the Vineland Social Maturity Scale and the Griffiths' Developmental Scale II. For language evaluation, the Reynell and the Peabody Picture Vocabulary Test can be useful. A newly developed neuropsychological test battery (the NEPSY (Korkman, 1988a, b, c)) may prove to be worthwhile in the evaluation of autism in childhood, but so far no systematic studies exist.

The WISC can only be used with children with autism aged 6–7 years or over and is particularly useful in cases with moderate or high-functioning autism (i.e. in those with IQ-levels above 50). In autism, the 'typical' profile is one in which verbal scores are lower than performance scores. Also, scores tend to be exceptionally low (relative to the child's other scores) for picture arrangement and comprehension (tests which, to a considerable degree, require the ability to reflect on other people's inner thoughts and to take account of context) and often exceptionally high for block design (a test which does not require the child to take account of context other than that provided by the visible patterns on the cubes).

The Leiter test is a non-verbal test which is often easy to administer (for a skilled psychologist) even in non-speaking children with autism. Many of the subtests of the Leiter reflect underlying abilities akin to those tested in the block design test of the WISC. Therefore, some children with autism will receive a high Leiter IQ, even when overall IQ (verbal and non-verbal) is not normal. Nevertheless, the Leiter has been shown to have relatively good correlation with other IQ-tests in many cases of autism and is widely used in the field.

The Vineland Social Maturity Scale is not an ordinary test but rather a structured interview with the closest carer. The examiner comes up with a social quotient, which, in autism, fairly well indicates the intelligence level also. The Vineland scale is therefore very useful in autism, especially in cases considered 'untestable'.

The Griffiths scale seems to be relatively useful in young children with autism (aged 2–7 years) in discriminating between those with IQ under 50 and those above. For a more detailed evaluation, the Griffiths scale seems relatively inadequate and usually has to be followed up with a WISC test during the early school years. Nevertheless, a characteristic test profile with relatively superior results on the gross motor and performance subscales and troughs on the hearing and language and practical reasoning subscales, usually emerges (Sandberg et al., 1993).

In making the diagnosis of autism as such, various questionnaires and other evaluation tools are available. The two currently most used manuals seem to be the CARS (Childhood Autism Rating Scale, Schopler, Reichler & Renner, 1988) and the ABC (Autism Behavior Checklist, Krug, Arick & Almond, 1980). The CARS has good reliability and validity at least in cases with clear-cut and obvious autism. The ABC can be seen rather as an interview contain-

ing 57 statements which can be used to elicit information about the child in about 30 minutes. It should not be used as the sole instrument for making a diagnosis of autism. The ADI (Autism Diagnostic Interview) (LeCouteur et al., 1989) and the ADOS (Autism Diagnostic Observation Schedule) (Lord et al., 1989) both appear to hold promise for more precise diagnosis in the field, but suffer from being very long and their requirement for extensive specific training.

For the educational evaluation, which can be seen as an important part of the neuropsychological work-up, the PEP (Psycho Educational Profile, Schopler & Reichler, 1979) is useful. It provides a concise picture of the child's current educational status in a number of areas and forms the basis for goal-directed educational interventions in the individual case. The PEP is intended to be used at regular intervals in an educational treatment programme in order to evaluate intervention effects.

Management, treatment and education

There can be no clear dividing-line between education, management and treatment in autism. Some cases of autism can be rationally treated (diet in PKU, autism, neurosurgery in tuberous sclerosis, autism/epilepsy to mention two) and helped by way of classic treatment, such as pharmacotherapy or psychotherapy or both. However, in the majority of cases, such measures do not produce sufficient change. Education and 'management' in a broad sense of that word, on the other hand, can lead to many worthwhile things. The crucial elements in any management/treatment programme for autism (or autistic-like conditions) are outlined in Table 6.6.

Specific treatments (including prevention)

PKU, if untreated, can cause autism. If PKU is appropriately treated with a diet from the first few days of life, autistic symptoms never develop. In fact, one is here dealing with prevention rather than cure, since the autistic symptoms

Table 6.6. *Management/intervention regimes in autism and autistic-like conditions*

Important component of intervention programme

- Clear diagnosis
- Individualized intervention programme
- Comprehensive work-up
- Information about diagnosis and work-up to parents/other carers
- Specific education about autism to parents, other relatives and other carers
- Specific treatments such as diets
- Rehabilitation team well acquainted with basic autism handicaps
- Home-based educational/behavioural intervention programme
- Structured environment including 'ritualizing' of everyday routines
- Continuity as regards people, place and interventions
- Graded change
- Physical exercise (including jogging and swimming)
- Education of child with emphasis on daily life activities and interest patterns which can form the basis for future work
- Pharmacotherapy in selected cases
- Psychotherapy by therapists well informed in matters relating to autism in selected cases
- Long-term (life-time) perspective

are never allowed to appear before treatment is started.

Other diet-treatments are possible in rare cases of autism. Coleman and Blass (1985) described lactic acidosis associated with autism and that, in such cases, dietary treatment could lead to the disappearance of autistic symptoms.

Herpes encephalitis can cause autism (DeLong *et al.*, 1981; Gillberg, 1986). There is a treatment for herpes encephalitis (an antiviral agent called Acyclovir), and, although not well researched in large populations, it seems that starting treatment very early in the course of herpes encephalitis (at the stage of mere suspicion rather than many hours later) can stop the otherwise often devastating brain destruction that can occur in herpes brain infection. If this is true, it would appear that it should be possible to prevent autistic symptoms from developing in this disease also.

Pharmacotherapy

Pharmacotherapy plays a minor, but important, role in the treatment of autism. There is no medication available in the treatment of autism for which benefits outweigh side effects in a majority of the cases. Nevertheless, some drugs, adequately tested in controlled studies, have clearly positive effects in a sufficient number of cases to warrant recommendation for treatment trials if there is a clinically felt need for pharmacological intervention. This is sometimes the case when thorough educational measures have not led to expected gains, when overactivity, destructiveness and/or self-injurious behaviour cause such turmoil that other interventions cannot be used at all, or when adolescent aggravation of symptoms (see below) prevents developmental progress. Drugs should never be used as the sole kind of intervention but should always be accompanied by educational and psychosocial approaches. Anti-epileptic pharmacotherapy is quite often indicated in autism with epilepsy.

The unspecific drugs most often used are vitamin B6, neuroleptics and sedating drugs. Lithium, naltrexone and clomipramine may be alternatives in the near future, but are still being investigated. In the treatment of epilepsy, carbamazepine and valproic acid appear to be drugs of first choice in many cases.

Vitamin B6 has been shown to have at least some positive effects in some relatively well-designed studies (Lelord *et al.*, 1981). It is given in doses of 300–900 mg/day and supplemented with magnesium in cases showing severe unspecific behaviour problems (including restlessness, aggressiveness, sleep problems and self-injurious behaviour).

Neuroleptics (particularly haloperidol and pimozide) have been examined in a number of double-blind placebo-controlled studies (Campbell, 1989). They seem to exert some positive effects on the basic problems associated with autism (social withdrawal, communication, learning and rigid behaviour patterns). However, it is difficult to recommend their use in the long-term because of the high incidence of severe or moderate extrapyramidal side effects (25–30% in most series). Neuroleptics can be of some value in breaking up 'vicious circles', particularly in adolescent symptom aggravation.

Sedative drugs are not indicated for more than short-term use (days–weeks). They are most often considered in the treatment of sleep problems. They often have 'paradoxical effects', the child reacting with even more hyperactivity and difficulty settling down in the evening. Benzodiazepines usually have extremely negative effects on behaviour and cognition in autism (Gillberg, 1991*b*) and should, if possible, be avoided.

In the treatment of epilepsy in autism, many drugs have detrimental side effects on behaviour and learning (Gillberg, 1991*b*). There are no well-controlled double-blind studies in the field, but a systematic survey of the literature and considerable clinical experience suggest that valproic acid and carbamazepine may be less negative than other drugs with respect to behavioural side effects. There are many different types of seizures in autism, complex partial seizures being perhaps the most prevalent. For this reason, carbamazepine and valproic acid are often considered drugs of first choice. Except for ethosuximide, other antiepileptic drugs have more negative effects on behaviour. The side effects of phenobarbital (irritability, hyperactivity, aggressive outbursts and decreased learning) are well known, but, at least in autism, the benzodiazepines (clonazepam in

particular) are often even worse. It is not uncommon for a child with complex partial seizures to appear autistic while on clonazepam but non-autistic as soon as he is taken off the drug.

Folic acid has been tried in the treatment of autism associated with fragile X (in doses ranging from 0.5–1.5 mg/kg/day). The findings so far are equivocal, but there appears to be a mild stimulant effect which can be useful in alleviating some of the unspecific symptoms such as concentration difficulties and hyperactivity.

Lithium may be an adjunct in controlling mood swings (and perhaps aggressiveness) occurring particularly during the adolescent period. Serum concentration should be kept at the lowest possible level (0.4–0.7 mEq/l).

Naltrexone and other opiate blockers have recently been tried in autism after the report of endogeneous opioid dysfunction in autism. Several double-blind-placebo controlled studies are currently in progress. One of these (Campbell *et al.*, 1993) showed only minor positive effects (specifically the reduction of hyperactivity) and minimal negative effects. Naltrexone seems to be a relatively safe drug, and might become more used in the future in autism, perhaps particularly if there is concomitant self-injurious behaviour. Several reports indicate a reduction of self-injurious behaviours (SIB) after treatment with opiate antagonists. Self-injurious behaviours in autism, on the other hand, have been reported to be associated with particularly high levels of CSF-endorphins (Gillberg, Terenius & Lönnerholm, 1985). The study by Campbell *et al.*, 1993 on 41 2–7 year-old children with autism did not produce a significant drop in the rate of SIB in the naltrexone as compared with the placebo group. However, there was a significantly more pronounced 'relapse' to pretreatment levels of SIB in the naltrexone group, indicating the possibility of a superior effect after all. Also, none of the individuals in the study by Campbell's group had extremely severe SIB. It is possible that very severe SIB might respond better to treatment with naltrexone. Further studies are needed in this field.

Fenfluramine, an anorexogenic drug with

serotonin-lowering properties, despite early enthusiastic reports, appears to have little place in the treatment of most cases of autism (Gadow, 1992).

For a good overview of medical treatment in autism, the reader is referred to Campbell, 1989.

Non-drug medical/biological treatments

Physical exercise is effective in reducing major behaviour problems (self-injurious behaviours, aggressiveness, hyperactivity and sleep problems) in autism (McGimsey & Favell, 1988; Haracopos, 1989) and should be used much more than is currently the case. Jogging programmes (2 half-hour sessions a day for instance) can be extremely helpful. Any type of physical activity which will lead to some degree of physical exhaustion on the part of the individual with autism is likely to cause some reduction of unspecific behaviour problems (Haracopos, 1989; Gillberg, 1992a).

Psychotherapy

In a wide sense of the word, there can be no autism treatment without psychotherapeutic elements. However, classical analytically oriented psychotherapy individually for children with autism has never been shown to have lasting or even positive effects in autism, and should not be used, unless as part of a systematic research trial, since there have been reports of negative effects both on the child and family (Gillberg, 1989a). If analytically oriented techniques are employed by somebody very experienced who also knows about the basic handicaps of autism (Tustin, 1981; Hobson, 1990), it is possible that, in some cases, such therapy can have some positive effects. Certainly, some of the high-functioning verbal people with autism, including many of those currently diagnosed as suffering from Asperger syndrome, do benefit from individual talks with somebody well acquainted with all the various aspects of autism, from around the time of puberty, when many of them begin to realize the extent to which they differ from other people.

Family therapy usually has no place in autism. However, regular contact with the family and teaching the family to become the child's best advocate (see below) should be essential parts of any good treatment/management programme.

Early diagnosis

To give autism a name as soon as possible can have far-reaching positive consequences. An early diagnosis can mean, for instance: (1) the discovery of treatable underlying conditions, (2) the identification of genetic disorders requiring genetic counselling, (3) getting the family out of a vicious circle including elements of self-blame, practical problems, loss of sleep and inappropriate behaviour management techniques, and (4) appropriate treatments and education for the child. Also, siblings can be better informed so that they may have a name for the deviant child's strange behaviours (Bågenholm & Gillberg, 1991).

There are now a number of screening devices that can be used in the well-baby clinic for the detection of autism. Two of these (Gillberg et al., 1990; Baron-Cohen, Allen & Gillberg, 1992) have been used in prospective studies. Of these, the CHAT (Checklist for Autism in Toddlers), is perhaps the simplest. It has been shown to be a reliable and valid autism screening instrument for children around 18 months of age (Table 6.7).

In a study of home videotapes of children's first year birthday parties, those children who later received a diagnosis of autism demonstrated little pointing, object showing, looking at others, and orientating to name, as compared with those who were later considered normal (Osterling & Dawson, 1994).

Home-based approaches

Howlin and colleagues in London (Howlin & Rutter, 1987) have shown that home based approaches to autism can have beneficial effects both for the child and family. Similar conclusions have been reached by Schopler's group in North Carolina (Schopler, 1989).

Table 6.7. *Checklist for autism in toddlers (CHAT)*

To be used by GPs or health visitors during the 18-month development check-up.

Child's name
Date of birth
Age
Child's address
Phone number

1. To record yes on this item, ensure the child has not simply looked at your hand, but has actually looked at the object you are pointing at.
2. If you can elicit an example of pretending in some other game, score a yes on this item.
3. Repeat this with 'Where's the teddy?' or some other unreachable object, if child does not understand the word 'light'. To record yes on this item, the child must have looked up at your face around the time of pointing.

Section A. Ask parent:

1. Does your child enjoy being   Yes   No
    swung, bounced on your knee,
    etc?
2. Does your child take an interest
    in other children?   Yes   No
3. Does your child like climbing on   Yes   No
    things, such as up stairs?
4. Does your child enjoy plaing   Yes   No
    peek-a-boo/hide-and-seek?
5. Does your child ever pretend,   Yes   No
    for example, to make a cup of
    tea using a toy cup and teapot,
    or pretend other things?
6. Does your child ever use his/her   Yes   No
    index figer to point, to ask for
    something?
7. Does your child ever use his/her   Yes   No
    index finger to point, to indicate
    interest in something?
8. Can your child play properly   Yes   No
    with small toys (e.g. cars or
    bricks) without just mouthing,
    fiddling, or dropping them?
9. Does your child ever bring   Yes   No
    objects over to you (parent), to
    show you something?

Section B. GP's or health visitor's observation:

i.   During the appointment, has the   Yes   No
     child made eye contact with
     you?
ii. Get child's attention, then point
     across the room at an interesting
     object and say 'Oh look! There's
     a [name a toy]!' Watch child's
     face.
     Does the child look across to see Yes   No
     what you are pointing at?

Table 6.7. (*cont.*)

iii.	Get the child's attention, then give child a miniature toy cup and teapot and say 'Can you make a cup of tea?' Does the child pretend to pour out tea, drink it, etc?	Yes	No
iv.	Say to the child 'Where's the light?', or 'Show me the light'. Does the child point with his/her index finger at the light?	Yes	No
v.	Can the child build a tower of bricks? (If so, how many?) (Number of bricks . . . .)	Yes	No

Parents should be regarded as co-therapists. All parents need to receive as much education as possible about autism, including symptoms, aetiology and treatments available. Seminars for groups of parents are often useful. The family should be informed about the existence of the National Autism Society. An integrated education/behaviour modification programme (including elements of 'graded change' (Howlin & Yates, 1989)) for the child should be planned in collaboration with the parents. Activities of daily life (such as feeding, hygiene and sleeping) should be the focus of home-based interventions. 'Institutional handling' of problems in this field usually do not generalize to the home situation without proper training at home.

Education

Ever since the days of Jean Itard (Itard, 1801), education has been felt to have particular merit in relation to autism. Education in autism is a vast and growing area (Schopler & Mesibov, 1988) beyond the scope of this volume. However, since education is currently considered the management of choice in autism, some brief comments are warranted.

Children with autism need a structured environment with as much predictability as possible. Their own need to insist on routine and 'sameness' should be met by adults introducing useful routines, which can be accepted by child and adult alike. Once routines have been taken over by adults in this way, the child with autism is more likely to stop introducing new, bizarre routines, and even to abandon some of the old ones. Whereas normal children, and indeed most mentally retarded children without autism, learn 'automatically' as they seek new experiences and interact with other people, children with autism do not get anything for free, and need to learn through training. Training needs to be planned, and this requires an evaluation tool. The PEP (Psycho Educational Profile) (Schople & Reichter, 1979) is a useful instrument for pinpointing individual skills and deficits in autism. The PEP can then also be used in the follow-up of management to document that the child has actually developed according 'to plan'.

Some principles of education in autism are essential. First, there is a need to individualize: in spite of similarities, people with autism are, first and foremost, individuals with different personalities, different IQ and different social background. Secondly, there is the need for structure and continuity in relation to time, place and teacher. In other words, the same thing should be trained at the same time in the same room by the same person. This style of structure might have to be applied with some rigour in the early stages of education, whereas the long-term goal might be to be able to gradually introduce a little more (perhaps not much more) flexibility. Thirdly, children with autism usually can harbour only one thought at a time, which means that instruction about several things cannot be given at once. Fourthly, and interconnected with the third point, is their deficient sense of time in most cases. This should be met, for instance, by seeing to it that all tasks are finished before the next task is introduced. Fifthly, but not least, education has to take account of the fact that children with autism, even those labelled high-functioning, usually have extremely deficient comprehension of spoken language and poor understanding of abstract symbols, but often relatively good visual or visuo-spatial skills. Spoken language has to be reduced to a minimum in interaction with people with autism, and one must find ways of ensuring that they actually understand your communications. Long sentences must be avoided in most cases as must most use of metaphorical language. Token and sign language can often be as difficult to cope with as spoken language. Pictures containing photos of concrete situations, which the child knows well, are often very helpful instead.

Special education and treatment facilities for people with autism

There is a need for special pre-schools, special class rooms, special job facilities and services planning work and special group homes for people with autism and autistic-like conditions. There is also the need for special facilities of this kind for people with other kinds of social and communicative impairments, most of whom are likely to have some kind of minor or major intellectual impairment. For some children with autism, the best option would be to be in a classroom specifically for children with autism, for others it would be a better placement to attend a classroom for the communication handicapped with or without autism and, for some, a classroom for the mentally retarded would be more suitable. Many children with autism do not need any of these special services, but they, and their families, might need the help

of an autism expert team to guide them through childhood, adolescence and adult life.

The special needs of people with autism and similar conditions can often not be well attended to in ordinary settings, which makes special services mandatory. The most important thing however, is that there exist true options for the child and family, and that no extreme philosophy of segregation or integration be allowed to be the only guideline for the kind of help and service that can be provided.

Outcome in autism

Most follow-up studies of autism agree that psychosocial outcome is variable but often quite poor. According to one recent survey of the literature (Gillberg, 1991c), the mortality rate seems to be increased. Almost 2% of all people with autism surviving the first two years of life, die before age 25 years. This increase in mortality is probably associated with the increased rate of severe neurological disorders found in autism. These neurological disorders, such as tuberous sclerosis, have a raised mortality as compared with the standardized mortality ratio of the general population.

Of those many people with autism who survive much longer, about 60% become totally dependent on other people for their everyday lives. Only a small number of these can hold even half-sheltered jobs. Another 25% show considerable progress, but still remain dependent on other people for many things. About 10% (recruited almost exclusively from the group with tested IQ > 60 in childhood) function independently and hold ordinary jobs, but may still be perceived as somewhat odd in their social interaction style. At most, about 5% in different follow-up studies have been considered 'cured' or rather as having grown out of symptoms associated with autism.

Outcome in autism is predicted by tested IQ around 5–7 years and the level of language competence at this age. Almost all cases with a (reliable) IQ of less than 50 and absence of spoken language at this age will belong in the psychosocially completely dependent adult outcome category (Rutter, 1970; Gillberg, 1991c). If tested full-scale IQ is above 70, it appears that about 50% may lead independent or semi-independent lives in adult age. The presence of a particular neurological disorder (such as the fragile X syndrome) will guide in suggesting a more fine-grained picture of the most likely outcome. The presence of epilepsy possibly increases the overall risk of poor outcome, but there are many exceptions to this rule. Structured education and early behavioural management promote adaptive behaviour skills, but do not affect ultimate cognitive functioning (Rutter, 1983).

About 10–20% of all children with autism deteriorate in adolescence and, as it appears, never regain their pre-adolescent level of functioning. Another 30% show symptom aggravation in adolescence. This aggravation may run a periodic course, but will usually become less of a problem at 25–30 years of age. The symptoms encountered in these pubertal change cases are often similar to those seen in the same child in the pre-school period, i.e. overactivity, aggressiveness, self-injurious behaviour, sleep problems, incoherent language, and bladder and bowel incontinence. A trial of lithium is indicated in some such cases (see above), and may occasionally be very helpful. Epilepsy is sometimes the first sign that deterioration may follow. On the other hand, there are deterioration cases which do not show association with onset of epilepsy, and also cases with the combination of epilepsy and symptom aggravation, which do not later develop deterioration. Unfortunately, the reason for deterioration is not known (even though in some instances progressive neurological/neurometabolic disorders are suspected) and there is usually no treatment available. Neuroleptics are often tried but, sometimes with little effect. Physical exercise more often yields positive results.

In adult age, three broad groups of people with autism can be discerned (Wing, 1989b): (1) those who remain autistic in many respects, (2) those who are passive and friendly and those who appear (3) active and odd. The second, passive group, quite often is not recognized as belonging in the autism category, unless a clear diagnosis of autism had been made in early childhood (and often not even then). The third group too is often not recognized as suffering from autism, but, because of the conspicuous problems they show (e.g. undressing or masturbating in public, touching other people in unexpected ways, etc.), they more often are brought to a psychiatrist who might be able to discern the original nature of the disorder.

The natural history in the individual case will also depend on the natural history of the particular associated medical condition (e.g. tuberous sclerosis, fragile X syndrome, etc.). Three aetiologically distinct subgroups of children with autism have been purported to have a relatively good outcome in respect of autistic symptomatology, i.e. those with Rett syndrome (Hagberg, 1993), infantile spasms (Riikonen & Amnell, 1981) and rubella embryopathy (Chess, 1977). In the case of Rett syndrome there is some, albeit slight, evidence that this may be true, but infantile spasms and rubella in autism have not been convincingly shown to have a better outcome than other autism cases. What is rarely appreciated in studies claiming a particularly good outcome for this or that subgroup is the fact that *most* children with autism improve over the years with regard to social withdrawal.

Finally, autism changes in symptomatology over the years, even in the subgroup that remains 'autistic'. Many clinicians are surprised when faced with a 10 year-old child given a diagnosis of autism at age 4 years. The child may no longer be gaze-avoidant (in fact he might never have been clearly *gaze-avoidant*, but perhaps only 'gaze-odd'), may accept the company of other people and even try to interact with them in a number of different ways. It is common for clinicians, seeing such children for the first time when the symptoms of autism are no longer so obvious, to confront the parents and other with the self-assured remark that 'This child does not have autism!' sometimes followed by 'And I do not think he ever had autism!' Autism symptomatology is not given once and for all.

It may need emphasizing that this is a relatively severe prognosis for a young child with autism in classical cases with mild–moderate or severe degrees of cognitive handicap (although not necessarily meeting criteria for mental retardation). With increasing awareness that the autism phenotype may be broader than previously believed (and may include some cases diagnosed as suffering from Asperger syndrome), percentages with poor outcome are likely to drop.

Atypical autism/autistic-like conditions

In clinical practice, one often comes across cases with almost, but not all of, the symptoms typical of autism. Also, some people with profound mental retardation show all the three clusters of symptoms considered necessary and sufficient to diagnose autism (Lorna Wing's triad, cf. above), but are difficult to classify as autism because there is a problem to decide whether the social, language and behavioural 'symptoms' are out of keeping with the degree of overall mental development or not. Finally, there is a group of boys and girls with deficits in attention, motor control and perception (see the section on syndromes attributed to minimal brain dysfunction) who show varying degrees of social, communication and behavioural problems, but who do not fit the full clinical picture of autism or Asperger syndrome.

At present, no adequate diagnostic category is available for all these cases. 'Pervasive developmental disorder not otherwise specified' is used for some of these cases by the DSM-III-R. This term is often seriously misleading, particularly when one is dealing with children of normal intelligence. 'Atypical autism' or 'autistic-like conditions' have been proposed by others to cover the group of 'autismlike' problems which do not fit readily into the classification systems. Some clinicians use the term 'autistic traits'.

Many children with so-called 'autistic traits' actually fulfil all currently accepted criteria for the full syndrome of autism, but, for some reason, do not receive the correct diagnosis of autism. This appears to be particularly common in cases where obvious brain dysfunction has been diagnosed at an early stage in the development of the child's problems, for instance, when there is hydrocephalus, infantile spasms, tuberous sclerosis or other well-known neurological disorders.

The prevalence of autistic traits is possibly much higher than that of autism proper. Wing's London studies of mentally handicapped individuals under age 15 years and Gillberg's Göteborg studies in the general 7 year-old population suggest that there are at least about 2–6 per 1000 children who exhibit severe autistic traits.

Some children do not show overt evidence of autism until after age 3 years. These can now be classified as suffering from 'autistic disorder' according to the DSM-III-R, but doubt remains whether they represent the same type of condition as autism with early onset or not. In some of these instances, a case can be made for diagnosing childhood disintegrative disorder or Heller dementia.

Childhood disintegrative disorder (Heller dementia infantilis)

Theodor Heller (1908) described six children who appeared to develop normally up until about the age of 3 to 4 years but who then dramatically regressed, became confused and hyperactive and were left, months later, in a more or less aloof and demented state. Recovery, if any, was very limited. More cases were reported (Heller, 1930) and some crude guidelines for diagnosis were detailed. These included (1) onset between 3 and 4 years of age, (2) progressive loss or marked impairment of spoken language followed by intellectual and behavioural deterioration, (3) associated behavioural and affective active symptoms such as hyperactivity and fear and (possibly) hallucinations, and (4) absence of neurological disorder. Heller proposed the term dementia infantilis. For many years the condition was known under this name or simply as 'Heller dementia'. Later authors (Rutter, 1977; Evans-Jones & Rosenbloom, 1978; Corbett, 1987) referred to disintegrative psychosis. The ICD-10 (WHO, 1992) now refers to other childhood disintegrative disorder ('other' to differentiate it from the other 'childhood disintegrative disorder', i.e. Rett syndrome). Other authors still have published data on this group while calling them 'pervasive disintegrative disorders' (Burd, Fisher & Kerbeshian, 1989).

Whatever the label, children with childhood disintegrative disorder (Volkmar, 1992; APA, 1994) are often clinically indistinguishable from those with autism once the regression period is over after 2–20 months. According to Volkmar (1992), only 77 relatively clear-cut cases of childhood disintegrative disorder have ever appeared in the literature. Of these, 29 were reported in the latest 15-year period. Virtually all of these cases had speech deterioration or complete loss, social disturbance, stereotypy or resistance to change and overactivity plus some affective symptomatology. The sex ratio in the sample reported during the latest 15-year-period was 8 to 1 males to females.

Some cases follow a gradually more downhill course. It can be extremely difficult to determine whether one is dealing with a case of 'late onset autism', that is classical autism but showing no major autism symptoms before about age 18 months, or childhood disintegrative disorder, with completely or almost normal development for at least 30–36 (sometimes as much as 50) months.

Outcome in the long-term perspective appears to be even worse in childhood disintegrative disorder than in autism. After the period of severe regression, there is often a static course and only minimal, if any, improvement. Less than 20% appear to be able to speak in sentences. Half of those that remain are completely mute and the other half uses single words. A relatively small subgroup appears to follow a progressive downhill course sometimes resulting in early death. Progressive neurological disorder may underlie such cases.

A few cases have been documented to have neurodegenerative conditions, but less is known about the aetiology of childhood disintegrative disorder than about that of autism. Heller, as noted, believed that no associated neurological disorder was ever present in 'his' cases. However, the assumption in later studies has usually been that the condition represents the behavioural manifestation of some, as yet usually unidentified, neurological condition. It has been reported in association with neurolipidosis (Malamud, 1959), tuberous sclerosis (Creak, 1963), subacute sclerosing panencephalitis (Rivinius et al., 1975), Addison-Schilder disease (Corbett et al., 1977), and progressive encephalopathy (Gillberg & Steffenburg, 1987). Major psychosocial events have been reported to show some temporal association with onset of symptoms of the disorder in a number of cases (Evans-Jones & Rosenbloom, 1978; Volkmar, 1992), but given that these events have included such trivial matters as 'birth of a sibling' and 'marital strife' (and control cases have not been included), it is very difficult to conclude what to make of the findings.

Childhood disintegrative disorder is obviously a very rare condition. The task force of the DSM-IV-committee reported that there are, at most, 80 cases in the literature going back to the beginning of this century (Campbell, personal communication, 1993). It has been estimated that its prevalence is about 11 in a million children born (Burd, Fisher & Kerbeshian, 1987; Volkmar, 1993, unpublished communication). In the author's experience, childhood disintegrative disorder constitutes about 1% of all autism/autistic-like conditions (a percentage which tallies well with the prevalence estimates for the general population). It is reported that it is very much more common in boys than in girls. However, some young girls with Rett syndrome show a clinical course which is similar to that described by Heller (Gillberg 1989b).

There is some controversy as to whether childhood disintegrative disorder should be regarded as a diagnostic category separate from autism or not. Some authors hold that the only clearly differentiating feature is that of age of onset, autism beginning in the first 2–3 years of life and childhood disintegrative disorder only after 2–4 years of normal development. Such a distinction, at one time, seemed reasonable. However, the demonstration that typical autism symptoms, indeed full-blown autistic syndromes, can occur after 4, 14 and even 31 years of normal development (DeLong *et al.*, 1981; Gillberg, 1986; Gillberg, I.C., 1991) has cast doubt on this notion. A recent report indicated that same high level of glial fibrillary acidic protein (GFA-protein) in the cerebrospinal fluid that has been found to be typical of autism (Ahlsén *et al.*, 1993), and not of Rett syndrome, may also be present in childhood disintegrative disorder. This finding, combined with the observation that even in 'clear-cut' disintegrative disorder, meticulous probing and history-taking may reveal that subtle abnormalities on the autism spectrum may have been present from infancy, could be taken to support the notion that the conditions are not clearly separate, and that underlying biological dysfunctions may be similar.

Furthermore, it is quite clear that there exist autism cases with gradual onset from infancy and others in which there is a setback after 18–30 months. This regression may follow after seemingly normal development in infancy. However, even in such cases, there is usually some indication that the child is not quite normal even before the setback occurs. The child may show little interest in other children, be more interested in objects than in human beings and throw tantrums if demands or approaches for social interaction are made. Whether it is clinically useful to distinguish such 'late onset' autism cases from childhood disintegrative disorder is doubtful. In research, however, it may be worthwhile to distinguish between the two, even though it is currently not quite clear on the basis of which exact criterion this distinction should be made.

Asperger syndrome

In 1944, the Austrian pediatrician Hans Asperger described what he considered to be an unusual personality variant in young children, most of whom were boys. He alluded to 'autistic psychopathy' but, after an influential paper by

Wing (1981*a*), the particular combination of problems that Asperger described is now generally referred to as Asperger syndrome.

Asperger syndrome is believed by many to be on a continuum with autism and autistic-like conditions but it is not yet clear whether it represents autism in people of generally good intelligence, or with a specific cognitive profile involving at least some areas of superior functioning, or whether there may exist other differentiating features. The ICD–10 (WHO, 1993) has taken the position that early language and language production must be grossly unaffected if Asperger syndrome is to be diagnosed (with evidence of two-word sentences by age 2 years and communicative sentences by age 3 years). However, this is not in keeping with Asperger's original writings (1944): both Ernst, K. and Hellmuth, L. (two of the four case histories reported by Asperger in his original paper) had early language and speech problems. Most authors in later years have included speech and language peculiarities and developmental language deviance in the definition of Asperger syndrome (Wing, 1981*a*; Gillberg & Gillberg, 1989*b*; Szatmari *et al.*, 1990). Also, it is common clinical knowledge that establishing *details* about early language development in retrospect in school age children (a time when many children with Asperger syndrome come to specialist attention) can be exceedingly difficult and, indeed, quite impossible. In summary therefore, it cannot be regarded as settled that autism and Asperger syndrome differ with respect to presence and absence of language problems.

Diagnosis and behavioural and physical phenotype

Diagnostic criteria have been proposed by the author (see Table 6.8). However, these should not be taken to implicate the existence of Asperger syndrome as clearly distinct from autism (the criteria for Asperger syndrome obviously overlap with those for autism). However, since they are the only criteria that have so far been tested for reliability and validity and have been applied in a population-based study

Table 6.8. *Diagnostic criteria for Asperger syndrome*

Diagnostic label	Reference	Diagnostic criteria
Asperger syndrome	Gillberg & Gillberg, 1989 Gillberg, 1991	Severe impairment in reciprocal social interaction, as manifested by at least two of the following four: • inability to interact with peers in a normal, reciprocal fashion • lack of desire to interact with peers • lack of appreciation of social cues • socially and emotionally inappropriate behaviour All-absorbing narrow interest, as manifested by at least one of the following three: • exclusion of other activities • repetitive adherence • more rote than meaning Imposition of routines and interests, as manifested by at least one of the following two: • imposition on self, in aspects of life • imposition on others Speech and language problems, as manifested by at least three of the following five: • delayed development of language • superficially perfect expressive language • formal, pedantic language • odd prosody, peculiar voice characteristics • impairment of comprehension including misinterpretations of literal/implied meanings Non-verbal communication problems, as manifested by at least one of the following five: • limited use of gestures • clumsy/gauche body language • limited facial expression • inappropriate expression • peculiar, stiff gaze Motor clumsiness, as documented by poor performance on neurodevelopmental examination
Asperger's syndrome	Szatmari *et al.*, 1989	Solitary, as manifested by at least two of the following four: • no close friends • avoids others • no interest in making friends • a loner Impaired social interaction, as manifested by at least one of the following five: • approaches others only to have own needs met • a clumsy social approach • one-sided responses to peers • difficulty sensing feelings of others • detached from feelings of others

Table 6.8. (*cont.*)

Diagnostic label	Reference	Diagnostic criteria
		Impaired non-verbal communication, as manifested by at least one of the following seven: ● limited facial expression ● unable to read emotion from facial expressions of child ● unable to give messages with eyes ● does not look at others ● does not use hands to express oneself ● gestures are large and clumsy ● comes too close to others
		Odd speech, as manifested by at least two of the following six: ● abnormalities in inflection ● talks too much ● talks too little ● lack of cohesion to conversation ● idiosyncratic use of words ● repetitive patterns of speech
		Does not meet criteria for autistic disorder
Asperger's syndrome	ICD–10 (WHO, 1993)	A lack of any clinically significant general delay in spoken or receptive language or cognitive development. Diagnosis requires that single words should have developed by two years of age or earlier and that communicative phrases be used by three years of age or earlier. Self-help skills, adaptive behaviour and curiosity about the environment during the first three years should be at a level consistent with normal intellectual development. Motor milestones may be somewhat delayed and motor clumsiness is usual (although not a necessary feature). Isolated special skills, often related to abnormal preoccupations, are common, but are not required for diagnosis
		Qualitative impairment in reciprocal social interaction (criteria as for autism, see Table 6.2)
		Restricted, repetitive, and stereotyped patterns of behaviour, interests and activities (criteria as for autism, see Table 6.2)
Asperger's disorder	DSM-IV (APA, 1994)	A. Qualitative impairment in social interaction, as manifested by at least two of the following: 1. marked impairment in the use of multiple nonverbal behaviors such as eye-to-eye gaze, facial expression, body postures, and gestures to regulate social interaction 2. failure to develop peer relationships appropriate to developmental level 3. a lack of spontaneous seeking to share enjoyment,

Table 6.8. (*cont.*)

Diagnostic label	Reference	Diagnostic criteria
		interests, or achievements with other people 4. lack of social or emotional reciprocity
		B. Restricted, repetitive, and stereotyped patterns of behaviour, interests, and activities as manifested by at least one of the following: 1. encompassing preoccupation with one or more stereotyped and restricted patterns of interest that is abnormal either in intensity or focus 2. apparently inflexible adherence to specific non-functional routines or rituals 3. stereotyped and repetitive motor mannerisms 4. persistent preoccupation with parts of objects
		C. Causes clinically significant impairment in social, occupational, or other important areas of functioning
		D. Lack of any clinically significant general delay in language (e.g. single words used by age two, communicative phrases used by age three)
		E. Lack of any clinically significant delay in cognitive development as manifested by the development of age-appropriate self-help skills, adaptive behaviour, and curiosity about the environment
		F. Does not meet criteria for another specific pervasive developmental disorder or schizophrenia

of Asperger syndrome (Ehlers & Gillberg, 1993), they are detailed here. The ICD–10 and DSM-IV criteria are also outlined for comparison. According to the Swedish prevalence study, slightly more cases will be diagnosed with the ICD–10 than with the Gillberg and Gillberg (1989b) criteria, at least if the language criterion is applied in more general terms (such as suggested by the diagnostic guidelines for the clinical version) rather than in the highly specific version requiring the precise documentation of a particular sequence of language development (as indicated in the research version). The very specific requirements about early language development of the ICD–10 are problematic in that they are usually impossible to ascertain convincingly in retrospect. Therefore, depending on exactly how this manual is used, many cases of Asperger syndrome may be withdrawn from diagnosis under the ICD–10 because it is impossible to check one of the criteria with certainty.

Perhaps the most distinctive feature of Asperger syndrome is the inability to conceptualize the mental states of other people. This inability (or severely restricted ability) to conceive of other people's minds (that is to spontaneously reflect on the thoughts, wishes, beliefs and feelings of others) is possibly not as pronounced as in autism. Some reflection on other people's 'inner' needs can usually be prompted by reminding the Asperger person about their existence, but the degree of empathy to be expected is generally low. That there actually is a partial lack of a 'theory of mind' in Asperger syndrome has recently been supported by a number of studies in experimental psychology (Frith, 1991), even though tests designed to tap this kind of dysfunction in school age children or adolescents have to be more complicated than the tests devised for demonstrating theory of mind deficits in classic autism, and tests tapping goal-direction and future orientation problems may have to be used instead (Ozonoff *et al.*, 1991). In autism, the salient feature is one of a severely restricted capacity for conceiving of other people's thoughts, feelings and even existence. This incapacity, or limited capacity, often never develops into anything resembling normality. In Asperger syndrome, a similar limitation in capacity may be present during the first several years. Later, however, some capacity usually develops and may even approach normal functional level (as evidenced, for instance, by improved picture arrangement results on the WISC with increasing age). Nevertheless, perhaps because the child with Asperger syndrome 'missed out' on social interaction, and hence on the possibility to educate skills in this domain, there may be persistent social interaction problems in adult life, in spite of good, or relatively good, empathy (or theory of mind) skills. Even when there is good *intellectual* capacity to conceive of other people's needs and emotions, intuitive use of this capacity in a real life setting may not occur. Disorders of empathy should not always be seen as static deficits. In general, they are probably better conceptualized as (usually very severe) developmental lags. It is interesting to note that many individuals with Asperger syndrome show general maturational lags. For instance, many Asperger people in adult age look considerably younger than their chronological age (Gillberg, unpublished data).

Several authors (Boucher & Lewis, 1992; Davies *et al.*, 1994) have remarked on the facial recognition problems encountered in Asperger syndrome. From the clinical point of view, this is indeed sometimes a very significant symptom: a teenager with Asperger syndrome may not recognize a well-known person unless he/she is wearing a particular garment or is driving his/her car (which is likely to be quickly identified). One report even considered the possibility that developmental prosopagnosia (the inability to recognize faces) might be the cause of Asperger syndrome in some cases (Kracke, 1994).

Asperger syndrome is sometimes evident as a restricted interest in social interaction already in the first year of life, but usually it is not until the second–fourth year (perhaps even later) that parents and others become concerned. Quite often there is worry about the apparent lack of need for playmates and relatively late language development (given the general family background) which, in turn, is often superseded by the development of formally impeccable, pedantic and prematurely adult-type language. Some cases do not attract attention until well into school age and then only because of extremely limited interests, motor clumsiness and lack of empathy. There is usually an odd prosody with a flat or staccato intonation or a shrill, monotonous quality. In certain cases, there is an exceptional tendency to cluttering. Speech therapists often refer to the speech and language problems as 'semantic–pragmatic disorder' (Bishop, 1989).

Because of their socially odd behaviour, peculiar, restricted interest patterns and unusual language characteristics, children with Asperger syndrome are variously perceived as 'odd', 'original', 'eccentric', 'the little professor', 'hilarious', 'cold', 'naive', 'lacking common sense', 'immature'. Some become the subject of mobbing at school, but most manage fairly well in this respect, possibly as a result of their "untouchability".

Asperger syndrome is usually associated with normal or above normal intelligence, but occasional typical cases in children with subnormal intelligence have been described. Associated handicaps/medical conditions are much less common than in autism but the available evidence suggests that the rate of epilepsy may be slightly higher than in the general population, and associated chromosomal abnormalities (e.g. fragile X, XYY) may not be altogether uncommon. A number of cases of Asperger syndrome (Gillberg, 1989*c*) in children with mild cerebral palsy have also been described.

The restricted interest pattern and reliance on an all-absorbing interest which is included as a diagnostic criterion of Asperger syndrome can sometimes be difficult to document, particularly in young children, who have not yet developed strong interests. Also, occasionally, the interest is of a more general type or may be perceived as 'normal', and hence may go unrecognized. For instance, the rote memory amassing of information about people, friends and family may well be an 'all-absorbing narrow interest', but may be thought of as reflecting a social interest and so will not be considered a possibly pathological symptom. Other examples of all-absorbing narrow interests which may go to extremes without other people reflecting on them as 'symptoms' is chess and the collection of stamps, usually, and usually appropriately, regarded as 'normal hobbies'.

From the clinical point of view it is important to note that unless obsessed with aspects of timing or with particular clocks or watches, many young people with Asperger syndrome – even those with superior intelligence – have enormous difficulty acquiring an 'internalized' sense of time. When asked, after a two-hour interview, how much time had elapsed since the interview began, a 16-year-old boy with Asperger syndrome responded: 'Oh, about six or seven minutes, I should guess.' His WISC IQ was 126.

Epidemiology

Asperger syndrome is believed to be about ten times more frequent in boys than in girls. Some authorities have hypothesized that a similar core condition might be present in girls but with a slightly different phenotype (Gillberg & Råstam, 1992).

The prevalence is likely to be at least 3 per 1000 children born (Gillberg & Gillberg, 1989b), but could be considerably higher. A recent study from a Swedish urban area (compatible with overall social class distribution in Sweden) found a prevalence in 8–16 year olds of at least 3.6 and possibly 7.1 per 1000 (Ehlers & Gillberg, 1993). Boys outnumbered girls by 'only' 3 to 1 in this study. Asperger syndrome might be underdiagnosed in girls because of the assumption that it is a typically male diagnosis, or because girls may have a slightly different behavioural phenotype than boys. It is often very difficult (if at all possible) to document early normal language development (which is required by the ICD–10 for a definite diagnosis of Asperger syndrome) once the child gets to be 7–10 years of age (which is the time at which a diagnosis of Asperger syndrome is often considered).

Background factors

Most cases are thought to be caused by genetic factors. Very often there is a close relative with similar problems or sometimes clear-cut autism. In the study by Gillberg (1989c) more than half the group had a first-degree relative with similar problems. In a matched comparison group diagnosed as high-functioning autism, the corresponding rate was relatively low.

Brain damage without a specific Asperger syndrome genetic predisposition can probably also cause the disorder (Wing, 1981a). Tuberous sclerosis, neurofibromatosis, the fragile X syndrome, perinatal brain insults, postnatal brain infections and congenital hypothyroidism are among the factors which have been reported to cause brain damage in children who later receive a diagnosis of Asperger syndrome (Gaffney et al., 1988; Gillberg, 1989c; Gillberg, Gillberg & Steffenburg, 1992). (See Fig. 6.3)

Differential diagnosis

The distinction of Asperger syndrome from sociopathy, severe antisocial behaviour ('psychopathy'), unsocialized conduct disorder, 'borderline conditions', various types of manipulating personality disorders and, possibly, childhood schizophrenia may present diagnostic problems. However, a distinction may often be made, based on the observation that, because of their limitations in conceiving of other people's minds, Asperger people do not have a well-developed capacity for cheating, lying, luring or manipulating other people. This

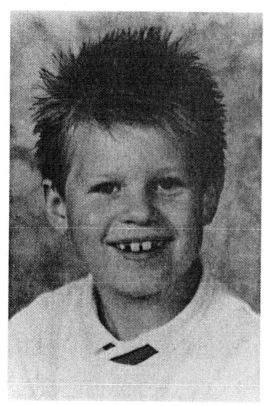

Fig. 6.3. 8-year-old boy with Asperger syndrome with possible semi-dominant semi-recessive mode of inheritance.

culture (including in a folic-acid depleted medium) is often called for to rule out the occasional co-occurrence of Asperger syndrome and the fragile X syndrome or other chromosomal syndromes (XXY and XYY syndromes in particular).

The WISC should be used in most cases, particularly if there is academic failure. Typically, there will be relatively lower results on comprehension, picture arrangement and similarities but in the highest functioning group even the most difficult tasks on these subtests may be too simple to be useful in differential diagnosis. Sometimes a more exhaustive neuropsychological work-up might be appropriate (such as when there appear to be specific auditory or visual perceptual problems, associated dyslexia, dyscalculia or dysgraphia). It appears that the Wisconsin Card Sorting Test (WCST) may be a useful addition to the neuropsychological work-up in Asperger syndrome. This 'frontal lobe' or 'executive function' test reveals moderate–severe impairments in Asperger syndrome (Ozonoff et al., 1991). Other tests of 'cognitive flexibility' (such as so-called Go–NoGo tasks) are also useful in identifying the rigid cognitive style of most individuals with Asperger syndrome (Ozonoff et al., 1994)

is quite unlike children and adults with the other types of problems listed. 'Borderline conditions' (a dubious notion anyway) are supposed to be characterized by intense swings in relationships with other people (love–hate: 'cannot live with you, cannot live without you'). This is the opposite of Asperger syndrome in which stability of 'relations' and behaviour over time is usually highly characteristic.

Medical and psychological work-up

The work-up in a child or adolescent suspected of suffering from Asperger syndrome is similar to that in high-functioning autism (see above). Thus, a screen for visual and hearing problems should be made in all cases. A chromosomal

Treatment

Specific treatment for Asperger syndrome or the problems associated with it is not available. The best approach according to current knowledge is to make a proper diagnosis, to give oral and written information to those concerned, and to offer educational and other measures intended to improve school adjustment and to follow-up (yearly if appropriate, more often if necessary). Attempts should be made to find interest areas that might eventually provide a basis for a good education and adult hobbies and to actively avoid (or consciously steer out of) areas that may hold potential danger ('violent' sports, etc). Medication makes little difference in most cases and may have harmful side effects. Psychotherapy is usually not indicated, but supportive talks on a regular basis with somebody knowledgeable in the field can be helpful, particularly in the teenage period when some insight into the situtaion is often gained and the experience of being different from 'the rest' can become overwhelming. Group sessions with Asperger youngsters can also be of value (Mesibov, 1990).

Parents often ask about the genetic risk, both for themselves, the Asperger child and his siblings. There is probably a considerable risk that more cases of Asperger syndrome will occur in the family (Bowman, 1988), unless there is no family history. At least half of all children with Asperger syndrome have a parent with the same (or very similar) condition. This should be acknowledged truthfully while at the same time emphasizing the relatively benign character of the problems. However, the possibility that Asperger syndrome might be genetically linked to classic autism makes counselling in this respect somewhat difficult at the present stage of knowledge. Unfortunately, risk estimates for siblings are not available. In a recent study of 23 children with Asperger syndrome, 1 boy had a brother with autism (and another brother with mild Asperger syndrome) and 1 girl had a sister with elective mutism (and Asperger traits) (Gillberg, 1989c).

Adult psychiatrists need to be aware of the existence of Asperger syndrome. In stressful situations in adult life, young adult people with Asperger syndrome are often referred to psychiatrists because of obsessiveness, feelings of helplessness and chaotic reactions. Because of limited facial expression, mimicry and gestures they will be diagnosed as perhaps depressed or paranoid and accordingly treated with antidepressants or neuroleptic drugs which usually do little to alter the cause of the disorder. Quite often, stress relief combined with the appreciation that this is only part of a lifelong condition will go a long way in reducing acute symptoms.

Outcome

Only a fraction of all children with Asperger syndrome ever apply for paediatric or psychiatric help specifically as a consequence of their 'Asperger problems'. Therefore, follow-up of cases seen in clinics will not necessarily yield a true picture of outcome. So far, the only studies of outcome available refer either to such populations or groups as assessed in adult psychiatric clinics and diagnosed retrospectively as possibly having suffered from Asperger syndrome from early childhood (Tantam, 1988). The overall impression is that many children with Asperger syndrome diagnosed in childhood, although not outgrowing the basic problems, manage fairly well in adult life, at least with respect to education, employment and marriage. Equally obvious, however, is the tendency for some to have severe psychiatric problems (often diagnosed as depression, paranoia, catatonia, pseudoneurotic schizophrenia or 'borderline' (Wing, 1981a), and commit suicide attempts, and for others to commit criminal offences (usually directly associated with one or other extreme interest, such as gun powder, poisonous chemicals, fires, etc.) (Baron-Cohen, 1989b, Everall & Le Couteur, 1990). However, it seems likely that the rate of criminal offences is not very high (Ghaziuddin, Tsai & Ghaziuddin, 1991). There has been at least one population-based follow-up report suggesting that alcoholism may be a common outcome in adolescents with Asperger syndrome (Hellgren, Gillberg & Gillberg, 1994).

Girls with social deficits and learning problems

There exists a group of girls with social deficits and learning problems for which no adequate diagnostic label seems to come to mind (Kopp & Gillberg, 1992). These girls usually have severe problems empathizing with the views of other people, and they appear to be lacking in theory of mind skills. They are often perceived as stubborn, negativistic and poorly motivated to participate in give-and-take activities and new learning situations. Unfortunately, for most of these cases, the diagnosis of autistic disorder or Asperger syndrome is probably never considered. However, it is quite common for such cases to fulfil autistic disorder criteria.

Girls in the general population develop relatively good speech and language skills at a younger age than do most boys (Wing, 1981b). They also have better 'superficial social skills' and show other types of interest patterns than boys (Gillberg, 1992a). Girls would be more interested in dolls and soft animals, playthings which are generally, though usually rather muddled-headedly, considered more 'symbolic laden' than model cars, trains and computer games which are often preferred by boys. Thus, if a boy has empathy problems, his symptoms are likely to be reflected in a typically 'boyish' way with severe language deficits, severe social deficits and rigid play patterns involving wheels of toy cars, computer games, etc. A girl with similar problems, unless she has severe and widespread brain damage, might have less obviously impaired language skills, might show fewer severe social interaction problems and might not be interested in the wheels of toy cars at all. On the other hand, she might have language skills but poor pragmatics, social interaction skills, but odd ways of interacting, and rigid play patterns characterized by endlessly putting her doll to bed, tucking her up, taking her out of bed, putting her back to bed, etc.

The autistic syndrome prototype might well have been modelled around a typical boy without paying attention to biological differences between boys and girls and hence the possibility that girls with core autism deficits (empathy problems) might show a different phenotype than boys.

Elective mutism

Some children do not speak to more than a very limited number of people from early childhood sometimes throughout the early school years and often into adolescence and adult age. It is not that they cannot speak, indeed, some of them can be verbally demanding and talkative when in their home environment. They do, however, refuse to say a word to most people outside of the immediate family (perhaps excluding even one or more members of the family). A few have one or two friends (even

though these friends could usually not be regarded as 'close') whom they will communicate verbally with. Some are mute most of the time, but will occasionally give up their complete silence to whisper or even say a few words silently. This group of children who can speak, but do so only with a very limited number of well-known people, are referred to as children with elective mutism (Browne, Wilson & Laybourne, 1963; Fundudis, Kolvin & Garside, 1979; Hayden, 1980; Kolvin & Fundudis, 1981; Fundudis, Kolvin & Garside, 1987). Many 'shy' children are temporarily silent on entering preschool or school. If their silence is of a transient nature, they should not be considered for a diagnosis of elective mutism.

The child with elective mutism probably can have normal language development but usually shows delay and deviance; there are often minor associated developmental disorders such as enuresis and slight motor delay; it appears that there may be a markedly increased rate of epilepsy; IQ tends to be lower than in the general population of children; typical symptoms usually appear before the child's third–fourth birthday; there is often a family history of psychiatric disorder, 'shyness' and elective mutism; and the outcome is variable but probably restricted. Many features of elective mutism are similar to those encountered in relatively high-functioning autistic-like conditions. Several authors have suggested that there may exist links with autism spectrum disorders, both at the clinical and familial level (Gillberg 1989c; Wolff et al., 1991; Gillberg, 1992a; Thomsen, 1993, 1994).

Children with elective mutism are usually shy, avoidant and sometimes clearly withdrawn. Also, many are described as being strong-willed and with outbursts of rage if demands or changes of routine are made. A recent report (see above) has mentioned the possible association of Asperger syndrome and elective mutism.

Elective mutism is rare, occurring in severe forms (with a duration of more than one year) in less than 1 in 5000 children. If problems of shorter duration are included, the prevalence may be a little higher (0.6 per 1000 7 year-olds in

Newcastle in the 1970s). The boy:girl ratio appears to be equal (or with a slight preponderance for females).

The psychological and medical work-up should include a cognitive test and a thorough clinical examination aimed at detecting hearing deficits and symptoms and signs suggestive of autistic disorder. The possibility of associated medical conditions should be entertained. The present author knows of two cases with the combination of elective mutism and neurofibromatosis.

Treatment in elective mutism has to focus on training of basic social skills and activities of daily life, such that the child/adolescent can accept the company of others and be able to express, at least in writing, his academic skills. Psychotherapeutic or psychopharmacological approaches have not been successful according to clinical experience.

Childhood onset schizophrenia

Autism and autistic-like conditions were long considered synonymous with childhood schizophrenia. Since about 1970, childhood schizophrenia is regarded as clearly separate from autism. Most authors agree that it is rare, the prevalence being just a tiny fraction of that of autism. Some authors have even questioned the existence of typical schizophrenia in childhood. In recent years however, some US authors have reintroduced the term to apply to conditions which are not exceptionally rare (Watkins, Asarnow & Tanguay, 1988). Spencer, Sanchez & Gillberg (1994) in citing the work of Burd et al. (1987) estimated that 0.19 per 10000 children in the general population (data from the North Dakota autism prevalence study) had childhood schizophrenia. Spencer et al. (1994) in citing the work of Gillberg and Steffenburg (1987) estimated that, at most, 0.16 per 10000 children in the general population (data from the Göteborg autism prevalence study) had schizophrenia, and presented some further data to suggest that it may be considerably less common.

It is now accepted that genetic factors are of major importance in early onset schizophrenia (Spencer et al., 1992). According to one recent study (Parnas et al., 1993) DSM-III-R schizophrenia occurred in 16% of offspring of mothers with schizophrenia. Another 19% had schizotypal personality disorder, indicating that this diagnosis may be part of the schizophrenia spectrum (whereas schizoid personality disorder, very infrequent in that study, would not be). One recent study reported a case of a boy with schizophrenia symptoms onset at age 9 years who had a translocation involving chromosomes 1 and 7 (46 × Y, t (1; 7) (p22; q22)) (Gordon et al., 1994).

Hospitalized patients aged 6–12 years in a New York child psychiatry department have been reported to meet criteria for childhood schizophrenia in quite a number of cases (Spencer et al., 1992). Over the latest 10 year-period at least 56 individuals aged 6–12 years meeting criteria for schizophrenia according to the DSM-III or the DSM-III-R have been reported from that centre. Clinically it is useful to know that some of these also fit diagnostic criteria for DAMP, ADHD, oppositional defiant disorder and conduct disorder (Spencer et al., 1994). It is unclear as to what proportion of all cases with 'schizophrenia' also meet criteria for other child psychiatric diagnostic categories (including major depression with psychotic features).

It is noteworthy that childhood schizophrenia is almost never diagnosed in Europe. Eggers made a prognostic study of childhood schizophrenia in Germany (Eggers, 1982) and had to cover a period of 30 years in order to come up with 57 cases, 30% of which were said to suffer from schizoaffective disorder. Also, most of the cases in Eggers's study were over age 10 years. McClellan, Werry & Ham (1993), in New Zealand, also performed a follow-up study of DSM-III-R schizophrenia with early onset but only found three cases under age 12 years. One can only speculate about the reasons for schizophrenia being probably more commonly diagnosed in the US than in Europe. A similar diagnostic discrepancy seems to apply in attention deficit syndromes as well. True prevalence differences, different diagnostic practice or sociocultural influences changing the clinical manifestations of similar types of underlying disorders might all be plausible reasons.

The term childhood schizophrenia should be taken to imply a severe disorder of affect and thought showing before 10 years of age with typical schizophrenic thought disorder, hallucinations and emotional bluntness. If applied in this way, it seems to be exceedingly rare, occurring in no more than two or three out of 100 000 children.

Some of the children with schizophrenia in the New York study met criteria for autism spectrum disorders. A few of the girls were similar to the girls described by Kopp and Gillberg (1992) with social deficits and learning disorders. At least one boy met criteria for pervasive developmental disorder not otherwise specified. A case could also be made for diagnosing some of the individuals in the New York childhood schizophrenia study as suffering from major affective disorder (including major depression with psychotic features). Some groups (including Watkins et al., 1988 and Frith & Frith, 1991) have proposed that schizophrenia and autism may not, in all cases, represent conditions as psychologically and biologically distinct as has been suggested by some authors (Rutter, 1985). Other groups (DeLong & Nohria, 1993) have suggested that autism and autistic-like conditions (including pervasive developmental disorder not otherwise specified) may be the earliest and most severe expression of a genetically determined major affective disorder. There is good evidence that when the presentation of major depression or mania in adolescence or childhood is accompanied by psychotic symptoms such as mood-congruent delusions or hallucination, the differential diagnosis from schizophrenia may be very difficult (Werry, 1992) since there is large overlap in schizophrenic and affective symptomatology (Carlson, 1990). The error appears to operate to misclassify mood disorder as schizophrenia (Bashir, Russell & Johnson, 1987; Carlson, 1990; Werry, 1992). This, in turn, may be assumed to misclassify more cases with early onset psychosis as having a poor prognosis, because schizophrenia is generally believed to have a poorer prognosis than mood disorders. However, according to a recent outcome study from Sweden, bipolar mood disorders with psychotic features may have at least as poor a prognosis as schizophrenia in the perspective from early–mid adolescence to age 30 years (Gillberg I.C., Hellgren & Gillberg, 1993).

Whatever its standing as a clinically relevant entity in child neuropsychiatry, schizophrenia with childhood onset is likely to be as muddled a concept as schizophrenia of adult age, which has always eluded straightforward definition and has an aetiology that remains mysterious. Most authors agree that, if schizophrenia is to be diagnosed in childhood, it should be according to the currently accepted diagnostic criteria for schizophrenia as it is outlined for adults. The DSM-IV criteria for schizophrenia is listed in Table 6.9.

As can be seen, making the diagnosis is complicated, as it involves several steps, exclusion criteria and subclassification of course and type. Of particular interest is the fact that, unlike autism, the diagnosis of schizophrenia cannot be made if it 'can be established that an organic factor initiated and maintained the disturbance'. This is a very problematic criterion, first of all because it would, at any rate, be difficult to prove that the organic factor *established*, much less *sustained* the disturbance, unless there was rational treatment available for the organic condition and the disappearance or amelioration of schizophrenic symptoms could be documented to coincide with the disappearance of the organic disorder. Also, it is incongruent with other parts of the DSM-III-R and the whole tradition of phenomenological diagnosis in psychiatry in suggesting, as it does, that a diagnosis cannot be made if there is a major associated organic factor. This is like saying that we know the aetiology of schizophrenia is not associated with any of these organic conditions, and *that* we certainly do *not* know. It is like saying that mental retardation, autism and ADHD cannot be diagnosed if there is a known organic condition associated with it. The DSM-III-R does not limit the diagnosis of these conditions to cases unassociated with

Table 6.9. *Diagnostic criteria for schizophrenia according to the DSM-III-IV*

Symptoms	Items/Specifics
A. Characteristic psychotic symptoms in the active phase for at least one week (unless the symptoms have been successfully treated) including:	two of the following: (a) delusions, (b) prominent hallucinations (throughout the day for several days or several times a week for several weeks, each hallucinatory experience not being limited to a few brief moments), (c) incoherence or marked loosening of associations, (d) catatonic behaviour, (e) flat or grossly inappropriate effect *or* one of the following: (a) bizarre delusions (such as thought broadcasting or being controlled by a dead person and which would be regarded by the person's culture as totally implausible), (b) prominent hallucinations, as above but including a voice with content having no apparent relation to depression or elation, or a voice keeping up a running commentary on the person's behaviour or thoughts, or two or more voices conversing with each other.
B. Social functioning (work, relations and self-care) is below the highest level achieved before onset of disturbance, or, in the case of children and adolescents, there is a failure to achieve expected level of social development.	
C. Continuous signs of the disturbance have been present for at least six months.	The six-month phase must include an active phase of at least one month (or less if there has been successful treatment) with symptoms as under A with or without a prodromal or residual phase
D. Schizo-affective and mood disorder with psychotic features have been ruled out.	
E. It cannot be established that an organic factor (such as a substance or a general medical condition) initiated and maintained the disturbance.	
F. If there is a history of autistic disorder, the additional diagnosis of schizophrenia is made only if prominent delusions or hallucinations are also present.	

There are five *types of courses*: 'subchronic', 'chronic', 'subchronic with acute exacerbation', 'chronic with acute exacerbation' and 'in remission'.
There are five *types of schizophrenia*: 'catatonic' (when the clinical picture is dominated by catatonic symptoms), 'hebephrenic' (when the clinical picture is dominated either by thought disorder or flat or grossly inappropriate affect), 'paranoid' (when there are delusions or auditor hallucinations on one particular theme and typical features of catatonic or hebephrenic type schizophrenia do not apply), 'undifferentiated' (other variants of schizophrenia not meeting criteria for the foregoing three) and 'residual' (in which at least two of residual symptoms from criterion D are present).

organic disorder, so why should it restrict the diagnosis of schizophrenia in this particular way?

Neuroleptics are likely to be more effective in childhood schizophrenia than in autism, and outcome is supposedly better. However, no good population-based follow-up studies exist, which means that the matter cannot be regarded as settled.

Paranoid disorder

Paranoid disorders are rare in children and adolescents. Most current child and adolescent psychiatry textbooks (Rutter & Hersov, 1985; Lewis, 1991) do not even mention their existence. Nevertheless, delusional thinking is generally included in the descriptions of childhood schizophrenia (Green *et al.*, 1984; Campbell *et al.*, 1991), and delusional thinking is the hallmark of the paranoid disorders.

In the author's experience, paranoid disorders have either occurred in isolation in adolescents, 13 years or older (some of the probands in the Gillberg *et al.* 1986 paper on teenage psychosis had paranoid disorders), or in parent/child dyads in which both parent and child share a similar type of system of delusional thinking. Such cases are sometimes referred to as *folie-à-deux*, on the assumption that delusional thinking of the parent is psychologically 'induced' in the child. The case for a *folie-à-deux* mechanism accounting for such parent/child dyads would be considerably strengthened if it could be shown that exposing the child to normal adults and minimizing the negative parental influence would lead to diminished levels of paranoid symptoms. To the author's knowledge, this has not been convincingly shown to be the case. Indeed, in some of the few cases followed by him, the paranoid symptoms in the young person have persisted, and even grown worse after separation from the parent. A genetic influence, rather than, or acting in conjunction with, psychological factors, might well be the reason for such persistence of paranoid symptoms.

The follow-up of young people with Asperger syndrome into adult age (Wing, 1981a; Gillberg & Steffenburg, in preparation) and the retrospective analysis of adult psychiatric patients (Tantam, 1991) suggest that paranoid problems may be relatively common in the course of this autism spectrum disorder. It is possible, but at the present stage purely speculative, that a shared deficiency in the development of empathy (or theory of mind) might underlie both Asperger syndrome and some variants of paranoid disorder (Gillberg, 1992a). Theory of mind skills may be present, not lacking altogether as is sometimes the case in severe cases of autism. However, they may only be accessible to the individual after conscious effort, unlike the situation in normals, who can access this system automatically in response to the social or communicative context.

References

Ahlsén, G., Rosengren, L., Belfrage, M., Palm, A., Haglid, K., Hamberger, A., Gillberg, C. (1993). Glial Fibrillary Acidic protein in the cerebrospinal fluid of children with autism and other neuropsychiatric disorders. *Biological Psychiatry*, **33**, 734–43.

Åkefeldt, A., Gillberg, C. (1991). Hypomelanosis of Ito in three cases with autism and autistic-like conditions. *Developmental Medicine and Child Neurology*, **33**, 737–43.

Akinsola, H.A., Fryers, T. (1986). A comparison of patterns of disability in severely mentally handicapped children of different ethnic origins. *Psychological Medicine*, **16**, 127–33.

American Psychiatric Association. (1980). *Diagnostic and Statistical Manual of Mental Disorders.* Washington, DC: APA.

American Psychiatric Association. (1987). *Diagnostic and Statistical Manual of Mental Disorders.* Third Edition – Revised. Washington, DC: APA.

American Psychiatric Association. (1994). *Diagnostic and Statistical Manual of Mental Disorders*, Fourth Edition. Washington, DC: APA.

Asperger, H. (1944). Die autistischen Psychopathen im Kindesalter. *Archiv für Psychiatrie und Nervenkrankheiten*, **117**, 76–136.

Aurnhammer-Frith, U. (1969). Emphasis and

meaning in recall in normal and autistic children. *Language and Speech*, **12**, 29–38.

Bågenholm, A., Gillberg, C. (1991). Psychosocial effects on siblings of children with autism and mental retardation: a population-based study. *Journal of Mental Deficiency Research*, **35**, 291–307.

Bailey, A., Bolton, P., Butler, L., Le Couteur, A., Murphy, M., Scott, S., Webb, T., Rutter, M. (1993). Prevalence of the Fragile X anomaly amongst autistic twins and singletons. *Journal of Child Psychology and Psychiatry*, **34**, 673–88.

Baird, G., Baron-Cohen, S., Bohman, M., Coleman, M., Frith, U., Gillberg, C., Gillberg, C., Howlin, P., Mesibov, G., Peeters, T., Ritvo, E., Steffenburg, S., Taylor, D., Waterhouse, L., Wing, L., Zappella, M. (1991). Autism is not necessarily a pervasive developmental disorder: letter. *Developmental Medicine and Child Neurology*, **33**, 363–4.

Baron-Cohen, S. (1988). Without a theory of mind one cannot participate in a conversation. *Cognition*, **29**, 83–4.

Baron-Cohen, S. (1989*a*). The autistic child's theory of mind: a case of specific developmental delay. *Journal of Child Psychology and Psychiatry*, **30**, 285–97.

Baron-Cohen, S. (1989*b*). Are autistic children behaviourists? An examination of their mental-physical and appearance-reality distinctions. *Journal of Autism and Developmental Disorders*, **19**, 579–600.

Baron-Cohen, S. (1990). Autism: a specific cognitive disorder of 'mind-blindness'. *International Review of Psychiatry*, **2**, 81–90.

Baron-Cohen, S. (1994). Origins of a theory of mind: the eye-direction detector, international *Journal of Psychology* (in press).

Baron-Cohen, S., Leslie, A.M., Frith, U. (1985). Does the autistic child have a theory of mind? *Cognition*, **21**, 37–46.

Baron-Cohen, S., Allen, J., Gillberg, C. (1992). Can autism be detected at 18 months? The needle, the haystack and the CHAT. *British Journal of Psychiatry*, **161**, 839–43.

Bartak, L., Rutter, M., Cox, A. (1975). A comparative study of infantile autism and specific developmental receptive language disorder. I. The children. *British Journal of Psychiatry*, **126**, 127–45.

Barthèlèmy, C., Bruneau, N., Jouve, J., Martineau, J., Muh, J.P., Lelord, G. (1989). Urinary dopamine metabolites as indicators of the responsiveness to fenfluramine treatment in children with autistic behavior. *Journal of Autism and Developmental Disorders*, **19**, 241–54.

Bashir, M., Russell, J., Johnson, G. (1987). Bipolar affective disorder in adolescence: a 10-year study. *Australian and New Zeeland Journal of Psychiatry*, **21**, 36–43.

Bayley, A. (1993). The biology of autism – editorial. *Psychological Medicine*, **23**, 7–11.

Bender, L. (1947). Childhood schizophrenia. *American Journal of Orthopsychiatry*, **17**, 40–56.

Bishop, D.V.M. (1989). Autism, Asperger's syndrome and semantic-pragmatic disorder: where are the boundaries? *British Journal of Communication*,

Bleuler, E. (1919). *Dementia Praecox or the Group of Schizophrenias*. Vienna: Translated by J. Zinkin. New York: International University Press.

Bohman, M., Bohman, I.L., Björk, P., Sjöholm, E. (1983). Childhood psychosis in a northern Swedish county: some preliminary findings from an epidemiological survey. *In* Schmidt, M.H.,Remschmith, H. (Eds.) *Epidemiological Approaches in Child Psychiatry*. Stuttgart: Georg Thieme.

Bolton, P., Rutter, M. (1990). Genetic influences in autism. *International Review of Psychiatry*, **2**, 67–80.

Boucher, J. (1981). Memory of recent events in autistic children. *Journal of Autism and Developmental Disorders*, **11**, 293–302.

Boucher, J., Lewis, V. (1989). Memory impairments and communication in relatively able autistic children. *Journal of Child Psychology and Psychiatry*, **29**, 4 33–445.

Boucher, J., Lewis, V. (1992). Unfamiliar face recognition in relatively able autistic children. *Journal of Child Psychology and Psychiatry*, **33**, 843–59.

Bowman, E.P. (1988). Asperger's syndrome and autism: the case for a connection. *British Journal of Psychiatry*, **152**, 377–82.

Browne, E., Wilson, V., Laybourne, P.C. (1963). Diagnosis and treatment of elective mutism in children. *Journal of the American Academy of Child and Adolescent Psychiatry*, **2**, 605–17.

Bryson, S., Smith, I.M., Eastwood, D. (1989). Obstetrical optimality in autistic children. *Journal of the American Academy of Child and Adolescent Psychiatry*, **27**, 418–22.

Burd, L., Fisher, W., Kerbeshian, J. (1987). A prevalence study of pervasive developmental disorders in North Dakota. *Journal of the American Academy of Child and Adolescent Psychiatry*, **26**, 704–10.

Burd, L., Fisher, W., Kerbeshian, J. (1989). Pervasive disintegrative disorder: are Rett syndrome and Heller dementia infantilis subtypes? *Developmental Medicine and Child Neurology*, **31**, 609–16.

Campbell, M. (1989). Pharmacotherapy in autism: An overview. *In* Gillberg, C. (Ed.) *Diagnosis and Treatment of Autism*. New York: Plenum.

Campbell, M., Anderson, L.T., Small, A.M., Adams, P., Gonzalez, N.M., Ernst, M. (1993). Naltrexone in autistic children: behavioral symptoms and attentional learning. in press.

Campbell, M., Kafantaris, V., Malone, R.P., Kowalik, S.C., Locascio, J.J. (1991). Diagnostic and assessment issues related to pharmacotherapy for children and adolescents with autism. *Behaviour Modification*, **15**, 326–54.

Carlson, G.A. (1990). Child and adolescent mania – diagnostic considerations. *Journal of Child Psychology and Psychiatry*, **31**, 331–41.

Chess, S. (1977). Follow-up report on autism in congenital rubella. *Journal of Autism and Childhood Schizophrenia*, 7, 68–81.

Chess, S., Korn, S.J., Fernandez, P.B. (1971). *Psychiatric Disorders of Children with Congenital Rubella*. New York: Brunner/Mazel.

Clark, P., Rutter, M. (1979). Task difficulty and task performance in autistic children. *Journal of Child Psychology and Psychiatry*, **20**, 271–85.

Coleman, M. (1989). Autism: Non-drug biological treatments. *In* Gillberg, C. (Ed.) *Diagnosis and Treatment of Autism*. New York: Plenum Press.

Coleman, M., Blass, J.P. (1985). Autism and lactic acidosis. *Journal of Autism and Developmental Disorders*, **15**, 1–8.

Coleman, M., Gillberg, C. (1985). *The Biology of the Autistic Syndromes*. New York: Praeger.

Cook, E.H. (1990). Autism: Review of neurochemical investigation. *Synapse*, **6**, 292–308.

Corbett, J. (1987). Development, disintegration and dementia. *Journal of Mental Deficiency Research*, **31**, 349–56.

Corbett, J., Harris, R., Taylor, E., Trimble, M. (1977). Progressive disintegrative psychosis of childhood. *Journal of Child Psychology and Psychiatry*, **18**, 211–19.

Creak, E.M. (1963). Childhood psychoses: a review of 100 cases. *British Journal of Psychiatry*, **109**, 84–9.

Dahlgren, S.O., Gillberg, C. (1989). Symptoms in the first two years of life. A preliminary population study of infantile autism. *European Archives of Psychiatry and Neurological Sciences*, **238**, 169–74.

Davies, S., Bishop, D., Manstead, A.S.R., Tantam, D. (1994). Face perception in children with autism and Asperger's syndrome. *Journal of Child Psychology and Psychiatry*, **33**, 1003–57.

Dawson, G., Fernald, M. (1987). Perspective-taking ability and its relationship to the social behavior of autistic children. *Journal of Autism and Developmental Disorders*, **17**, 487–98.

Dawson, G., McKissick, F.C. (1984). Self-recognition in autistic children. *Journal of Autism and Developmental Disorders*, **14**, 383–94.

DeLong, G.R., Beau, S.C., Brown, F.R. (1981). Acquired reversible autistic syndrome in acute encephalopathic illness in children. *Archives of Neurology*, **38**, 191–4.

DeLong, R., Nohria, C. (1993). Psychiatric family history and neurological disease in autism spectrum disorders. *Developmental Medicine and Child Neurology*, **36**, 441–8.

Eggers, C. (1982). Psychoses in childhood and adolescence. *Acta Paedopsychiatrica*, **48**, 81–98.

Ehlers, S., Gillberg, C. (1993). The epidemiology of Asperger syndrome. A total population study. *Journal of Child Psychology and Psychiatry*, **34**, 1327–50.

Evans-Jones, L.G., Rosenbloom, L. (1978). Disintegrative psychoses in childhood. *Developmental Medicine and Child Neurology*, **20**, 462–70.

Everall, I.P., LeCouteur, A. (1990). Firesetting in an adolescent boy with Asperger's syndrome. *British Journal of Psychiatry*, **157**, 284–7.

Folstein, S., Rutter, M. (1977). Infantile autism: a genetic study of 21 twin pairs. *Journal of Child Psychology and Psychiatry*, **18**, 297–321.

Friedman, E. (1969). The autistic syndrome and phenylketonuria. *Schizophrenia*, **1**, 249–61.

Frith, U. (1989*a*). Autism and 'theory of mind'. *In* Gillberg, C. (Ed.) *Diagnosis and Treatment of Autism*. New York: Plenum Press.

Frith, U. (1989*b*). *Autism: Explaining the Enigma*. Oxford: Basil Blackwell.

Frith, U. (Ed.) (1991). *Autism and Asperger Syndrome*. Cambridge: Cambridge University Press.

Frith, C.D., Frith, U. (1991). Elective Affinities in Schizophrenia and Childhood Autism. *In* Babbington, P. (Ed.) *Social Psychiatry: Theory, Methodology and Practice*. New Brunswick, New Jersey: Transactions.

Fundudis, T., Kolvin, I., Garside, R.F. (1979). *Speech Retarded and Deaf Children: Their Psychological Development*. London: Academic Press.

Fundudis, T., Kolvin, I., Garside, R. (1987). *Speech Retarded and Deaf Children: Their Psychological Development.* New York: Academic Press.

Gadow, K.G. (1992). Pediatric psychopharmacotherapy: a review of recent research. *Journal of Child Psychology and Psychiatry,* 33, 153–95.

Gaffney, G.R., Kuperman, S., Tsai, L.Y., Minchin, S. (1988). Morphological evidence for brainstem involvement in infantile autism. *Biological Psychiatry,* 24, 578–86.

Ghaziuddin, M., Tsai, L., Ghaziuddin, N. (1991). Violence in Asperger syndrome: a critique. *Journal of Autism and Developmental Disorders,* 21, 349–54.

Gillberg, C. (1984). Infantile autism and other childhood psychoses in a Swedish urban region. Epidemiological aspects. *Journal of Child Psychology and Psychiatry,* 25, 35–43.

Gillberg, C. (1986). Brief report: Onset at age 14 of a typical autistic syndrome. A case report of a girl with herpes simplex encephalitis. *Journal of Autism and Developmental Disorders,* 16, 369–75.

Gillberg, C. (1989a). Habilitation for children with autism: a Swedish example. *In* Gillberg, C. (Ed.) *Diagnosis and Treatment of Autism.* New York: Plenum Press.

Gillberg, C. (1989b). The borderland of autism and Rett syndrome: five case histories to highlight diagnostic difficulties. *Journal of Autism and Developmental Disorders,* 19, 545–59.

Gillberg, C. (1989c). Asperger syndrome in 23 Swedish children. *Developmental Medicine and Child Neurology,* 31, 520–31.

Gillberg, C. (1990a). Epidemiologi. *In* Gillberg, C.,Hellgren, L. (Eds.) *Lärobok i barn- och ungdomspsykiatri.* Stockholm: Natur och Kultur. (In Swedish.)

Gillberg, C. (1990b). Medical work-up in children with autism and Asperger syndrome. *Brain Dysfunction,* 3, 249–60.

Gillberg, C. (1900c) What is autism? *International Review of Psychiatry,* 2, 61–6.

Gillberg, C. (1991a). Debate and argument: Is autism a pervasive developmental disorder? *Journal of Child Psychology and Psychiatry,* 32, 1169–70.

Gillberg, C. (1991b). The treatment of epilepsy in autism. *Journal of Autism and Developmental Disorders,* 21, 61–77.

Gillberg, C. (1991c). Outcome in autism and autistic-like conditions. *Journal of the American Academy of Child and Adolescent Psychiatry,* 30,
375–82.

Gillberg, C. (1992a). The Emanuel Miller Memorial Lecture 1991: Autism and autistic-like conditions: subclasses among disorders of empathy. *Journal of Child Psychology and Psychiatry,* 33, 813–42.

Gillberg, C. (1992b). Subgroups in autism: are there behavioural phenotypes typical of underlying medical conditions? *Journal of Intellectual Disability Research,* 36, 201–14.

Gillberg, C. (1993). Autism and related behaviours. *Journal of Intellectual Disability Research,* 37, 343–72.

Gillberg, C. (1994). The prevalence of autism and autism spectrum disorders. *In* Verhulst, F.C.,Koot, H.M. (Eds.) *The Epidemiology of Child and Adolescent Psychopathology.* Oxford: Oxford University Press.

Gillberg, C., Coleman, M. (1992). *The Biology of the Autistic Syndromes.* 2nd edition. London, New York: Mac Keith Press, Cambridge University Press.

Gillberg, C., Forsell, C. (1984). Childhood psychosis and neurofibromatosis – more than a coincidence? *Journal of Autism and Developmental Disorders,* 14, 1–8.

Gillberg, C., Gillberg, I.C. (1983). Infantile autism: a total population study of reduced optimality in the pre-, peri-, and neonatal period. *Journal of Autism and Developmental Disorders,* 13, 153–66.

Gillberg, C., Gillberg, I.C. (1991). Note on the relationship between population-based and clinical studies: the question of reduced optimality in autism: letter. *Journal of Autism and Developmental Disorders,* 21, 251–3.

Gillberg, C., Råstam, M. (1992). Do some cases of anorexia nervosa reflect underlying autistic-like conditions? *Behavioural Neurology,* 5, 27–32.

Gillberg, C., Steffenburg, S. (1987). Outcome and prognostic factors in infantile autism and similar conditions: a population-based study of 46 cases followed through puberty. *Journal of Autism and Developmental Disorders,* 17, 273–87.

Gillberg, C., Svennerholm, L. (1987). CSF monoamines in autistic syndromes and other pervasive developmental disorders of early childhood. *British Journal of Psychiatry,* 151, 89–94.

Gillberg, C., Winnergård, I., Wahlström, J. (1984). The sex chromoomes – one key to autism? An XYY case of infantile autism. *Applied Research in Mental Retardation,* 5, 353–60.

Gillberg, C., Terenius, L., Lönnerholm, G. (1985). Endorphin activity in childhood psychosis. Spinal fluid levels in 24 cases. *Archives of General Psychiatry*, **42**, 780–3.

Gillberg, C., Wahlström, J., Forsman, A., Hellgren, L., Gillberg, I.C. (1986). Teenage psychoses–epidemiology, classification and reduced optimality in the pre-, peri- and neonatal periods. *Journal of Child Psychology and Psychiatry*, **27**, 87–98.

Gillberg, C., Steffenburg, S., Jakobsson, G. (1987). Neurobiological findings in 20 relatively gifted children with Kanner-type autism or Asperger syndrome. *Developmental Medicine and Child Neurology*, **29**, 641–9.

Gillberg, C., Ehlers, S., Schaumann, H., Jakobsson, G., Dahlgren, S.O., Lindblom, R., Bågenholm, A., Tjuus, T., Blidner, E. (1990). Autism under age 3 years: a clinical study of 28 cases referred for autistic symptoms in infancy. *Journal of Child Psychology and Psychiatry*, **31**, 921–34.

Gillberg, C., Schaumann, H., Steffenburg, S. (1991*a*). Is autism more common now than 10 years ago? *British Journal of Psychiatry*, **158**, 403–9.

Gillberg, C., Steffenburg, S., Wahlström, J., Gillberg, I.C., Sjöstedt, A., Martinsson, T., Liedgren, S., Eeg-Olofsson, O. (1991*b*). Autism associated with marker chromosome. *Journal of the American Academy of Child and Adolescent Psychiatry*, **30**, 489–94.

Gillberg, C., Gillberg, I.C., Steffenburg, S. (1992). Siblings and parents of children with autism. A controlled population based study. *Developmental Medicine and Child Neurology*, **34**, 389–98.

Gillberg, I.C. (1991). Autistic syndrome with onset at age 31 years. Herpes encephalitis as one possible model for childhood autism. *Developmental Medicine and Child Neurology*, **33**, 920–4.

Gillberg, I.C., Gillberg, C. (1989*a*). Children with preschool minor neurodevelopmental disorders. IV: Behaviour and school achievement at age 13. *Developmental Medicine and Child Neurology*, **31**, 3–13.

Gillberg, I.C., Gillberg, C. (1989*b*). Asperger syndrome – some epidemiological considerations: a research note. *Journal of Child Psychology and Psychiatry*, **30**, 631–8.

Gillberg, C., Gillberg, I.C., Steffenburg, S. (1992). 'Siblings and parents of children with autism. A controlled population based study.' *Developmental Medicine and Child Neurology*, **34**, 389–98.

Gillberg, I.C., Hellgren, L., Gillberg, C. (1993).

Psychotic disorders diagnosed in adolescence. Outcome at age 30 years. *Journal of Child Psychology and Psychiatry*, **34**, 1173–85.

Gillberg, I.C., Gillberg, C., Ahlsén, G. (1994). Autistic behaviour and attention deficits in tuberous sclerosis. A population-based study. *Developmental Medicine and Child Neurology*, **36**, 50–6.

Goodman, R., Ashby, L. (1990). Delayed visual maturation and autism. *Developmental Medicine and Child Neurology*, **32**, 808–19.

Gordon, A.G. (1993). Interpretation of auditory impairment and markers for brain damage in autism. *Journal of Child Psychology and Psychiatry*, **34**, 587–92.

Green, W.H., Campbell, M., Hardesty, A.S., Grega, D.M., Padron-Gayol, M., Shell, J., Erlenmeyer-Kimling, L. (1984). A comparison of schizophrenic and autistic children. *Journal of the American Academy of Child Psychiatry*, **23**, 399–409.

Griffiths, R. (1970). *The Abilities of Young Children*. London: Child Research Centre.

Hagberg, B. (Ed.) (1993). *Rett Syndrome – Clinical & Biological Aspects*. London: Mac Keith Press.

Hagerman, R.J. (1989). Chromosomes, genes and autism. *In* Gillberg, C. (Ed.) *Diagnosis and Treatment of Autism*. New York: Plenum Press.

Hagerman, R.J. (1992). Fragile-X syndrome: advances and controversy. Annotation. *Journal of Child Psychology and Psychiatry*, **33**, 1127–39.

Happé, F., Frith, U. (1991). Is autism a pervasive developmental disorder? Debate and argument: How useful is the 'PDD' label? *Journal of Child Psychology and Psychiatry*, **32**, 1167–8.

Happé, F. (1994). Annotation: current psychological theories of autism: the 'theory of mind' account and rival theories. *Journal of Child Psychology and Psychiatry*, **35**, 215–29.

Haracopos, D. (1989). Comprehensive treatment program for autistic children and adults in Denmark. *In* Gillberg, C. (Ed.) *Diagnosis and Treatment of Autism*. New York: Plenum Press.

Haslam, J. (1809). *Observation of Madness and Melancholy*. London: Hayden.

Hayden, T.L. (1980). The classificaiton of elective mutism. *Journal of the American Academy of Child and Adolescent Psychiatry*, **19**, 118–33.

Heller, T. (1908). Dementia infantilis. *Zeitschrift für die Erforschung und Behandlung des jugendlichen Schwachsinns (Journal for Research and Treatment of Juvenile Feeblemindedness)*, **2**, 17–28.

Heller, T. (1930). Über Dementia infantilis.

Zeitschrift für Kinderforschung, **37**, 661–7.

Hellgren, L., Gillberg, C., Gillberg, I.C. (1994). Children with Deficits in attention, motor control and perception (DAMP) almost grown up: The contribution of various background factors to outcome at age 16 years. *European Child & Adolescent Psychiatry*, **3**, 1–15.

Hermelin, B., O'Connor, N. (1970). *Psychological Experiments with Autistic Children*. Oxford: Pergamon Press.

Hermelin, B., O'Connor, N. (1990). Factors and primes: a specific numerical ability. *Psychological Medicine*, **20**, 163–9.

Hertzig, M.E., Snow, M.E., New, E., Shapiro, T. (1990). DSM-III and DSM-III-R diagnosis of autism and pervasive developmental disorder in nursery school children. *Journal of the American Academy of Child and Adolescent Psychiatry*, **29**, 123–6.

Hobson, P.R. (1990). On psychoanalytic approaches to autism. *American Journal of Orthopsychiatry*, **60**, 324–36.

Hobson, R.P. (1984). Early childhood autism and the question of egocentrism. *Journal of Autism and Developmental Disorders*, **14**, 85–104.

Hobson, R.P. (1986a). The autistic child's appraisal of expressions of emotions. *Journal of Child Psychology and Psychiatry*, **27**, 321–42.

Hobson, R.P. (1986b). The autistic child's appraisal of expressions of emotions: a further study. *Journal of Child Psychology and Psychiatry*, **27**, 671–80.

Hobson, R.P. (1987). The autistic child's recognition of age- and sex-related characteristics of people. *Journal of Autism and Developmental Disorders*, **17**, 63–79.

Hobson, R.P., Ouston, J., Lee, A. (1988). Emotion recognition in autism: coordinating faces and voices. *Psychological Medicine*, **18**, 911–23.

Hogrefe, G.J., Wimmer, H., Perner, J. (1986). Ignorance versus false believe: a developmental lag in attribution of epistemic states. *Child Development*, **57**, 567–82.

Howlin, P. (1982). Echolalic and spontaneous phrase speech in autistic children. *Journal of Child Psychology and Psychiatry*, **23**, 281–93.

Howlin, P., Rutter, M. (1987). *Treatment of autistic children*. London: John Wiley & Sons.

Howlin, P., Yates, P. (1989). Treating autistic children at home. A London based programme. *In* Gillberg, C. (Ed.) *Diagnosis and Treatment of Autism*. New York: Plenum.

Hunt, A., Dennis, J. (1987). Psychiatric disorder among children with tuberous sclerosis.

Developmental Medicine and Child Neurology, **29**, 190–8.

Hunt, A., Shepherd, C. (1993). A prevalence study of autism in tuberous sclerosis. *Journal of Autism and Developmental Disorders*, **23**, 323–39.

Itard, J.M.G. (1801). Mémoire et rapport sur Victor de l'Aveyron. *In* Malson, L. (Ed.) *Les Enfants Sauvages:*. Paris (1964): Union Générale d'Editions.

Kanner, L. (1943). Autistic disturbances of affective contact. *Nervous Child*, **2**, 217–50.

Kerbeshian, J., Burd, L., Randall, T., Martsolf, J., Jalal, S. (1990). Autism, profound mental retardation and atypical bipolar disorder in a 33-year-old female with a deletion of 15q12. *Journal of Mental Deficiency Research*, **34**, 205–10.

Kolvin, I., Fundudis, T. (1981). Elective mute children: psychological development and background factors. *Journal of Child Psychology and Psychiatry*, **22**, 219–32.

Komoto, J., Udsui, S., Otsuki, S., Terao, A. (1984). Infantile autism and Duchenne muscular dystrophy. *Journal of Autism and Developmental Disorders*, **14**, 191–5.

Kopp, S., Gillberg, C. (1992). Girls with social deficits and learning problems: autism, atypical Asperger syndrome or a variant of these conditions. *European Child & Adolescent Psychiatry*, **1**, 89–99.

Korkman, M. (1988a). NEPSY – An adaptation of Luria's investigation for young children. *The Clinical Neuropsychologist*, **2**, 375–92.

Korkman, M. (1988b). *NEPSY – A neuropsychological test battery for young developmentally disabled children*. Helsinki University.

Korkman, M. (1988c). *NEPSY. A proposed neuropsychological investigation for children – Revised version*. Helsinki: Psykoligien kustannus.

Kracke, I. (1994). Developmental prosopagnosia in Asperger syndrome: presentation and discussion of an individual case. *Developmental Medicine and Child Neurology*, **36**, 873–86.

Krug, D.A., Arick, J., Almond, P. (1980). Behavior checklist for identifying severely handicapped individuals with high levels of autistic behavior. *Journal of Child Psychology and Psychiatry*, **21**, 221–9.

Le Couteur, A., Rutter, M., Lord, C., Rios, P., Robertson, S., Holdgrafer, M., McLennan, J. (1989). Autism diagnostic interview: a standardized investigator-based instrument. *Journal of Autism and Developmental Disorders*, **19**, 363–87.

Lelord, G., Muh, J.P., Barthélémy, C., Martineau, J., Garreau, B., Callaway, E. (1981). Effects of pyridoxine and magnesium on autistic symptoms – initial observations. *Journal of Autism and Developmental Disorders*, 11, 219–30.

Leslie, A.M. (1987). Pretence and representation: the origins of a 'theory of mind'. *Psychological Review*, **94**, 412–26.

Leslie, A.M., Frith, U. (1988). Autistic children's understanding of seeing, knowing and beleiving. *British Journal of Developmenting Psychology*, 4, 315–24.

Lewis, M. (Ed.) (1991). *Child and Adolescent Psychiatry. A Comprehensive Textbook.* Baltimore, Maryland: Williams & Wilkins.

Lockyer, L., Rutter, M. (1970). A five to fifteen year follow-up study of infantile psychosis. IV: Patterns of cognitive ability. *British Journal of Social and Cognitive Ability*, 9, 152–63.

Lord, C., Rutter, M., Goode, S., Heemsbergen, J., Jordan, J., Mawhood, L., Schopler, E. (1989). Autism diagnostic observation schedule: a standardized observation of communicative and social behavior. *Journal of Autism and Developmental Disorders*, 19, 185–212.

Lotter, V. (1966). Epidemiology of autistic conditions in young children. I. Prevalence. *Social Psychiatry*, 1, 124–37.

Lotter, V. (1967). *The Prevalence of the Autistic Syndrome in Children.* London: University of London Press.

Mahler, M.S. (1952). On child psychoses and schizophrenia: autistic and symbiotic infantile psychoses. *Psychoanalytic Study of the Child*, 7, 286–305.

Malamud, N. (1959). Heller's disease and childhood schizophrenia. *American Journal of Psychiatry*, 116, 215–18.

Maltz, A. (1981). Comparison of cognitive deficits among autistic and retarded children on the Arthur Adaption of the Leiter International Performance Scale. *Journal of Autism and Developmental Disorders*, 11, 413–26.

Martineau, J., Garreau, B., Barthelemy, C., Callaway, E., Lelord, G. (1981). Effects of vitamin B6 on averaged evoked potentials in infantile autism. *Biological Psychiatry*, 16, 627–41.

Masterton, B.A., Biederman, G.B. (1983). Proprioceptive versus visual control in autistic children. *Journal of Autism and Developmental Disorders*, 13, 141–52.

McEvoy, R.E., Roger, S.J., Pennington, B.F. (1993). Executive function and social communication deficits in young autistic children.

Journal of Child Psychology and Psychiatry, **34**, 563–78.

McGimsey, J.F., Favell, J.E. (1988). The effects of increased physical exercise on disruptive behavior in retarded persons. *Journal of Autism and Developmental Disorders*, **18**, 167–9.

McClellan, J.M., Werry, J.S., Ham, M. (1993). A follow-up study of early onset psychosis: comparison between outcome diagnoses of schizophrenia, mood disorders, and personality disorders. *Journal of Autism and Developmental Disorders*, 23, 243–62.

Mesibov, G.B. (1990). Perceptions of popularity among a group of high-functioning adults with autism. *Journal of Autism and Developmental Disorders*, 20, 33–44.

Mirenda, P.L., Donnellan, A.M., Yoder, D.E. (1983). Gaze behaviour: a new look at an old problem. *Journal of Autism and Developmental Disorders*, 13, 397–409.

Nydén, A., Ehlers, S., Gillberg, C. (1994). Cognitive problems in Asperger Syndrome and other disorders on the autism spectrum. *Submitted*,

O'Connor, N., Hermelin, B. (1990). The recognition failure and graphic success of idiot-savant artists. *Journal of Child Psychology and Pychiatry*, **31**, 203–15.

Ohta, M. (1987). Cognitive disorders of infantile autism: A study employing the WISC, spatial relationship conceptualization, and gesture imitation. *Journal of Autism and Developmental Disorders*, 17, 45–62.

Ornitz, E. (1989). Early symptoms of autism. Paper presented at Biological Psychiatry Conference. Jerusalem, April.

Ornitz, E.M., Guthrie, D., Farley, A.J. (1977). The early development of autistic children. *Journal of Autism and Childhood Schizophrenia*, 7, 207–29.

Oshima-Takana, Y., Benaroya, S. (1989). An alternative view of pronominal errors in autistic children. *Journal of Autism and Developmental Disorders*, 19, 73–85.

Osterling, J., Dawson, G. (1994). Early recognition of children with autism: a study of first birthday home videotapes. *Journal of Autism and Developmental Disorders*, 24, 247–57.

Ozonoff, S., Pennington, B.F., Rogers, S.J. (1991). Executive function deficits in high-functioning autistic individuals: relationships to theory of mind. *Journal of Child Psychology and Psychiatry*, **32**, 1081–105.

Ozonoff, S., Strayer, D.L., McMahon, M., Filloux, F. (1994). Executive function abilities in autism and Tourette syndrome: an information processing approach. *Journal of Child Psychology and Psychiatry*, **35**, 1015–32.

Parnas, J., Cannon, T.D., Jacobsen, B., Schulsinger, H., Schulsinger, F., Mednick, S.A. (1993). Lifetime DSM-III-R diagnostic outcomes in the offspring of schizophrenic mothers. Results from the Copenhagen High-Risk Study. *Archives of General Psychiatry*, **50**, 707–14.

Piven, J., Simon, J., Chase, G.A., Wzorek, M., Landa, R., Gayle, J., Folstein, S. (1993). The etiology of autism: pre-, peri-, and neonatal factors. *Journal of the American Academy of Child and Adolescent Psychiatry*, **6**, 1256–63.

Premack, D., Woodruff, G. (1978). Does the chimpanzee have a 'theory of mind? *Behavioural and Brain Sciences*, **4**, 515–26.

Pring, L., Hermelin, B. (1993). Bottle, tulip and wineglass: semantic and structural picture processing by savant artists. *Journal of Child Psychology and Psychiatry*, **34**, 1365–85.

Prior, M., Dahlstrom, B., Squires, T.-L. (1990). Autistic children's knowledge of thinking and feeling states in other people. *Journal of Child Psychology and Psychiatry*, **31**, 587–601.

Rank, B. (1949). Adaptation of the psycho-analytic technique for the treatment of young children with atypical development. *American Journal of Orthopsychiatry*, **19**, 130–9.

Reiss, A.L., Feinstein, C., Rosenbaum, K.N., Borengasser-Caruso, M.A., Goldsmith, B.M. (1985). Autism associated with Williams syndrome. *Journal of Paediatrics*, **106**, 247–9.

Riikonen, R., Amnell, G. (1981). Psychiatric disorders in children with earlier infantile spasms. *Developmental Medicine and Child Neurology*, **23**, 747–60.

Rivinius, T.M., Jamison, D.L., Graham, P.J., *et al.* (1975). Childhood organic neurlogic disease presenting as a psychiatric disorder. *Archives of Disease in Childhood*, 115–19.

Rumsey, J.M., Creasey, H., Stepanek, J.S., Dorwart, R., Patronas, N., Hamburger, S.D., Duara, R. (1988). Hemispheric assymetries, fourth ventricular size, and cerebellar morphology in autism. *Journal of Autism and Developmental Disorders*, **18**, 127–37.

Rumsey, J.M., Hamburger, S.D. (1988). Neuropsychological findings in high-functioning men with infantile autism, residual state. *Journal of Clinical and Experimental Neuropsychology*, **10**, 201–21.

Rutter, M. (1970). Autistic children: Infancy to Adulthood. *Seminars in Psychiatry*, **2**, 435–50.

Rutter, M. (1977). Infantile autism and other childhood psychoses. *In* Rutter, M.,Hersov, L. (Eds.) *Child Psychiatry. Modern Approaches.* Oxford: Blackwell Scientific.

Rutter, M. (1978). Diagnosis and definition. *In* Rutter, M.,Schopler, E. (Eds.) *Autism. A Reappraisal of Concepts and Treatment.* New York: Plenum Press.

Rutter, M. (1983). Cognitive deficits in the pathogenesis of autism. *Journal of Child Psychology and Psychiatry*, **24**, 513–31.

Rutter, M. (1985). Diagnosis and definition. *In* Rutter, M.,Hersov, L. (Eds.) *Child and Adolescent Psychiatry: Modern Approaches.* Oxford: Blackwell Scientific.

Rutter, M., Hersov, L. (Eds.) (1985). *Child and Adolescent Psychiatry. Modern Approaches.* Oxford: Blackwell Scientific.

Sandberg, S., Rutter, M., Giles, S., Owen, A., Champion, L., Nicholls, J., Prior, V., McGuinness, D., Drinnan, D. (1993). Assessment of psychosocial experiences in childhood: methodological issues and some illustrative findings. *Journal of Child Psychology and Psychiatry*, **34**, 879–96.

Schopler, E., Reichler, R.J. (1979). *Psychoeducational Profile (PEP).* Austin, TX: Pro-Ed.

Schopler, E., Reichler, R.J., Lansing, M. (1980). *Teaching Strategies for Parents and Professionals.* Austin, TX: Pro-Ed.

Schopler, E. (1989). Principles for directing both educational treatment and research. *In* Gillberg, C. (Ed.) *Diagnosis and Treatment of Autism.* New York: Plenum.

Schopler, E., Mesibov, G. (Eds.) (1988). *Diagnosis and Assessment in Autism.* New York: Plenum.

Schopler, E., Reichler, R.J., Renner, B.R. (1988). *The Childhood Autism Rating Scale (CARS).* Revised. Los Angeles: Western Psychological Services, Inc.

Shah, A., Frith, U. (1983). An islet of ability in autistic children: a research note. *Journal of Child Psychology and Psychiatry*, **24**, 613–20.

Sigman, M., Mundy, P. (1989). Social attachments in autistic children. *Journal of the American Academy of Child and Adolescent Psychiatry*, **28**, 74–81.

Sigman, M., Ungerer, J.A. (1984). Cognitive and language skills in autistic, mentally retarded, and normal children. *Developmental Psychology*, **20**, 293–302.

Sigman, M., Mundy, P., Sherman, T., Ungerer, J. (1986). Social interactions of autistic, mentally retarded and normal children and their caregivers. *Journal of Child Psychology and Psychiatry*, **27**, 647–56.

Smith, I., Beasley, M.G., Wolff, O.H., Ades, A.E. (1988). Behavior disturbance in 8-year-old children with early treated phenylketonuria. *Journal of Pediatrics*, **112**, 403–8.

Spencer, E.K., Kafantaris, V., Padron-Gayol, M.V., Rosenberg, C.R., Campbell, M. (1992). Haloperidol in schizophrenic children: early findings from a study in progress. *Psychopharmacology Bulletin*, **28**, 183–6.

Spencer, E., Sanchez, L., Gillberg, C. (1994). Comorbidity patterns in childhood schizophrenia. *Submitted*,

Steffenburg, S. (1990). *Neurbiological correlates of autism*. MD Thesis. University of Göteborg.

Steffenburg, S. (1991). Neuropsychiatric assessment of children with autism: a population-based study. *Developmental Medicine and Child Neurology*, **33**, 495–511.

Steffenburg, S., Gillberg, C., Hellgren, L., Andersson, L., Gillberg, I.C., Jakobsson, G., Bohman, M. (1989). A twin study of autism in Denmark, Finland, Iceland, Norway and Sweden. *Journal of Child Psychology and Psychiatry*, **30**, 405–16.

Stubbs, E.G. (1978). Autistic symptoms in a child with congenital cytomegalovirus infection. *Journal of Autism and Childhood Schizophrenia*, **8**, 37–43.

Szatmari, P. (1992). The validity of autistic spectrum disorders: a literature review. *Journal of Autism and Developmental Disorders*, **22**, 583–600.

Szatmari, P., Brenner, R., Nagy, J. (1989). Asperger's syndrome: a review of clinical features. *Canadian Journal of Psychiatry*, **34**, 554–60.

Szatmari, P., Boyle, M.H., Offord, D.R. (1993). Familial aggregation of emotional and behavioral problems of childhood in the general population. *American Journal of Psychiatry*, **150**, 1398–403.

Szatmari, P., Offord, D.R., Siegel, L.S., Finlayson, M.A.J., Tuff, L. (1990). The clinical significance of neurocognitive impairments among children with psychiatric disorders: diagnosis and situational specificity. *Journal of Child Psychology and Psychiatry*, **33**, 287–99.

Tantam, D. (1988). Asperger's syndrome. *Journal of Child Psychology and Psychiatry*, **29**, 245–55.

Tantam, D. (1991). Asperger syndrome in adulthood. *In* Frith, U. (Ed.) *Autism and Asperger syndrome*. Cambridge: Cambridge University Press.

Thomsen, P.H. (1993). Obsessive–compulsive disorder in children and adolescents. Self-reported obsessive symptoms and trait in Danish pupils. *Acta Psychiatrica Scandinavia*, **88**, 212–17.

Thomsen, P.H. (1994). Obsessive–compulsive disorder in children and adolescents: a study of phenomenology and family functioning in 20 consecutive Danish cases. *European Child & Adolescent Psychiatry*, **3**, 29–36.

Tinbergen, N., Tinbergen, E.A. (1983). *Autistic Children. New Hope for a Cure*. London: Allen & Unwin.

Treffert, D.A. (1989). *Extraordinary People*. New York: Harper & Row.

Tustin, F. (1981). *Autistic State in Children*. London: Routledge & Kegan Paul.

Tsai, L.Y. (1989). Recent neurobiological findings in autism. *In* Gillberg, F. (Ed.) *Diagnosis and Treatment of Autism*. New York: Plenum Press.

van Bourgondien, M.E., Mesibov, G. (1987). Humor in high-functioning autistic adults. *Journal of Autism and Developmental Disorders*, **17**, 417–24.

Verkerk, A.J.M.H., Pieretti, M., Sutcliffe, J.S. *et al.* (1991). Identification of a gene (FMR-1) containing a CGG repeat coincident with a breakpoint cluster region exhibiting length variation in fragile X syndrome. *Cell*, **65**, 905–14.

Volkmar, F.R. (1992). Childhood disintegrative disorder: Issues for DSM-IV. *Journal of Autism and Developmental Disorders*, **22**, 625–42.

Volkmar, F.R., Bregaman, J., Cohen, D.J., Cicchetti, D.V. (1988). DSM-III and DSM-III-R diagnoses of autism. *American Journal of Psychiatry*, **145**, 1404–8.

Volkmar, F.R., Cohen, D.J. (1989). Disintegrative disorder or 'late onset' autism? *Journal of Child Psychology and Psychiatry*, **30**, 717–24.

von Knorring, A.-L. (1991). Outcome in autism. *Svensk Medicin*, **23**, 34–6.

von Knorring, A.-L., Hägglöf, B. (1993). Autism in Northern Sweden. A population based follow-up study: Psychopathology. *European Child & Adolescent Psychiatry*, **2**, 91–7.

Waterhouse, L., Fein, D. (1989). Social or cognitive or both? *In* Gillberg, C. (Ed.) *Diagnosis and Treatment of Autism*. New York: Plenum Press.

Watkins, J.M., Asarnow, R.F., Tanguay, P.E. (1988). Symptom development in childhood onset schizophrenia. *Journal of Child Psychology and Psychiatry*, **29**, 865–78.

Welsch, M.C., Pennington, B.F., Grossier, D.B. (1991). A normative-developmental study of executive function: a window of prefrontal function in children. *Developmental*

Neuropsychology, 7, 131–49.

Werry, J.S. (1992). Child and adolescent (early onset) schizophrenia: a review in light of DSM-III-R. *Journal of Autism and Developmental Disorders*, **22**, 601–24.

Whitehouse, D., Harris, J.C. (1984). Hyperlexia in infantile autism. *Journal of Autism and Developmental Disorders*, **14**, 281–9.

WHO (1992). *The ICD–10 Classification of Mental and Behavioural Disorders. Clinical descriptions and guidelines*. Geneva: Author.

WHO (1993). *The ICD–10 Classification of Mental and Behavioural Disorders. Diagnostic Criteria for Research*. Geneva: Author.

Wing, J.K. (1966). Diagnosis, epidemiology, aetiology. *In* Wing, J.K. (Ed.) *Early Child Autism*. Oxford: Pergamon Press.

Wing, L. (1980). Childhood autism and social class: A question of selection. *British Journal of Psychiatry*, **137**, 410–17.

Wing, L. (1981*a*). Asperger's syndrome: a clinical account. *Psychological Medicine*, **11**, 115–29.

Wing, L. (1981*b*). Sex ratios in early childhood autism and related conditions. *Psychiatry Research*, **5**, 129–37.

Wing, L. (1989*a*). The diagnosis of autism. *In* Gillberg, C. (Ed.) *Diagnosis and Treatment of Autism*. New York: Plenum Press.

Wing, L. (1989*b*). Autistic adults. *In* Gillberg, C. (Ed.) *Diagnosis and Treatment of Autism*. New York: Plenum Press.

Wing, L. (1991). The relationship between Asperger's syndrome and Kanner's autism. *In* Frith, U. (Ed.) *Autis m and Asperger syndrome*. Cambridge: Cambridge University Press.

Wing, L. (1992). Brief note: Is autism a pervasive developmental disorder? *European Child & Adolescent Psychiatry*, **1**, 130–31.

Wing, L. (1993). The definition and prevalence of autism: A review. *European Child & Adolescent Psychiatry*, **2**, 1–14.

Wing, L., Gould, J. (1979). Severe impairments of social interaction and associated abnormalities in children: epidemiology and classification. *Journal of Autism and Developmental Disorders*, **9**, 11–19.

Wolff, S., Townsend, R., McGuire, R.J., Weeks, D.J. (1991). Schizoid personality in childhood and adult life. II: Adult adjustment and the continuity with schizotypal personality disorder. *British Journal of Psychiatry*, **159**, 620–9.

Zappella, M. (1992). The Rett girls with preserved speech. *Brain & Development*, **14**, 98–101

Zetterström, R. (1983). Infantile Autism – Neuropsychological Correlates. Paper read at Sävstaholm Conference on Autism. May, Uppsala, Sweden.

7 Disorders involving obsessions and compulsions (including Tourette syndrome and eating disorders)

Obsessive and compulsive phenomena are common in child and adolescent psychiatric disorders. They are part and parcel of Asperger syndrome and occur at a very high rate in Tourette syndrome, to mention but two disorders in which obsessions, ritualistic phenomena and repetitive activities comprise the clinical picture. Obsessions and compulsions in adults are usually reported to be egodystonic, i.e. they are perceived by the individual affected by them as negative phenomena which they would like to be rid of. This egodystonic quality is often reported not to be present in children and adolescents, who may well consider their 'symptoms' to represent normal phenomena.

It has recently been suggested that not only are autism and the other disorders on the autism spectrum associated with severe empathy deficits, but that such problems may be of crucial importance in some cases subsumed under other phenomenological diagnostic labels (Gillberg, 1992). These have been suggested to include obsessive–compulsive personality disorders and subgroups of the eating disorders.

Obsessive–compulsive personality disorder

As with all so-called personality disorders, a diagnosis of obsessive–compulsive personality disorder (OCPD) cannot be made appropriately until an individual's 18th birthday. However, the concept of 'personality disorder' is muddled. It is not clear to what extent some terms, such as narcissistic and histrionic personality disorder, represent 'disorder' rather than 'personality constitution'. Furthermore, 'personality', whatever it is, can certainly be perceived long before 18 years of age (Chess & Thomas, 1977; Thomas & Chess, 1977).

Among the so-called personality disorders, a few, including obsessive compulsive personality disorder have the 'gestalt' of a true disorder. Just by looking at the criteria (Table 7.1), one senses the presence of a severe psychiatric problem with social dysfunction and severe empathy problems that would suggest a categorization with the autism spectrum group (Gillberg, 1992). Whether it is appropriate to group this type of problem behaviour among the personality disorders, or whether it would more appropriately be grouped with the developmental disorders, is open to debate. The DSM-III-R criteria for OCPD (at least the first, second, third, fourth, sixth, seventh and ninth) are all compatible with a diagnosis of Asperger syndrome or high-functioning autism. Only systematic study will reveal to what extent the OCPD concept overlaps with that of autism spectrum disorders generally, and with Asperger syndrome in particular. The DSM-IV criteria for OCPD (APA, 1994) are very similar to those of the DSM-III-R except that criteria 5 and 7 of the latter manual have been removed and 'rigidity and stubbornness' is included instead. In the DSM-IV only four out of eight criteria have to be met for a diagnosis to be made.

OCPD in the DSM-III-R is grouped with avoidant, dependent and passive–aggressive personality disorder in the so-called 'cluster C personality disorders'. Looking at the criteria for these disorders, it makes considerable sense

Table 7.1. *Diagnostic criteria for obsessive–compulsive personality disorder (OCPD) according to the DSM-III-R (see text for comparison with DSM-IV)*

A pervasive pattern of perfectionism and inflexibility, beginning by early adulthood and present in a variety of contexts, as indicated by at least five of the following:

(1) perfectionism that interferes with task completion, e.g., inability to complete a project because own overly strict standards are not met
(2) pre-occupation with details, rules, lists, order, organization, or schedules to the extent that the major point of the activity is lost
(3) unreasonable insistence that others submit to exactly his or her way of doing things, or unreasonable reluctance to allow others to do things because of the conviction that they will not do them correctly
(4) excessive devotion to work and productivity to the exclusion of leisure activities and friendships (not accounted for by obvious economic necessity)
(5) indecisiveness: decision making is either avoided, postponed, or protracted, e.g. the person cannot get assignments done on time because of ruminating about priorities (do not include if indecisiveness is due to excessive need for advice or reassurance from others)
(6) over-conscientiousness, scrupulousness, and inflexibility about matters of morality, ethics, or values (not accounted for by cultural or religious identification)
(7) restricted expression of affection
(8) lack of generosity in giving time, money, or gifts when no personal gain is likely to result
(9) inability to discard worn-out or worthless objects even when they have no sentimental value

to group the three first of these disorders, because clinically they share severe social interaction and obsessive–compulsive/ritualistic phenomena. However, with regard to passive–aggressive personality disorder, there is a less convincing case for grouping it with the others. Social interaction problems do not appear to be as prominent, and ritualistic phenomena are not mentioned.

OCPD is over-represented in populations suffering from anorexia nervosa (Dally, 1969; Gartner *et al.*, 1989; Råstam, 1992). Some young adults with Asperger syndrome meet full DSM-III-R criteria for OCPD, and a clinical decision has to be made which of the two labels should be pronounced to be the major diagnosis. In some cases, with anorexia nervosa, Asperger syndrome may be diagnosed in the adolescent period, and OCPD may be the main diagnosis in early adult life (Gillberg, I.C., Råstam & Gillberg, 1994*a*).

The distinction of OCPD from obsessive–compulsive disorder (OCD) is sometimes the subject of clinical debate. Often this confusion arises from a misunderstanding: OCPD and OCD are not synonymous. Most individuals with OCD do not have OCPD, and it is unlikely

that they will ever develop it. Most persons with OCPD experience their social withdrawal, rigid routines, need for orderliness, hoarding behaviours and indecisiveness as ego-syntonic. Many persons with OCD (though not all and particularly not the very young) define their obsessions and compulsions as markedly ego-dystonic. Most persons with OCPD do not experience severe compulsions, or, at least, are not substantially impaired by them. Furthermore, their impairments stem more from a stable pattern of functioning than from any exacerbation of isolated symptoms, which is common in OCD. Also, the 'cold' social interaction and lack of generosity, typical of many individuals with OCPD is definitely not the rule in OCD. List making and rigid scheduling behaviours are characteristic of OCPD, but are uncommon compulsive phenomena in OCD (Rasmussen & Tsuang, 1986).

Obsessive–compulsive disorder with and without tics

In recent years, obsessive–compulsive disorders commencing in childhood have been the subject of a substantial number of publications (Flament et al., 1988; Swedo et al., 1989; Riddle et al., 1990). So far, the majority of the studies published have originated in a few centres, and we must await studies by other groups before we can safely make conclusions in this field. Nevertheless, it is already clear that obsessive compulsive disorder (OCD) is a relatively common complaint among child psychiatric clinic attenders (Rapoport, 1988), and it appears that some of the symptoms are amenable to psychopharmacological treatment (Green, 1991). It is also evident that it shows considerable overlap with other neuropsychiatric disorders, including Tourette syndrome (APA, 1987; Comings, 1990), anorexia nervosa (Råstam, 1992) and autism (Ghaziuddin et al., 1992, 1993). Finally, there is some evidence that OCD has major biological roots.

Prevalence

The prevalence of OCD is not known. So far, only a few representative population studies of the disorder have been performed, and, as far as the author is aware, no OCD prevalence studies have been performed outside the US. According to the available data at least 1–1.9% of adolescents have current or life-time diagnoses of OCD (Flament et al., 1989; Whitaker et al., 1990), although the rate depends heavily on exactly where the line is drawn between normality and disorder. For instance, in the study by Flament et al. (1988), 'only' 0.35% had current OCD according to direct psychiatric interview, but this figure rose to 1% if weightings of individual symptoms similar to those used in the so-called Epidemiological Catchment Area survey of psychiatric disorders in adults were applied. These observations reflect the fact that normal (subthreshold) obsessional concerns or compulsive behaviours are not easily differentiated from OCD. It is essential that a clinical diagnosis of OCD is not made unless there is some degree of functional impairment. This point needs to be kept in mind particularly at a time when effective pharmacological treatment has become available so that large numbers of children and adolescents with 'non-handi-capping' obsessions and compulsions are not offered medication. Subclinical obsessions and compulsions appear to be stable phenomena that do not significantly interfer with normal psychological development (Flament et al., 1988).

Diagnosis

OCD is diagnosed according to the DSM-III-R as outlined in Table 7.2. It should be noted here (see above) that OCD and OCPD are separate 'conditions' and the OCPD does not necessarily predispose to the development of OCD or vice versa. OCD in the DSM-IV is virtually identical except that the diagnosis can be made even if the individual does not presently recognize that the obsessions and compulsions are excessive or unreasonable, but did so at some point in the past. Also, in the DSM-IV, obsessions are required to have caused anxiety at least at some time during the course of the disorder.

Unfortunately, OCD is still classified with the anxiety syndromes, in spite of the fact that the word anxiety is not a central symptom in the elaboration of the diagnostic criteria and that there has been no well-controlled study supporting its link to generalized anxiety disorder or panic disorder.

Clinical picture

The clinical symptoms in OCD are variable and dependent both on the age at which the individual presents for help, and what type of obsession(s)/compulsion(s) is/are involved. Nevertheless, one of the striking features of child and adolescent OCD is its strong similarity to OCD in adults. OCD is characterized by recurrent obsessional thoughts or impulses which are initially, at least, experienced as senseless or intrusive; or by compulsive (i.e. repetitive, purposeful and intentional) behaviours which are perfumed in response to an obsession, certain rules or in a stereotyped fashion. The obsessions or compulsions must lead to significant interference with the individual's life or marked distress or be time consuming. Most young patients report a shifting

Table 7.2. *Diagnostic criteria for obsessive–compulsive disorder (OCD) according to the DSM-III-R (see text for comparison with DSM-IV)*

A. Either obsessions or compulsions:
    Obsessions: (1), (2), (3), and (4):
    (1) recurrent and persistent ideas, thoughts, impulses, or images that are experienced, at least initially, as intrusive and senseless, e.g. a parent's having repeated impulses to kill a loved child, a religious person's having recurrent blasphemous thoughts
    (2) the person attempts to ignore or suppress such thoughts or impulses or to neutralize them with some other thought or action
    (3) the person recognizes that the obsessions are the product of his or her own mind, not imposed from without (as in thought insertion)
    (4) if another Axis I disorder is present, the content of the obsession is unrelated to it, e.g. the ideas, thoughts, impulses, or images are not about food in the presence of an eating disorder, about drugs in the presence of a psychoactive substance, or guilty thoughts in the presence of a major depression

    Compulsions: (1), (2), (3), and (4):
    (1) repetitive, purposeful, and intentional behaviours that are performed in response to an obsession, or according to certain rules or in a stereotyped fashion
    (2) the behavior is designed to neutralize or to prevent discomfort or some dreaded event or situation; however, either the activity is not connected in a realistic way with what it is designed to neutralize or prevent, or it is clearly excessive
    (3) the person recognizes that his or her behaviour is excessive or unreasonable (this may not be true for young children; it may no longer be true for people whose obsessions have evolved into overvalued ideas)

B. The obsessions or compulsions cause marked distress, are time-consuming (take more than an hour a day), or significantly interfere with the person's normal routine, occupational functioning, or usual social activities or relationships with others.

symptom pattern over time with a particular constellation being predominant for months or years before yielding to a different pattern. OCD symptoms also may show variation throughout the day and according to setting. Stress may exacerbate symptoms. Just as in Tourette disorder, children and adolescents suffering from OCD may work hard to inhibit or control symptoms in school or other social situations, only to engage in them even more in the privacy of their own room. Both parents and teachers can sometimes be unaware of some relatively severe OCD symptoms.

Onset can be as early as age 2 or 3 years, but is most often after age 7 years. In one study (Swedo *et al.*, 1989) only 11% of all OCD cases had onset under age 7 years. Males may have slightly earlier onset than females.

Washing rituals (mostly hand washing or showering) are by far the most common symp-toms (Table 7.3.). A considerable number of children and adolescents use chemicals to clean their hands and bodies and provoke dermatitis in so doing. Other common compulsions include going in and out through doors, rising from, and sitting down in, chairs, and checking locks, stove, electricity, etc. Obsessions are considerably less common and, when present, deal primarily with contamination danger, symmetry or moral issues. 'Pure' obsessives are uncommon; there is usually a combination of obsessions and compulsions. Compulsions, on the other hand, often exist in the absence of obsessions.

There is usually some other associated psychiatric problem warranting a diagnosis. Tourette disorder, depression, anxiety and eating disorders are all commonly associated with OCD. For instance, a life-time history of tics may be present in almost 60% in an adolescent

Table 7.3. *Presenting symptoms in OCD*

Symptom	US (Rapoport et al., 1992) (% affected)	Symptom	Denmark (Thomsen, 1993) (% affected)
Obsessions		*Obsessions*	
Concerns with dirt, germs or environmental toxins	40	Contamination	50
Something terrible happening	24	Past	40
Symmetry, order or exactness	17	Aggression	35
Scrupulosity	13	Somatic	25
Lucky or unlucky numbers	9	Religious	20
Forbidden, aggressive or pervasive sexual thoughts, images or impulses	4	Magic	15
Concern with household items	3	Death	35
Washing/intrusive nonsense sound, words or music	1	*Compulsions*	
		Repeating	60
Compulsions		Washing	60
Excessive or ritualized hand-washing, showering, bathing, toothbrushing or grooming	86	Counting	30
		Checking	25
Repeating rituals	51	Ordering and arranging	15
Checking	46		
Miscellaneous rituals	26	*Associated behaviours*	
Rituals to remove contact with contaminants	23	Pathological doubting	65
Touching	20	Avoidance	65
Counting	19	Indeciseveness	45
Ordering or arranging	17	Responsibility	45
Measure to prevent harm to self or others	16		
Hoarding or collecting rituals	11		
Rituals of cleaning household or inanimate objects	6		

Note: Each individual can present with several different types of obsessions and compulsions.

OCD population. Conversely, 20–80% of patients with clear Tourette disorder have been reported to have obsessive compulsive symptoms or OCD (Frankel *et al.*, 1986; Pauls & Leckman, 1986; Leonard *et al.*, 1992, 1993). At least in the case of Tourette disorder, anxiety and eating disorder, the associations may suggest common underlying basal ganglia dysfunction, given that, in all three of these disorders, neurological fine motor dysfunction has been demonstrated (Comings, 1990; Shaffer *et al.*, 1985; Råstam, 1992).

There seems to be relatively little overlap of OCD with obsessive–compulsive personality disorder (OCPD). Only 20% of a child and adolescent sample with OCD were judged to have OCPD (Rapoport, Swedo & Leonard, 1992).

The similarity of some of the symptoms of Asperger syndrome to those of OCD (including various kinds of rituals) indicates the need for study of 'comorbidity' patterns in these disorders.

Background factors

The studies by Rapoport and her colleagues have tried to elucidate the neurobiology of OCD. It seems that there may be specific, or at least syndrome-associated, dysfunctions of portions of the basal ganglia with cerebral blood flow reduction in the putamen and globus pallidus (Swedo et al., 1989). Frontal lobe and caudate nuclei abnormalities have been implicated in MRI and CT scan studies (Garber et al., 1989; Luxenberg et al., 1988). Also, one study of oculomotor performance (on adults with OCD) showed major abnormalities, at least in males, and this finding is compatible with basal ganglia dysfunction (Tien et al., 1992). However, oculomotor dysfunction could also result from frontal lobe and brainstem dysfunction. It is of interest that some of the brain areas that have been implicated in the neurobiological studies of OCD are similar, or identical, to those identified in autism.

There is inferential support for basal ganglia dysfunction in OCD coming from the studies of obsessive compulsive symptoms in well-documented basal ganglia disorder. In Sydenham's chorea, which is caused by auto-immune cross reaction to *Streptococcus A/B*, the caudate and putamen are affected. Obsessive–compulsive symptoms have been well documented in this disorder. Tourette syndrome, Segawa's dystonia and post-encephalitic Parkinson's disease are all believed to be associated with, or caused by, basal ganglia dysfunction, and all of these have been shown or purported to be associated with high levels of obsessive–compulsive behaviours.

An interesting finding in a few studies has been the elevated CSF concentrations of oxytocin and vasopressin in young people with OCD (Altemus et al., 1990; Swedo et al., 1992). A few reports have maintained that the administration of oxytocin can produce obsessive and compulsive symptoms in patients with OCD.

Laplane et al. (1989) have proposed a theory for the development of OCD and associated symptomatology. Motor stereotypies (such as tics) and mental stereotypies (such as thinking about the same thing over and over again) and more complex obsessive–compulsive behaviours are seen as existing on a continuum and resulting from impaired inhibitory abilities due to lesions in the basal ganglia with the site of the lesion determining the type of symptom expressed. Baxter (1990) suggested that striatal dysfunction of a particular type may result in reduced ability to suppress adventitious thoughts, sensations, and actions which, instead, have to be processed by more inefficient cortical pathways leading to both psychic distress and repetitive behaviour patterns.

It has also been hypothesized that OCD may be related to hyperactivity or increased receptor sensitivity of some serotonin pathways in the brain and that serotonin re-uptake blockers may exert their beneficial effects by interfering with this overactive state (Piacentini et al., 1992). In a double-blind, placebo-controlled study of adult patients with OCD and controls, the administration of a serotonin agonist, metachlorphenylpiperazine, but not of placebo, led to a transient, but marked exacerbation of obsessive–compulsive symptoms. These findings, too, are consistent with a particular role for serotonin in OCD psychopathology (Zohar & Insel, 1987; Zohar et al., 1988).

Familiality is common in OCD, and particularly so in cases with very early onset. In a sample of 46 consecutive childhood onset cases, Lenane et al. (1990) reported that 25% had a first-degree relative with OCD according to personal structured interview.

There is also overlap between Tourette syndrome and OCD, not only at the phenomenological level but also in terms of familial clustering of both disorders. There is a high rate of Tourette syndrome (1.8%) and tics (14%) in the first degree relatives of young patients with OCD according to one study (Leonard et al., 1992). Conversely, there is a very high rate of OCD problems in the families of patients with Tourette syndrome (Pauls & Leckman, 1986).

Thus, at the present stage, it seems that at least a considerable proportion of childhood/adolescent onset OCD might be linked to genetically determined basal ganglia dysfunction.

Treatment

Before the 1980s, OCD was often treated along psychoanalytical lines. However, since then, a virtual shift of treatment emphasis has occurred. Today, most young patients presenting with severe OCD symptoms are first treated with tricyclic antidepressants or similar drugs. Clomipramine, especially, has been systematically tested in young OCD patients, and has been shown to be considerably more effective than placebo in alleviating obsessive–compulsive symptoms (Flament et al., 1985). Controlled trials of a number of new serotonin re-uptake blockers are currently being performed, but there is still no consensus regarding their usefulness in OCD. Nevertheless, it seems that fluoxetine may become the preferred drug in the next several years, because of its tendency to be associated with fewer and less severe side effects (Piacentini et al., 1992). However, the fact that clomipramine is a considerably better researched drug which has been used for several decades, and that fluoxetine represents a relatively recent addition to the psychopharmacological treatment options, indicates the need to retain a cautious attitude. Whether or not to treat all young OCD patients psychopharmacologically is not quite such a straightforward issue as it might seem, however. The decision to treat depends, among other things, on (1) the degree of incapacitation, (2) the expected degree of compliance with treatment, (3) the type and degree of associated symptoms (such as tics, empathy and attention deficits) and (4) the nature and degree of possible side effects. Also, behavioural modes of interventions may be equally effective in children and adolescents as in adults with OCD. This possibility needs elucidation in the near future. Perhaps behavioural treatment can be used alone or its effect be augmented by the simultaneous treatment with psychopharmacological agents.

It is important to understand the extent to which the availability of effective treatments for a particular disorder influences the frequency with which the disorder is diagnosed (see also above under 'Prevalence'). In a study from a university hospital in Boston, Massachusetts, the rate of diagnosed OCD rose from 0.2% of all inpatients in the 1970s to 0.8% in the 1980s. This increase was paralleled by a corresponding increase in the rate of publications on OCD, and particularly in papers relating to OCD treatment (Stoll, Tohen & Baldessarini, 1992). Increases of this kind may represent a treatment-oriented diagnostic bias in which clinicians more readily diagnose a condition for which there is effective treatment. It seems clear that OCD was under-diagnosed before 1980. Whether it is currently over-diagnosed remains open to speculation.

Outcome

The outcome in OCD is uncertain. The follow-up studies that exist are all short term, and the prognosis into adult age is not known.

However, some conclusions regarding outcome seem to be appropriate. First, the clinical course of the disorder may be chronic or episodic, and spontaneous remissions, even after many years, may occur (Karno et al., 1988). Secondly, about half of clinically referred childhood OCD cases either do poorly or still qualify for an OCD diagnosis many years after initial presentation (Hollingsworth et al., 1980; Zeitlin, 1983, Flament et al., 1990). Finally, in spite of the availability of effective treatment, it has not been possible to demonstrate a *long-term* beneficial effect of vigorous behavioural or drug treatment so far (Leonard et al., 1988).

Tourette syndrome

The French neurologist, Gilles de la Tourette in 1885, described the constellation of multiple motor tics and coprolalia, and concluded that this was a neuropsychiatric disorder with a chronic course and a variable, but often gloomy, outcome. It now appears that Tourette described only part of a continuum of tic disorders involving the combination of multiple motor and vocal tics, which, in turn, might be seen as being on a continuum with motor tics generally. Exactly where on the continuum to

Table 7.4. *Diagnostic criteria for Tourette syndrome/disorder according to the DSM-III-R (APA 1987) (see text for comparison with DSM-IV)*

Diagnostic criteria
Both multiple motor and one or more vocal tics present at some time during the illness, though not necessarily concurrently
Tics occur many times a day (usually in bouts) nearly every day or intermittently throughout a period of more than one year
Location, number, frequency, complexity and severity of tics change over time
Onset before age 21 years
Not exclusively occurring during intoxication with psychoactive substances or CNS disease such as Huntington chorea or postviral encephalitis

draw the line in differential diagnosis and decide that this is 'Tourette syndrome' and this is not is currently the subject of considerable controversy. This is one of the reasons why reliable population prevalence rates for Tourette syndrome are not available.

Prevalence

Simple motor tics are extremely common phenomena, occurring at some time during the late pre-school and early school years in at least 10% of all children (Comings, 1990). Full-blown Tourette syndrome, on the other hand, is relatively rare, but mild–moderate degrees of the combination of motor tics (e.g. in the upper parts of the body: blinking, nodding or shaking of head or shrugging of shoulders) and vocal tics (ranging from repetitive throat-clearing and snorting, convulsive-like sounds variously described as 'barking', roaring or shouting) may exist in per cent rather than per mille and most such cases would nowadays possibly be diagnosed as suffering from Tourette syndrome. In a recent study of 16–17 year-old Israeli youngsters screened for induction into the Israel Defence Force, the point prevalence of DSM-III-R Tourette disorder was 0.49 per 1000 in males and 0.31 per 1000 in females (Apter *et al.*, 1993). This study was very thorough, but is likely to have produced an underestimate, given the well-known clinical observation that many patients with Tourette syndrome can control their tics in situations where it is absolutely 'necessary' to do so. It is hard to imagine a situation in which an individual would be more motivated both to suppress tics and deny them on a questionnaire than at induction of this kind. In a recent Swedish study of all 7–16 year-old school children in a Swedish industrial urban area, the minimum prevalence of Tourette syndrome was 0.07–2.1 per 1000, depending on the definition of the distinction of motor tics from motor stereotypies (Ehlers & Gillberg, 1993, Ehlers & Gillberg, unpublished data).

Onset of Tourette syndrome is usually in the 5–8 year-old age range (Corbett *et al.*, 1969). Tics usually affect facial muscle groups first and then, with time, tend to show downwards spread to affect muscles of the neck, trunk, arms and, rarely, legs.

Diagnosis

The criteria for diagnosing Tourette syndrome according to the DSM-III-R (American Psychiatric Association, 1987) are outlined in Table 7.4. The combination of multiple motor and vocal tics is required but other symptoms, such as coprolalia (the urgent need to say out loud 'dirty words') echolalia (the often 'meaningless' repetition of phrases or parts of phrases), attention problems, fidgetiness and obsessiveness may, or may not, be present. In the DSM-IV, onset before age 18 years is required. There is also a requirement for either marked distress or significant functional impairment.

Behavioural and physical phenotype

The motor and vocal tics are the *sine qua non* for a Tourette syndrome diagnosis. According to some authors, some degree of obsessive–compulsive behaviours are also so common as to be almost part and parcel of the full-blown syndrome (Comings, 1990; Robertson *et al.*, 1993), although others maintain that less than half the Tourette syndrome group meet all criteria for OCD (Apter *et al.*, 1993). It is clear that ADHD (see Chapter 8) is often a concomitant of Tourette syndrome but there are cases with few or no attention deficit symptoms. Also, it is unclear to what extent the possible underlying attentional deficit of ADHD is of the same quality as that encountered in Tourette syndrome. In the former syndrome there is often extreme distractibility, fidgetiness, unfocused attention and poor activity control. The clinical attention problems encountered in Tourette syndrome are often, though not necessarily, associated with various types of obsessive thoughts and an overfocus on these rather than on the tasks that need to be completed. Also, distractibility may not be as marked. Rather, there may be a high degree of fast (not necessarily loose) associations. Disinhibition may, however, be a hallmark of both 'classical' ADHD and 'classical' Tourette syndrome, suggesting some shared neurobiological problem (possibly associated with frontal lobe dysfunction). Full-blown ADHD is possibly only mildly over-represented as compared with the general population (Apter *et al.*, 1993). Obsessively recurrent thoughts or compulsions (e. g. to touch things in passing) seem to be even more common. Recent surveys (Shapiro *et al.*, 1988; Comings, 1990) have indicated that a number of other problems are commonly associated with Tourette syndrome, problems as diverse as maths difficulties (> 50% of cases), severe conduct problems, and compulsive touching of (common) or even public exposure of genitals (< 10% of cases). A few studies have suggested a connection between Tourette syndrome, on the one hand, and autism, Asperger syndrome and anorexia nervosa on the other (e. g. Råstam *et al.*, 1994). One study found self-injurious behaviours to be extremely common, affecting as many as one-third to a severe degree (Robertson, 1989). Head banging, life-time or present, was the most common self-injurious behaviour encountered in Tourette syndrome. It affected 16% of the whole group. Some of the head-bangers had cavum septum pellucidum on CT scans (which are otherwise usually normal in Tourette syndrome).

Pathogenesis

The aetiology of tics and Tourette syndrome remains obscure, but hereditary factors play an essential part in the pathogenetic chain of events (Comings, 1990). The study of large family trees has implicated a genetic link between Tourette syndrome, tics and obsessive–compulsive disorders. One model for interpretation of this data is that obsessive–compulsive disorders without tics and tics with or without obsessive–compulsive problems are outward manifestations of the same underlying genetically determined trait.

From the neuroanatomical point of view, the basal ganglia (and perhaps the frontal lobes) are the brain structures most often implicated in the genesis of Tourette syndrome (Chappell *et al.*, 1992). The basal ganglia are widely considered the brain regions associated with a variety of movement disorders, including Parkinson and Huntington disease and tardive dyskinesia. The presence and type of abnormal movements in Tourette syndrome, the suggestive neuropathological findings from some cases, and pharmacological data, implicate midbrain structures. In addition, the recent demonstration of caudate/frontal dysfunction in OCD (Baxter *et al.*, 1987; Swedo *et al.*, 1989) and the association of Tourette syndrome with OCD, further supports a possible link of basal ganglia abnormality and Tourette syndrome. The type of disinhibited behaviour so often associated with the classical Tourette syndrome phenotype suggests frontal lobe dysfunction in addition to basal ganglia abnormality.

Differential diagnosis

It is important to consider the possibility of Tourette syndrome in any child who shows, even mild, tics at physical examination. To some extent, even major tics can be suppressed voluntarily for a limited amount of time.

Tourette syndrome or multiple tics are sometimes the underlying cause of symptoms such as conduct problems and obsessions, and physicians have to be aware of its existence and systematically enquire about it. In Tourette's original writings, he surmised that outcome was often poor with intellectual deterioration in many cases. This now seems to be the exception rather than the rule. Nevertheless, it is important to consider the possibility of underlying neurological disorder and, occasionally, it can be difficult to decide whether tic–like movements are really tics or myoclonic jerks.

Work-up

Medical and psychological work-up in a child with clear or suspected Tourette syndrome must include a detailed medical/neurobiological/psychological/developmental history, sometimes an EEG (to exclude epilepsy which, very occasionally, can present differential diagnostic problems in childhood) and neuropsychological examination with the WISC (usually yielding a characteristic profile with low results on arithmetics and block design against an overall background of normal or above normal results), and some more specific neuropsychological battery in cases where there is associated academic failure.

Treatment

Dopamine blockers, perhaps particularly dopamine 2 antagonists (such as pimozide), have been shown effectively to reduce tics (Comings, 1990), and should be tried in cases where specific treatment is sought. Dosage is often much lower than when 'antipsychotic' action is requested. Pimozide, for instance, can often be effective in doses of 1–4 mg/day in school-age children (usually divided into morning and afternoon medication). However, the majority of patients with multiple tics and Tourette syndrome do not require 'specific treatment', either pharmacologically or psychologically. The best approach at the present time is usually to make a correct diagnosis, to inform parents and child that this is not primarily a psychological problem and that, in most cases, the tics do not indicate an underlying severe psychiatric or neurological disorder.

Certain other drugs, such as clonidine and sulpiride, have also been shown to have some positive effects, and the dopamine hypothesis in relation to tics remains an intriguing possibility rather than scientific fact.

Supportive psychotherapeutic techniques are often useful in the management of Tourette patients. Long-term outcome has received little study, but the evidence that exists supports the notion of a chronic disorder with a rather stable course, only rarely remitting altogether and only rarely carrying a clearly negative prognosis. Tics without associated neuropsychiatric symptomatology, on the other hand, usually requires no other intervention than diagnosis and often have a self-limiting course.

Outcome

The outcome is usually relatively good in Tourette syndrome and tics generally. This does not mean that all 'ticquers cease to tic' at a certain age (even though quite a large proportion stop having tics before adolescence), but rather that most of them can learn to live with the problem without too much embarrassment. However, depending on the associated symptoms, such as obsessive–compulsive conduct or attention deficit problems, outcome can be much less favourable, even though, in general, this is not related to the tics as such.

Anorexia nervosa

Anorexia nervosa is the best known of the so-called eating disorders. The literature on such disorders continues to grow at a rate of more than one thousand publications per year (Lask

Table 7.5 *Diagnostic criteria for anorexia nervosa according to the DSM-III-R (see text for comparison with DSM-IV)*

Criterion
1. Refusal to maintain bodyweight above a minimum weight for age and height, e.g. a weight loss of more than 15% under expected weight, or failure to achieve normal weight gain during period of growth so that weight is more than 15% below the expected level.
2. A strong fear of gaining weight or growing fat even in the face of underweight.
3. Disturbed body image concerning body weight, proportion or shape, e.g. claims to be fat in spite of extreme emaciation or that part of the body is 'too fat' in spite of obvious underweight.
4. For women, amenorrhoea (primary or secondary) comprising at least three consecutive cycles when normal menstruation should have been present. (Amenorrhoea is considered to be present if menstruation occurs only after hormone treatment, such as with oestrogen.)

& Bryant-Waugh, 1992). However, only a fraction of the published literature in the field relates to anorexia nervosa research in young people. This is all the more surprising, given the now well-established fact that the overwhelming majority of all anorexia nervosa cases have teenage onset of the disorder.

Controversy over the aetiology of anorexia nervosa has prevailed almost throughout the twentieth century. Psychological, sociocultural, family and hormonal factors have all been suggested to contribute to the development or, at least, the manifestations of the disorder (Råstam, 1992). From time to time, and particularly in recent years, intrinsic personality factors have been highlighted. Thus, Caspar, Hedeker & McClough (1992) and Råstam (1992) both found rather stable personality traits in a large subgroup with anorexia. Genetic factors have been implicated both in studies of twins and of non-twin siblings. It is conceivable that what is inherited in a subgroup of people suffering from the anorexia nervosa syndrome is a particular type of personality. Gillberg has proposed that empathy dysfunction, similar but more subtle than the type of dysfunction encountered in autism, might be a common underlying trait in anorexia nervosa with a particular type of personality make-up (Gillberg, 1992). In studies from Göteborg, the Råstam group (Gillberg & Råstam, 1992; Gillberg et al., 1994a) found empathy deficits to be significantly more frequent in the anorexia

group than in a carefully matched control group.

It is in this perspective that anorexia nervosa is included in the present textbook. The disorder is reviewed here with a special emphasis on underlying personality problems, some of which appear to be on a continuum with autism spectrum disorders.

Definition

Anorexia nervosa, according to the DSM-III-R, consists of a set of four symptoms which are outlined in Table 7.5. The DSM-IV criteria are almost identical. According to this manual, the type of anorexia nervosa (i.e. 'restricting' or 'binge-eating/purging') has to be specified.

These criteria may be difficult to apply in the youngest age group (under age 14 years). For instance, amenorrhoea cannot apply when menarche has not occurred. Also, the normal immaturity of young children has to be taken into account as it can modify the clinical presentation considerably. Criteria set out by Lask and Bryant-Waugh (1992) and modified by them from those originally set out by Morgan and Russell (1975) may seem more reasonable for the prepubertal group. These criteria are outlined in Table 7.6.

There are a number of other eating disorders in children, but these will not be particularly dealt with here. They include food avoidance emotional disorder (similar to anorexia but not

Table 7.6. *Diagnostic criteria for prepubertal anorexia nervosa suggested by Lask and Bryant-Waugh (1992) and adapted from Morgan and Russell (1975)*

Criterion

1. Determined food avoidance.
2. Weight loss or failure to gain weight during the period of pre-adolescent accelerated growth[a] and the absence of any physical or mental illness (other than the anorexia)[b].
3. Any two or more of the following:
   (a) pre-occupation with body weight
   (b) pre-occupation with energy intake
   (c) distorted body image
   (d) fear of fatness
   (e) self-induced vomiting
   (f) extensive exercising
   (g) laxative abuse.

Notes:
[a] this period restricted to 10-14 year age period by Lask and Bryant-Waugh, but such accelerated growth can occur in considerably younger children
[b] brackets information inserted by present author

meeting all criteria and being part only of another emotional disorder), pervasive refusal syndrome (in which food, drinking, talking, etc. are all restricted) and various kinds of food fads (including isolated selective eating in teenagers).

Prevalence

There has only been one unequivocally population-based study of anorexia nervosa in children and adolescents so far. It looked at the accumulated prevalence up to, and including, age 15 years in a Swedish urban area. In girls, 0.9% of the total population met, or had previously met DSM-III-R criteria for anorexia nervosa. In boys, the prevalence in the Swedish study was 0.1%. These figures are likely to be very close to the true prevalence, given that all 4400 individuals in the general population were examined with their clothes removed, and that they completed an eating disorders screening questionnaire and had their growth charts examined in detail. The population was followed up to include ages 16 and 17 years, and the prevalence rose to a minimum of 1.1% for females (and remained at 0.1% in the males).

The vast majority of the individuals in the Swedish study were teenagers and the peak age of onset was 14–15 years. New cases appearing after age 25 years are very rare and possibly constitute less than 3–5% of all cases (Theander, 1970; Garfinkel & Garner, 1982). However, it seems that a condition very similar to adolescent anorexia nervosa can have its onset considerably later (even at 48 years of age as in the study by Boast, Coker & Wakeling, 1992).

Almost all other epidemiological reports relating to anorexia nervosa have presented lower rates. For instance, in one of the best studies to date (Whitaker *et al.*, 1990), a lifetime prevalence of 0.2% (estimated on the basis of new cases appearing in the 13–18 year-old age range) was reported from New York. Nevertheless, the findings of the Swedish study are likely to be the most reliable, given the completeness of the screening survey and case finding.

There have been claims for a (relatively steep) prevalence increase in anorexia nervosa during the past two decades. Unfortunately, this issue cannot be addressed properly by any meta-analysis of older and new research in the field because all the older studies are non-population based. Råstam (1992) showed that only a minority of a population-based group of cases of anorexia nervosa attended clinics during the early stages of the disorder, and that, even in a perspective of several years follow-up, many were not seen by doctors or diagnosed by practitioners as suffering from an eating disorder. In particular, child psychiatrists were consulted by less than half the total anorexia group. Gynaecologists, internists, surgeons and general practitioners often treat young individuals with anorexia nervosa for a number of different ailments without ever making a diagnosis of the basic underlying disorder (Gillberg, 1993).

Anorexia nervosa is purportedly a disorder of industrialized, well-fed societies/populations. Recently, there have been reports of the disorder occurring in developing countries (Davis & Yager, 1992), but it still seems likely that it is considerably less common in such countries than in some of the western societies.

Sex ratios

The sex ratio in anorexia nervosa is unlike that in most other neuropsychiatric conditions of childhood in that girls are very clearly overrepresented. Very few neurodevelopmental or psychiatric disorders affect only one of the sexes. Some authors have argued that anorexia nervosa belongs in this small category of disorders. However, most would agree that boys/males may be affected and that, with the exception of amenorrhoea, all the typical symptoms may be present. In Råstam's population sample, 10% of all cases were male (Råstam, Gillberg & Garton, 1989). In that study, as in several other that have included males, social dysfunction appeared to be particularly pronounced in boys. There is presently general consensus that 5–10% of all individuals affected by anorexia nervosa are male. In the very young age group (with onset under age 14 years) the female dominance may be less pronounced and the female:male ratio about 1:4 (Lask & Bryant-Waugh, 1992).

The clinical picture in anorexia nervosa

Even though anorexia nervosa, just like autism, is a fairly distinct condition, there can be no doubt that it is not *one* disease, and that there are a wide variety of clinical presentations.

Mode of onset can be acute or insidious. In the first instance, there is very often a history of a close friend, relative or casual acquaintance commenting that the child/adolescent is (sometimes slightly) overweight or that there is a need for people in general to be more careful about matters relating to nutrition. Sometimes acute onset of anorexia nervosa is immediately preceded by some major stressful life event. Rarely, the disorder is ushered in by a severe or moderately severe febrile (including viral) illness. In more insidious cases, it is sometimes difficult to decide with any certainty the approximate date of onset. The first sign that anorexia nervosa is slowly developing is sometimes the loss of previously regular menstruations. In other cases still, vegetarianism in a family not otherwise practising vegetarianism, may be an important early marker for the later development of a severe eating disorder. In the youngest age group, the disorder often begins after a period of complete and 'obstinate'/oppositional refusal to eat, drink or even talk.

Preoccupation with physical appearance, calories, any aspect conceivable relating to food, obsessive and compulsive thinking about, and watching over, eating patterns of other family members then come to the forefront. Dieting and loss of menstruation may precede, coincide with, or follow, this behaviour and experiential pattern. Weight loss may be slow and gradual, but may sometimes be dramatic and amount to 5–10 kg per week. In such extreme cases, extreme levels of exercising, purging (including pathological use of laxatives and diuretics) and bingeing/vomiting are usually present early in the disorder. In yet other cases, such behaviours make their gradual appearance over a period of many months. Various degrees of bulimic behaviours are present in at least 60% of a population sample of anorexia nervosa patients two years after the onset of the primary eating disorder (Råstam,

Gillberg & Gillberg, 1994). It may need emphasizing here that there is a much greater number of young people who develop bulimic symptoms and meet DSM-III-R criteria for bulimia nervosa who never meet criteria for anorexia nervosa or show severe anorectic symptoms (Whitaker *et al.*, 1990). Anorexia nervosa is sometimes subdivided into *restricting and bingeing* variants. The proposed criteria for the DSM-IV (APA, 1994) suggest that anorexia nervosa be classified in restricting and binge-eating/purging subtypes (DaCosta & Halmi, 1992; Garner, 1993). However, these categories may not be generally useful, because so many patients with anorexia nervosa would qualify for a diagnosis of both variants.

Increased physical activity, including excessive work-out, ballet-dancing, training of various kinds and extremes of motor restlessness are the rule in anorexia nervosa. Such behaviours may antedate the actual weight loss, or may develop only after some months of dieting.

Social relationships quickly deteriorate, but the extent to which social interaction has been deficient long before the onset of ritualistic eating behaviours is seldom fully appreciated. A careful history-taking including a detailed account of the developmental course during the first few years, with both parents present, is often overlooked in the original diagnostic procedure. This may mean the failure to document an autistic-like empathy deficit with infancy or early childhood onset. Such failure, in turn, might lead to the inappropriate diagnosis of a disorder with (even sudden) teenage onset (anorexia nervosa), when, in fact, a lifelong rigidity and obsessive/ritualistic style of social interaction have hampered the child's development, and the obsessive/compulsive eating behaviours are but one aspect of a chronically disabling autistic-like condition. It is not that, in such cases, the diagnosis of anorexia nervosa is incorrect or useless. However, by not recognizing the 'premorbid' problems, what is only an exacerbation of the insistence on sameness and dependence on rituals, there is a great risk that the eating disorder will be considered as an exclusive teenage phenomenon (with, implicitly, a much better prognosis).

With the advent of the abnormal eating behaviours, there is often a feeling of emptiness, lack of control (which can only be regained or maintained by living up to the standards set by the patient for optimal weight control) and, very often, severe depression. Many authorities have discussed the possibility that anorexia nervosa might be best considered as a depressive phenomenon and part of a depressive syndrome. The study by Råstam (1992) seems to indicate that depression is not an antecedent, but rather a consequence of the eating disorder, perhaps of the starvation as such. Nevertheless, the possibility that, at least in some cases, anorexia nervosa can be regarded as a 'depressive equivalent' needs to be entertained, so that, if necessary, appropriate antidepressant treatment can be started.

The severe depression, which so often accompanies anorexia nervosa, is likely to cause most problems as weight is gradually restored. With the cessation of starvation, initiative, which has often been at a low in the acute weight losing stage, is usually rapidly regained, and suicidal attempts may result if depressive feelings have not yet lifted. This risk must be acknowledged and, indeed, taken very seriously in the long-term management of anorexia nervosa. The suicide attempt may come as a total surprise if only the abnormal eating patterns are the focus of attention. Depression is part and parcel of the anorectic syndrome and needs to be taken into account in all cases.

It is also appropriate to discuss briefly the concept of anorexia nervosa as a dependence disorder. The eating patterns, relationship to food, weight and calories and manipulations in order to maintain the bizarre eating behaviour encountered in anorexia nervosa is strikingly similar to the behaviour patterns seen in alcoholism and drug dependence. It is sometimes only when considered in this light that some of the most incomprehensible aspects of anorexia nervosa eating and other behaviour patterns including outright lies and manipulations become more intelligible. In this context there have been theoretical discussions concerning the role of brain endorphins in anorexia nervosa, but, the empirical evidence for or against a crucial import of endogenous opioids is still lacking.

The manipulative behaviours encountered in anorexia nervosa are clinically reminiscent of similar behaviours in alcoholism and Asperger syndrome/high-functioning autism. They relate only to the circumscribed interest patterns (food in anorexia, alcohol in alcoholism or, in the case of autism, any particular, unusual interest which may be taking up the individual's time), and do not extend to other areas. This means that, in most circumstances, the affected person can be expected to be telling the truth (in fact she/he may often be particularly conscientious in this respect).

Preoccupation with thoughts of food, calories, weight, scales, etc. are almost always present and may linger for many years (sometimes perhaps throughout life) even after weight has been restored to normal. However, such preoccupation is often stubbornly denied by the patient, who may, for instance, continue to negate the daily use of a scale (or vomiting) in the face of overwhelming evidence to the contrary.

Background factors

The aetiology of anorexia nervosa is still largely unknown, but several important leads exist. The search for a single cause has mostly been abandoned in research, and the disorder tends to be viewed as multiply determined.

Genetic factors are likely to play a considerable role in the pathogenetic chain of events, although the exact mode by which they operate remains in doubt. It has been known for a long time that siblings are affected more often than would be expected on the basis of chance alone (Strober *et al.*, 1990). Monozygotic twins, according to one study, are concordant for anorexia nervosa in 56%, while dizygotic pairs both have anorexia only in 5% (which is similar to the general sibling rate) (Holland, Sicotte & Treasure, 1988). Even though this issue has not been properly and thoroughly addressed in research so far, it is possible that what is inherited in anorexia nervosa is not a propensity to the eating disorder *per se* but to a particular

personality profile which may predispose to the development of obsessive–compulsive eating behaviours. Twin studies of bulimia nervosa also indicate that genetic factors may be important in some cases with this disorder, but it appears that their contribution to the whole spectrum of this prevalent group of disorder might be considerably smaller.

It appears that there might be a familial loading of affective disorders in the families of young people with anorexia nervosa (Cantwell *et al.*, 1977; Hendren, 1983; Gershon *et al.*, 1984; Toner, Garfinkel & Garner, 1988; Hsu, Crisp & Callender, 1992; Råstam *et al.*, 1994). A few reports have indicated that autism and anorexia nervosa may cluster in certain families (Gillberg, 1985; Comings, 1990; Råstam, 1992). It is also possible that obsessive–compulsive personality disorder and disorders of empathy other than autism (such as Asperger syndrome) may cluster in at least a subgroup of the population with anorexia nervosa, but research in this field is only just beginning.

Several studies do suggest an increased rate of obsessive–compulsive problems (obsessive–compulsive disorder (OCD) or obsessive–compulsive personality disorder (OCPD)) in the actual individuals with anorexia nervosa (e.g. Dally, 1969; Råstam, 1992). In a recent follow-up study of anorexia nervosa from age 16–22 years, obsessive–compulsive personality disorder was diagnosed in more than 30% of the anorexia cases but in only 4% of the comparison cases (diagnoses at age 22 years were made blind to the original case/control status of the individuals). A majority of these OCPD cases also showed moderate–severe empathy problems suggestive of dysfunction within the autism spectrum. Wechsler Adult Intelligence Scale Revised (WAIS-R) profiles in many such cases were similar to profiles encountered in high-functioning autism (Gillberg, 1993). Such empathy problems also occurred in some of the non-OCPD anorexia cases, but very rarely in the comparison group. Gillberg and Råstam (1992) have suggested that in some cases (30–50% of the whole group), anorexia nervosa in females could be the most striking outward manifestation of an empathy disorder, milder

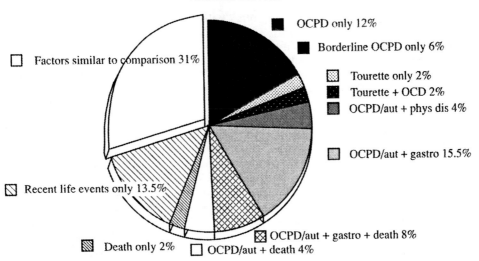

Fig. 7.1. Background factors in anorexia nervosa.

than classic autism, but similar in many other respects, encompassing social interaction problems from early childhood, insistence on sameness, ritualistic behaviours and deficient development of 'theory of mind' skills. Given that an association of anorexia nervosa and autistic-like problems has only been reported by one group so far, the suggestion of a true connection must be regarded as tentative at the present stage.

The study by Råstam and Gillberg (1992) suggested that several different types of background factors could be presumed to be individually more important than others in individual cases. Thus, an 'empathy disorder' (autistic-like conditions, Asperger syndrome, obsessive–compulsive personality disorder), possibly genetic or at least partly 'biologically determined', was present in slightly less than half the cases. Recent stressful life events (rape by stranger, physical assault) and death of first degree relatives were considered important background factors in other subgroups (Fig. 7.1.). In the whole group of anorexia cases, family problems were more common than in the comparison group, but the type of family dysfunction ('enmeshment, rigidity, lack of conflict resolution and overprotectiveness' (Minuchin et al., 1975) popularly believed to be a major

cause of anorexia was not more common. According to Lask and Bryant-Waugh (1992) 'there is no evidence to indicate that family dysfunction causes eating disorders'.

Biological/hormonal/neuroendocrine dysfunction (including hypothalamic dysfunction (Newman & Halmi, 1989; Kaye, Gwirtsman & George, 1989) and zinc deficiency (Lask et al., 1993) has been established in several reports on (very often emaciated) anorexia subjects (Nishizawa et al., 1991), but it is still not known whether the various changes reported are of primary importance in causing anorexia nervosa or a reflection of the starvation state of the patients. Many dysfunctions have been shown to be reversible with weight gain, at least in a large proportion of cases. Nevertheless, it is clear that *not all* individuals recover from all biological problems. Thus, for instance, whereas cerebral atrophy with ventricular dilatation documented on computed tomographic brain scans (Datlof et al., 1986; Krieg et al., 1988) usually reverts to normal when weight is gained, there are cases in which it does not. This also appears to be true of EMG-changes and morphological muscle changes demonstrated by biopsy (Alloway et al., 1988).

An interesting link between delayed gastric emptying (which is known to occur in anorexia nervosa), excess activity of cholecystokinin (CCK) at the local gastric receptor level (which is known to induce slowing of gastric emptying) and correspondingly abnormal influence of CCK on central (hypothalamic) receptors (which, theoretically could lead to behavioural and experiential effects, including, perhaps, a distortion of body image), has been suggested by Lask and Bryant-Waugh (1992).

A wide variety of cultural and psychosocial background factors, other than those referred to, have all been implicated as important background factors in anorexia nervosa. Societal ideals of female slimness have been held responsible for the purported (but unproven) increase in anorexia prevalence. Norms within subcultures, such as at ballet schools and certain private schools, have also been implied as factors contributing to high rates of eating disorders in such institutions (Szmukler *et al.*, 1986; Crisp, 1980; Råstam *et al.*, 1989). It is quite possible that such factors do play an important role in the causation of some cases of anorexia nervosa, but there is equally a need to appreciate the possibility that pupils with a particular personality profile, and hence perhaps a liability to develop restricting anorexia nervosa, may well select such institutions themselves without the school atmosphere itself contributing to the increased rate of disorder in such schools.

Work-up in anorexia nervosa

Neuroimaging of one kind or another (CT or MRI) is required in patients with anorexia nervosa because (a) occasionally a hypothalamic tumour (craniopharyngeoma, pinealoma) can present with classic symptoms of anorexia, and (b) the brain atrophy which often develops has to be 'monitored' as early as possible in the disorder and then followed up in order to document reversion to normal with weight recovery. It may also be appropriate to perform an X-ray of the oesophagus and stomach in order to rule out a tumour or other restricting processes (including superior mesenteric artery syndrome (Elbadawy, 1992)) in these organs. Otherwise, the medical work-up in the patient

with anorexia nervosa depends on the degree of starvation present. Anything from nothing more than the X-ray examinations mentioned to a comprehensive medical and laboratory work-up including blood (protein, electrolytes, zinc, haemoglobin, haematocrite, white blood cell count, thyroid hormones, HIV-serology, and tests of liver and kidney function) and urine (concentration ability, protein) tests, CSF tests (monoamines when extreme depletion is suspected either on the grounds of severe emaciation or clinical major depression or both, protein separation when the clinical picture is atypical and primary brain disorders might be suspected), ECGs (to (a) follow the development of electrolyte imbalance including potassium depletion or intracellular hyperkalaemia both of which often show in the ECG when serum potassium may be completely normal and (b) to monitor the possible appearance of cardiac arrhythmias), EEGs (to (a) distinguish severely anorectic behaviour in encephalitis with characteristic encephalitic EEG-changes from anorexia nervosa and (b) to establish an early diagnosis of severe brain dysfunction in anorexia nervosa with extreme emaciation in order to take appropriate action in various kinds of psychotherapeutic interventions so that not too much or too little is demanded of the patient) and further X-ray (including repeated CT scans and upper intestinal X-ray) examinations might be called for.

The recent demonstration of bone abnormality in anorexia nervosa is likely to become one of the most important associated biological conditions in need of monitoring in the follow-up of patients with eating disorders. Osteoporosis, it appears, may develop after starvation in connection with anorexia nervosa after only 6 months of malnourishment (Rigotti *et al.*, 1984) and may persist for years after weight recovery (Biller *et al.*, 1989).

The neuropsychological work-up in anorexia nervosa can usually be limited to a WISC-III-test, or, if the patient is older than 16 years, a WAIS-R. A test of this kind can be of importance because it may reveal that the patient is 'only' of normal intelligence in the face of superior results in academic performance. The result of the formal test, in itself, can go some way in explaining the breakdown of the teenager: obsessive and perfectionistic goals of superior achievement cannot be fulfilled against a background of only average intelligence and one of the few ways open for escape without perceived disgrace is through fasting, dieting or weight loss which will detract from the impending academic failure. There is, unfortunately, a widespread clinical belief that anorexia nervosa is associated with superior intelligence. The limited available systematic evidence suggests that anorexia nervosa patients and anorexia nervosa individuals in the general population have an average IQ of barely 100, and that the number of very gifted individuals is not particularly great (Dura & Bornstein, 1989; Gillberg, I.C. *et al.*, 1994*a, b*). Once it becomes accepted that most patients with anorexia nervosa are of normal (or even subnormal) intelligence, expectations and explanations of causation are likely to become more reasonable.

In the future, the WISC or the WAIS might become more useful tools in delineating the subgroup of individuals with anorexia nervosa that suffers from a disorder of empathy. Subtests of comprehension, picture arrangement and similarities may prove particularly valuable, and poor results on these could predict, not only an empathy problem, but, in addition, a more restricted prognosis with social interaction problems well into adult age, perhaps chronically (Gillberg & Råstam, 1992; Gillberg, I.C. *et al.*, 1994*a, b*).

The various psychometric devices specifically designed for the purpose of studying anorexia nervosa (such as the Eating Attitudes Test/EAT (Garner & Garfinkel, 1979) appear to have little or no value in the clinical assessment procedure in anorexia nervosa (Lask & Bryant-Waugh, 1992).

Treatment

There is, of course, no one comprehensive treatment model for all cases of a multifactorially caused disorder such as anorexia nervosa. Unfortunately, simple comprehensive treatment strategies for anorexia nervosa have been proposed over and over again without any scientific evidence in their support.

After years of debate, there now seems to be consensus that the most important primary aspect of treatment in anorexia nervosa must be the restoration of weight or, at the very least, the cessation of further weight loss. This is because starvation may cause irreversible damage to the brain, the bones, the muscles and endocrine system, not to mention the risk that the child/adolescent may die from acute starvation. The need to consider the weight aspect in anorexia nervosa takes precedence over any (however important) psychological considerations that might seem appropriate.

There may be gains from psychopharmacological treaments but some authorities (including Vandereycken, Kog & Vanderlinden, 1989) oppose such interventions with fervour. The number of well-designed placebo-controlled studies in the field are surprisingly few.

Clomipramine treatment has been advocated by some (Weltzin *et al.*, 1990), and if there is a severe obsessive–compulsive disorder or perfectionism within the bounds of obsessive compulsive personality disorder, this drug might be tried at doses ranging from 50–200 mg/day (partly age-dependent), beginning with 10 mg in one daily dose, and increasing gradually by 10 mg every three days until dryness of the mouth or other side-effects limit further increase. Clomipramine may be particularly useful if severe depressive symptomatology is also present. Clomipramine has a blocking effect on serotonin re-uptake, purportedly leading to increased serotonin effect in brain cells. Serotonin functioning can be altered both in anorexia nervosa (Kaye *et al.*, 1991) and depression (Gillberg, 1985), and serotonin turnover may be altered in obsessive compulsive disorder as well (Piacentini *et al.*, 1992). Thus, there seems to be a reasonable theoretical rationale for using drugs that enhance serotonin function in anorexia nervosa. In consequence, it is possible that newer, more specific serotonin uptake blocking drugs (Gwirtsman *et al.*, 1990; Kaye *et al.*, 1991), may eventually obtain a place in the treatment of certain cases of anorexia nervosa. However, so far, there is only anecdotal evidence in support of positive effects of such drugs.

Neuroleptic drugs (notably thioridazine) were used with some success in obtaining weight gain in studies performed several decades ago (e.g. Dally, 1969). In the author's view, they should be used with great caution, given the relatively high risk of extrapyramidal side effects, perhaps particularly in populations with severe brain dysfunction (which is almost definitely present in severely emaciated anorexia nervosa cases).

Halmi (1987) reported beneficial effects, including increased weight gain, of treatment with cyproheptadine.

Zinc has been advocated as everything from a specific anorexia nervosa treatment to a trace element which, because of starvation effects, needs to be supplemented in anorexia nervosa (Safai-Kutti, 1990; Katz et al., 1987). There is some systematic support for the use of zinc in anorexia nervosa, even though in one study zinc supplementation did not appear to influence the outcome (Lask et al., 1993). However, given that, with starvation, zinc deficiency is likely to develop in long-standing cases with anorexia nervosa, it is probably reasonable to provide zinc supplementation in cases with a duration of six months or more, at least if the patient is treated in an out-patient setting in which it is difficult to monitor nourishment intake. Also, zinc deficiency in itself causes nausea and anorexia, thereby possibly further contributing to the problem of refeeding in anorexia nervosa. There is, however, currently no support for the notion that zinc deficiency contributes in the original causation chain of events in anorexia nervosa.

Some sort of psychoptherapeutic intervention is almost always required in anorexia nervosa. However, it is far from clear what form this intervention should take.

Sometimes individual counselling in a cognitive psychotherapy setting including advice as to how to behave around matters such as food, meals and excercise may be sufficient, particularly if a teenager presents for treatment in his/her late teens.

In other instances, parental counselling without the patient present may be more effective (Russell et al., 1992). This intervention should focus on how to get the daughter/son to eat or decrease exercise or both, while providing emotional support for the parents who may (or may not) be severely disturbed or upset by the eating disorder.

Conjoint family therapy has been shown to be more effective than individual psychotherapy in anorexia nervosa affecting children and adolescents under age 18 years and with a duration of the disorder of less than 3 years in a well-designed study from London, UK (Russell et al., 1987). In this study, parental counselling along the lines suggested above, was included as an important component of the family therapy.

Individual psychotherapy is occasionally requested by the teenager her/himself. There is no convincing evidence that such therapy is effective, but individual talks should be offered when the patient feels the need for them. Also, when there is a suspicion that sexual abuse or other psychologically traumatizing incidents have occurred, individual talks are essential in trying to help the young person formulate her/himself so that appropriate measures can then be taken to alleviate ongoing external threats or problems.

It is possible that group therapies similar to those found helpful with adults suffering from alcoholism, adipositas and bulimia nervosa might be useful in anorexia nervosa as well. However, systematic research in this field has, so far, been very limited.

In a recent study by Schmidt, Tiller & Treasure (1993), self-therapy including a minor 'behavioural self-report hand-book' on bulimia nervosa, was shown to be surprisingly effective in reducing bulimic symptoms. A similar approach may well be helpful in anorexia nervosa also, but controlled studies are only just being started and there is no systematic data to support its use yet.

In cases with extreme emaciation, intensive medical care is occasionally, indeed quite often, required. Several things need to be kept in mind when providing therapy of this kind. In severe chronic cases (usually older than 18 years) a complete intravenous nutrition programme might be necessary and can indeed be quite effective even after five to ten years of anorexia nervosa with extreme emaciation (Nishizawa *et al.*, 1991). However, intravenous treatment should be seen as the last resort and should always comprise a detailed programme including every type of nutritional element necessary. It should never be given 'light-heartedly' in the form of hypertonic carbohydrate solutions, which might well cause acute electrolyte imbalance, cardiac arrhythmias and arrest. Occasionally, the cause of death in anorexia nervosa is just such over-ambitious intravenous drop treatment. Supplements of small doses of some kind of nourishing drink (5–15 ml every 5–10 minutes) through a gastric tube is often to be preferred over intravenous treatment in acute stages of treatment. The risk of inducing electrolyte imbalance is probably quite small using this procedure.

There is often a clinical problem in deciding when to admit the patient with an eating disorder for intensive medical care (beyond that contained in an ordinary out- or inpatient psychiatric facility). In the opinion of the present author, the following guidelines should be followed: (1) Any patient with anorexia nervosa who is psychotic (that is confused, delusional or hallucinating in areas which do not relate to food), delirious or comatose or who has (2) a severely deranged EEG which has developed during the course of the eating disorder must be immediately considered for referral to an intensive care unit. The same holds if the patient has (3) a body temperature less than 34.5°C, (4) a heart rate less than 42–44, (5) an ECG indicating atrioventricular block, (6) peripheral petechial bleedings or widespread mucous haemorrhages or (7) generalized oedema (not only affecting the lower legs, which is quite common even in relatively 'well-nourished' cases).

Outcome

The outcome in anorexia nervosa is highly variable, ranging from excellent to poor (and even early death). Reviewing all the outcome studies to date is a sad venture, yielding, as it does, an overall picture strikingly reminiscent of autism. A minority, albeit larger than in the case of autism and amounting to about one third of all cases in the most positive studies, do relatively well after a follow-up period of one to ten years. However, the vast majority (two-thirds or more in most studies) have a poor outcome with either persistence of severe eating disorders or deplorable social functioning (Theander, 1985; Crisp *et al.*, 1992). Added to this negative outcome picture is the extremely high rate of early death in anorexia nervosa, ranging from 5 to 18% depending on the length of the follow-up period. It is possible that the very high death rate reported in the earliest follow-up studies is a reflection of the clinic bias in the original case selection, but, for the moment, this can only be a tentative suggestion, given that follow-up of more recent, less biased samples, is only in its infancy.

Concluding remarks

Although anorexia nervosa has been on the 'medical map' for well over a century (Gull, 1874) and has been documented in the medical literature for more than 300 years (Morton, 1689), there is still little in the way of general consensus regarding its aetiology and treatment. There is growing recognition that it represents a syndrome of multiple aetiologies, and that starvation effects may be so serious that weight restoration must be the most important primary object of treatment. It affects at least 1 in 100 females. Certain personality characteristics are commonly encountered in anorexia nervosa and are likely to have some bearing on the development of the disorder. There is the possibility that childhood empathy problems on the autism spectrum may be particularly important antecedents of the disorder in a large subgroup of patients. Outcome is variable and socially poor in a large minority. The rate of premature death from suicide or from causes directly related to the eating disorder and starvation (including over-enthusiastic treatment) is clearly increased. There is a great need for concerted research efforts on representative (population-based) samples of individuals with anorexia nervosa in order

Table 7.7. *Diagnostic criteria for bulimia nervosa according to the DSM-III-R*

A.   Recurrent episodes of binge eating (rapid consumption of a large amount of food in discrete period of time)
B.   A feeling of lack of control over eating behaviour during the eating binges
C.   The person regularly engages in either self-induced vomiting, use of laxative or diuretics, strict dieting or fasting, or vigorous exercise in order to prevent weight gain
D.   A minimum average of two binge eating episodes a week for at least three months
E.   Persistent overconcern with body shape and weight

better to understand the many facets of this puzzling disorder leading to immeasurable human suffering and enormous costs for industrialized societies.

Bulimia nervosa and other eating disorders

There is little evidence that the other eating disorders (bulimia nervosa and binge eating disorder, for instance) are to be regarded as neuropsychiatric disorders of childhood and adolescence. Bulimia nervosa has received very little research attention from the neurobiological point of view. It appears that, in certain families there may be considerable support for a connection between anorexia and bulimia nervosa in that some members may be affected by one and others by the other of these eating disorders. This could argue in favour of some kind of common neurobiological dysfunction. Also anorexia nervosa often transforms into bulimia nervosa and less severe variants of bulimic behaviour as time goes by. However, the opposite development, that of bulimia nervosa later developing into anorexia nervosa, appears to be rare.

It should be kept in mind that bulimia nervosa is an extremely common problem, and that familial clustering with anorexia nervosa could be due to this fact rather than to any intrinsic biological abnormality.

Several studies have suggested a link between bulimic eating behaviours and a history of childhood sexual abuse (Folsom *et al.*, 1993). However, firm conclusions must await further study. So far, all that seems to be clear is that bulimia nervosa is associated with an equally high rate of reported childhood sexual abuse as

are other psychiatric disorders requiring treatment (Steiger & Zanko, 1990; Folsom *et al.*, 1993), and that the rate is very much higher than in anorexia nervosa (for which disorder rates may actually be lower than in the general population).

Whether seen to represent a neuropsychiatric disorder or a cultural/psychological phenomenon, it appears that individuals with bulimia nervosa might benefit from treatment with drugs that reduce obsessional behaviours (including clomipramine and desipramine) (Halmi, 1987; Garfinkel & Garner, 1987; Hughes *et al.*, 1986). The combination of such psychopharmacological intervention and group therapy might be particularly helpful in reducing the number of binge eating episodes, purging and vomiting. Just recently, Schmidt and Treasure (1993) presented preliminary evidence that a 'survival kit' self-help book might be particularly useful in reducing binge-eating and other abnormal eating behaviours in bulimia nervosa. Table 7.7 lists the diagnostic criteria for bulimia nervosa according to the DSM-III-R. The DSM-IV criteria are very similar.

References

Alloway, R., Shur, E., Obrecht, R., Russell, G.F. (1988). Physical complications in anorexia nervosa. Haematological and neuromuscular changes in 12 patients: published erratum appears in *British Journal of Psychiatry* 1988 Dec; 153:854:. *British Journal of Psychiatry*, **153**, 72–5.

Altemus, M., Pigott, T.A., Kalogeras, K., Demitrack, M.A., Dubbert, B., Murphy, D.L., Gold, P.W. (1990). Arginine vasopressin secretion in obsessive compulsive disorder. *Neuroendocrinological Letter*, **12**, 318.

American Psychiatric Association (1987). *Diagnostic and Statistical Manual of Mental Disorders*. Third Edition – Revised. Washington, DC: APA.

American Psychiatric Association. (1994). *Diagnosis and Statistical Manual of Mental Disorders*, Fourth Edition. Washington, DC: APA.

Apter, A., Pauls, D.L., Bleich, A., Zohar, A.H., Kron, S., Ratzoni, G., Dycian, A., Kotler, M., Weizman, A., Gadot, N., Cohen, D.J. (1993). An epidemiologic study of Gilles de la Tourette's syndrome in Israel. *Archives of General Psychiatry*, **50**, 734–8.

Baxter, L.R. (1990). Brain imaging as a tool in establishing a theory of brain pathology in obsessive-compulsive disorder. *Journal of Clinical Psychiatry*, **51**, 22–5.

Baxter, L.R., Phelps, M.E., Mazziotta, J.C., Guze, B.H., Schwartz, J.M., Selin, C.E. (1987). Local cerebral glucose metabolic rates in obsessive–compulsive disorder. *Archives of General Psychiatry*, **44**, 211–18.

Biller, B.M.K., Saduxe, V., Herzog, D.B., Rosenthal, D.I., Holzman, S., Klibanski, A. (1989). Mechanisms of osteoporosis in adult and adolescent women with anorexia nervosa. *Journal of Clinical Endocrinology and Metabolism*, **68**, 548–54.

Boast, N., Coker, E., Wakeling, A. (1992). Anorexia nervosa of late onset. *British Journal of Psychiatry*, **160**, 257–60.

Cantwell, D.P., Sturzenberger, S., Burroughs, J., Salkin, B., Green, J.K. (1977). Anorexia nervosa: an affective disorder? *Archives of General Psychiatry*, **37**, 1087–93.

Casper, R.C., Hedeker, D., McClough, J.F. (1992). Personality dimensions in eating disorders and their relevance for subtyping. *Journal of the American Academy of Child Adolescent Psychiatry*, **31**, 830–40.

Chappell, P., Leckman, J.F., Riddle, M.A., Anderson, G.M., Listwack, S.J., Ort, S.I., Hardin, M.T., Schahill, L.D., Cohen, D.J. (1992). Neuroendocrine and behavioral effects of naloxone in Tourette syndrome. *Advances in Neurology*, **58**, 253–62.

Chess, S., Thomas, A. (1977). Temperamental individuality from childhood to adolescence. *Journal of the American Academy of Child Psychiatry*, **16**, 218–26.

Comings, D. (1990). *Tourette Syndrome and Human Behavior*. Duarte, CA: Hope Press.

Corbett, J.A., Mathews, A.M., Connell, P.H. & Shapiro, D.A. (1969). Tics and Gilles de la Tourette's syndrome: a follow-up study and critical review. *British Journal of Psychiatry*, **115**, 1229–41.

Crisp, A.H. (1965). A treatment regime for anorexia nervosa. *British Journal of Psychiatry*, **112**, 505–12.

Crisp, A.H. (1980). *Anorexia Nervosa: Let Me Be*. London: Academic Press.

Crisp, A.H., Callender, J.S., Halek, C., Hsu, G.L.K. (1992). Long-term mortality in anorexia nervosa. A 20-year follow-up study of the St George's and Aberdeen cohorts. *British Journal of Psychiatry*, **161**, 104–7.

DaCosta, M., Halmi, K.A. (1992). Classification of anorexia nervosa: questions of subtypes. *International Journal of Eating Disorders*, **11**, 305–13.

Dally, P. (1969). *Anorexia Nervosa*. London: William Heineman Medical Books.

Datloff, S., Coleman, P., Forbes, G., Kreipe, R. (1986). Ventricular dilatation on CAT scans of patients with anorexia nervosa. *American Journal of Psychiatry*, **143**, 96–8.

Davis, C., Yager, J. (1992). Transcultural aspects of eating disorders: a critical literature review. *Culture, Medicine and Psychiatry*, **16**, 377–94.

Dura, J.R., Bornstein, R.A. (1989). Differences between IQ and school achievement in anorexia nervosa. *Journal of Clinical Psychology*, **45**, 433–5.

Ehlers, S., Gillberg, C. (1993). The epidemiology of Asperger syndrome. A total population study. *Journal of Child Psychology and Psychiatry*, **34**, 1327–50.

Elbadawy, M.H. (1992). Chronic superior mesentric artery syndrome in anorexia nervosa. *British Journal of Psychiatry*, **160**, 552–4.

Flament, M., Rapoport, J.L., Berg, C.J., Sceery, W., Kilts, C., Mellstrom, B., Linnoila, M. (1985). Clomipramine treatment of childhood obsessive compulsive disorder; a double blind controlled study. *Archives of General Psychiatry*, **42**, 977–83.

Flament, M.F., Whitaker, A., Rapoport, J.L., Davies, M., Berg, C.Z., Kalikow, K., Sceery, W., Shaffer, D. (1988). Obsessive compulsive disorder in adolescence: an epidemiological study. *Journal of the American Academy of Child and Adolescent Psychiatry*, **27**, 764–71.

Flament, M.F., Rapoport, J.L., Davies, M., *et al.* (1989). An epidemiological study of obsessive compulsive disorder in adolescence. *In* Rapoport, J.L. (Ed.) *Obsessive Compulsive Disorder in*

Children and Adolescents. Washington,: American Psychiatric Press.

Flament, M.F., Koby, E., Rapoport, J.L., Berg, C.J., Zahn, T., Cox, C., Denckla, M., Lenane, M. (1990). Childhood obsessive-compulsive disorder: a prospective follow-up study. *Journal of Child Psychology and Psychiatry*, **31**, 363–80.

Folsom, V., Krahn, D., Nairn, K., Gold, L., Demitrack, M.A., Silk, K.R. (1993). The impact of sexual and physical abuse on eating disordered and psychiatric symptoms: a comparison of eating disordered and psychiatric inpatients. *International Journal of Eating Disorders*, **13**, 249–57.

Frankel, M., Cummings, J.L., Robertson, M.M., Trimble, M.R., Hill, M.A. (1986). Obsessions and compulsions in Gilles de la Tourette's syndrome. *Neurology*, **36**, 378–82.

Garber, H.J., Anath, J.V., Chiu, L.C., Griswold, V.J., Oldendorf, W.H. (1989). Nuclear magnetic resonance study of obsessive–compulsive disorder. *American Journal of Psychiatry*, **146**, 1001–5.

Garfinkel, P.E., Garner, D.M. (1982). *Anorexia Nervosa: A Multidimensional Perspective*. New York: Brunner/Mazel.

Garfinkel, P.E., Garner, D.M. (1987). *The Role of Drug Treatments for Eating Disorders*. New York: Mazel.

Garner, D.M. (1993). Pathogenesis of anorexia nervosa. *Lancet*, **341**, 1631–5.

Garner, D.M., Garfinkel, P.E. (1979). The Eating Attitudes Test: an index of the symptoms of anorexia nervosa. *Psychological Medicine*, **9**, 273–9.

Gartner, A.F., Marcus, R.N., Halmi, K., Loranger, A.W. (1989). DSM-III-R personality disorders in patients with eating disorders. *American Journal of Psychiatry*, **146**, 1585–91.

Gershon, E.S., Schreiber, J.L., Hamovit, J.R., Dibble, E.D., Kaye, W.H., Nurnberger, J.I., Andersen, A., Ebert, M.H. (1984). Clinical findings in patients with anorexia nervosa and affective illness in their relatives. *American Journal of Psychiatry*, **141**, 1419–22.

Ghaziuddin, M., Tsai, L., Ghaziuddin, N. (1992). Comorbidity of autistic disorder in children and adolescents. *European Child & Adolescent Psychiatry*, **1**, 209–13.

Ghaziuddin, N., Metler, L., Ghaziuddin, M., Tsai, L. & Giordani, B. (1993). Three siblings with Asperger syndrome: A family case study. *European Child & Adolescent Psychiatry*, **2**, 44–9.

Gillberg, C. (1985). Anorexia Nervosa – Current Research in Sweden. Seminars in Biological Psychiatry. University of North Carolina.

Gillberg, C. (1992). The Emanuel Miller Memorial Lecture 1991: Autism and autistic-like conditions: subclasses among disorders of empathy. *Journal of Child Psychology and Psychiatry*, **33**, 813–42.

Gillberg, C. (1993). Empathy disorders: basic problems in severe psychiatric handicap conditions. *Läkartidningen*, **90**, 467–70 (In Swedish).

Gillberg, C., Råstam, M. (1992). Do some cases of anorexia nervosa reflect underlying autistic-like conditions? *Behavioural Neurology*, **5**, 27–32.

Gillberg, C., Rastam, M. (1993). Vart är forskningen på väg (inom anorexia och bulimia nervosa)? *Läkartidningen*, **90**, 3061–8 (in Swedish).

Gillberg, C., Carlström, G., Rasmussen, P., Waldenström, E. (1983). Perceptual, motor and attentional deficits in seven-year-old children. Neurological screening aspects. *Acta Paediatrica Scandinavica*, **72**, 119–24.

Gillberg, I.C., Råstam, M., Gillberg, C. (1994a). Anorexia nervosa 6 years after onset. Part I. Personality disorders. *Comprehensive Psychiatry*, in press.

Gillberg, I.C., Råstam, M., Gillberg, C. (1994b). Anorexia nervosa outcome: Six year controlled longitudinal study of 51 cases including a population cohort. *Journal of the American Academy of Child and Adolescent Psychiatry*, **32**, 729–39.

Green, W.H. (1991). *Child and Adolescent Clinical Psychopharmacology*. Baltimore: Williams and Wilkins.

Gull, W.W. (1874). Anorexia nervosa (apepsia hysterica, anorexia hysterica). *Translations of the Clinical Society of London*, **7**, 22–8.

Gwirtsman, H.E., Guze, B.H., Yager, J., Gainsley, B. (1990). Fluoxetine treatment of anorexia nervosa: an open clinical trial. *Journal of Clinical Psychiatry*, **51**, 378–82.

Halmi, K.A. (1987). Anorexia nervosa and bulimia. *Annual Review of Medicine*, **38**, 378–80.

Hendren, R.L. (1983). Depression in anorexia nervosa. *Journal of the American Academy of Child Psychiatry*, **22**, 59–62.

Holland, A.J., Sicotte, N., Treasure, J. (1988). Anorexia nervosa: Evidence for a genetic basis. *Journal of Psychosomatic Research*, **32**, 561–71.

Hollingsworth, C.E., Tanguay, P.E., Grossman, L., Pabst, P. (1980). Long-term outcome of obsessive-compulsive disorder in childhood. *Journal of the American Academy of Child Psychiatry*, **19**, 134–44.

Hsu, L.K., Crisp, A.H., Callender, J.S. (1992).

Psychiatric diagnoses in recovered and unrecovered anorectics 22 years after onset of illness: a pilot study. *Comprehensive Psychiatry*, **33**, 127-.

Hughes, P.L., Wells, L.A., Cunningham, C.J., Ilstrup, D.M. (1986). Treating bulimia with desipramine. *Archives of General Psychiatry*, **43**, 182–6.

Karno, M., Golding, J.M., Sorenson, S.B., Burnam, M.A. (1988). The epidemiology of obsessive-compulsive disorder in five US communities. *Archives of General Psychiatry*, **45**, 1094–9.

Katz, R.L., Keen, C.L., Litt, I.F., Hurley, L.S., Kellams-Harrison, K.M., Glader, L.J. (1987). Zinc deficiency in anorexia nervosa. *Journal of Adolescence and Health Care*, **8**, 400–6.

Kaye, W.H., Gwirtsman, H.E., George, D.T. (1989). The effect of bingeing and vomiting on hormonal secretion. *Biological Psychiatry*, **25**, 768–80.

Kaye, W.H., Gwirtsman, H.E., George, D.I., Ebat, M.N. (1991). Altered serotonin activity in anorexia nervosa after long-term weight restoration. Does elevated cerebrospinal fluid 5-hydroxyindoleacetic acid level correlate with rigid and obsessive behaviour? *Archives of General Psychiatry*, **48**, 556–62.

Krieg, J., Pirke, K., Laves, C., Backmund, H. (1988). Endocrine, metabolic and cranial computed tomographic findings in anorexia nervosa. *Biological Psychiatry*, **23**, 377–87.

Laplane, E., Levasseur, M., Pillon, B., *et al.* (1989). Obsessive–compulsive and other behavioral changes with bilateral basal ganglia lesions. *Brain*, **112**, 699–725.

Lask, B., Bryant-Waugh, R. (1992). Early-onset anorexia nervosa and related eating disorder. *Journal of Child Psychology and Psychiatry*, **33**, 281–300.

Lask, B., Fosson, A., Rolfe, U., Thomas, S. (1993). Zinc deficiency and childhood-onset anorexia nervosa. *Journal of Clinical Psychiatry*, **54**, 63–6.

Lenane, M.C., Swedo, S.E., Leonard, H., Pauls, D.L., Sceery, W., Rapoport, J.L. (1990). Psychiatric disorders in first degree relatives of children and adolescents with obsessive compulsive disorder. *Journal of the American Academy of Child and Adolescent Psychiatry*, **29**, 407–412.

Leonard, H.L., Swedo, S.E., Rapoport, J.L., Coffey, M.L., Cheslow, D.L. (1988). Treatment of childhood obsessive compulsive disorder with clomipramine and desmethylimipramine: a double blind crossover comparison. *Psychopharmacological Bulletin*, **24**, 93–5.

Leonard, H.L., Lenane, M.C., Swedo, S.E., Rettew, D.C., Gershon, E.S., Rapoport, J.L. (1992). Tics and Tourette disorder: a 2 year to 7-year follow-up of 54 obsessive-compulsive children. *American Journal of Psychiatry*, **149**, 1244–51.

Leonard, H.L., Swedo, S.E., Lenane, M.C., Rettew, D.C., Hamburger, S.D., Bartko, J.J., Rapoport, J.L. (1993). A 2- to 7-year follow-up study of 54 obsessive-compulsive children and adolescents. *Archives of General Psychiatry*, **50**, 429–39.

Luxenberg, J.S., Swedo, S.E., Flament , M.F., Friedland, R.P., Rapoport, J., Rapoport, S.I. (1988). Neuroanatomical abnormalities in obsessive-compulsive disorder detected with quantitative X-ray computed tomography. *American Journal of Psychiatry*, **145**, 1089–93.

Minuchin, S., Baker, L., Rosman, B., Liebman, R., Milman, L., Todd, T. (1975). A conceptual model of psychosomatic illness in children. *Archives of General Psychiatry*, **32**, 1031–8.

Morgan, H.G., Russell, G.F.M. (1975). Value of family background and clinical features as predictors of long-term outcome in anorexia nervosa: four-year follow-up study of 41 patients. *Psychological Medicine*, **5**, 355–71.

Morton, R. (1689). *Phtisiologia – or A Treatise of Consumption*. London: Smith.

Newman, M.M., Halmi, K.A. (1989). Relationship of bone density to estradiol and cortisol in anorexia nervosa and bulimia. *Psychiatry Research*, **29**, 105–12.

Nishizawa, M., Okui, K., Ishii, T., Mashima, Y. (1991). Parenteral nutrition in malnutrition (emaciation). *Nippon Rinsho*, **49**, Suppl:561–5.

Pauls, D.L., Leckman, J.F. (1986). The inheritance of Gilles de la Tourette's syndrome and associated behaviors: evidence for autosomal dominant transmission. *New England Journal of Medicine*, **315**, 993–7.

Piacentini, J., Jaffer, M., Gitow, A., Graae, F., Davies, S.O., Del Bene, D., Liebowitz, M. (1992). Psychopharmacologic treatment of child and adolescent obsessive compulsive disorder. *Pediatric Psychopharmacology*, **15**, 87–107.

Rapoport, J.L. (1988). The neurobiology of obsessive-compulsive disorder: clinical conference. *JAMA*, **260**, 2888–90.

Rapoport, J.L., Swedo, S.E., Leonard, H.L. (1992). Childhood obsessive compulsive disorder. *Journal of Clinical Psychiatry*, **53**, 11–16.

Rasmussen, S.A., Tsuang, M.T. (1986). Clinical characteristics and family history in DSM-III obsessive-compulsive disorder. *American Journal of Psychiatry*, **143**, 317–22.

Råstam, M. (1992). Anorexia nervosa in 51 Swedish adolescents. Premorbid problems and comorbidity. *Journal of the American Academy of Child and Adolescent Psychiatry*, **31**, 819–29.

Råstam, M., Gillberg, C. (1992). Background factors in anorexia nervosa. A controlled study of 51 teenage cases including a population sample. *European Child & Adolescent Psychiatry*, **1**, 54–65.

Råstam, M., Gillberg, C., Garton, M. (1989). Anorexia nervosa in a Swedish urban region. A population-based study. *British Journal of Psychiatry*, **155**, 642–6.

Råstam, M., Gillberg, C., Trygstad, O., Foss, I. (1990). Anorexia nervosa and urinary excretion of peptides and protein-associated peptide complexes. *Child and Youth Psychiatry. European Perspectives*, **1**, 54–8.

Råstam, M., Gillberg, C., Gillberg, I.C. (1994). Anorexia nervosa 6 years after onset. Part II. Comorbid psychiatric problems. *Comprehensive Psychiatry*, in press.

Riddle, M.A., Scahill, L., King, R., Hardin, M.R., Towbin, K.E., Ort, S.I., Leckman, J.F., Cohen, D.J. (1990). Obsessive compulsive disorder in children and adolescents: phenomenology and family history. *Journal of the American Academy of Child and Adolescent Psychiatry*, **29**, 766–72.

Rigotti, N.A., Nussbaum, S.R., Herzog, B.D. & Neer, R.M. (1984). Osteoporosis in women with anorexia nervosa. *New England Journal of Medicine*, **311**, 1601–6.

Robertson, M.M. (1989). The Gilles de la Tourette Syndrome: the Current Status. *British Journal of Psychiatry*, **154**, 147–69.

Robertson, M.M., Channon, S., Baker, J. & Flynn, D. (1993). The psychopathology of Gilles de la Tourette's syndrome. A controlled study. *British Journal of Psychiatry*, **162**, 144–17.

Russell, G.F.M., Szmukler, G.I., Dare, C., Eisler, I. (1987). An evaluation of family therapy in anorexia nervosa and bulimia nervosa. *Archives of General Psychiatry*, **44**, 1047–56.

Russell, J.D., Kopec-Schrader, E., Rey, J.M., Beumont, P.J. (1992). The Parental Bonding Instrument in adolescent patients with anorexia nervosa. *Acta Psychiatrica Scandinavica*, **86**, 236–9.

Safai-Kutti, S. (1990). Oral zinc supplementation in anorexia nervosa. *Acta Psychiatrica Scandinavica. Supplement 361*, **82**, 14–17.

Schmidt, U., Treasure, J. (1993). *Getting Better Bit(e). by Bit(e)*. Lawrence Erlbaum.

Schmidt, U., Tiller, J., Treasure, J. (1993). Self-treatment of bulimia nervosa: a pilot study. *International Journal of Eating Disorders*, **13**, 273–7.

Shaffer, D., Schonfeld, I., O'Connor, P., Stokman, C., Trautman, P., Shafer, S., Ng, S. (1985). Neurological soft signs. Their relationship to psychiatric disorder and intelligence in childhood and adolescence. *Archives of General Psychiatry*, **42**, 342–51.

Shapiro, A.K., Shapiro, E.S., Young, J.G., Feinberg, T.E. (Eds.) (1988). *Gilles de la Tourette Syndrome*. New York: Raven Press.

Sharp, C.W., Freeman, C.P.L. (1993). The medical complications of anorexia nervosa. *British Journal of Psychiatry*, **162**, 452–62.

Szmukler, G.I., McCane, C., McCrone, L., Hunter, D. (1986). Anorexia nervosa: a psychiatric case register study from Aberdeen. *Psychological Medicine*, **16**, 49–58.

Steiger, H., Zanko, M. (1990). Sexual traumata among eating-disordered, psychiatric, and normal female groups. *Journal of Interpersonal Violence*, **5**, 74–86.

Steinhausen, H.-C., Rauss-Mason, C., Seidel, R. (1991). Follow-up studies of anorexia nervosa: a review of four decades of outcome research. *Psychological Medicine*, **21**, 447–54.

Stoll, A.L., Tohen, M., Baldessarini, R.J. (1992). Increasing frequency of the diagnosis of obsessive-compulsive disorder: see comments in: Am J Psychiatry 1993 Apr;150(4):682–3. *American Journal of Psychiatry*, **149**, 638–40.

Strober, M., Morrell, W., Lampert, C., Burroughs, J. (1990). Relapse following discontinuation of lithium maintenance therapy in adolescents with bipolar I illness: a naturalistic study. *American Journal of Psychiatry*, **147**, 457–61.

Swedo, S.E., Schapiro, M.B., Grady, C.L., Cheslow, D., Leonard, H.L., Kumar, A., Friedland, R., Rapoport, S.I., Rapoport, J. (1989). Cerebral glucose metabolism in childhood-onset obsessive compulsive disorder. *Archives of General Psychiatry*, **46**, 518–23.

Swedo, S.E., Leonard, H.L., Kruesi, M.J.P., Rettew, D.C., Listwak, S.J., Berrettini, W., Stipetic, M., Hamburger, S., Gold, P.W., Potter, W.Z., Rapoport, J.L. (1992). Cerebrospinal fluid neurochemistry in children and adolescents with obsessive-compulsive disorder. *Archives of General Psychiatry*, **49**, 29–36.

Theander, S. (1970). Anorexia nervosa: a

psychiatric investigation of 94 female patients. *Acta Psychiatrica Scandinavica*, Suppl. 214.

Theander, S. (1985). Outcome and prognosis in anorexia nervoxa and bulimia: some results of previous investigations compared to those of a Swedish long-term study. *Journal of Psychiatric Research*, **19**, 493–508.

Thomas, A., Chess, S. (1977). *Temperament and development*. New York: Brunner/Mazel.

Tien, R.D., Kucharczyck, J., Bessette, J., Middleton, M. (1992). MR imaging of the pituitary gland in infants and children: changes in size, shape and MR signal with growth. *American Journal of Roentgenology*, **183**, 347–54.

Toner, B.B., Garfinkel, P.E., Garner, D.M. (1988). Affective and anxiety disorders in the long-term follow-up of anorexia nervosa. *International Journal of Psychiatry in Medicine*, **18**, 357–64.

Vandereyken, W., Kog, E., Vanderlinden, J. (1989). *The Family Approach to Eating Disorders*. New York: PMA: Publishing Corp.

Weltzin, T.E., Kaye, W.H., Hsu, L.K.G., Sobkiewics, T. (1990). Fluoextine impacts outcome in anorexia nervosa. Paper presented at the 143rd Annual Meeting of the American Psychiatric Association, Nr 497.

Whitaker, A., Johnson, J., Shaffer, D., Rapoport, J.L., Kalikow, K., Walsh, B.T., Davies, M., Braiman, S., Dolinsky, A. (1990). Uncommon troubles in young people: prevalence estimates of selected psychiatric disorders in a nonreferred adolescent population. *Archives of General Psychiatry*, **47**, 487–96.

Zeitlin, H. (1983). *The Natural History of Psychiatric Disorder in Childhood*. University of London.

Zohar, J., Insel, T.R. (1987). Obsessive compulsive disorder: psychobiological approaches to diagnosis, treatment, and pathophysiology. *Biological Psychiatry*, **22**, 667–87.

Zohar, J., Insel, T.R., Zohar-Kadouch, R.C., Hill, J.L., Murphy, D.L. (1988). Serotonergic responsivity in obsessive-compulsive disorder: effects of chronic treatment. *Archives of General Psychiatry*, **45**, 167–72.

8 Deficits in attention, motor control and perception, and other syndromes attributed to minimal brain dysfunction

Over the last 30 years, a number of behavioural and learning disorders have been lumped together under the uninformative label of 'minimal brain dysfunction' (MBD). Even long before that, MBD was used as a blanket term to cover children with hyperactivity and learning problems who, it was often taken for granted, had 'minimal brain *damage*'. The roots of this unfortunate diagnostic etiquette are to be found at the beginning of this century, when, on the basis of studies of children with encephalitis, it was surmised that a characteristic syndrome of over-activity often developed as a consequence of brain damage sustained *in utero* or in early childhood. Reciprocally, the notion gradually emerged that over-activity was in itself a sign that the child was brain damaged. Subsequent empirical study has shown that (a) over-activity is *usually* not a sign of brain damage and (b) brain damage does not *usually* lead to over-activity (Rutter, 1982).

Synonyms

A comprehensive survey of all the many synonyms and partly overlapping concepts used in this field is beyond the scope of this book. However, a list of some of the most common diagnostic labels is appropriate, as an introduction to a description of the symptom profiles encountered in children who have been given the, often inappropriate, label of minimal brain dysfunction (MBD) over the last 30 years (see Table 8.1).

The array of labels outlined in the table testify to the confusion in the field. Unfortunately, it does not appear that it is yet time for consensus. In North America, inflectional versions of the attention deficit disorder – attention deficit hyperactivity disorder (ADD–ADHD) spectrum are mostly used. In the British Isles, the 'hyperkinesis' and 'clumsy child' concepts seem to be more popular. In Scandinavia and Central Europe yet other concepts are emerging.

Attention deficit disorder (ADD) became obsolete almost before it was introduced, partly as a result of its hopeless inherent tautology: it must be either attention deficit *or* attention disorder, not both. One good thing about the ADD diagnostic category was that it allowed the presence of normoactivity and hypoactivity. No study has yet shown that attention deficit is invariably associated with hyperactivity. In point of fact, most children diagnosed as hyperactive, are probably not pathologically hyperactive and do not show excessive motor activity when compared with other same-sexed age-matched children. However, they are perceived as showing attention and activity which is inappropriate in a particular setting, in which attending to a task may be required.

Attention deficit hyperactivity disorder (ADHD) is the term used in the DSM-III-R (and it seems likely that it will be included in the DSM-IV as well, even though a subdivision into cases with predominant motor overactivity and cases with predominant attention deficit may be introduced). It is currently the diagnostic label most often cited in the literature. However, its meaning is far from clear, and it has not been

138

Table 8.1. *Syndromes attributed to so-called ADHD/MBD. Synonyms and partly overlapping concepts*

Diagnostic label	Comments
MBD (minimal brain dysfunction)	Once referred to minimal brain *damage* (before *c.* 1960), now to minimal brain *dysfunction*. Almost universally used until *c.* 1980. Still in *clinical* use in many countries. Usually refers to various combinations of attention and motor/learning problems. Inappropriate in that it implies brain dysfunction on phenotypical grounds and in its use of the word 'minimal'.
ADD (Attention Deficit Disorder)	DSM-III-label (APA, 1980). Widespread use in US. Semantically confusing (should be 'deficit' or 'disorder'). Diagnostic criteria very loose and subjective. Pervasiveness not required. With or without motor/learning problems.
ADHD (Attention Deficit Hyperactivity Disorder)	DSM-III-R-label (APA, 1987). Does not account for cases without clear hyperactivity. If categorized as 'severe', then pervasiveness required. With or without motor/learning problems.
ADHD (Attention Deficit Hyperactivity Disorder, predominantly inattentive type or predominantly hyperactive–impulsive type, or combined type)	DSM-IV label (APA, 1994). Accounts for cases without clear hyperactivity but does not make it clear how the two types are inter-related (if at all)
DAMP (Deficits in Attention, Motor control and Perception)	Accepted term in Nordic countries. Umbrella concept covering various combinations of motor control and perceptual problems in conjunction with attentional problems encountered in children who do not show mental retardation or cerebral palsy
Hyperkinetic disorders	Mostly used in the UK. Usually refers to a syndrome of pervasive hyperactivity. In the past, this diagnosis was often made only if there were not major associated conduct problems. The syndrome was then regarded as exceedingly rare. As used in the late 1980s, it has become obvious that it is not quite so rare, that conduct disorders often coincide, and that motor/speech/learning problems are the rule.
MND (minor neurological dysfunction)	Sometimes used to describe summary score for minimal motor/neurological problems or 'soft neurological signs'.
MCD (minimal cerebral dysfunction)	Rarely used concept. Refers mostly to over-riding concept of cerebral dysfunctions rather than to any specific clinical syndrome.
Clumsy child syndrome	UK concept. Highlights only one aspect of what is usually a multi-faceted syndrome.
Motor–perceptual handicap	Common Scandinavian concept. Attention problems are common in this group.
Organic brain syndrome	Central European concept. Highlights certain behavioural features, but essentially similar to MBD.
OBD (organic brain dysfunction)	Used particularly by groups that stress the importance of neonatal reflexes in the genesis of learning and attention problems.

studied *in depth* in population-based studies. It is generally accepted that attention deficit syndromes are often associated with other problems and that motor control, perceptual and learning problems are common. Unfortunately, this widespread realization is rarely reflected in the study of ADHD, and concomitant neuropsychological and motor coordination problems are often overlooked or not reported at all.

Not in the table, but certainly on the map of confusion in the field, is the concept of dyslexia which shows considerable overlap with all the named 'syndromes'. Reading and writing difficulties are almost part and parcel of many of the so-called MBD syndromes. Dyslexia is also problematic in itself in that most currently used definitions are conceptually unsound.

Further complication stems from the fact that many other neuropsychiatric syndromes (autism, many of the mental retardation syndromes and Tourette syndrome to mention but a few) often comprise elements of the 'MBD synonym group'. At present, the most common practice seems to be to diagnose only one syndrome. For instance, if a boy of ten years suffers from the combination of multiple motor and vocal tics, pervasive attention deficit problems and dyslexia, it is quite common to diagnose only Tourette syndrome, in spite of the fact that a case could be made for diagnosing Attention Deficit Hyperactivity Disorder (ADHD) and dyslexia as well. This should become less of a problem once it becomes generally clinically accepted that 'co-morbidity' is common in child neuropsychiatry, just as it is in child neurology.

Attention deficits

Attention deficit hyperactivity disorder

Normally (or slightly subnormally) intelligent but impulsive, distractible and (sometimes) hyperactive children have long been a burdensome problem to themselves, parents and teachers. More recently, school health officers, child psychiatrists, paediatricians and psychologists have taken an interest in this group. In spite of thousands and thousands of articles published in the field over the last 20 years, there is still no consensus as to what should be regarded as the boundaries, much less the aetiology of syndromes associated with impulsivity and distractibility. Currently, the most widespread label used for syndromes in this field is attention deficit hyperactivity disorder (ADHD), the DSM-III-R and DSM-IV diagnostic criteria of which are shown in Table 8.2. It should be noted already at this point that (a) it is not clear that 'attention deficits' (whatever problems are inferred by this term) constitute the basis of the syndrome, and (b) hyperactivity is not a salient feature of the behavioural cluster usually associated with so-called attention deficits.

Disturbances of attention are inferred in the syndrome of ADHD. Most of the brain is involved in subserving attentional functions (Colby, 1991). Frontal control dysfunction (Chelune et al., 1986), locus ceruleus dysfunction (Mefford & Potter, 1989), striatal (Lou et al., 1989) and cortico-striato-nigro-thalamo-cortical loop dysfunction (Voeller, 1991) have all been proposed to account for the behavioural and functional problems demonstrated by those affected. Also, dopamine and noradrenaline (e.g. Voeller, 1991) imbalance and generalized resistance to thyroid hormone (Ciaranello, 1993) have been suggested to be at the neurochemical root of (at least some cases with) ADHD. However, as yet, the evidence for any one of these models is limited.

There is neuropsychological evidence that impulsivity in cognitive functioning may be a salient feature of so-called ADHD. In several experiments, Trommer, Hoeppner & Zecker (1991) examined the hypothesis that the go–no go test is pathological in ADHD. This test requires the subject to emit a simple motor response to one cue (the go stimulus) while inhibiting this response in the presence of another cue (the no go stimulus). In frontal tumours and other frontal brain lesions, results on this test are poor, and the most common error type is the commission error, resulting from failure to inhibit the response to the no go

Table 8.2. *The DSM-III-R and DSM-IV criteria for attention-deficit hyperactivity disorder (ADHD)*

Diagnostic manual	Diagnostic criteria
DSM-III-R (APA, 1987)	*Note:* Consider a criterion met only if the behaviour is considerably more frequent than that of most people of the same mental age.

A. A disturbance of at least six months during which at least eight of the following are present.
1. often fidgets with hands or feet or squirms in seat (in adolescent, may be limited to subjective feelings of restlessness)
2. has difficulty remaining seated when required to do so
3. is easily distracted by extraneous stimuli
4. has difficulty awaiting turn in game or group situations
5. often blurts out answers to questions before they have been completed
6. has difficulty following through on instructions from others (not due to oppositional behaviour or failure of comprehension), e.g. fails to finish chores
7. has difficulty sustaining attention in tasks or play activities
8. often shifts from one uncompleted activity to another
9. has difficulty in playing quietly
10. often talks excessively
11. often interrupts or intrudes on others, e.g. butts into other children's games
12. often does not seem to listen to what is being said to him or her
13. often loses things necessary for tasks or activities at school or at home (e.g. toys, pencils, books, assignments)
14. often engages in physically dangerous activities considering possible consequences (not for the purpose of thrill-seeking), e.g. runs into street without looking

Note: The above items are listed in descending order of discriminating power based on data from a national field trial of the DSM-III-R criteria for disruptive behaviour disorders.

B. Onset before the age of seven.

C. Does not meet the criteria for a pervasive developmental disorder.
Criteria for severity of attention-deficit hyperactivity disorder:
Mild: Few, if any, symptoms in excess of those required to make the diagnosis *and* only minimal or no impairment in school and social functioning.
Moderate: Symptoms or functional impairment intermediate between 'mild' and 'severe'.
Severe: Many symptoms in excess of those required to make the diagnosis *and* significant and pervasive impairment in functioning at home and school and with peers.

DSM-IV (APA, 1994)	A. Either 1. or 2.

1. six (or more) of the following symptoms of *inattention* have persisted for at least 6 months to a degree that is maladaptive and inconsistent with developmental level:

Table 8.2. (*cont.*)

Diagnostic manual	Diagnostic criteria
	Inattention (a) often fails to give close attention to details or makes careless mistakes in schoolwork, work, or other activities (b) often has difficulty sustaining attention in tasks or play activities (c) often does not seem to listen when spoken to directly (d) often does not follow through on instructions and fails to finish schoolwork, chores or duties in the workplace (not due to oppositional behaviour or failure to understand instructions) (e) often has difficulty organizing tasks and activities (f) often avoids, dislikes, or is reluctant to engage in tasks that require sustained mental effort (such as schoolwork or homework) (g) often loses things necessary for tasks or activities (e.g. toys, school assignments, pencils, books, or tools) (h) is often easily distracted by extraneous stimuli (i) is often forgetful in daily activities 2 six (or more) of the following symptoms of hyperactivity–impulsivity have persisted for at last 6 months to a degree that is maladaptive and inconsistent with development level: *Hyperactivity* (a) often fidgets with hands or feet or squirms in seat (b) often leaves seat in classroom or in other situations in which remaining seated is expected (c) often runs about or climbs excessively in situations in which it is inappropriate (in adolescents or adults, may be limited to subjective feelings or restlessness) (d) often has difficulty playing or engaging in leisure activities quietly (e) is often 'on the go' or often acts as if 'driven by a motor' (f) often talks excessively *Impulsivity* (g) often blurts out answers before questions have been completed (h) often has difficulty awaiting turn (i) often interrupts or intrudes on others (e.g. butts into conversations or games) B. Some hyperactive–impulsive or inattentive symptoms that caused impairment were present before the age 7 years. C. Some impairment from the symptoms is present in two or more settings (e.g. at school [or work] and at home). D. There must be clear evidence of clinically significant impairment in social, academic, or occupational functioning. E. The symptoms do not occur exclusively during the course of a pervasive developmental disorder, schizophrenia, or other psychotic disorder and are not better accounted for by another mental disorder (e.g. mood disorder, anxiety disorder, dissociative disorder, or a personality disorder).

Table 8.2. (*cont.*)

Diagnostic manual	Diagnostic criteria
	Code based on type: *Attention-deficit/hyperactivity disorder, combined type:* if both Criteria A1 and A2 is/are met for the past 6 months *Attention-deficit/hyperactivity disorder, combined type: predominantly inattentive type:* if Criterion A1 is met but Criterion A2 is not met for the past 6 months *Attention-deficit/hyperactivity disorder, combined type:* if Criterion A2 is met but Criterion A1 is not met for the past 6 months Coding note: For individuals (epecially adolescents and adults) who currently have symptoms that no longer meet full criteria, 'In partial remission' should be specified.

stimulus. Omission errors (i.e. failure to respond to the go stimulus) suggest inattention. The rate of commission errors was particularly high in the attention deficient group without hyperactivity, but it was high in the ADHD group also. Methylphenidate (in a double-blind, placebo-controlled study), in moderate doses (0.15–0.30 mg/kg) improved performance on the go-no go test.

Hyperkinetic syndrome/disorder

In the UK, hyperkinetic syndrome, or, more recently hyperkinetic disorder, has been the preferred term and object of study in the field of disorders associated with motor overactivity, inattentiveness and impulsivity. Motor overactivity, as the term hyperkinetic disorder suggests, is conceptualized as the most salient feature of this disorder.

In a recent study by Taylor *et al.* (1991), a high score on the Conners' Classroom Rating Scale (Conners, 1969) (Table 8.3) together with a high score on the parental account of children's symptoms (PACS) interview (Taylor *et al.*, 1986) provided the basis for diagnosing hyperkinetic disorder. In a two-stage epidemiological study of all non-severely-learning-disabled 6–7 year-old boys in one school district (Newham, $n = 2462$) using the Rutter teacher and parent scales for initial screening, they

found a point-prevalence for hyperkinetic disorder (roughly equivalent to the ICD-10 diagnosis) of 1.7% for boys in this age group. This finding is similar to that reported by Gillberg, Carlström & Rasmussen (1983*a*) who found persistent pervasive hyperkinesis in 1.3% of all boys in Göteborg, Sweden. More than 40% of the UK group of children met criteria for conduct disorder. Less than 20% of the boys in the Swedish group met such criteria. The difference in this respect might well be accounted for by stricter criteria for diagnosing conduct disorder in the Swedish study.

The distinction of attention deficits from conduct disorder

In most studies to date, ADHD/hyperkinetic disorder/hyperkinetic syndrome and conduct disorder have not been separated well enough to make a decision regarding the extent of overlap of the two 'syndromes' or concerning the nature of the possible link between them.

In meta-analyses of the research on attention deficits, it is often concluded that there may not be enough validation of ADHD (or similar constructs) as a separate syndrome, and that attention deficit may better be conceptualized as a dimensional problem which cuts across a number of other syndromes (e.g. autism, anxiety disorders) which may, or may not, in

Table 8.3. *The Conners' Classroom Rating Scale*

Item	Not at all	Just a little	Quite a bit	Very much
1. Sits fiddling with small objects				
2. Hums and makes other odd noises				
3. Falls apart under stress of examination				
4. Coordination poor				
5. Restless or overactive				
6. Excitable				
7. Inattentive				
8. Difficulty in concentrating				
9. Oversensitivity				
10. Overly serious or sad				
11. Daydreams				
12. Sullen or sulky				
13. Selfish				
14. Disturbs other children				
15. Quarrelsome				
16. 'Tattles'				
17. Acts 'smart'				
18. Destructive				
19. Steals				
20. Lies				
21. Temper outbursts				
22. Isolates himself from other children				
23. Appears to be unaccepted by group				
24. Appears to be easily led				
25. No sense of fair play				
26. Appears to lack leadership				
27. Does not get along with opposite sex				
28. Does not get along with same sex				
29. Teases other children or interferes with their activities				
30. Submissive				
31. Defiant				
32. Impudent				
33. Shy				
34. Fearful				
35. Excessive demands for teacher's attention				
36. Stubborn				
37. Overly anxious to please				
38. Uncooperative				
39. Attendance problem				

themselves have considerably better validation (Thorley, 1984; Gillberg & Hellgren, 1994).

In many studies 'conduct disorder symptoms' (verbal and non-verbal aggressiveness, destructiveness and peer interaction problems) are not clearly separated from those of 'attention deficits'. Even in the DSM-III-R, some of the symptoms included in the diagnostic set for ADHD are suggestive of conduct rather than inattention–hyperactivity problems. It seems clear that much of the literature on ADHD and conduct disorder is confounded by this failure to distinguish the two and to provide in-depth account of the extent of possible overlap. For instance, many of the US follow up studies of children with ADHD, who have been treated with stimulants, may have included disproportionate numbers of cases with a proclivity for criminal activity (Gittelman et al., 1985; Mannuzza et al., 1989) making it difficult to tease out the extent to which treatment has affected the attentional dysfunction or the conduct problems or both. Similar lines of reasoning may well account for some of the discrepant findings in the follow-up literature, in which 'ADHD' children from New York seem to have a greater risk for criminal behaviour than 'ADHD' children in Canada (Klein & Mannuzza, 1991; Weiss, 1991).

Lower IQ is associated with more pronounced hyperactivity and attention deficits (e.g. Sonuga-Barke et al., 1994), but not with conduct disorder. In fact for girls, it appears that the rate and intensity of conduct problems may go up with higher IQ.

Specific developmental disorders

Communications disorders

Language and speech disorders are part and parcel of a number of child neuropsychiatric disorders (autism, Asperger syndrome, DAMP, Landau–Kleffner syndrome, etc.) and childhood behavioural problems (Cantwell, Baker & Rutter, 1978; Cantwell et al., 1989; Richman, Stevenson & Graham, 1982). Delayed language development and semantic–pragmatic disorders, in particular, seem to be extremely common concomitants of early onset child psychiatric problems (see further, page 158).

Motor skills disorder/motor perception dysfunction ('clumsy child syndrome')/developmental coordination disorder

Motor control problems are sometimes referred to as 'clumsy child syndrome', 'motor perception dysfunction (MPD)' or, in the terminology of the DSM-III-R 'motor skills disorder'/DSM-IV 'developmental coordination disorder' (DCD). There is a considerable literature

suggesting that such problems may be much more common than suggested by chance alone in child and adolescent psychiatric disorders (Gillberg, 1983; Shaffer et al., 1985; Hellgren, Gillberg, Enerskog, 1987; Losse et al., 1991; McKinlay, 1993). However, unfortunately, neurodevelopmental problems of this kind have only rarely been specifically examined in the study of child psychiatric disorders. The Swedish DAMP studies (see below) suggest that motor skills disorder is an integral part of many attention deficit syndromes, and specifically those attention deficits with a poor outcome in the ten-year perspective from age 6 to 16 years (Hellgren et al., 1993).

The type of motor control problems encountered are not commonly of the type that one would associate with outright neurological disorder, but rather appear to represent immaturities of the central nervous system in children with above normal, normal or near normal intelligence. The motor deficiencies cannot be explained in terms of poor overall functioning. Motor control and motor performance is often appropriate to that of a considerably younger child. Thus it is appropriate to speak of 'specific' motor skills disorder. Nevertheless, the motor skills disorder usually overlaps with language and speech disorder and with ADHD. This, prognostically relevant, constellation of symptoms is referred to below as deficits in attention, motor control and perception (DAMP).

There is also a considerable number of individuals in the general population who are clumsy but who do not show attention deficit problems to any marked degree. These are children with potentially much better outcomes than those with a full-blown DAMP syndrome. However, their outlook is worse than that for children with early onset ADHD without motor control problems (Hellgren et al., 1993).

The types of motor control problems encountered in motor skills disorder are (a) overall gross motor clumsiness, including clumsy and awkward gait, difficulty in acquiring age-appropriate skills such as riding a bicycle, learning to swim, etc., (b) difficulty in standing and hopping on one leg, (c) bilateral dysdiadochoki-

nesis without specific localizing signs, (d) difficulty in performing the Fog's test (Fog & Fog,
1963) and (e) difficulty in performing in an age-
appropriate fashion in a maze-tracing task (Bishop, 1980). Any one or several (including all) of
these may be present in addition to a whole host
of other minor neurodevelopmental problems.
These symptoms and signs have been described
in more detail in Touwen (1979), Rasmussen *et
al.*, (1983) and Gillberg, Gillberg & Groth
(1989), Lunsing *et al.*, 1992*a, b*). Simple screening tools for motor skills disorders are available
from the author and have been published previously (Gillberg *et al.*, 1983*b*).

I would like to suggest that *all* child and
adolescent psychiatric clinic attenders, whether
in an in- or outpatient setting be examined with
a view to disclosing some of the neurodevelopmental problems mentioned in the foregoing
(plus several more whenever the examination
suggests the need for this).

Academic skills disorder/learning disorders without mental retardation

Academic skills disorders of various kinds (particularly dyslexia or specific reading retardation, slightly less commonly writing difficulties)
are very common, affecting almost 10% of a
whole school age population (Dockrell &
McShane, 1993). They appear to be closely
linked to behaviour problems of the ADHD
type. They will be considered below in a special
section on dyslexia, dysgraphia and dyscalculia.

DAMP (deficits in attention, motor control and perception)

Definition of DAMP

Surveying the literature on so-called MBD, it
became apparent that the types of problems
mostly inferred were perceptual, motor and
attention deficits in various combinations in
children without mental retardation or cerebral
palsy (Gillberg *et al.*, 1982). The concept of
DAMP was therefore launched in the mid–
1980s to cover most of the syndromes pre-

viously referred to as 'MBD' but without any
implicit aetiological meaning (Gillberg *et al.*,
1989). This label has now been accepted as an
umbrella definition in the Nordic countries
(Airaksinen *et al.*, 1990).

DAMP is defined here as the combination of
motor coordination/perception dysfunction
(MPD/motor perception dysfunction, roughly
equivalent to the DSM-IV concept 'developmental coordination disorder') and pervasive
attention deficit (ADD/attention deficit disorder) in any child of normal or low normal
intelligence who does not meet criteria for cerebral palsy. This syndrome is referred to as
MPDADD in Table 8.4. There are also children
with MPD only and ADD only.

Attention deficits have to be present in
several observational settings such as at home,
in school and in the peer group. Reliable and
valid rating scales are available. The most
widely used is that of Conners (Conners, 1969),
which exists in a 39-item version (Table 8.3) and
a 10-item version designed for use either by
parents or by teachers. The minimum requirement for diagnosing attention deficit is that the
child is rated as abnormal on a rating scale of
this kind by at least two independent observers
(e.g. parent and teacher). Not all children with
attention deficit are hyperactive. Some are
rather hypoactive and many fluctuate between
hyper- and hypoactivity. Many are best described as disorganized in their activity. This is
one of the many reasons why the 'hyperactivity'
label as a cover-all blanket term is inadequate.
Unfortunately, the DSM-III-R does not
include a diagnostic category for children with
attention deficit without hyperactivity. This is
going to be remedied in the DSM-IV which
proposes categories for ADHD primarily with
attention dysfunction, and ADHD primarily
with hyperactivity.

The motor coordination problems are
usually best described as immature performance on a number of different neurological/
neuromotor tests such as diadochokinesis,
finger tapping, alternating movements, standing and skipping on one leg, walking on lateral
sides of feet and various fine motor performance tests such as tracing in a maze, cutting

Table 8.4. *Diagnostic criteria for DAMP*

DAMP

MPDADD	A.	ADD as manifested by

MPDADD A. ADD as manifested by
      (a) severe problems in at least one or moderate problems in at least two of the following areas: attention span, activity level, vigilance and ability to sit still, and
      (b) cross-situational problems in the areas mentioned under (a), documented at two or more of the following: psychiatric, neurological, psychological evaluation and maternal report
    B. MPD as manifested by marked
      (a) gross motor dysfunction according to detailed neurological examination (see Rasmussen *et al.*, 1983), or
      (b) fine motor dysfunction according to detailed neurological examination (see Rasmussen *et al.*, 1983), or
      (c) perceptual dysfunction according to testing with SCSIT (Ayres 1974) and defined in Gillberg *et al.*, (1982)
    C. Problems not accounted for or associated with MR or CP.
    All of A–C have to be met.
    Severity is rated in the following way: severe MPDADD (s-MPDADD) is diagnosed in a child who meets all of the criteria A–C and in addition, meets all of the subcriteria (a)–(c) under B, and in addition shows SLD; mild–moderate MPDADD (m-MPDADD) is diagnosed in all other cases meeting criteria for MPDADD.

ADD A. ADD as for MPDADD
    B. Problems not accounted for or associated with MPD, MR or CP.
    Both A and B have to be met.

MPD A. MPD as for MPDADD
    B. Problems not accounted for, or associated with, ADD, MR or CP.
    Both A and B have to be met.

ADD = Attention Deficit Disorder; MPD = Motor Perception Dysfunction; MR = Mental Retardation; CP = Cerebral Palsy.

out paper, etc. These problems show in everyday settings and are evident as overall clumsiness, poor table manners, difficulties with dressing and tying shoe-laces, difficulties with learning to draw, write, ride a bicycle, swim, ski and skate. Many children with such motor coordination problems are poor at games, particularly ball-games and especially if such games involve small balls. The Touwen manual for examination of the child with minor neurological dysfunction (Touwen, 1979) is helpful to the clinician wanting to acquire the skills necessary to perform and age-adequate neuromotor evaluation in this field. However, exact age norms are not available in this manual. There are a number of different other 'manuals' available (Denckla, 1985; Gillberg I.C., 1987,

Whitmore & Bax, 1986; Michelsson & Ylinen, 1987), all of which have at least some face validity.

There are problems pertaining to the diagnosis of ADD/ADHD and MPD. One of the most important of these is the difficulty of mapping the behavioural descriptions on to relevant neurological substrates and behaviours. Thus, for example, a neurological model would discriminate locomotor hyperactivity, akathisia and stereotypy, all of which could 'result' in behavioural hyperactivity. Akathisia is characterized by restless, fidgety, overactive movements and would temporally be associated with an inner sense of restlessness. Exploratory locomotor hyperactivity, on the other hand, is characterized by a high level of walking about (perhaps even running), particularly in a new environment. Stereotypy involves high-frequency, repetitive movements. Akathisia and exploratory locomotor hyperactivity seem to be subserved by closely related, yet distinct neuronal circuits. Lesions at various points in the dopamine-containing mesolimbic pathways can produce one or the other types of symptoms with a differential response pattern to stimulant drug medication. Stereotypy is linked to the dopaminergic system, is induced by amphetamine, and is completely blocked by certain lesions in the caudate–putamen–globus pallidus. All of these behaviours comprise the behavioural descriptor of 'hyperactivity'. This example is just one of many possible illustrations of the many ways in which attention deficit/hyperactivity symptoms and syndromes may elude objective definition and remain in the realm of subjectively defined clinical syndromes in spite of ever more specific requirements for diagnosis in the diagnostic manuals.

The perceptual problems appear on formal tests (such as the performance part of the WISC (block design, picture completion and object assembly are often problematic), the SCSIT (Southern California Sensory Integration Tests (Ayres, 1974)) and in specific tests of perception which may vary from one country to another). There are often perceptual problems in several domains (visual, auditory, tactile, etc.) but most tests focus on visual–perceptual tasks, and it is sometimes difficult to determine whether one is dealing with a pure visual–perceptual problem, a fine motor problem, a dysfunction of eye–hand coordination, or combinations of these. Clinically, the perceptual problems often show in impaired perception of form, space and shape, in drawing and writing immaturities and in severe problems acquiring automatic reading skills. Disturbance of body image (with difficulty judging the location of body and body parts in space, possibly contributing to problems such as having problems judging the appropriate distance from other people during social interactions) is also a common consequence of various perceptual difficulties.

Children with DAMP often also show various types of speech and language problems, some of which can be regarded as belonging in the motor group of problems (some articulation problems, hypotonia of mouth and certain variants of stuttering), others of which mirror auditory perceptual problems (some articulation problems, failure to adjust volume and pitch of voice to auditory feed-back demands), and still others which must be seen as related to some more basic and specific language deficit (overall delay in language development, semantic–pragmatic disorder).

MPDADD can be subdivided into *severe cases*, i.e. those with MPDADD who show all five of (1) attention, (2) gross motor, (3) fine motor, (4) perceptual and (5) speech language dysfunction, and *mild cases*, i.e. those with MPDADD who do not show all of these five dysfunctions.

It is quite common for children with severe DAMP to show comorbid autistic features and even the full-blown clinical picture of Asperger syndrome. The interrelationships between (mild and severe) DAMP, AD(H)D, MPD and autistic features (including Asperger syndrome) are shown in Fig. 8.1.

An adequate working diagnosis in severe cases (i.e. a formulation in diagnostic terms which can serve as a basis for intervention suggestions), requires the collaboration of the paediatrician (or a child psychiatrist) with a clinical neuropsychologist and, optimally, a speech therapist, all of whom should make independent evaluations, and then combine their data in a consensus fashion. In mild–moderate cases, the paediatrician (or school doctor) will have to do most of the diagnostic work himself, considering the high prevalence of the disorder and the relative lack of diagnostic resources.

Epidemiology

DAMP (MPDADD) in severe form is present in about 1.2% of all 7 year-old children, whereas milder variants are present in another 3–6% according to various different Nordic studies (Gillberg *et al.* 1982, Gillberg, Winnergård & Gillberg, 1993; Landgren *et al.*, 1993).

Social class and IQ are generally a little lower

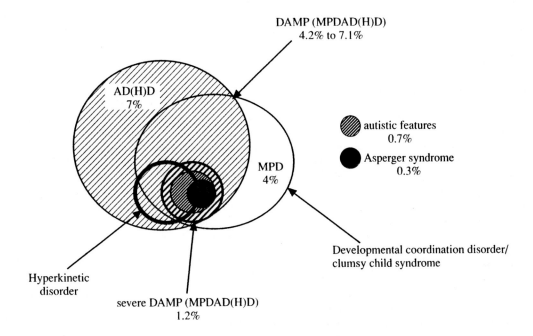

Fig. 8.1. The overlap of (mild–moderate and severe) DAMP (MPD + AD(H)D) and autistic features – Asperger syndrome in the general population of 7 year olds (data from Gillberg, 1983 and Gillberg & Gillberg, 1989a) and the possible overlap with hyperkinetic syndrome and developmental coordination disorder/clumsy child syndrome.

in DAMP than in the general population, but children with DAMP come from all social classes and some have very high IQs. It has been queried whether DAMP might not reflect simply slightly lowered IQ. However, many children with high IQ have DAMP problems, and a simple linear effect between declining IQ and increasing DAMP problems does not exist (Gillberg & Hellgren, 1994).

Sex ratios

There are many more boys than girls with MPDADD, ADD and MPD. According to the longitudinal Swedish study, the overall male-:female ratio is about 2–3:1, cohorts of severe cases showing an even stronger skewing (Gillberg et al., 1982). However, boys and girls, as separate groups, develop in accordance with different schemata for brain evolution. Thus

pre-school age boys appear to be superior to girls on some skills requiring good visuo-motor performance, whereas in all other respects (except sheer physical strength) girls tend to develop faster than boys. If boys and girls are treated as one group this will inevitably lead to a situation in which boys will outnumber girls in any epidemiological study defining deficits in attention, motor control and perception on the basis of some 'pooled' cut-off. In other words, if boys were compared with boys and girls were compared with girls, sex ratios of disordered boys over girls might not be as inflated as currently held.

Background factors

According to the Swedish studies, DAMP is 'idiopathic' in about 10% of cases, mainly hereditary in one-third of cases, mainly associated with pre-, peri-, or postnatal brain damage in another third and by combinations of hereditary and potentially brain damaging factors in 20% of cases (Gillberg & Rasmussen, 1982). Some of the variance attributed to brain damage could be due to hereditary factors (cf. Chapter 4 under 'Borderline intellectual functioning'). A recent twin study of hyperactivity is compatible with a model for the development of DAMP in which hereditary factors are of dominating importance (Goodman & Stevenson 1989a, b). Also, twin studies of dyslexia (Stevenson & Graham, 1993) suggest high genetic loading for reading and spelling problems, and a strong link between dyslexia and hyperactivity (Stevenson, 1991), suggesting that the whole of the clinical DAMP complex might have even stronger genetic contributions than previously appreciated. DAMP is associated with overall lower IQ, even though any level of intellectual functioning (above IQ 70) is possible (Gillberg & Rasmussen, 1982). There is considerable evidence that, even within a wider group of 'normally intelligent' pre-school children, hyperactivity/attention deficit is much more common in those with relatively lower IQ (Sonuga-Barke et al., 1994).

Whatever the basic cause, there is considerable direct and indirect evidence that DAMP (and some of the ADHD or hyperkinetic syndromes) may be associated with a lack of, or deficiency in automatization skills, both in attentional and motor domains (Lou, Henriksen & Bruhn, 1984; Lou et al., 1989; Lou et al., 1990a, b; Gillberg, 1992a). It is not that motor functions in themselves are qualitatively abnormal (as is the case, for instance in cerebral palsy) in most cases. The child can perform the particular motor action required (e.g. hopping on one leg), but only if conscious cognitive control is exercised (e.g. counting out loud "one', 'two', 'three', 'four', etc. in order not to stop the repeated action of hopping up and down). Thus, it would be inappropriate to be speaking of abnormal motor function, but quite appropriate to infer abnormal *control* of motor function. Hypoperfusion of frontal and striatal areas in DAMP/ADHD has been demonstrated in studies examining regional cerebral blood flow (Lou et al., 1984). An MRI study of

school-age boys with ADHD revealed smaller posterior (splenial) Corpus calossum regions than controls (Semrud-Clikeman et al., 1994). Girls with ADHD may have reduced brain metabolism as compared with boys according to a recent PET study (Ernst et al., 1994).

Eye movements are usually abnormal in DAMP (Rasmussen et al., 1983). The interaction among the large number of brain structures involved in the control of eye movements and attention is a striking example of how the brain can achieve a balance between reflexive (data-driven) and goal-orientated (knowledge-driven) behaviours. Different neural mechanisms come into play depending on whether the object of information selected for attentional processing is external (a current sensory stimulus) or internal (a representation of a previous stimulus). Right-sided frontal striatal dysfunction might be responsible for the specific impulsivity symptoms associated with ADHD, while the motor restlessness may reflect frontal lobe dysfunction due to impairment of the mesocortical dopamine system (Heilman, Voeller & Nadeau, 1991). There are cortico-striatal-nigro-thalamo-cortical loops that can activate other regions of the brain. These multiple, parallel, segregated loops link the basal ganglia with the cortex and constitute 'miniloops' that emanate from, and end in, a single cortical column or possible a small set of columns (Goldman-Rakic & Selemon, 1990). When these loops are disrupted, for whatever reason, they may inactivate remote areas that are anatomically quite distant (Voeller, 1991). This, in turn, could well be the cause of breakdown of control, both of attentional, eye movements and other motor control functions.

Many experimental studies (on animals, some in humans) support the notion of right hemisphere dysfunction in DAMP. Among these are the findings of inattention and defective response inhibition in adults with right-sided brain damage, 'neglect' of the left side in children with ADHD (Heilman et al., 1991), and the common finding in children with ADHD of a particular WISC-test profile (poor results on the arithmetic, comprehension, information and digit span subtests) believed to reflect right hemisphere dysfunction.

Several studies of monkeys have shown that certain subcortical structures (the caudate nucleus, substantia nigra, superior colliculus and thalamus) are crucially involved in the automatic regulation of eye movements and shifts of attention. If these structures are blocked in their action (such as occurs after the injection of a GABA agonist into the anatomic structure), reaction time is prolonged and the outward behavioural manifestation is inattention. Competition between left- and right-brain structures in the control of attention has also been well documented (Colby, 1991).

Some evidence for the crucial role played by subcortical midbrain structures in the pathogenesis of attention deficits and motor control problems in humans comes from the, unfortunately unreplicated, studies by Lou et al. (1984). Reduced blood flow in the caudate nucleus (and frontal cortex) was found in children with attention deficits and dysphasia.

Clinical course and outcome

The diagnosis of DAMP requires the presence of both attention and motor–perception dysfunction. There are also children with attention problems only and others who show motor–perception problems without attention deficits. According to one major Swedish study (Gillberg, & Gillberg, 1989b), there are about as many children with attention problems only as there are children with DAMP, who, in turn, are about twice as many as those with motor–perception dysfunction only. Follow-up studies suggest that it is the group of children with the combination of problems which requires treatment and interventions of various kinds and that the outcome for the other two groups, in broad terms, is relatively good. Also, the identification of 'pervasively hyperkinetic' children (Sandberg, Rutter & Taylor, 1978), as opposed to 'situationally hyperkinetic' children, has revealed that motor–perceptual and speech–language problems are almost universal in this group, which argues for the clinical separation of a diagnostic category with the combination of attention and motor–perceptual dysfunction, as distinct from groups with only one of the two types of dysfunction.

Situational attention deficit or hyperactivity can be a sign of psychological problems specific to a particular situation. Follow-up of children with situational as contrasted with pervasive hyperkinesis (Gillberg & Gillberg, 1988) has shown that outcome in the six-year perspective is much better and not too dissimilar to that of children without attention deficits of any kind.

Isolated motor–perceptual difficulties sometimes cause considerable academic problems, particularly during the first school years. Nevertheless, limited systematic follow-up and clinical experience suggest that, in this group also, outcome is usually considerably better than if there is the combination of attention problems and motor–perceptual difficulties.

In the following, reference will often be made to the longitudinal study of more than 100 children with DAMP (and comparison children without DAMP) examined from early childhood through age 20 years in the city of Göteborg, Sweden (e.g. Gillberg, I.C. 1987). However, the account also takes into consideration the considerable data bank which exists in neighbouring fields (e.g. Taylor, 1986).

The infant period

Retrospective analysis of case histories from children diagnosed as suffering from DAMP at age 4–6 years provides important clues to the clinical picture of DAMP in infancy.

There may be at least two clinically distinct subgroups within the DAMP group with respect to infant development: (1) the hyperactive group and (2) the hypo- or normoactive group.

The hyperactive group usually show sleep problems, feeding difficulties, 'colicky' stomach pains and a generally high level of motor activity even from the first months of life. They often start walking before 10 months of age. From that time on (and sometimes even before), parents often have to change their domestic habits dramatically: anything movable will have to be removed, not only from the level of the child's reach, but completely out of sight.

The infant hypoactive/normoactive group of children with DAMP often were suspected of a more negative prognosis. Their slowness was thought to indicate low IQ. These children are regarded by parents as 'good', sometimes even 'exceptionally good' infants. Some of them show repetitive behaviours from a very early age (head rolling, even head banging and repetitive sounds).

Some studies have tried to relate early visual recognition memory (VMR) to later cognitive functioning (Bornstein & Sigman, 1986). Convincing evidence is now accumulating that VMR may indeed be a potent predictor of later cognitive and academic success (Benasich & Bejar, 1992). Poor auditory temporal processing (i.e. poor performance on tests designed to monitor the ability to rapidly process changing non-verbal auditory stimuli) in children of about 6 months of age has been suggested to be related to later DAMP/dyslexia type problems (Benasich & Tallal, 1993). These experimental findings might well be closely linked to the inability/decreased ability to attend to relevant auditory stimuli (and sometimes visual stimuli) that is very often reported by parents of young children who later develop the full-blown clinical picture of DAMP, attention disorders without motor clumsiness and learning disorders, including so-called dyslexia.

The pre-school years

From about the age of starting to walk, the two subgroups, for a number of years, often appear to be indistinguishable from each other. Both appear hyperactive, or at least inattentive. Parents may worry because their children just do not seem to listen, and they have noticed that shouting may be the only way of attracting the children's attention. Motor coordination problems may surface already around age 2–4 years, but are often obscured by the high activity level and lack of appropriate fear, which is also very common. Speech and language is delayed in something like two-thirds of the cases, but only in about half of these is the delay severe enough to warrant consultation. Towards the end of the pre-school years, the child's 'unwillingness' to draw and paint and the constant clashes in games with age-peers usually become a major source of concern, but also of increasing scolding.

The early school years

Many children with DAMP can manage fairly well through infancy and the pre-school years but their behavioural and academic performance almost invariably deteriorate during the first few years at school. They are likely to have difficulties concentrating, sitting still, listening, interacting in an age-appropriate fashion with peers, participating in games and physical education and, sometimes almost insurmountable, difficulties acquiring basic automatic reading and writing skills. All of these problems peak in the 7–10 year-old age period in a vast majority of DAMP cases, and cause emotional upset in the child, parents and teachers. Problems will be especially difficult to cope with if information that the child is suffering from a handicapping condition (and not just a bad streak of naughtiness) has not been given to anyone involved.

If one identifies a DAMP group of children around age 6 years (as was done in the Göteborg studies), by definition all will have motor control problems, and all will have pervasive attention deficits. At around age 10 years, this same group of children will have motor difficulties only in about half the cases, and the attentional problems will also have subsided to a considerable degree. Unfortunately, however, psychiatric–behavioural problems will have increased from just over 60 to 80% and dyslexia/dysgraphia will be present in 80% of all cases. In a comparison group of age-peers without DAMP, these same rates will be at a very much lower level (Table 8.5.).

Pre-adolescence and adolescence

Many pre-adolescent and adolescent children with DAMP experience persistent difficulties concentrating. Many are described by their teachers (and sometimes parents) as daydreaming. Dyslexia is a very common complaint. The motor clumsiness is often (though not always) less conspicuous than it used to be. According to several studies by Hadders-Algra and her group, minor neurological dysfunction decreases with the onset of puberty, but that, in

Table 8.5. *Outcome in DAMP. Figures in brackets refer to age-matched population without DAMP*

| Area of dysfunction | Percentage showing dysfunction at age | | | |
	7	10 (years)	13	16
Attention/hyperkinesis	100(0)	45(4)	19(3)	–
Motor control	100(0)	55(4)	30(2)	36(5)
Perception/reading–writing	69(0)	76(16)	73(8)	74(5)
Psychiatric/behavioural	69(10)	81(20)	64(25)	64(11)
Specialist treatment	40(4)	50(4)	52(5)	70(5)
Accidents requiring hospital treatment	12(2)	–	–	25(5)

the subgroup whose dysfunction was believed to be caused by perinatal (rather than constitutional) factors, minor neurological dysfunction tended to persist (Hadders-Algra *et al.*, 1992; Soorani-Lunsing *et al.*, 1993). However, other follow-up studies have not provided support for this notion, but rather that minor neurological dysfunction may subside *before* puberty and not change much in adolescence (Hellgren *et al.*, 1993). There is a considerable risk for various types of psychiatric problems. Furthermore, if a child with DAMP attends a clinic for the first time in teenage, there is the very substantial risk that the psychiatric disorder is seen as primary and a 'new' problem, not specifically associated with DAMP. If this is the case, then the child's problems run the risk of not being put in a reasonable perspective and suggestions for intervention might well be inappropriate.

Psychiatric problems in DAMP

On the whole, one can discern three main groups of psychiatric problems in DAMP: (1) depression, (2) conduct disorders and (3) autistic traits. Quite often, there are other psychiatric problems as well, including anxiety and so called psychosomatic symptoms (headaches, gastrointestinal symptoms, etc.), but these do not appear to be more common than in the general population of children without DAMP (Gillberg, 1983).

Depression and feelings of low self-esteem are common already during the first school years, but appear to peak around age 10 years, when they often coincide with various kinds of conduct problems. The child with DAMP often becomes increasingly aware of his/her 'otherness' during the school years. Feeling that 'there is nobody to help', the child often becomes depressed and even contemplating suicide (which is decidedly uncommon in groups without DAMP). In the midst of depression there is also often much anger and resentment which may show outwardly as a clinical conduct disorder. The risk is then that the child's predicament is mistaken for 'antisocial problems with an outlook to psychopathy'. Personal interview alone with the child will soon reveal, however, that this is, usually, not a 'hardened' criminal-to-be, but rather an immature and sad child who needs to have his basic learning problems recognized. Nevertheless, there are also cases with DAMP and severe conduct problems who have a very gloomy outlook with respect to later antisocial activities including criminality (Thorley, 1984; Taylor *et al.*, 1991; Gillberg, 1992*b*).

The conduct problems encountered in DAMP can be of any kind; stealing, fire-setting, lying, bullying, running away from home and drug/alcohol abuse. In the pre-school years, there is often considerable aggression towards other children in connection with inadvertent disruption of play and games. About 10% of all

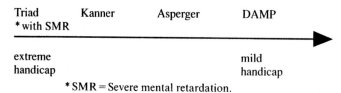

Fig. 8.2. Autism spectrum disorders.

children with DAMP show severe conduct disorders already on school entry. This figure
increases to about 50% at around age 10 years,
but seems to fall back to about 30% during the
teenage years.

In severe cases of DAMP, autistic features
are present in at least half the cases. These
comprise (a) motor stereotypies and stereotypic
activities including hand-flapping, finger-flic-
king, finger-picking, body rocking, head-bang-
ing, repetitive and monotonous production of
sounds (in an almost tic-like fashion), (b) preoccupations with certain topics, objects or parts
of objects, (c) peculiarities of language (pro-
noun reversal, repetitive questioning and
immaturities of grammar and poor sentence
structure), (d) abnormalities in the production
of speech (abnormalities of pitch and volume,
odd prosody and little speech or incessant questioning), (e) non-verbal communication
problems with a restricted repertoire of gesticu-
lation and mimicry, (f) occasionally the full-
blown clinical picture of semantic–pragmatic
disorder and (g) similar, but milder, social
interaction problems as in autism. 'Naïve'
forms of empathy deficits are often prominent,
children asking embarrassing questions of people they know in front of strangers, etc. Children with mild DAMP usually do not exhibit
major autistic type features. It is sometimes
impossible to make a clear distinction between
DAMP and Asperger syndrome (Gillberg &
Gillberg, 1989a; Ehlers & Gillberg, 1993). Very
occasionally, there is even a case for making a
diagnosis of autistic disorder in severe variants
of the DAMP syndrome, but the latter diagnosis should be made clinically only in those for
which the symptomatology is not better
accounted for by the term autistic disorder.

Gillberg and Gillberg (1989b) and Wing

(1991) have suggested that severe DAMP may
exist on a continuum with Wing's triad, Kanner
autism and Asperger syndrome (Fig. 8.2.).

In adolescence, there is a high rate of personality disorder, including a number of such disorders invariably involving social withdrawal
or negativism (paranoid, schizotypal, schizoid,
avoidant or obsessive-compulsive) (Hellgren et
al., 1994). It also appears that bipolar disorders
may emerge at a rate considerably higher than
in the general population.

Intervention and treatment

There is, of course, no one treatment for a
group of disorders as heterogeneous as those
belonging under the DAMP label.

A Swedish study of a representative group of
children receiving various kinds of intervention
at age 6–7 years (Gillberg I.C. et al., 1993),
suggested the positive effect of establishing a
diagnosis, and informing the child, parents and
teachers. Outcome in the three-year perspective
in matters relating to school adjustment and
achievement and behaviour both at school and
at home was better than for children who had
not received information about the diagnosis as
such (according to parental interview).

The most important part of any treatment
plan for a child with DAMP is the physical,
psychiatric and neuromotor/neuropsychologi-
cal examination followed by oral and written
information to parents, child, siblings and (in
collaboration with the family) teachers, about
the type of problems the child exhibits and their
possible aetiology. This usually alleviates some
of the feeling of self-blame which has been
experienced both by parents and children.
Secondary emotional problems tend to be minimized if information is given in this way.

Many children with DAMP need special education measures. Most need individualized education some hours every day (i.e. they need to be alone, or almost alone, with one teacher) in order to be able to acquire new academic skills. A minority need special physical education or the help of a physiotherapist. Most importantly, the physical education teacher has to be informed about the child's handicap so as not to scapegoat him/her in an unnecessary, often quite unwitting, way.

The vast majority of children with DAMP face severe problems acquiring reading and writing skills and in maintaining an academic achievement level appropriate to their overall IQ-level (e.g. Gillberg, I.C. 1987). They may need all sorts of particular attention and intervention measures to remedy these 'dyslexia-associated' problems. Specific programmes for this type of problems are sometimes available in local schools, and some of the essential features of such programmes should be included in all intervention plans for children with the extremely common combination of DAMP and dyslexia (see below in the section on dyslexia, dysgraphia and dyscalculia).

Some children with DAMP should be tried on stimulants (Taylor, 1986). Both D-amphetamine (10–40 mg/day given in two to three doses with three-hour intervals in order to last through the school day) and methylphenidate (40–200 mg/day given in the same fashion) have been shown to be very effective in the amelioration of hyperactivity, concentration difficulties, some learning problems, feelings of low self-esteem and family interaction problems (Barkley, 1990). Both drugs have also been shown to be relatively free of major side effects. Relatively common side effects are loss of appetite, a tendency, questioned by many, to increase the likelihood of tics in DAMP, reduced mimicry, and ultimate height decreased by 1 cm if treatment is continued throughout puberty. The risk for increasing doses and developing drug dependence and abuse appears to be non-existent. Side effects are much less pronounced than with the commonly used tricyclic antidepressants. The risk of provoking epileptic seizures is small, particularly with amphetamine. Nevertheless, pres-

cribing stimulants to children is a delicate matter (Taylor *et al.*, 1991). Therefore, and perhaps also because the possible long-term benefits of using stimulants have been poorly examined, stimulant treatment should be selected only for children with very severe DAMP problems and no major psychosocial problems. Stimulants should never be given as the only mode of treatment!

Various motor training programmes have not been documented to have a lasting effect on the overall clinical problems associated with DAMP. For most children with DAMP, the motor coordination problems are those with the best prognosis, even without treatment. Therefore, it seems unwise to focus too much energy on this domain. In the long term (see below), problems associated with reading and writing are the most handicapping, and every effort should therefore be spent on trying to reverse the negative development in this field.

Long-term follow-up

In early adult life, it appears that quite a few of those who once had DAMP have overcome most or all of the severe problems. Nevertheless, at least about half of all cases have severe persisting problems of one or other kind. Criminal offences seem to be common as do major psychiatric problems requiring in- or outpatient psychiatric treatment. Even among the many who outwardly appear to be doing relatively well, low self-esteem is common.

Severe dyslexia, quite uncommon in adult age in those who never had DAMP, is possibly present in 30–50% of all cases. Even though the motor control problems appear to have the best prognosis of all, a substantial minority (probably about 1 in 5) continue to have important problems with motor clumsiness well into adult age.

The hyperkinetic syndrome

In the Isle of Wight population study in the 1960s, the 'pure' hyperkinetic syndrome was encountered in less than 1 in 2000 10–11 year-olds without 'neuro-epileptic' disorders attending normal schools (Rutter, Graham & Yule, 1970). In marked contrast, 7% of all children with 'neuro-epileptic' disorders and children excluded from school because of severe mental subnormality were considered to suffer from a hyperkinetic syndrome. The notion that hyperkinesis is extremely uncommon has lingered in Europe, in spite of the fact that in the US several per cent of all school children were described as hyperactive/hyperkinetic (Wender, 1971). It was not until the early 1980s, when a re-analysis of the Isle of Wight material revealed that about 2% of the population showed hyperactive behaviour both at home and at school, that it became more accepted that hyperactivity, even pervasive forms, is a common problem in school age children. Up until then, European children tended to be diagnosed as hyperactive/hyperkinetic only if hyperactivity was their only (or at least main problem). In clinical practice there is very often overlap between hyperactivity/attention problems and conduct disorders. It is now becoming more common to make dual and triple diagnoses in child psychiatry. As a consequence, rates of hyperkinetic syndromes reported from Europe and the US are no longer so extremely discrepant. Nevertheless, there does still appear to be a difference, which it is more difficult to account for.

The concept of hyperactivity has become linked with attention deficit. It is not yet clear that attention deficit underlies hyperactivity in the majority of the cases. Attention deficits are quite often associated with normoactive behaviours, hypoactivity and fluctuating degrees of activity. The hyperkinetic syndrome as a disorder of pervasive behaviour problems (Taylor et al., 1991) has come a long way from its anecdotal and flimsical status 20 years ago. It is not yet anywhere near the status of other child psychiatric diagnoses such as anorexia nervosa, elective mutism, school refusal or autism as far as distinctiveness, reliability and validity are concerned. It is possible that, in the next ten years, pervasive hyperkinesis may emerge as a distinct clinical entity. However, it does not appear to be the umbrella term needed in the field of DAMP.

In the US literature, attention deficits (ADD and ADHD) have become broad, inclusive terms comprising a very large proportion of the child population showing disruptive and oppositional–defiant behaviours (Barkley, 1990).

Stimulant treatment (see above) is often recommended for the treatment of hyperkinetic syndromes. Such treatment should, in the opinion of the author, be reserved for very specific cases with severe DAMP, who also meet criteria for severe ADHD and additional requirements (such as educational and behavioural interventions having failed to produce optimal gains), and should never be seen as the solution to the 'problem of hyperactivity in childhood'.

Dyslexia, dysgraphia and dyscalculia

Dyslexia, regardless of associated problems, constitutes one of the most challenging problems in child neuropsychiatry in that it constitutes an invisible handicapping condition with far-reaching consequences for the emotional well-being of the individual affected.

Prevalence

At least 5–10% of a school age population of children are affected by dyslexia/dysgraphia. In a UK study, 4% had 'specific reading difficulties' and another 2% had such problems plus 'specific arithmetic difficulties'. The figures are likely to be somewhat, though not much, lower in the adult population. The male:female ratio is similar to that in most neuropsychiatric disorders of childhood, i.e. 2–4:1 in different studies.

Definitions and overlap with other neuropsychiatric problems

Dyslexia – 'reading disorder' according to the DSM-IV (APA, 1994) – and dysgraphia – 'disorder of written expression' according to the DSM-IV – are often collectively referred to as dyslexia, which is quite inadequate, considering that spelling and other writing problems do not necessarily overlap with reading problems and vice versa. Also, one twin study (Stevenson *et al.*, 1987) suggests that spelling problems may have a considerably stronger genetic load than reading backwardness, which would be a point in favour of keeping reading and spelling problems as two separate conditions. (However, one of the reasons for a failure to document a strong genetic component in reading as compared with spelling problems, in that twin study, could be the mean age of the twins (early adolescence), leading to spelling problems being the most obvious outward sign of a common underlying dyslexia/dysgraphia disorder which would have shown in the early school years as clear outward reading problems as well, see also below). Nevertheless, the two are usually treated as one, and it is, of course, very common for the two to occur together. Dyscalculia – 'mathematics disorder' according to the DSM-IV is sometimes, though probably less frequently, associated with dyslexia. Dyscalculia and dyslexia often seem to constitute separate conditions. One study demonstrated the strong correlation of DAMP problems with dyscalculia but not with dyslexia (Rosenberger, 1989).

Dyslexia (and dysgraphia) very often develop during the school years in children diagnosed as suffering from DAMP. Such children, in turn, have very often shown early language delays and speech and language abnormalities before the whole 'syndrome' of DAMP developed. Extrapolating from the results of the Göteborg studies, it would appear that almost half of all children with severe dyslexia have a DAMP background. Of children still showing severe dyslexic/dysgraphic problems in early teenage, the majority had DAMP diagnosed already in the pre-school period. Clinical experience indicates that the true number of children with dyslexia/dysgraphia/dyscalculia who also have attention–motor–perception problems may be even greater, and that it is quite uncommon for a child to have isolated dyslexia/dysgraphia/dyscalculia without associated attention–motor problems.

Phonological awareness problems are believed to be a precursor of dyslexia in a majority of all cases (Lundberg, Olofsson & Wall, 1980; Höjen & Lundberg, 1990). However, it is clear that dyslexia is not always a 'pure culture' disorder affecting only one aspect of brain functioning. Very often there are associated visuo-motor problems (see above in relation to DAMP), problems of visual orientation in space (leading to spelling and writing problems, for instance, because the child does not automatically know where to start writing a particular letter; at the bottom, the top or 'in the middle') and even (albeit of controversial significance) oculomotor dysfunction).

Dyslexia (or specific reading retardation) is often defined as a reading level two years below grade (or below the level expected on the basis of IQ results). It is extraordinary that this illogical definition has managed to survive almost uncriticized. It goes without saying that being two years behind at age 7 is very different (minus 29%) from being two years behind at age 13 (minus 15%) years.

The only more reasonable way of defining dyslexia would be on the basis of some sort of quotient conceptually similar to that used in defining overall intelligence. For instance, a 'reading quotient' more than 20 (or 30) points below that expected on the basis of general IQ, might be one possible definition. However, even such definitions have their critics. Stanovich (1994) concludes that the evidence for a distinct cause of a reading disorder defined by the degree of reading – IQ discrepancy is scant. He proposes that the reading disabilities field must seriously consider whether the term is not best dispensed with.

Another important diagnostic issue is whether to relate the reading problems to full-scale IQ or to performance IQ only. It is self-evident that, if verbal IQ measures are included in the basis for assigning IQ level in a child with dyslexia, the level is likely to be lower than if only non-verbal subtests are included.

Pathogenetic factors

Most recent authors in the field regard dyslexia as a biological/developmental problem. Nevertheless, a number of studies have demonstrated a relationship between dyslexia, on the one hand, and low socioeconomic status and being later born in a large sibship, on the other. These associations most likely reflect both genetic and environmental influences (Rutter & Madge, 1976). Dyslexia, like DAMP, tends to cluster in families and this has been taken as evidence for a genetic model. It seems indisputable that many cases of dyslexia are 'purely' genetic in the sense that they run in families and affect large numbers of family members on different branches of the family tree. However, some of the tendency for dyslexia to run in families could be accounted for by certain social factors (Stevenson *et al.*, 1984, 1987), such as low availability of books, and low interest in reading in the parents and siblings.

Spelling disability appears to be particularly associated with genetic factors in young adolescents (Stevenson & Graham, 1993). In adolescence, spelling disability is often the only clear 'outward' remnant of a phonological processing disorder (Lundberg *et al.*, 1980; Bryant *et al.*, 1989), which may be predictive of, and show as, language delay and articulation disorder in preschool age, and as dyslexia (with reading delay, slow reading and reading comprehension problems) in the early school years. Thus, dyslexia may only be found to correlate with genetic factors in the 7–11 year-old age-range (Pennington, 1990). The failure to reproduce this finding in adolescence should not be taken to mean that dyslexia does not have genetic roots. To the contrary, the persistence of spelling disability, and its strong link with genetic factors, provides further support for genetic mechanisms in dyslexia.

A very thought-provoking study was recently published by Stevenson and Graham (1993). They studied a general population sample of 213 pairs of 13 year-old same-sex twins. The rate of co-morbidity of specific spelling retardation and antisocial behaviour was almost 2.5 times greater than expected by chance alone. The heritability of spelling disability was shown to be high whilst that for antisocial behaviour was not. Co-morbidity of the two types of problem could not be accounted for by a common genetic factor, nor with either condition leading to the other. However, further refinement of the analyses suggested that the co-morbidity arose as a result of genetic factors leading to spelling disability being associated with environmental factors leading to antisocial behaviour. The most likely mechanism was suggested to be one whereby fathers genetically predisposed to spelling disability genetically transmit this disability while, at the same time in certain cases creating an environment leading to antisocial behaviour in their children.

During the late 1980s, a number of different studies (brain autopsies and magnetic resonance *in vivo* imaging) suggested that abnormalities of corticogenesis (microdysgenesis, microhamartomata) in the planum temporale of the brain might be specifically associated with dyslexia (Galaburda *et al.*, 1985; Hynd *et al.*, 1990). Several of the findings (including the absence of normal asymmetry, left hemisphere considerably larger than the right, in the region of planum temporale) are in need of replication before firm conclusions can be drawn in this field. It is interesting to note that children with focal epilepsies attending normal schools have poorer reading skills than those without epilepsy (Stores & Hart, 1976).

Dyscalculia

Dyscalculia ('developmental dyscalculia', 'specific arithmetic difficulties', or 'mathematical disorder' according to the DSM-IV) can occur singly, or in combination with other learning disorders, including dyslexia and DAMP. If a child suffers from isolated dyscalculia (and hence does not show signs of other learning disorders), he/she may well not be referred for assessment because such a disability is more socially acceptable than dyslexia. It is not considered to be (or be associated with/lead to) a severe educational (or emotional) people. As has been pointed out by Gordon (1992), people will often say, even with a degree of pride: 'I was never any good at maths'.

It has been estimated that about 6% of school-age children may have serious problems with arithmetic (Badian & Ghublikan, 1982). A more recent study (from the UK) showed a prevalence of 1.3% specific arithmetic difficulties plus 2.3% arithmetic and reading difficulties among 9–10 year-olds (Lewis, Hitch & Walker, 1994). Boy:girl ratios appear to be about 1:1 in dyscalculia.

Several different types of dyscalculia may exist (Badian, 1983). There is considerable evidence for the presence of at least one of these, i.e. spatial dyscalculia. Oral mathematics and numerical reasoning may be less impaired, indeed well functioning, and the main problems arise in written arithmetics with horizontal and vertical confusion. There is often disorganisation when arranging rows and columns of figures. Individuals suffering from this type of spatial dyscalculia often have great difficulty telling the time. They confuse the hands of the clock and often also seem to have a poor internal sense of time. On the digit span test of the WISC, they often have the most problems with numbering digits backwards. Clinical experience suggests that this type of spatial dyscalculia may be particularly common in Asperger syndrome.

A particular form of dyslexia for numbers also probably exists with syntactical difficulties relating to numbers. Children affected tend to reverse the position of numbers and add extra zeros which, in turn, impairs their skills in arithmetic.

Dysarithmetica involves mixing up the procedures involved in addition, subtraction and multiplication. There are also problems of memory.

Children with DAMP and ADHD often exhibit attention-sequential dyscalculia, in which there is difficulty learning and recalling multiplication tables and putting decimal points in the right place.

Mixed types of dyscalculia are probably common, but the evidence is very limited.

Right hemisphere dysfunction has been suggested to be important in dyscalculia. There is certainly indirect support for its association with spatial dyscalculia, given the localization of some spatial abilities to the right hemisphere and the high rate of impaired visual attention to exact detail in many cases of dyscalculia (Badian, 1983). In a study by Rourke and Finlayson (1978) 9 to 14 year-old children were studied. Three groups were included: (1) overall learning disabled, (2) better in arithmetic than reading and spelling and (3) poor arithmetic skills in spite of good reading and spelling. The third group had considerably more problems with visuo-perceptual and visuo-spatial skills than the first two, who, in turn, showed poorer performance on verbal and auditory-perceptual abilities.

Verbal and other left-hemisphere skills may also be important in dyscalculia. For instance, the dyslexic child with low reading speed and comprehension problems will have a major problem achieving in arithmetic in spite of, perhaps, superior understanding in arithmetic.

It is essential that the problem of dyscalculia be recognized in the work-up of children with learning disorders, regardless of whether there are several or isolated problems in the field of arithmetic.

It is only recently that the social characteristics of some individuals with dyscalculia have attracted attention. As mentioned in the foregoing, individuals with Asperger syndrome often have isolated academic problems in arithmetics. Some young people with Tourette syndrome have similar problems (Comings, 1990). Individuals with the fragile X syndrome often exhibit severe specific difficulties with arithmetic. Weintraub and Mesulam (1983) have described a syndrome of right hemisphere dysfunction which is particularly interesting as it suggests links between all of the mentioned disorders. Affected children are reported to suffer from problems with mathematics and visuo-spatial disturbances, shyness, emotional and interpersonal difficulties, poor eye-contact, absence of gesture and deficient speech prosody. In addition, there may be right–left confusion, poor sense of direction and difficulty with motor tasks, including learning to ride a bicycle. Social maturity is said to be very low.

Management

Various approaches to the remediation of dyslexia and dysgraphia (less in the field of dyscalculia) have been suggested. No approach that did not focus on the training of such skills *per se* has been shown to be reliably effective so far. An almost unbelievable array of claims regarding the efficacy of various programmes have been made, but the fact remains that, in order to achieve better reading and writing skills, reading and writing have to be trained. Several studies have demonstrated that, if parents of pre-school children can be encouraged to listen to their children reading on a regular basis, this has some preventative effect on the development of reading problems.

Enhancing phonemic analysis and increasing phonemic awareness, including increasing the speed of reading nonsense phonemes, all appear to increase reading skills (Williams, 1980; Richardson, 1984; Bradley & Bryant, 1985; Lundberg, Frost & Petersen, 1988; Hurford, 1990). A pre-school training programme, consisting of exercises of phonemic awareness and preliminary grapheme-phoneme conversions on a two-letter syllable level, for children with specific language impairments (who are generally at risk for developing specific reading problems/dyslexia) has been shown to be quite effective in preventing severe dyslexic problems, at least during the first school year (Korkman & Peltomaa, 1991).

It would seem that, on the basis of the considerable evidence favouring phonemic/ phonological awareness training in language- and reading-disordered children, such intervention should be made available to all pre-school and school children who can be demonstrated on testing to have, in addition to language and/ or reading/writing problems, specific problems in the field of auditory phonological awareness.

Computer-based reading and spelling programmes are valuable aids for many children with dyslexia/dysgraphia. Computers as such have the added advantage of allowing the dysgraphic child to have as 'beautiful' a written output (on the screen or on the printed paper) as the child without dysgraphia. Also, computers do not take offence (like teachers and parents can) when the child makes mistakes, which makes 'interactions' less emotionally stressful.

The interest in pharmacological approaches to the treatment of dyslexia has recently increased with the advent of studies of piracetam (derived from GABA) in children with dyslexia (e.g. Tallal et al., 1986; Wilsher et al., 1987). Even before that, limited benefits of stimulant medication (in combination with reading remediation) had been reported (Gittelman, Klein & Feingold, 1983), but the effects appeared to be more on attention problems than on reading as such. Piracetam, on the other hand, seems to have a modest, but clear, positive effect on reading skills in many children with dyslexia regardless of associated attention problems. The mechanism of action is unknown, but limited neuropsychological evidence seems to point to an enhancement of certain left cortical hemisphere abilities. The drug is exceptionally well tolerated in most cases (Wilsher & Taylor, 1994). So far, in many countries, piracetam has not been registered for the treatment of dyslexia, but it appears to hold promise, and may eventually come to be included as an adjunct in the multifaceted management of severe dyslexia. The amount of gain in reading skills to expected with piracetam medication is not large enough to make remedial education unnecessary. In no way does such pharmacological treatment constitute a 'cure'.

Outcome

Bearing the reservations about definitions and delineation from other disorders in mind, it is clear that dyslexia has a tendency to become chronic. Even though there is, with appropriate remediation, usually a gradual amelioration of some of the most severe reading and writing problems, many dyslexic children become slow readers and poor spellers in adult life. Dyslexia is often associated with an increase in behaviour problems which can lead to a poor psychosocial adjustment. In a review of the best follow-up studies in the field, Schonaut and Satz (1983) concluded that outcome in dyslexia is variable, but poor, in respect of reading skills and psychosocial adjustment.

The Swedish DAMP studies suggested that there may be a very strong correlation between the development of psychiatric disorder in DAMP and the appearance of reading and spelling problems (Hellgren et al., 1994): once reading problems developed in DAMP, psychiatric disorder increased in prevalence and severity, and was closely linked to the further development of the reading and spelling problems as such.

Hyperlexia

Hyperlexia, a term first used by Silberberg and Silberberg (1967), is by some regarded as a specific variant of dyslexia. Others consider it to be on the opposite end of a spectrum of proficiencies in reading ability, dyslexia representing the lowermost and hyperlexia the uppermost portions of this spectrum of normally distributed skills. Yet other authors regard hyperlexia as a specific symptom of the 'savant' syndrome (see Chapter 6) or even of autistic disorder (Patti & Lupinetti, 1993). Hyperlexia in children refers to a highly developed word recognition skill in the presence of little or no comprehension of the words recognized. Similar to the findings in dyslexia, some hyperlexic children respond better to visual configurations of printed letters than to their phonetic constructions (Cobrinik, 1982). The frequent co-occurrence of autism (a disorder with severe language impairment) and hyperlexia (with its connotations of, at least superficially, excellent language skills) indirectly suggests the taking over of certain cognitive functions by the right side of the brain. When exceptional reading ability is coupled with overall cognitive superiority, hyperlexia should not be diagnosed and should definitely not be seen as a pathological trait. Nevertheless, even in individuals with this combination of assets, motor coordination problems and hypotonia may be common and antedate the development of a personality profile typical of Asperger syndrome (Gillberg 1989, 1991a). Thus, extremely early development of lexical skills should always prompt the search for autistic type symptomatology.

Speech and language disorders

Disorders of speech and language are part of all severe DAMP syndromes and are very common generally in children with perceptual–motor–attention deficits. In fact, delayed language development and other disorders of speech are among the most common early signs that the child might be at risk for the development of neuropsychiatric or psychological problems (Richman, Stevenson & Graham, 1982). There is also a very strong correlation between speech–language problems in early childhood and dyslexia/dysgraphia in school-age. Thus, the trajectory is often one of DAMP showing in early life as language delay (with or without significant behaviour problems), later as abnormalities of speech production, motor clumsiness and attention problems and in school-age as behaviour problems, dyslexia and other learning problems.

Prevalence

Abnormalities of speech and language development are very common. They affect several per cent of children in the 3–6-year-old age range, the prevalence varying as a consequence of the definition used.

Sex ratios

Boys are much more frequently affected than girls, at ratios of 2:1 to 4:1 (Shriberg *et al.*, 1986; Silva, 1987; Robinson, 1991). However, it is difficult to determine whether this much higher rate in boys only reflects higher rates of pathology in boys (as compared with boys) than in girls (as compared with girls) or whether our standards for normal language development tend to be based on the norm for girls (or possibly girls and boys combined).

This presentation, after reviewing some of the possible mechanisms underlying language and speech disorders, will briefly survey a few problem areas, i.e. developmental language delay (isolated), stuttering, abnormalities of pitch, semantic–pragmatic disorder and Landau–Kleffner syndrome.

Pathogenetic mechanisms

There is, of course, no single and simple explanation for all language and speech deficits encountered in children and adolescents. There is not only a variety of possible causes; more than one factor often appears to operate in the individual child. Furthermore, the causes of, for instance stuttering and semantic pragmatic disorders, although possibly overlapping to some extent, are likely to be different in many cases.

Robinson (1991) recently summarized the background factors in a series of 82 7–13 year-old children with severe and persistent 'specific' speech and language disorders. He, like all other authors in the field, found a male excess (of 3.8:1) and familial loading (siblings of language disordered children having a language disorder in 19%). He also found a high rate (about one-quarter) of associated medical disorders (including Klinefelter syndrome in 5% of the boys), seizures (21%), left-handedness (29%), clumsiness (90%) and late walking (18%). Interestingly, there was also a higher than expected rate of twinning. All of these findings are closely parallel to those published by Steffenburg (1991) in the field of autism. Even the increased rate of twinning has been suggested to be associated with autism (Gillberg *et al.*, 1991). Robinson also found a higher than expected rate of male siblings, a finding supported by Gillberg, Gillberg & Steffenberg (1992) in DAMP (a 'disorder' comprising speech–language problems, clumsiness and attention deficits). This could suggest the operation of immunoreactive factors, male foetuses being antigenetically more dissimilar to the mother than female foetuses, thus provoking an attack on the brain which could lead to neuro-developmental problems including language disorders (Gualtieri & Hicks, 1985).

There is some evidence of lower regional cerebral blood flow in the left temporofrontal region in children with developmental language disorders (Lou *et al.*, 1990*a*, *b*). This, and the findings from Robinson's study, suggest that interference with normal cerebral lateralization may be important in disorders involving language and speech. The hypothesis advanced by Geschwind and Galaburda (1985*a*, *b*, *c*) may be relevant in this context. This hypothesis is briefly summarized here. Most individuals have asymmetry of brain structure and function dating from foetal life. The left hemisphere is pre-

programmed to handle language and some fine motor skills. Genetic and intra-uterine (including testosterone) influences probably underlie this specialization of the left hemisphere. The left hemisphere, because of the influence of testosterone, matures more slowly in *utero* than the right, and this is possibly more marked in the male (Taylor, 1969). The brain is more vulnerable to noxious agents during maturation, and the more slowly maturing left hemisphere is therefore vulnerable for longer than the right (and particularly in males). Genetic, or other, factors which either contribute to further slowing of left hemisphere development or damage it in the process of maturation may cause any of: (1) 'anomalous' cerebral dominance, with or without left-handedness, (2) specific disorders of language, and (3) other neurological abnormalities including fine motor problems, delayed motor milestones and epilepsy.

An extensive literature exists on the types of difficulties encountered by these individuals, but only a small body of work has been published that deals with psychological and biological models that explain language (and speech) impairments in terms of impairment in particular aspects of cognitive processing or biological functioning. According to Bishop (1992), there are at least six different models that have been developed to account for the development of specific language impairment: (1) output problems in children who have normal underlying linguistic competence, (2) auditory perception problems which influence the course of language acquisition, (3) isolated impairment of specific linguistic mechanisms, (4) conceptual problems that impinge on, but is not restricted to, language processing, (5) learning strategies are deficient and (6) reduction of speed and capacity of the information-processing system. According to Bishop, there is considerable evidence that (2) auditory perception problems are common in language impaired children. There is also evidence of (6) limited processing capacity. Bishop argues that the fundamental deficit in specific language impairment could be a slowed rate of information-processing and that this could lead to dysfunction in any task requiring processing/integration of rapidly presented information. Processing of auditory stimuli would then be more obviously impaired because of the brief and sequential nature of auditory stimuli. Visual processing would not be as obviously affected because of the more persistent nature of visual stimuli. Thus the underlying problem is not restricted to auditory perception, but it leads to disproportionately negative effects on the processing and integration of auditory/language stimuli compared to those in other modalities.

Developmental language delay including expressive language disorder, mixed receptive–expressive language disorder and phonological disorder

Developmental language delay is often treated as a separate diagnostic category, clearly different from autistic-like conditions, DAMP and behaviour problems. It is said to occur in about 1 in 2000 children and to affect expressive rather than receptive language skills. However, the available evidence runs counter to this notion of an isolated syndrome of specific expressive developmental language delay. In fact, almost all studies which have included behavioural/psychiatric measures as well as aspects of language development have shown that there is a very strong correlation between 'isolated' language delay and all sorts of rather severe behavioural problems, including autistic traits, elective mutism, aggression and other conduct problems (Cantwell & Baker, 1985). Also, the receptive language problems of children diagnosed as suffering from expressive delay have often been sadly neglected. Finally, the language delay is usually associated with other developmental delays, including phonological/articulation dysfunction and DAMP problems as well. Therefore, before making a diagnosis of isolated developmental language delay, considerable caution is warranted.

Stuttering

Stuttering involves the outbursts of repetitions of consonants and word-blocking. It usually starts around 3–4 years of age. Most children show some degree of sound/word production reminiscent of stuttering, but only about 3% (4% of boys and 2% of girls) have problems which take on a clinical dimension (Barker, 1979; Graham, 1986). The course is often chronic even though the problems for most affected children tend to diminish with age. Stuttering is thought to be genetic in origin. It is not specifically associated with psychiatric problems, either in the individual or in the family, but, in severe forms, it does lead to great anxiety and distress.

Stuttering is managed differently from one clinic to another. Most children who stutter do not need any kind of treatment other than encouragement to ignore the stuttering as such. Parents and siblings need to be informed at some length regarding the devastating emotional effects that can come from being teased mercilessly for many years. In severe cases, it is often helpful to advise the child to tell other people about the stuttering (before they have started to tease or react negatively in other ways).

Various psychological techniques (including bio-feedback) have been used, but the effectiveness has yet to be demonstrated.

Occasionally, Tourette syndrome can present as stuttering. This will be evident if gradually more severe motor and vocal tics emerge. However, one must also keep in mind the possibility that someone who stutters, and wants to control the stuttering, can develop facial movements which can be misinterpreted as grimaces or tics.

Abnormalities of pitch and volume

The reason for including a special small section on abnormalities of pitch in this text is that it is a very common symptom in child neuropsychiatry and one that is usually overlooked. Abnormalities of pitch do not constitute a special subclass of disorders, but should be thought of as a possible lead to other syndromes, and as a symptom which might be important in the management of some behaviour problems in childhood.

The inability to adjust the tone or volume of voice to varying circumstances is typical of many children with DAMP, autism, autistic-like conditions (including Asperger syndrome) and semantic pragmatic disorder (see following section). Many children with DAMP have a monotonous, rather too loud voice, which can cause considerable irritation at dinner tables or in classroom settings. Verbal children with autism and those with Asperger syndrome almost invariably exhibit abnormalities of pitch, such as exaggerated shrillness, half-whispering huskiness, etc., usually in the context of a monotonous speech production.

Some of these abnormalities may reflect motor coordination problems in the larynx, whereas others are possibly caused by auditory feedback difficulties leading to problems in the timing of adjusting level of voice to the prevailing situation. In still other cases, more fundamental deficits in the understanding of the meaning of spoken language for communication could underlie the problems in regulating pitch.

Semantic–pragmatic disorders

Disorders of semantics and pragmatics have only recently come to the attention of doctors and speech therapists. Their boundaries are not yet clear, and there are currently no good tests available for establishing a clear diagnosis. Clinical experience has not yet reached a sufficient level of sophistication to allow even the suggestion of operationalized diagnostic criteria. In spite of this, it is already quite clear that semantic–pragmatic disorder(s) will be an important sub-branch of child neuropsychiatry research and clinical activity in the coming 10 years.

Some children have specific difficulties applying the rules of grammar when interacting with other people. They may rely too heavily on certain grammatical rules. Others may seem to ignore such rules to the extent that their language becomes very self-centered. They may have mild, moderate or severe problems in producing readily comprehensible spoken sentences. These are children with semantic problems.

Some children have specific problems in applying their sometimes excellent language skills in situations of social interaction. They may sound 'more like a book than a human being' as one teacher put it. They more often initiate conversation than respond to or acknowledge the interlocutor (Bishop, Hartley & Weir, 1994). They may ask endless questions and sometimes upset the persons being asked by giving evidence that they know all the answers. One of the reasons for their asking these questions about things they already know about is that they cannot divine that other people might know things that they themselves do not know anything about. Because of this they will not be able to formulate questions suitable for unknown answers.

Many children have both semantic and pragmatic problems. On closer inspection, such children will often demonstrate severe problems comprehending spoken language. These same children may have less (or indeed no) problems comprehending a written text.

Recently, many clinicians and researchers have become increasingly concerned with the distinction of semantic–pragmatic disorder (Rapin & Allen, 1983; Lister-Brook & Bowler, 1992; Bishop, Hartley & Weir, 1994) from Asperger syndrome (Bishop, 1989). It is obvious that the two very often overlap. The two outstanding questions are: (1) are there Asperger persons without semantic–pragmatic disorder and (2) are there persons with semantic–pragmatic disorders without other symptoms of Asperger syndrome? Given the kinds of definition for Asperger syndrome currently in use, it seems unlikely that Asperger syndrome could exist without, at the very least, severe pragmatic problems. However, the second issue has not been resolved. Given the enormous importance in social interaction of being able to use language for smooth communication, it would seem likely that most children with semantic–pragmatic disorder would show at least some signs of social interaction problems, even if not filling criteria for Asperger syndrome.

In treatment of semantic–pragmatic disorder one has to take into account the full clinical picture of possible associated behavioural difficulties and social oddities. Role-play and video-taped sessions with 'play-back feed-back' are currently used in some centres, but it is yet too early to decide their efficacy as specific treatment tools.

Acquired aphasia with EEG abnormalities

Landau–Kleffner syndrome

The Landau–Kleffner syndrome is an uncommon disorder of language and speech which often (always?) coincides with social and developmental abnormalities reminiscent of those encountered in autism, and for which a case can often be made to diagnose childhood disintegrative disorder. It is often seen first by speech pathology therapists which may account for its inclusion among speech- and language disorders rather than autism and autism spectrum problems. An alternative explanation may be that boys referred to child psychiatrists are likely to be diagnosed with childhood disintegrative disorder, and that girls and boys referred to phoniatric departments or neuropediatricians are more likely to be given a diagnosis of Landau–Kleffner syndrome.

Prevalence

Its prevalence is not known. It is uncommon, but occurs often enough for a diagnosis to be made with some regularity in a child neuropsychiatric clinic admitting about 300 new cases each year.

Sex ratios

In the author's experience, Landau–Kleffner syndrome has been more commonly diagnosed in girls, but this could be an artefact of boys with a similar/identical disorder being given diagnoses of Heller syndrome.

Behavioural and physical phenotype

The onset of Landau–Kleffner syndrome ('acquired aphasia', 'epileptic aphasia') is usually at age 3–5 (–9) years and is relatively abrupt (though occasionally more gradual).

Aphasia (usually ushered in by receptive problems (mainly in the domain of verbal auditory discrimination), then quickly followed by expressive difficulties) after normal or almost normal language development in association with typical EEG abnormalities (spike foci in the posterior temporal and parietal regions, usually bilateral, asynchronous with a left-sided predominance; sometimes the EEG changes take on the shape of continuous spike-wave discharges during slow sleep, also referred to as ESESS (electrical status epilepticus of slow sleep), and characterized by the presence of diffuse bilateral slow (<2 Hz) spike-wave complexes that occupy more than 85% of the slow sleep time (Tassinari et al., 1985)) are the hallmarks of the disorder. It has a doubtful prognosis, even though, after the first several weeks–months after onset, it usually becomes 'quiet' and does not lead to further regression. Clinical epilepsy may, or may not, be associated with the disorder. It has been reported that about 80% of children have convulsive seizures (Aicardi, 1992).

Emotional and behavioural symptoms are the rule. Some of these can be seen as anxiety reactions in a child suddenly bereft of the understanding of spoken language. In other instances, some of the symptoms are reminiscent of those seen in typical autism cases.

The Landau–Kleffner syndrome is highly heterogeneous (Deonna et al., 1977). Occasionally, one comes across the type of child who could be said to fit both the criteria for childhood disintegrative disorder (Heller dementia) and Landau–Kleffner syndrome (Nass, Heier & Walker, 1993). In still other instances, the onset of major epileptic seizures can be so dramatic as to conceal the gradual emergence of a typical Landau–Kleffner syndrome.

No specific physical abnormalities or characteristics of children with Landau Kleffner syndrome have been reported to date.

Diagnosis

The diagnosis is made on the basis of (1) a typical history of normal or almost normal development (including normal language development) followed by (2) a relatively abrupt loss of expressive language skills, which is usually later found to have followed (3) a prodromal stage of verbal discrimination receptive language problems; (4) typical EEG changes are documented at EEG examination and epileptic seizures may or may not ensue (occasionally they may be the first obvious sign that the child is developing abnormally).

Pathogenesis

The pathogenesis of Landau–Kleffner syndrome is unknown. The disorder appears to be sporadic and no known genetic influences have been documented to date. However, this possible background factor has not been well examined in previous research into the mechanisms underlying the disorder, and so no definitive conclusions may be drawn. The EEG changes have been thought to reflect severe underlying brain dysfunction, which, in turn have been assumed to cause the language and socioemotional abnormalities. These hypotheses have led to the attempt to surgically treat patients with the disorder by multiple bilateral temporal transections (Morrell, Whisler & Bleck, 1989).

Work-up

Several EEGs should be performed (including during sleep) over a period of six to twelve months once a diagnosis of Landau–Kleffner syndrome has been made. A full neuropsychological work-up including an IQ-test and several language tests as well as taped and videotaped recordings of spoken language and social and communicative interactions should be obtained at first presentation and at yearly follow-ups in order to monitor regressions and positive developments that may occur (but that may be blurred by the dramatic negative changes suggesting a downhill course or a plateau when there may, in fact, be considerable improvements in some areas).

Treatment

Most children with this disorder are tried on anticonvulsant treatment (perhaps most often carbamazepine), but it is unclear whether it does have any effect on anything but clinical seizures. It has not even been clearly demonstrated that the effect on seizures is very good, and the paroxysmal EEG changes usually do not disappear with anticonvulsant treatment.

Corticosteroids are often used also (Lerman & Lerman-Sagie, 1989), but their efficacy has not been properly evaluated. This is, of course, very difficult to achieve in such a rare disorder. A trial of corticosteroids may well be indicated in the initial stages of the disorder if the symptoms are dramatic.

Outcome

The EEG abnormalities show a tendency to wax and wane spontaneously. In many, if not most, cases, the EEG abnormalities (and epileptic seizures) disappear before mid- to late adolescence (Dulac, Billard & Arthius, 1983). The language difficulties persist even when there has been considerable improvement. It is common for adults who had the syndrome as children to still show mild–moderate deficits in verbal communication (Bishop, 1985).

Many children with Landau–Kleffner syndrome are suspected of being deaf. It is essential that a clear diagnosis be established early so that they can benefit from special education in classrooms for children with aphasia or high-functioning autism/learning disorders.

References

Aicardi, J. (Ed.) (1992). *Diseases of the Nervous System in Childhood. Clinics in Developmental Medicine, No. 115/118.* London: Mac Keith Press.
Airaksinen, E., Bille, B., Carlström, G., Diderichsen, J., Ehlers, S., Gillberg, C., Gillberg, I.C., Gunnarsson, S., Hellgren, L., Herrgård, E., Hundevadt, L., Jansen, J., Kadesjö, B., Korkman, M., Lie, H., Lindahl, E., Lundberg, A., Michelsson, K., Nettelbladt, U., Nordin, V., Ramberg, C., Rasmussen, P., Ruud, E., Strand,

G., Trillingsgaard, A., Westerberg, B. (1990). Barn och ungdomar med DAMP/MBD (Children and adolescents with DAMP/MBD). *Läkartidningen*, **88**, 714 (in Swedish).

American Psychiatric Association. (1980). *Diagnostic and Statistical Manual of Mental Disorders*. Washington, DC: APA.

American Psychiatric Association. (1987). *Diagnostic and Statistical Manual of Mental Disorders*. Third Edition – Revised. Washington, DC.: APA.

American Psychiatric Association (1994). *Disgnostic and Statistical Manual of Mental Disorders*. Fourth Edition. Washington, DC: APA.

Ayres, A.J. (1974). *Southern California Sensory Integration Test*. Los Angeles: Western Psychological Services.

Badian, N.A. (1983). Developmental dyscalculia. *In* Myklebust, H.R. (Ed.) *Progress in Learning Disability*. New York: Grune & Stratton.

Badian, N.A., Ghublikian, M. (1982). The personal–social characteristics of children with poor mathematical computation skills. *Journal of Learning Disabilities*, **16**, 154–7.

Barker, P. (1979). *Basic Child Psychiatry*. London: Granada Publishing.

Barkley, R.A. (1990). *Attention Deficit Hyperactivity Disorder*. New York: Guilford Press.

Benasich, A.A., Bejar, I.I. (1992). The Fagan test of infant intelligence: A critical review. *Journal of Applied Developmental Psychology*, **13**, 153–71.

Benasich, A.A., Tallal, P. (1993). An operant conditioning paradigm for assessing auditory temporal processing in 6- to 9-month-old infants. *Annals of the New York Academy of Sciences*, **682**, 312–14.

Bishop, D.V.M. (1980). Handedness, clumsiness and cognitive ability. *Developmental Medicine and Child Neurology*, **22**, 569–79.

Bishop, D.V.M. (1985). Age of onset and outcome in 'acquired aphasia with convulsive disorder' (Landau–Kleffner syndrome). *Developmental Medicine and Child Neurology*, **27**, 705–12.

Bishop, D.V.M. (1989). Autism, Asperger's syndrome and semantic-pragmatic disorder: where are the boundaries? *APHASIA*.

Bishop, D. (1992). The underlying nature of specific language impairment. *Journal of Child Psychology and Psychiatry*, **33**, 3–66.

Bishop, D., Hartley, J., Weir, F. (1994). Why and when do some language-impaired children seem talkative? A study of initiation in conversations of children with semantic–pragmatic disorder. *Journal of Autism and Developmental Disorders*, **24**, 177–97.

Bornstein, M.H., Sigman, M.D. (1986). Continuity in mental development from infancy. *Child and Development*, **57**, 251–74.

Bradley, L., Bryant, P. (1985). Rhyme and reason in reading and spelling (International Academy for Research in Learning Disabilities Series). Ann Arbor: University of Michigan Press.

Bryant, P.E., Bradley, L., McLean, M., Crossland, J. (1989). Nursery, rhymes, phonological skills and reading. *Journal of Child Language*, **16**, 407–28.

Cantwell, D.P., Baker, L. (1985). Speech and language: development and disorders. *In* Rutter, M.,Hersov, L. (Eds.) *Child and adolescent psychiatry. Modern approaches*. Second Edition. Oxford: Blackwell Scientific Publications.

Cantwell, D., Baker, L., Rutter, M. (1978). A comparative study of infantile autism and specific developmental receptive language disorder – IV. Analysis of syntax and language function. *Journal of Child Psychology and Psychiatry*, **19**, 351–62.

Cantwell, D.P., Baker, L., Rutter, M., Mawhood, L. (1989). Infantile autism and developmental receptive dysphasia: A comparative follow-up into middle childhood. *Journal of Autism and Developmental Disorders*, **19**, 19–31.

Chelune, G.J., Ferguson, W., Koon, R., Dickey, T.O. (1986). Frontal lobe disinhibition in attention deficit disorder. *Child Psychiatry and Human Development*, **16**, 221–34.

Ciaranello, R. (1993). Editorial. *New England Journal of Medicine*, **328**, 1038–9.

Cobrinik, L. (1982). The performance of hyperlexic children on an 'incomplete words' task. *Neuropsychologia*, **20**, 569–77.

Colby, C.L. (1991). The neuroanatomy and neurophysiology of attention. *Journal of Child Neurology*, **6 (Suppl.)**, S90-S118.

Comings, D. (1990). *Tourette Syndrome and Human Behavior*. Duarte, CA: Hope Press.

Conners, C.K. (1969). A teacher rating scale for use in drug studies with children. *American Journal of Psychiatry*, **126**, 884–8.

Denckla, M.B. (1985). Neurological examination for subtle signs (PANESS). *Psychopharmacology Bulletin*, **21**, 773–800.

Deonna, T., Beaumanoir, A., Gaillard, P., Assal, G. (1977). Acquired aphasia in childhood with seizure disorder: a heterogeneous syndrome. *Neuropädiatrie*, **8**, 263–73.

Dockrell, J., McShane, J. (1993). *Children's*

Learning Difficulties. Oxford: Blackwell.

Dulac, O., Billard, C., Arthuis, M. (1983). Aspects électroencéphalographiques et évolutifs de l'épilepsie dans e syndrome aphasie-épilepsie. *Archives Françaises de Pédiatrie*, **40**.

Ehlers, S., Gillberg, C. (1993). The epidemiology of Asperger syndrome. A total population study. *Journal of Child Psychology and Psychiatry*, **34**, 1327–50.

Ernst, M., Liebenauer, L.L., King, A.C., Fitzgerald, G., Cohen, R.M., Zametkin, A.J. (1994). Reduced brain metabolism in hyperactive girls. *Journal of the American Academy of Child and Adolescent Psychiatry*, **33**, 858–68.

Fog, E., Fog, M. (1963). Cerebral Inhibition Examined by Associated Movements. *In* Bax, M.,Mac Keith, R. (Eds.) *Minimal Cerebral Dysfunction. Clinics in Developmental Medicine No. 10*. London: S.S.M.E.I.U./William Heinemann Medical Books Ltd.

Galaburda, A.M., Sherman, G.F., Rosen, G.D., Aboitiz, F., Geschwind, N. (1985). Developmental dyslexia: four consecutive patients with cortical anomalies. *Annals of Neurology*, **18**, 222–32.

Geschwind, N., Galaburda, A.M. (1985a). Cerebral lateralization. Biological mechanisms, associations, and pathology: I. A hypothesis and a program for research. *Archives of Neurology*, **42**, 428–59.

Geschwind, N., Galaburda, A.M. (1985b). Cerebral lateralization. Biological mechanisms, associations, and pathology: II. A hypothesis and a program for research. *Archives of Neurology*, **42**, 521–52.

Geschwind, N., Galaburda, A.M. (1985c). Cerebral lateralization. Biological mechanisms, associations, and pathology: III. A hypothesis and a program for research. *Archives of Neurology*, **42**, 634–54.

Gillberg, C. (1983). Perceptual, motor and attentional deficits in Swedish primary school children. Some child psychiatric aspects. *Journal of Child Psychology and Psychiatry*, **24**, 377–403.

Gillberg, C. (1989). Asperger syndrome in 23 Swedish children. *Developmental Medicine and Child Neurology*, **31**, 520–31.

Gillberg, C. (1991a). Clinical and neurobiological aspects of Asperger syndrome in six family studies. *In* Frith, U. (Eds.) *Autism and Asperger Syndrome*. Cambridge: Cambridge University Press.

Gillberg, C. (1991b). Outcome in autism and autistic-like conditions. *Journal of the American Academy of Child and Adolescent Psychiatry*, **30**, 375–82.

Gillberg, C. (1992a). Deficits in attention, motor control and perception and other syndromes attributed to minimal brain dysfunction. *In* Aicardi, J. (Ed.) *Child's Nervous System*. London: Mac Keith Press.

Gillberg, C. (1992b). The Emanuel Miller Memorial Lecture 1991: Autism and autistic-like conditions: subclasses among disorders of empathy. *Journal of Child Psychology and Psychiatry*, **33**, 813–42.

Gillberg, C., Hellgren, L. (1994). Outcome of attention disorders. *In* Sandberg, S. (Ed.) *Hyperactivity Disorders*. Cambridge: Cambridge University Press.

Gillberg, C., Rasmussen, P. (1982). Perceptual, motor and attentional deficits in seven-year-old children: background factors. *Developmental Medicine and Child Neurology*, **24**, 752–70.

Gillberg, C., Rasmussen, P., Carlström, G., Svenson, B., Waldenström, E. (1982). Perceptual, motor and attentional deficits in six-year-old children. Epidemiological aspects. *Journal of Child Psychology and Psychiatry*, **23**, 131–44.

Gillberg, C., Carlström, G., Rasmussen, P. (1983a). Hyperkinetic disorders in seven-year-old children with perceptual, motor and attentional deficits. *Journal of Child Psychology and Psychiatry*, **24**, 233–46.

Gillberg, C., Carlström, G., Rasmussen, P., Waldenström, E. (1983b). Perceptual, motor and attentional deficits in seven-year-old children. Neurological screening aspects. *Acta Paediatrica Scandinavica*, **72**, 119–24.

Gillberg, C., Gillberg, I.C., Steffenburg, S. (1990). Reduced optimality in the pre-, peri-, and neonatal periods is not equivalent to severe peri- or neonatal risk: a rejoinder to Goodman's technical note [comment]. Comment on: *Journal of Child Psychology and Psychiatry 1990, Jul 31, 5, 809–12. Journal of Child Psychology and Psychiatry*, **31**, 813–15.

Gillberg, C., Gillberg, I.C., Steffenburg, S. (1992). Siblings and parents of children with autism. A controlled population based study. *Developmental Medicine and Child Neurology*, **34**, 389–98.

Gillberg, C., Steffenburg, S., Wahlström, J., Gillberg, I.C. Sjöstedt, A., Martinsson, T., Liedgren, S., Eeg-Olofsson, O. (1991). Autism associated with marker chromosome. *Journal of the American Academy of Child and Adolescent Psychiatry*, **30**, 489–94.

Gillberg, I.C. (1987). *Deficits in Attention, Motor Control and Perception: Follow-up from Pre-School to Early Teens*. MD Thesis. University of Uppsala.

Gillberg, I.C., Gillberg, C. (1988). Generalized hyperkinesis: follow-up study from age 7 to 13 years. *Journal of the American Academy of Child and Adolescent Psychiatry*, **27**, 55–9.

Gillberg, I.C., Gillberg, C. (1989a). Asperger syndrome – some epidemiological considerations: a research note. *Journal of Child Psychology and Psychiatry*, **30**, 631–8.

Gillberg, I.C., Gillberg, C. (1989b). Children with preschool minor neurodevelopmental disorders. IV: Behaviour and school achievement at age 13. *Developmental Medicine and Child Neurology*, **31**, 3–13.

Gillberg, I.C., Gillberg, C., Groth, J. (1989). Children with preschool minor neurodevelopmental disorders. V: Neurodevelopmental profiles at age 13. *Developmental Medicine and Child Neurology*, **31**, 14–24.

Gillberg, I.C., Winnergård, I., Gillberg, C. (1993). Screening methods, epidemiology and evaluation of intervention in DAMP in preschool children. *European Child & Adolescent Psychiatry*, **2**, 121–35.

Gittelman, R. (1985). Controlled trials of remedial approaches to reading disability. *Journal of Child Psychology and Psychiatry*, **26**, 843–6.

Gittelman, R., Klein, D.F., Feingold, I. (1983). Children with reading disorders – II. Effects of methylphenidate in combination with reading remediation. *Journal of Child Psychology and Psychiatry*, **24**, 193–212.

Gittelman, R., Mannuzza, S., Shenker, R. & Bonagura, N. (1985). Hyperactive boys almost grown up: I. Psychiatric status. *Archives of General Psychiatry*, **42**, 937–47.

Goldman-Rakic, P.S., Selemon, L.D. (1990). New frontiers in basal ganglia research. Introduction :see comments: Comment in: *Trends Neurosci* 1991 Feb;14(2):55–9. *Trends in Neuroscience*, **13**, 241–4.

Goodman, R., Stevenson, J. (1989a). A twin study of hyperactivity – I. An examination of hyperactivity scores and categories derived from Rutter teacher and parent questionnaires. *Journal of Child Psychology and Psychiatry*, **30**, 671–89.

Goodman, R., Stevenson, J. (1989b). A twin study of hyperactivity – II. The aetiological role of genes, family relationships and perinatal adversity. *Journal of Child Psychology and Psychiatry*, **30**, 691–709.

Gordon, N. (1992). Children with developmental dyscalculia. *Developmental Medicine and Child Neurology*, **34**, 459–63.

Graham, P. (1986). *Child Psychiatry. A Developmental Approach*. Oxford: Oxford Medical Publications.

Gualtieri, C.T., Hicks, R.E. (1985). An immunoreactive theory of selective male afflication. *Behavioral and Brain Science*, **8**, 427–41.

Hadders-Algra, M., van Eykern, L.A., Klip-van den Nieuwendijk, A.W., Prechtl, H.F.R. (1992). Developmental course of general movements in infancy. 2: EMG correlates. *Early Human Development*, **28**, 231–52.

Heilman, K.M., Voeller, K.K.S., Nadeau, S.E. (1991). A possible pathophysiologic substrate of attention deficit hyperactivity disorder. *Journal of Child Neurology*, **6 (Suppl.)**, S76–81.

Hellgren, L., Gillberg, C., Enerskog, I. (1987). Antecedents of adolescent psychoses: a population-based study of school health problems in children who develop psychosis in adolescence. *Journal of the American Academy of Child and Adolescent Psychiatry*, **26**, 351–5.

Hellgren, L., Gillberg, C., Gillberg, I.C., Enerskog, I. (1993). Children with Deficits in Attention, Motor control and Perception (DAMP) almost grown up. General health at age 16 years. *Developmental Medicine and Child Neurology*, **35**, 881–92.

Hellgren, L., Gillberg, I.C., Bågenholm, A., Gillberg, C. (1994). Children with Deficits in Attention, Motor control and Perception (DAMP) almost grown up: psychiatric and personality disorders at age 16 years. *Journal of Child Psychology and Psychiatry*, **35**, 1255–71.

Hurford, D.P. (1990). Training phonemic segmentation ability with a phonemic discrimination intervention in second- and third-grade children with reading disabilities. *Journal of Learning Disabilities*, **23**, 564–9.

Hynd, G.W., Semrud-Clikeman, M., Lorys, A.R., Novey, E.S., Eliopulos, D. (1990). Brain morphology in developmental dyslexia and attention deficit disorder/hyperactivity. *Archives of Neurology*, **47**, 919–26.

Højen, T., Lundberg, I. (1990). *Dysleksi*. Oslo: Gyldendals förlag.

Klein, R.G., Mannuzza, S. (1991). Long-term outcome of hyperactive children: a review. *Journal of the American Academy of Child and Adolescent Psychiatry*, **30**, 383–7.

Korkman, M., Peltomaa, K. (1991). A pattern of test findings predicting attention problems at school. *Journal of Abnormal Child Psychology*, **19**, 451–67.

Landgren, M., Pettersson, R., Kjellman, B., Gillberg, C. (1993). DAMP/MBD hos 6–7-

åringar, metodik för BVC och preliminära resultat. Läkarstämman. Stockholm. (In Swedish.)

Lerman, P., Lerman-Sagie, T. (1989). Early steroid therapy in Landau-Kleffner syndrome. *Advances in Epileptology*, **17**, 330–2.

Lewis, C., Hitch, G.J., Walker, P. (1994). The prevalence of specific arithmetic difficulties and specific reading difficulties in 9–10 year-old boys and girls. *Journal of Child Psychology and Psychiatry*, **35**, 283–92.

Lister-Brook, S., Bowler, D. (1992). Autism by another name? Semantic and pragmatic impairments in children. *Journal of Autism and Developmental Disorders*, **22**, 61–82.

Losse, A., Henderson, S.E., Elliman, D., Hall, D., Knight, E., Jongmans, M. (1991). Clumsiness in children – do they grow out of it? A 10-year follow-up study. *Developmental Medicine and Child Neurology*, **33**, 55–68.

Lou, H.C., Henriksen, L., Bruhn, P. (1984). Focal cerebral hypoperfusion in children with dysphasia and/or attention deficit disorder. *Archives of Neurology*, **41**, 825–9.

Lou, H.C., Henriksen, L., Bruhn, P., Börner, H., Nielsen, J.B. (1989). Striatal dysfunction in attention deficit and hyperkinetic disorder. *Archives of Neurology*, **46**, 48–52.

Lou, H.C., Henriksen, L., Bruhn, P. (1990a). Focal cerebral dysfunction in developmental learning disabilities. *Lancet*, **335**, 8–11.

Lou, H., Henriksen, L., Greisen, G., Schneider, S. (1990b). Redistribution of cerebral activity during childhood. *Brain Development*, **12**, 301–5.

Lundberg, I., Olofsson, Å., Wall, S. (1980). Reading and spelling skills in the first school years predicted from phonemic awareness skills in kindergarten. *Scandinavian Journal of Psychology*, **21**, 159–73.

Lundberg, I., Frost, J., Petersen, O.-P. (1988). Effects on an extensive program for stimulating phonological awarness in preschool children. *Reading Research Quarterly*, **23**, 263–84.

Lunsing, R.J., Hadders-Algra, M., Huisjes, H.J., Touwen, B.C.L. (1992a). Minor neurological dysfunction from birth to 12 years. I: Increase during late school-age. *Developmental Medicine and Child Neurology*, **34**, 399–403.

Lunsing, R.J., Hadders-Algra, M., Huisjes, H.J., Touwen, B.C.L. (1992b). Minor neurological dysfunction from birth to 12 years. II: Puberty is related to decreased dysfunction. *Developmental Medicine and Child Neurology*, **34**, 404–9.

Mannuzza, S., Klein, R.G., Konig, P.H.,

Ciampino, T.L. (1989). Hyperactive boys almost grown up. IV. Criminality and its relationship to psychiatric status. *Archives of General Psychiatry*, **46**, 1073–9.

McKinley, I. (1993). What children have what forms of developmental disorders? Meeting on Specific Learning Disorders. Wallingford, Oxford, December.

Mefford, I.N., Potter, W.Z. (1989). A neuroanatomical and biochemical basis for attention deficit disorder with hyperactivity in children: a defect in tonic adrenaline mediated inhibition of locus coeruleus stimulation. *Medical Hypotheses*, **29**, 33–42.

Michelsson, K., Ylinen, A. (1987). A neurodevelopmental screening examination for five-year-old children. *Early Child Development and Care*, **29**, 9–22.

Morrell, F., Whisler, W.W., Bleck, T.P. (1989). Multiple subpial transection: a new approach to the surgical treatment of focal epilepsy. *Journal of Neurosurgery*, **70**, 231–9.

Nass, R., Heier, L., Walker, R. (1993). Landau–Kleffner syndrome: temporal lobe tumor resection results in good outcome. *Pediatric Neurology*, **9**, 303–5.

Patti, P.J., Lupinetti, L. (1993). Brief report: implications of hyperlexia in an autistic savant. *Journal of Autism and Developmental Disorders*, **23**, 397–405.

Pennington, B.F. (1990). The genetics of dyslexia. *Journal of Child Psychology and Psychiatry*, **31**, 193–201.

Rapin, I., Allen, D. (1983). Developmental language disorders. In Kirk, V. (Ed.) *Neuropsychology of Language, Reading and Spelling*. New York: Academic Press.

Rasmussen, P., Gillberg, C., Waldenström, E., Svenson, B. (1983). Perceptual, motor and attentional deficits in seven-year-old children: neurological and neurodevelopmental aspects. *Developmental Medicine and Child Neurology*, **25**, 315–33.

Richardson, E. (1984). The impact of phonemic processing instruction on the reading achievement of reading-disabled children. *Annals of the New York Academy of Sciences*, **433**, 97–118.

Richman, N., Stevenson, J., Graham, P. (1982). *Pre-School to School: A Behavioural Study*. London: Academic Press.

Robinson, R.J. (1991). Causes and associations of severe and persistent specific speech and language disorders in children. *Developmental Medicine and Child Neurology*, **33**, 943–62.

Rosenberger, P.B. (1989). Perceptual–motor and attentional correlates of developmental dyscalculia. *Annals of Neurology*, **26**, 216–20.

Rourke, B.P., Finlayson, M.A. (1978). Neuropsychological significance of variations in patterns of academic performance: verbal and visual-spatial abilities. *Journal of Abnormal Child Psychology*, **6**, 121–33.

Rutter, M. (1982). Syndromes attributed to minimal brain dysfunction in childhood. *American Journal of Psychiatry*, **139**, 21–33.

Rutter, M., Madge, N. (1976). *Cycles of Disadvantage: A Review of Research*. London: Heinemann Educational.

Rutter, M., Graham, P., Yule, W. (1970). *A Neuropsychiatric Study in Childhood*. London: S.I.M.P./William Heinemann Medical Books Ltd.

Sandberg, S.T., Rutter, M., Taylor, E. (1978). Hyperkinetic disorder in psychiatric clinic attenders. *Developmental Medicine and Child Neurology*, **20**, 279–99.

Schonhaut, S., Satz, P. (1983). Prognosis for children with learning disabilities. *In* Rutter, M. (Ed.) *Developmental Neuropsychiatry*. New York: Guilford Press.

Semrud-Clikeman, M., Filipek, P.A., Biederman, J., Steingard, R., Kennedy, D., Renshaw, P., Bekken, K. (1994). Attention-deficit hyperactivity disorder: magnetic resonance imaging morphometric analysis of the corpus callosum. *Journal of the American Academy of Child and Adolescent Psychiatry*, **33**, 875–81.

Shaffer, D., Schonfeld, I., O'Connor, P.A., Stokman, C., Trautman, P., Shafer, S., Ng, S. (1985). Neurological soft signs. Their relationship to psychiatric disorder and intelligence in childhood and adolescence. *Archives of General Psychiatry*, **42**, 342–51.

Shriberg, L.D., Kwiatkowski, J., Best, S., Hengst, J., Terselic-Weber, B. (1986). Characteristics of children with phonologic disorders of unknown origin. *Journal of Speech and Hearing Disorders*, **51**, 140–61.

Silberberg, N.E., Silberberg, M. (1967). Hyperlexia: Specific word recognition skills in young children. *Exceptional Children*, **34**, 41–2.

Silva, P.A. (1987). Epidemilogy, longitudinal course, and some associated features: an update. *In* Yule, W.,Rutter, M. (Eds.) *Language Development and Disorders. Clinics in Developmental Medicine, Nos. 101/102*. London: Mac Keith Press with Blackwell Scientific.

Sonuga-Barke, E.J.S., Lamparelli, M., Stevenson, J. Thompson, M., Henry A. (1994). Behaviour problems and pre-school intellectual attainment: the associations of hyperactivity and conduct problems. *Journal of Child Psychology and Psychiatry*, **35**, 949–60.

Soorani-Lunsing, R.J., Hadders-Algra, M., Huisjes, H.J., Touwen, B.C. (1993). Minor neurological dysfunction after the onset of puberty: association with perinatal events. *Early Human Development*, **33**, 71–80.

Stanovich, K.E. (1994). Annotation: does dyslexia exist? *Journal of Child Psychology and Psychiatry*, **35**, 579–95.

Steffenburg, S. (1991). Neuropsychiatric assessment of children with autism: a population-based study. *Developmental Medicine and Child Neurology*, **33**, 495–511.

Stevenson, J. (1991). Which aspects of processing text mediate genetic effects? *Reading and Writing*, **3**, 249–69.

Stevenson, J., Graham, P. (1993). Antisocial behaviour and spelling disability in a population sample of 13 year old twins. *European Child & Adolescent Psychiatry*, **2**, 179–91.

Stevenson, J., Graham, P., Fredman, G., McLoughlin, V. (1984). The genetics of reading ability. *In* Turner, C. (Ed.) *The Biology of Human Intelligence*. London: Eugenics Society.

Stevenson, J., Graham, P., Fredman, G., McLoughlin, V. (1987). A twin study of genetic influences on reading and spelling ability and disability. *Journal of Child Psychology and Psychiatry*, **28**, 229–47.

Stores, G., Hart, J. (1976). Reading skills of children with generalised or focal epilepsy attending ordinary school. *Developmental Medicine and Child Neurology*, **18**, 705–16.

Tallal, P., Chase, C., Russell, G., Schmitt, R.L. (1986). Evaulation of the efficacy of piracetam in treating information processing, reading and writing disorders in dyslexic children. *International Journal of Psychophysiology*, **4**, 41–52.

Tassinari, C.A., Bureau, M., Dravet, C., Dalla Bernardina, B., Roger, J. (1985). Epilepsy with continuous spikes and waves during slow sleep. *In* Roger, J., Dravet, C., Bureau, M., Dreifus, F.E.,Wolf, P. (Eds.) *Epileptic Syndromes in Infancy, Childhood and Adolescence*. London: John Libbey.

Taylor, D.C. (1969). Differential rates of cerebral maturation between sexes and between hemispheres: evidence from epilepsy. *Lancet*, **ii**, 140–2.

Taylor, E. (1986). Childhood hyperactivity. *British*

Journal of Psychiatry, **149**, 562–73.

Taylor, E., Schachar, R., Thorley, G., Wieselberg, M. (1986). Conduct disorder and hyperactivity: I. Separation of hyperactivity and antisocial conduct in British child psychiatric patients. *British Journal of Psychiatry*, **149**, 760–7.

Taylor, E., Sandberg, S., Thorley, G., Giles, S. (1991). *The Epidemiology of Childhood Hyperactivity*. London: Institute of Psychiatry.

Thorley, G. (1984). A pilot study to assess behavioural and cognitive effects of artificial good colours in a group of retarded children. *Developmental Medicine and Child Neurology*, **26**, 56–61.

Touwen, B.C.L. (1979). *Examination of the Child with Minor Neurological Dysfunction*. 2nd Edition. London: S.I.M.P./William Heinemann Medical Books Ltd.

Trommer, B.L., Hoeppner, J.-A.B., Zecker, S.G. (1991). The go-no test in attention deficit disorder is sensitive to methylphenidate. *Journal of Child Neurology*, **6 (Suppl.)**, S128–31.

Voeller, K.K.S. (1991). Clinical management of attention deficit hyperactivity disorders. *Journal of Child Neurology*, **6 Suppl**, S51-S65.

Weintraub, S., Mesulam, M.M. (1983). Developmental learning disabilities of the right hemisphere. *Archives of Neurology*, **40**, 464–8.

Weiss, G. (1991). Attention deficit hyperactivity disorder. *In* Lewis, M. (Ed.) *Child and Adolescent Psychiatry. A Comprehensive Textbook.* Baltimore, Maryland: Williams & Wilkins.

Wender, P.H. (1971). *Minimal Brain Dysfunction in Children*. New York: Wiley.

Whitmore, K., Bax, M. (1986). The school entry medical examination. *Archives of Diseases in Childhood*, **61**, 807–17.

Williams, J.P. (1980). Teaching decoding with an emphasis on phoneme analysis and phoneme blending. *Journal of Educational Psychology*, **72**, 1–15.

Wilsher, C.R., Taylor, E.A. (1994). Piracetam in developmental reading disorders: A review. *European Child & Adolescent Psychiatry*, **3**.

Wilsher, C.R., Bennett, D., Chase, C.H., Conners, C.K., DiIanni, M., Feagans, L., Hanvik, L.J., Helfgott, E., Koplewicz, H., Overby, P., *et al.* (1987). Piracetam and dyslexia: effects on reading tests. *Journal of Clinical Psychopharmacology*, **7**, 230–7.

Wing, L. (1991). The relationship between Asperger's syndrome and Kanner's autism. *In* Frith, U. (Ed.) *Autism and Asperger syndrome*. Cambridge: Cambridge University Press.

9 Sleep and elimination disorders

Disorders of sleep and elimination are extremely common in infancy and childhood. At least 10% of all primary school children have sleep disorders, enuresis or encopresis or a combination of these (Graham, 1986). Depending on definitions, younger children have even higher rates of disorder in these domains.

In pre-school children, jactatio capitis nocturna and night terrors are among the most frequent complaints (although not often initially recognized as night terrors) leading to consultation by a whole host of different specialists, including child neurologists and psychiatrists. Sleep walking is also a common sleep disorder, affecting many adolescents and often not properly diagnosed. Many severe sleep disturbances are described simply as 'frequent night waking' (Minde *et al.*, 1993). 'Good' sleepers wake up as frequently as 'poor' sleepers, but they manage to soothe themselves back to sleep without disturbing anyone, at least during the pre-school years. Poor sleepers have more behaviour problems, a more difficult temperament and may have suffered more perinatal insults than those who are regarded as good sleepers.

Enuresis is one of the most common symptoms of early school-age children. It is regarded as an isolated specific developmental disorder which, in itself, should not be regarded as a psychiatric disorder. However, it is often associated with psychiatric disorder, and it often causes emotional and behavioural problems. Encopresis is also a specific developmental disorder. It is associated with severe psychopathology more often than enuresis. Many children who suffer from encopresis also have enuresis, but only a minority of those with enuresis have encopresis.

Jactatio capitis (nocturna)

Pre-pubertal children, and infants in particular, often engage in rhythmic body movements and rhythmic vocalizations, such as head banging, head rocking, body rocking and rhythmic humming. This type of behaviour is comprehensively referred to as jactatio capitis (with the addition of 'nocturna', if the behaviour occurs mostly, or exclusively, at night).

Prevalence

Jactatio capitis occurs in about 5 to 15% of children who are perceived as normal. It is likely that a considerable proportion of these will go on to develop symptoms of developmental disorders, including DAMP and Tourette syndrome, but these diagnoses are usually not suspected at the time when the head rolling is the most intensive.

Sex ratios

Boys are much more often affected by jactatio capitis than are girls. The male:female ratio is likely to be at least in the 3:1 range.

Behavioural and physical phenotype

The typical movements (rapid head rolling, slow rhythmic head wagging from side to side, rhythmic head banging) and vocalizations may occur at any time during the day, but almost always at times of decreased wakefulness or when deliberately trying to go off to sleep. Most of these behaviours diminish by age 3 years, but some individuals go on to head bang, head roll or hum for many years, even into adult age. Nocturnal head bobbing/banging or lateral movements occurring in connection with falling asleep in a rhythmical manner are known as jactatio capitis.

Pathogenesis

The pathogenesis of jactatio capitis is completely unknown. However, the repetitive quality of its symptoms and the fact that, at least in retrospective studies, a link with Tourette disorder has been demonstrated suggests that it may be associated with the same types of brain dysfunction or variation that occur in that syndrome. It is possible that jactatio capitis is a heritable disorder, which would be further strengthened by its association with Tourette disorder, but clear evidence for genetic factors is lacking.

Treatment

No treatment, other than re-assurance, is usually needed. It is important not to contribute to further problems by suggesting that the behaviour may have psychological roots. The author has come across a teenager who had been in regular weekly psychotherapy for three years (and whose parents had been in parental counselling for the same amount of time) for jactatio capitis (with no improvement).

Behavioural intervention may be useful in extreme cases continuing through adolescence. The teenager is encouraged to listen to his own humming and record it (in a special diary) or to interrupt his head rolling and record every occasion on which it occurs, with a gradual diminution of symptoms most likely accomplished within weeks. The reward consists only of the normalization of what is perceived, at least by standers-by, as an extremely abnormal behaviour.

Outcome

Outcome in jactatio capitis is excellent. Most cases are asymptomatic after age 3 years, and only a few per cent continue to head bang throughout adolescence and into adult life.

Pavor nocturnus (night terrors)

Night terrors, or pavor nocturnus, appear to be unrelated to nightmares.

Prevalence

Pavor nocturnus affects 1–4% of all pre-school children. If more abortive forms of the condition are included, the prevalence is likely to be considerably higher than that.

Behavioural and physical phenotype

The condition consists of repeated episodes of 1–20 minutes' duration of sudden 'awakening' (without becoming clearly awake), usually associated with screams, shouting, talking aloud in a confused way or some such similar phenomenon, occurring 30–180 minutes after going to sleep. The child may talk about pains in the legs or just generally in a way which appears to be driven by anxiety and which, at least in the beginning, is likely to inspire anxiety, even terror, in the parents. Thus, in a sense, the night terrors are not the child's but rather affect the parents.

The child exhibits a number of signs of activation of the autonomic nervous system. There is almost always associated confusion, disorganized behaviour and perseverative body movements (such as plucking at a blanket or a cushion). The next morning, the child has total amnesia.

Onset is often in the 3–7 year-old age-range.

Pathogenesis

The aetiology is unknown, but there is indirect evidence that oxygen deprivation or a failure to change from nasal to oral breathing might be involved (Agrell & Axelsson, 1972). The clinical manifestations are associated with partial arousal from deep slow sleep (stages III and IV).

Treatment

Empirical study indicates that there is often a dramatically positive effect of removing the nasal adenoids in pavor nocturnus, even in cases where the adenoids do not appear enlarged (Agrell & Axelsson, 1972). This, unfortunately, is not well known among paediatricians, psychiatrists or oto-laryngologists. Therefore, many children with night terrors do not receive adequate help. Medication is often tried, but usually without much success. If removal of nasal adenoids is not considered necessary, positive reassurance should be given that the problem is not a potentially dangerous one and that the child most likely will grow out of it before adolescence (one-half have normal sleep at age 8 years, two-thirds at adolescence).

Outcome

Long-term outcome is good, but some affected children develop somnambulism in later childhood. Many children with night terrors undergo time-consuming, worrying and expensive examinations under the suspicion that they might be suffering from epilepsy. Differential diagnosis is usually easy if a thorough medical history is taken.

Sleep walking

Sleep walking appears to be closely related to pavor nocturnus in that episodes usually occur 30–180 minutes after going to sleep and that they coincide with non-REM-sleep (Dunn, 1980). The child rises up out of his/her bed and wanders about for up to 20–30 minutes. Total amnesia on awakening in the morning is the rule. If awakening occurs directly in association with the episode, confusion and disorientation may be obvious for seconds or minutes. The

point prevalence at any time during the school years is around 5%, but as many as 15% of all children have walked in their sleep at one or other time during childhood or adolescence (Steffenburg, 1990). The onset of this sleep disturbance is usually in the age range following the peak age of onset for pavor nocturnus, i.e. at any age from 6–12 years.

Occasionally onset is in adult age. Boys are affected much more often than girls.

Pavor nocturnus and sleep walking often occur in the same individual and familial loading is common (Kales et al., 1980). Immaturity of the central nervous system or an autosomally dominant hereditary condition have both been proposed as underlying aetiologies. Psychic and physical stress may increase the frequency of sleep walking.

Parents of children who walk in their sleep should be informed about the nature of the child's condition and be encouraged not to subject the child to extra stress immediately before going to bed. Hypnotics should not be given. The parent should, if possible, stay with the child during the episode and lead him/her back to bed. Windows and dangerous stairs should be checked. The generally held notion that nothing dangerous can happen during sleep walking is unsupported by the empirical evidence.

Outcome is generally good. Few people sleep walk in adult age, but there are exceptions to this general rule.

Narcolepsy

Narcolepsy is characterized by inappropriate sleep attacks (most often during monotonous activities) in association with hypnogogic hallucinations, sleep paralysis or/and cataplexy (the sudden loss of muscle tone, precipitated by laughter or excitement).

Prevalence

Only small paediatric series of individuals with narcolepsy are on record (Young et al., 1988;

Dahl, Holttum & Trubnick, 1994). However, the syndrome is likely to be common, given that most adults with the disorder report that they have had the condition since childhood. Nevertheless, it probably occurs with the typical tetrad of symptoms (narcolepsy, cataplexy, hypnagogic hallucinations and sleep paralysis) in fewer than 1 in 1000 children.

Sex ratios

Narcolepsy is probably as common in girls as in boys. However, in the author's clinical experience, the over-representation of boys has been marked. This could be due to referral bias associated with the fact that severely neuropsychiatrically disordered cases are preferentially referred to a neuropsychiatric clinic. Such neuropsychiatrically disordered child cases are more likely to be boys. Most of the children with narcolepsy, examined by the author, have suffered from other neuropsychiatric disorders.

Behavioural and physical phenotype

Narcolepsy comprises irrepressible sleep episodes occurring (on average) three to five times a day, with or without the associated phenomena of cataplexy, hypnagogic hallucinations and sleep paralysis. The basic disturbance might be a more general continuous sleepiness. The attacks most often last for a few minutes and sleep is not usually clinically very deep. At least half of all patients are easy to awaken even in the middle of an attack. However, the younger the patient, the more likely that the episodes may turn into 'day naps' and last for half an hour to several hours. This, in turn, will often lead to nocturnal insomnia.

Most children and adolescents have only narcolepsy, and the associated phenomena only occur later in life.

The symptoms are typical of rapid eye movement (REM) sleep episodes occurring inappropriately during the day, on entering sleep, on arousal during the day or in the morning. Narcolepsy is probably an abnormality of the brainstem property of REM sleep and takes precedence over the right-brain function of

wakefulness (vigilance). However, not all sleep episodes are associated with early onset REM (Aldrich, 1990).

It appears that narcolepsy may be misdiagnosed as, or associated with, severe psychiatric disorder including major depression and ADHD (Dahl, Holttum & Trubnick, 1994).

Pathogenesis

It appears that in many cases, narcolepsy might be dominantly inherited (Douglass, Harris & Pazderka, 1989). A gene for the susceptibility of developing symptoms of narcolepsy may exist on the short arm of chromosome 6. Narcolepsy may also be genetically related to some instances of idiopathic hypersomnia (Parkes & Lock, 1989).

There are clearly also cases of narcolepsy that are due to acquired brain damage (Rivera *et al.*, 1986; Aldrich & Naylor, 1989). The area of the brain most often implicated in such cases is the hypothalamus, and coma or excessive hypersomnia is the rule.

The sleep attack behaviour usually begins in childhood. Sleep paralysis may begin in adolescence. Cataplexy is a phenomenon of adult age in most cases. Early onset REM activity during night-time recordings or during day-time multiple sleep latency tests is typical.

Diagnosis

The neuropsychiatrist will have to ask specifically about symptoms associated with narcolepsy. This is because most children and adolescents will not volunteer this information, either to their parents or a doctor.

Work-up

An EEG should be performed in all cases because of the risk of misdiagnosis in relation to epilepsy. Amnesic automatisms, simulating epilepsy, are common (Aldrich, 1990). A neurodevelopmental screening, for motor control problems, and a general neuropsychiatric evaluation, to determine whether comorbid problems (such as DAMP, mental retardation or autism spectrum disorders) are present or not, should always be accomplished.

Treatment

Stimulant medication is the preferred treatment for severe narcolepsy which interferes significantly with daily life (Honda & Hishikawa, 1980). However, there is always a risk of abuse. It is also common for the drug to lose its effect after some time. Thus, intermittent treatment might be required. Active treatment for three months might be followed by drug holidays of 1–2 months. In cases with significant cataplexy or hypnagogic hallucinations, an REM-sleep suppressant medication (e.g. protriptyline) may be used to control symptoms (Dahl, Holttum & Trubnick, 1994).

It is important to reassure the patient and family that this is not a psychological problem or a sign that the patient is suffering from a chronic, deteriorating condition.

Outcome

The course of narcolepsy is life-long. Except in cases with severe brain damage associated with other hypothalamic symptoms, there is no evidence that the disorder is strongly associated with other severe neuropsychiatric morbidity or with increased mortality rates. However, the very real risk that the individual with narcolepsy might fall asleep while riding a bike (or later in life while driving a car, which, at times, can be a very monotonous activity) should lead to a very cautious attitude in discussions concerning prognosis. Only after careful evaluation and long-term personal follow-up should recommendations be made in this area.

Enuresis

Enuresis (night- or day-time wetting) is defined differently in different cultures, depending on societal practice and expectations. In most western societies, it is often defined as persistent wetting unaccompanied by obvious physical disorder in children over age 5 years. Boys are much later than girls in acquiring bladder control, and there could be a case for differential age criteria across the sexes in diagnosing enuresis.

There are at least two subtypes of enuresis, primary and secondary. Primary enuresis encompasses children who have never achieved continence, while secondary enuresis comprises cases who do achieve continence, only to lose it at some point in time after having maintained continence a year or more. The two subtypes can be further subdivided into nocturnal (night-time) and diurnal (day-time).

Prevalence

Nocturnal enuresis (night-time wetting) has been reported to occur in 10% of 5 year-olds and in 5% of 10 year-olds (Stein & Susser 1965). In the Isle of Wight study, at age 10–11 years, 6.7% of boys and 3.3% wet their bed at least once a week (Rutter, Yule & Graham, 1973). The corresponding figures at 14 years were 1.2% and 0.5%, respectively. In a study of 8 year-olds in New Zealand, 3.3% had primary and 4.1% secondary enuresis (Ferguson, Horwood & Shannon, 1986). In a study from Finland, 9.8% of 7 year-olds had enuresis. Nocturnal enuresis accounted for 65% of this prevalence. Purely diurnal and mixed variants contributed 16–18% each to the total rate.

At least 2% of 5 year-olds wet in the day-time more than once a week and at least 8% at least once a month (De Jounge, 1973). These figures both drop to about 1% around age 10 years. Three-quarters of children with daytime enuresis also have problems with night-time wetting (Blomfield & Douglas, 1956).

About 2% of the population continue to have similar problems through adolescence. Modern studies of the prevalence in adult age are lacking. This is all the more surprising given that the available data from 50 years ago suggest that as many as 1% of the whole population persist into adult age (Thorne, 1944).

Sex ratios

The sex ratio in enuresis is usually in the order of 2:1 male:female, almost regardless of what age group is being studied. Although the rate of enuresis in adult life has been poorly researched, it appears that the male:female ratio may be even higher in older subjects.

Behavioural and physical phenotype

There is no particular behavioural or physical phenotype typical of enuresis. Enuresis should never be taken as an indication that the child has a psychiatric disorder. Nevertheless, it is associated with such disorder more often than would be expected on the basis of chance alone. However, the nature of the behavioural disturbance in enuresis is non-specific (Mikkelsen *et al.*, 1980). It appears to be stronger for secondary enuresis (McGee *et al.*, 1984), but the difficulty of separating 'pure' secondary cases from those with only primary enuresis can be considerable, and many of those with apparently secondary problems could have been diagnosed as suffering from primary enuresis at a younger age. Therefore, conclusions in this regard can only be tentative at the present stage. When children with enuresis attending a child psychiatric clinic were compared with other child psychiatric clinic attenders, the only major differences were an increased rate of developmental delays and a decreased frequency of eating disorders and 'specific neurotic patterns' (Steinhausen & Göbel, 1989) in the former group.

Many studies (Essen & Peckham, 1976; Shaffer, Gardner & Hedge, 1984; Mimouni *et al.*, 1985; Shaffer *et al.*, 1984, Steinhausen & Göbel, 1989) agree that developmental delays are common in enuresis. Bone age was significantly reduced in one controlled study (Mimouni *et al.*, 1985).

Whatever the nature of the association between enuresis and behavioural/emotional problems, it should come as no surprise that the affected child suffers from a symptom which may lead to social and emotional problems. The appropriate and thoughtful treatment of enuresis should be able to contribute to the secondary prevention of at least some emotional and psychiatric problems.

Diagnosis

The diagnosis of enuresis should be made whenever there is repeated involuntary or intentional voiding of urine during the day or night into bed or clothes, after an age at which continence is expected (DSM-III-R, APA, 1987; DSM-IV, APA, 1994). As has already been suggested, this age might, at least clinically, be allowed to vary depending on sex, and on the cultural setting in which the child is examined. It is usually not relevant to make a diagnosis of enuresis unless treatment is sought (usually by child or parents) or considered. No child should be diagnosed with enuresis under age 5 years (6 years may be more appropriate for boys). Secondary enuresis can be diagnosed at any age so long as the child has been reliably continent for a period of more than 1 year. However, the usual age of onset appears, at least on the basis of results obtained in the Isle of Wight study, to be 5–7 years (Rutter, 1989).

Pathogenesis

The incidence of obstructive and other lesions in the urinary tracts of children with enuresis has been the subject of considerable study (for a review see Shaffer, 1985). Cohen (1975) found the rate of such obstructive lesions to be 3.7% in a primary care paediatric setting. He concluded that contrast studies would only be indicated in enuresis when there is evidence of anatomical or functional pathology by history or examination.

The aetiology and pathogenesis of enuresis is unknown. However, there is strong evidence that familial/hereditary factors play a crucial role. In the study from Finland, the risk that a child would suffer from enuresis was seven times greater if the father had had enuresis after age 4 years and five times greater if the mother had had enuresis after this age. The finding of decreased bone age suggests that enuresis may be associated with generally (or at least more widespread) delayed maturation of CNS regulatory functions (Mimouni *et al.*, 1985). The fact of the occurrence of enuresis during sleep has sparked a whole host of theories relating enuresis to various sleep stages or abnormalities of arousal (Pierce *et al.*, 1961; Broughton, 1968; Ritvo *et al.*, 1969). However, more recent studies have failed to provide evidence for these hypotheses (Mikkelsen *et al.*, 1980). Sleep studies combined with cystometry (Nrgaard *et al.*, 1989) might help provide a firmer basis for some of these hypotheses regarding enuresis aetiology.

Day-time enuresis is occasionally clearly triggered by emotional upset. It is sometimes, although rarely, temporally associated with the birth of a sibling, and may, in such cases, be regarded as a regressive psychological phenomenon.

In other cases still, constipated children and children with primary encopresis may fail to differentiate bowel and bladder control and may be unable to control bladder sphincter function in times of acute defaecation needs (while just managing to control bowel sphincter tonus). In such cases, a diagnosis of secondary enuresis may only help obscure pathogenetic mechanisms and withdraw the child from appropriate intervention, i.e. the treatment of constipation/encopresis.

Work-up

Urinary tract infection must always be considered as a differential (or associated) diagnosis in the work-up of children with symptoms of enuresis. Rarely, other underlying metabolic or hormonal disorders (diabetes mellitus, diabetes insipidus and hyperthyroidism) and constipation can lead to urine incontinence and masquerade as enuresis.

Other than a thorough physical examination, and a careful history taking in combination with a urinary test for bacteria, glucose and osmolality), there is no need for an exhaustive work-up in the routine diagnostic procedure in enuresis.

Treatment

Enuresis has prompted considerable research effort with regard to intervention, but it is still not accepted as the major cause for concern and intervention that it is likely to warrant. Untreated enuresis carries many potential hazards, including poor self-esteem. Enuresis should alert the neuropsychiatrist to the need for intervention in order to reduce secondary psychiatric disorder.

Nocturnal enuresis over age 6 years should be treated with an enuresis alarm if the child and family are well motivated, and if there is a nurse or a team available who can administer the treatment. The usual form of alarm is one consisting of a two wire-mesh bed mats, connected to a bell or buzzer which goes off when electrical contact is made by the child wetting. According to a large review by Werry (1966), the success rate using this approach is about 75%. This is in keeping with later studies (Berg, Forsythe & McGuire, 1982). The results of studies of retention-control training have been equivocal, and the current tendency is to discourage its use because of the many unwanted 'side effects', such as having parents and children arguing over it every evening. Buzzer ulcers are extremely rare, but they do occur and parents need to be warned about this possibility (Diez & Beger, 1988).

Tricyclic antidepressants are often tried, with some beneficial effects in the short term but relatively little success in the long term. Most children will respond with some degree of improvement on doses of imipramine of 75–125 mg (Mikkelsen & Rapoport 1980). However, in the opinion of this author, these drugs have too many potential side effects to warrant widespread use for enuresis.

For night wetters who want to stay the night with their best friend or go to a camp, the use of a nasal Minirin spray (desmopressin acetate, an oxytocin analogue) may be very helpful in reducing urine volume for 6–10 hours, thereby minimizing the risk that the child wets. Some authorities now advocate long-term desmopressin treatment of nocturnal enuresis (Rew & Rundle, 1989). So far, no hormonal or haematological side effects of such treatment for more than one year have been reported.

Various bladder training programmes may be effective for some day-time wetters.

Outcome

There is a very high rate of spontaneous remission of both nocturnal and diurnal forms of enuresis at most ages between 5 and 12 years. The rate will continue to drop after this age (even in the absence of any treatment), but the speed at which this is achieved may be slower in adolescence and early adult life. Again, it needs to be pointed out that many adults do suffer from enuresis.

Encopresis

Encopresis is defined as the 'repeated involuntary passage of faeces into places not appropriate for that purpose' (APA, 1987). It can also occur intentionally, although this would be much rarer. It should have occurred at least once a month for a period of at least 6 months, and the mental age of the child (chronological age in normally intelligent children) should be at least 4 years. As with enuresis, there are at least two subtypes of encopresis, primary (when the child has never managed complete bowel control for a period of six months or more) and secondary encopresis (when encopresis occurs after there has been appropriate bowel control for a year or more).

Prevalence

In a Swedish study in the 1960s, Bellman (1966) found a rate of encopresis of 1.5% of all 7–8 year-olds. In the Isle of Wight study, Rutter found that 0.8% of all 10–12 year-olds soiled at least once a month (Rutter, Tizard & Whitmore, 1981). That study, as many others, found a significant correlation between the occurrence of encopresis and enuresis.

Sex ratios

The sex ratio in encopresis is usually reported to be in the range of 3–4:1 male:female (Bellman, 1966; Rutter *et al.*, 1981).

Behavioural and physical phenotype

There is no particular physical or behavioural phenotype typical of children with encopresis. However, the disorder is more common in mentally retarded children and possibly, although not undisputedly, more common in children with conduct and emotional problems (Bellman, 1966). There are at least two subtypes of primary and secondary encopresis, i.e. retentive and non-retentive. The retentive subtype is characterized by several days of retention, painful expulsion of faeces and then another period of retention. There may, or may not, be associated stercoral diarrhoea, i.e. there may be leakage around an accumulating faecal mass with consequent faecal staining of the underwear.

Hersov (1985) suggested that encopresis could be subdivided according to another type of categorization: (a) appropriate bowel control with volitional depositing of faeces in inappropriate places, (b) inappropriate bowel control with or without awareness of soiling and (c) soiling due to excessive fluid either as a consequence of diarrhoea, anxiety or a retention overflow as described previously. According to Hersov (1985), the retention overflow would be the most common mechanism in category (c). Some authors would dispute this categorization on the basis that diarrhoea may be a physical disorder which could adequately account for the soiling. However, in most other respects, Hersov's subclasses make clinical sense and are useful when trying to explain the symptom and its associations to parents.

Diagnosis

The diagnosis of encopresis should be made in children over age 4 years (or, in mentally retarded children, if mental age is over 4 years) who, for a period of more than 6 months and at a rate of at least once a month, pass faeces into places that are not appropriate for that purpose, and in whom there is no associated physical disorder which could reasonably account for the behaviour. Encopresis can occur alone, but is encountered more commonly in children with mental retardation, autism and hyperkinetic disorder than in the general population of children.

Pathogenesis

Psychodynamic speculation about the origins of encopresis has been abundant over the years (Bellman, 1966). However, apart from the observations by Freud and Burlingham (1943) of a high rate of soiling in children separated from their parents during World War II, very little empirical data exists to support the notion of psychological factors being at the root of encopresis. Bemporad and Halloway (1987) identified a small subgroup of children with encopresis which was largely intractable, and they proposed the term 'chronic neurotic encopresis' for this group.

Taylor (1992) described two children in whom encopresis appeared to have a particular psychological meaning and in whom a reasonable case could be made for psychological factors being clearly at the root of the disorder.

Recent research has focused more on the physiological basis for encopresis (Wald et al., 1986; Loening-Baucke & Cruickshank, 1986; Loening-Baucke, 1987). It seems that children with encopresis may have specific problems relaxing the anal sphincter. In one study Loening-Baucke (1987) found that more than half of a group of children with encopresis were unable to defaecate rectal balloons and that most of these were non-responsive to treatment. In contrast, a majority of those who managed to defaecate the rectal balloon had recovered with, or without, treatment a year later. Measures of behaviour/behaviour problems and social competence were also included in one study reported by this group. Outcome was closely correlated with physiological measures (poor outcome in the group with inability to relax the anal sphincter) but not at all with psychological findings. However, the girls who could not defaecate the balloons had lower social competence than those who could. This might well be a result of the encopresis or encopresis, and social dysfunction could be associated because of an underlying common problem.

Work-up

A thorough history from the parent and child should be elicited both for investigative purposes and because the careful history taking may lead to a better understanding of associated characteristics, specific situational triggers and how best to handle/avoid these on the part of the parent (and child). IQ-testing is indicated whenever there is suspicion that the child may be of subnormal intelligence. Hirschprung's disease, smooth muscle disease, endocrine abnormalities (including thyroid disease) and stenosis of the anus or rectum must always be ruled out before a diagnosis of encopresis is made.

Treatment

In the treatment of encopresis it is usually important to meet the parents and child as a group and to provide education about the symptom and bowel function in order to diffuse psychological tension which is likely to exist in the family after the symptom of encopresis has been present for weeks or months (or even years). Behaviour therapy has been shown to be effective in treating encopresis (Young & Goldsmith 1972; Wright, 1977; Wright & Walker, 1978). A routine of daily timed intervals on the toilet is introduced with, or without, the concomitant use of daily doses of a mild laxative (to allow the painless passing of faeces). Reinforcement is used and involves training the parent to praise the child or to provide a conditioned reinforcer when the child passes faeces appropriately. It may be necessary to deliver a reinforcer for the approximation of appropriate behaviours, e.g. rewarding the child for passing faeces in the pants while in the bathroom. This type of intervention has been shown effectively to eliminate encopresis, but it usually takes 3–5 months, and the length itself of this duration may be sufficient to discourage many parents from persisting in applying the treatment.

According to one study (Levine, Mazonson & Bakow, 1980), the success rate may be almost 80% with this procedure. Because of its comparatively limited intrusiveness, this method might be regarded as 'intervention of first choice'. Imipramine treatment (25–75 mg per day) has also been reported to be helpful in the treatment of encopresis in some cases (Siomopoulos, 1976).

Outcome

Outcome in encopresis appears to be good in most cases with normal IQ (Mikkelsen, 1991), and it is definitely rare for encopresis to persist into the teens or adult age. However, to the best of the author's knowledge, no longitudinal study that followed the probands into adult age has been published. Thus, definite conclusions regarding the rate of persistence of encopresis in adult age need to be cautious.

In conditions such as autism and mental retardation with or without hyperkinetic disorder, encopresis may well persist into adolescence and adult age. In most cases, this state of affairs could have been positively affected by the early introduction of a behaviour modification approach. In fact, a behaviour modification paradigm for the treatment of encopresis in disorders, such as autism, is one of the most important aspects of intervention. From the practical and social points of view, quality of life is likely to be very much better in an individual with autism who has bowel control than in one who does not.

References

Agrell, I.-G., Axelsson, A. (1972). The relationship between pavor nocturnus and adenoids. *Acta Paedopsychiatrica*, **39**, 46–53.

Aldrich, M.S. (1990). Narcolepsy. *New England Journal of Medicine*, **323**, 389–94.

Aldrich, M.S., Naylor, M.W. (1989). Narcolepsy associated with lesions of the diencephalon. *Neurology*, **39**, 1505–8.

American Psychiatric Association. (1980). *Diagnostic and Statistical Manual of Mental Disorders*. Washington, DC: APA.

American Psychiatric Association. (1987). *Diagnostic and Statistical Manual of Mental Disorders*. Third Edition – Revised. Washington, DC: APA.

American Psychiatric Association (1994). *Diagnostic and Statistical Manual of Mental Disorders*. Fourth Edition. Washington, DC: APA.

Bellman, M. (1966). Studies on encopresis. *Acta Paediatrica Scandinavica*, **55**, Suppl. 170, 1.

Bemporad, J.R. & Halloway, E. (1987). Advances in the treatment of disorders of elimination. *In* Noshpitz, J.D., Call, J.D., Cohen, R.L., *et al.* (Eds.) *Basic Handbook of Child Psychiatry*. New York: Basic Books.

Berg, I., Forsythe, I., McGuire, R. (1982). Response of bedwetting to the enuresis alarm. Influence of psychiatric disturbance and maximum functional bladder capacity. *Archives of Diseases of Childhood*, **57**, 394–6.

Blomfield, J.M., Douglas, J.W.B. (1956). Bedwetting – prevalence among children age 4–7. *Lancet*, **i**, 850–2.

Broughton, R.F. (1968). Sleep disorders: Disorders of arousal? *Science*, **159**, 1070–8.

Cohen, M. (1975). Enuresis. *Pediatric Clinics of North America*, **22**, 545–60.

Dahl, R.E., Holttum, J., Trubnick, L. (1994). A clinical picture of child and adolescent narcolepsy. *Journal of the American Academy of Child and Adolescent Psychiatry*, **33**, 834–41.

De Jounge, G.A. (1973). Epidemiology of enuresis. A survey of the literature. *In* Kolvin, I., MacKeith, R.C., McAdow, S.R. (Eds.) *Bladder Control and Enuresis. Clinics in Developmental Medicine. Nos 48/49*. London: Heineman/S.I.M.P.

Diez, F.J., Berger, T.G. (1988). Scarring due to an enuresis blanket. *Pediatric Dermatology*, **5**, 58–60.

Douglass, A.B., Harris, L., Pazderka, F. (1989). Monozygotic twins concordant for the narcoleptic syndrome. *Neurology*, **39**, 140–1.

Dunn, J. (1980). Feeding and sleeping. *In* Rutter, M. (Ed.) *Scientific Foundations of Developmental Psychiatry*. London: Heinemann Medical.

Essen, J., Peckham, C. (1976). Nocturnal enuresis in childhood. *Developmental Medicine and Child Neurology*, **18**, 577–89.

Ferguson, D.M., Horwood, L.J., Shannon, F.T. (1986). Factors related to the age of attainment of nocturnal bladder control: An 8-year longitudinal study. *Pediatrics*, **78**, 884–90.

Freud, A., Burlingham, D.T. (1943). *War and Children*. New York: Medical War Book.

Graham, P. (1986). *Child Psychiatry. A*

Developmental Approach. Oxford: Oxford Medical Publications.

Hersov, L. (1985). Faecal Soiling. *In* Rutter, M.,Hersov, L. (Eds.) *Child and Adolescent Psychiatry. Modern Approaches.* London: Blackwell Scientific Publications.

Honda, Y., Hishikawa, Y. (1980). A long-term treatment of narcolepsy and excessive daytime sleepiness with pemoline (Betanime®). *Current Therapeutic Research,* **27**, 429–41.

Kales, A., Soldatos, C.R., Bixler, E.O., Ladda, R.L., Charney, D.S., Webber, G., Schweitzer, P.K. (1980). Hereditary factors in sleepwalking and night terrors. *British Journal of Psychiatry,* **137**, 111–18.

Levine, M.D., Mazonson, P., Bakow, H. (1980). Behavioral symptom substitution in children cured of encopresis. *American Journal of Diseases of Children,* **134**, 663–7.

Loening-Baucke, V.A. (1987). Factors responsible for persistence of childhood constipation. *Journal of Pediatric Gastroenterology and Nutrion,* **6**, 915–22.

Loening-Baucke, V.A., Cruikshank, B.M. (1986). Abnormal defecation dynamics in chronically constipated children with encopresis. *Journal of Pediatrics,* **108**, 562–6.

McGee, R., Makinson, T., Williams, S., Simpson, A. & Silva, P.A. (1984). A longitudinal study of enuresis from five to nine years. *Aust Paediatr,* **20**, 39–42.

Mikkelsen, E.J. (1991). Modern approaches to enuresis and encopresis. *In* Lewis, M. (Ed.) *Child and Adolescent Psychiatry. A Comprehensive Textbook.* Baltimore, MD: Williams & Wilkins.

Mikkelsen, E.J., Rapoport, J.C. (1980). Enuresis: psychopathology, sleep stage, and drug response. *Urologic Clinics of North America,* **7**, 361–77.

Mikkelsen, E.J., Rapoport, J.L., Nee, L., Gruenau, C., Mendelson, W., Gillin, J.C. (1980). Childhood enuresis. *Archives of General Psychiatry,* **37**, 1139–44.

Mimouni, M., Shuper, A., Mimouni, F., Grünebaum, M., Vatsano, T. (1985). Retarded skeletal maturation in children with primary enuresis. *European Journal of Pediatrics,* **144**, 234–5.

Minde, K., Popiel, K., Leos, N., Falkner, S., Parker, K., Handley-Derry, M. (1993). The evaluation and treatment of sleep disturbances in young children. *Journal of Child Psychology and Psychiatry,* **34**, 521–33.

Nrgaard, J.P., Hansen, J.H., Wildschitz, G., Söresen, S. Rittig, S. & Djurhuus, J.E. (1989).

Sleep cystometries in children with nocturnal enuresis. *Journal of Urology,* **141**, 1156–9.

Parkes, J.D., Lock, C.B. (1989). Genetic factors in sleep disorder. *Journal of Neurology, Neurosurgery and Psychiatry,* **52 (Suppl.)**, 101–8.

Pierce, C.M., Whitman, R.M., Mass, J.W., *et al.* (1961). Enuresis and dreaming. Experimental studies. *Archives of General Psychiatry,* **4**, 116–70.

Rew, D.A., Rundle, J.S. (1989). Assessment of the safety of regular DDAVP therapy in primary nocturnal enuresis. *British Journal of Urology,* **63**, 352–3.

Ritvo, E.R., Ornitz, E.M., Gottlieb, F., Poussaint, A.F., Maron, B.J., Ditman, K.S., Blinn, K.A. (1969). Arousal and nonarousal enuretic events. *American Journal of Psychiatry,* **126**, 77–84.

Rivera, V.M., Meyer, J.S., Hata, T., Ishikawa, Y., Imai, A. (1986). Narcolepsy following cerebral hypoxic-ischemia. *Annals of Neurology,* **19**, 505–8.

Rutter, M. (1989). Isle of Wight revisited: twenty-five years of child psychiatric epidemiology. *Journal of the American Academy of Child and Adolescent Psychiatry,* **28**, 633–53.

Rutter, M., Graham, P., Yule, W. (1970). *A Neuropsychiatric Study in Childhood.* London: S.I.M.P./William Heinemann Medical Books Ltd.

Rutter, M., Yule, W., Graham, P. (1973). Enuresis and behavioural deviance. *In* Kolvin, I., MacKeith, R.,Meadow, S.R. (Eds.) *Bladder Control and Enuresis. Clinics in Developmental Medicine. Nos. 48/49.* London: Heinemann/S.I.M.P.

Rutter, M., Tizard, J., Whitmore, K. (1981). *Education, Health and Behavior.* New York: Krieger, Huntington.

Shaffer, D. (1985). Enuresis. *In* Rutter, M.,Hersov, L. (Eds.) *Child and Adolescent Psychiatry: Modern Approaches.* London: Blackwell Scientific Publications.

Shaffer, D., Gardner, A., Hedge, B. (1984). Behavior and bladder disturbance of enuretic children: A rational classification of a common disorder. *Developmental Medicine and Child Neurology,* **26**, 781–92.

Siomopoulos, V. (1976). Psychogenic encopresis treated with imipramine. *JAMA,* **235**, 1842.

Steffenburg, S. (1990). Enures och enkopres. *In* Gillberg, C.,Hellgren, L. (Eds.) *Barn- och ungdomspsykiatri.* Stockholm: Natur och Kultur. (In Swedish.)

Stein, Z.A., Susser, M.W. (1965). Socio-medical study of enuresis among delinquent boys. *British Journal of Preventive and Social Medicine,* **19**, 174–81.

Steinhausen, H.D., Göbel, D. (1989). Enuresis in child psychiatric clinic patients. *Journal of the American Academy of Child and Adolescent Psychiatry*, **28**, 279–81.

Taylor, D.C. (1992). Real life soilers: holding on and giving up encopresis. *European Child & Adolescent Psychiatry*, **1**, 100–4.

Thorne, F.C. (1944). The incidence of nocturnal enuresis after the age of 15 years. *American Journal of Psychiatry*, **100**, 686–9.

Wald, A., Chandra, R., Chiponis, D., Gabel, S. (1986). Anorectal function and continence mechanisms in childhood encopresis. *Journal of Peadiatrics and Gastroenterological Nutrion*, **5**, 346–51.

Werry, J. (1966). The conditioning treatment of enuresis. *American Journal of Psychiatry*, **123**, 226–9.

Wright, L. (1977). Conceptualizing and defining psychosomatic disorders. *Annals of Psychology*, **32**, 625–8.

Wright, L. Walker, C.E. (1978). Case histories and shorter communications: a simple behavioural treatment program for pscyhogenic encopresis. *Behavioral Research Therapy*, **16**, 209–12.

Young, D., Zorick, F., Wittig, R., Roehrs, T., Roth, T. (1988). Narcolepsy in a pediatric population. *American Journal of Diseases of Children*, **142**, 210–13.

Young, I., Goldsmith, A. (1972). Treatment of encopresis in a day treatment program. *Psychotherapy Theory Research Practice*, **9**, 231–5.

10 Specific syndromes not otherwise referred to

There are a number of named syndromes, for which there is now a small and growing literature outlining the 'behavioural phenotype', i.e. the particular profile/constellation of behaviours which is believed to be typical of the underlying, usually genetically determined, disorder. The body of evidence underpinning the particular behavioural and emotional styles and problems varies from one syndrome to another. Also, some of the syndromes have been relatively securely mapped on to the human genome, whereas several more, at the time of publication of this book, have no clear gene localization. For these reasons, the amount of information presented for each named syndrome in this chapter varies considerably. The syndromes will be described in alphabetical order. Most of these syndromes are known only by their 'person's name label'. Although the policy in this respect varies, and is viewed differently, by different investigators, for purposes of coherence, syndromes named after one or other individual will be presented primarily in their 'named' variant. However, in the case of, for instance, neurofibromatosis and tuberous sclerosis, also known as von Recklinghausen disease and Bourneville disease, the former 'names' will be used, because these are now the ones most widely accepted.

The alphabetical listing may lead to some (hopefully slight) logical confusion, such as with tuberous sclerosis, neurofibromatosis and Ito's hypomelanosis, which are otherwise often grouped together in a section on 'neurocutaneous disorders'. However, with the expansion of knowledge in the field of molecular biology, a case could equally be made for one, two or all three of these disorders being grouped according to their particular associations with genetic defects on particular chromosomes. In view of this, it is hoped that the logic of putting the syndromes in 'alphabetical order' will be acceptable to the reader.

Aicardi syndrome and other syndromes including corpus callosum agenesis/dysgenesis

Dysgenesis of the corpus callosum is probably a relatively common brain abnormality, sometimes associated with more specific neuropsychiatric symptoms and then awarded the status of a separate syndrome. Thus, callosal dysgenesis can be sub-divided into non-syndromic and syndromic forms. Aicardi syndrome is the most common of these 'subsyndromes' of corpus callosum dysgenesis/agenesis.

Prevalence

Callosal agenesis was found in 2.3% of all brain CT scans ($n = 1447$) surveyed in one centre (Jeret *et al.*, 1985–1986). However, CT scans are most often performed in individuals with clear or suspected neurological disorder indicating that the true frequency of callosal agenesis/dysgenesis is not known.

Sex ratios

Among the syndromic forms of callosal agenesis, girls are over-represented. Some of these

syndromes (Aicardi syndrome, oro-facio-digi-
tal syndrome) are seen only in girls.

Behavioural and physical phenotype

There is no specific physical or behavioural
phenotype associated with callosal dysgenesis
in all cases, but in the non-syndromic forms,
which are the most common as a group, mental
retardation, psychiatric/behavioural disorder
(including severe OCD, autistic-type and intermittent explosive behaviours), seizures, macrocephaly and hypertelorism are very frequent
features. 'Cerebral palsy' is often diagnosed as
well. There is often remarkable preservation of
inter-hemispheric transfer (Jeeves & Temple,
1987). Endocrine disturbances are possibly
over-represented (Smith et al., 1986). In a recent
study of ADHD, the posterior parts of the
callosum were reduced (Semrud-Clikeman et
al., 1994).

In Aicardi syndrome (Chevrie & Aicardi,
1986), which is probably caused by an X-linked
dominant mutation (and only reported in girls),
there are infantile spasms (complex) partial
seizures, ocular abnormalities, severe mental
retardation, vertebrocostal abnormalities and
split-brain EEG. Multiple heterotopias and
micropolygyrias in the brain have been
reported (Hamano et al., 1989).

Pathogenesis

In non-syndromal forms of corpus callosum
agenesis, genetic transmission is rare, although
a few dominant (Aicardi, Chevrie & Baraton,
1987), autosomal recessive and X-linked recessive variants (Menkes, Philappart & Clark,
1964) have been described. A variety of chromosomal defects (including trisomies of chromosomes 18, 13 and 8) are on record. Foetal
alcohol exposure has been reported to be associated with corpus callosum agenesis (Jones et
al., 1973). Metabolic disorders may be
concurrent.

There may be complete agenesis or partial
dysgenesis. In the latter case, the posterior part
is usually missing. However, anterior dysgenesis has also been described. The absent callosal
commissure is usually replaced by two longitudinal bundles. Enlargement of the occipital
horn (colpocephaly) is common, as are a multitude of CNS malformations (heterotopias,
abnormalities of gyration, etc. (Jellinger et al.,
1981; Jeret et al., 1987). It is believed that, in
most instances, these associated abnormalities,
rather than the corpus callosum abnormality as
such, are responsible for most of the clinical
manifestations.

Several of the syndromic variants are genetic.
These syndromes too (like Aicardi syndrome)
are often associated with other abnormalities of
brain development, including heterotopias and
cysts.

Diagnosis

The diagnosis of corpus callosum agenesis/
dysgenesis is made on the combined evidence
from ultrasonography, CT scan and/or MRI
scan of the brain. MRI scans are particularly
sensitive in the diagnosis of partial agenesis.

Antenatal diagnosis is now possible from
about the twentieth week of gestation
(Klingensmith & Cioffi-Ragan, 1986). However, normal development seems to be common
in some individuals with callosal agenesis. For
instance, Blum and co-workers found half of a
group of 12 infants with a prenatal diagnosis of
corpus callosum agenesis to be developing normally at 2–8 years of age. If there was associated
chromosomal abnormality, outcome was poor
(Blum et al., 1990). Thus, in order to provide the
best possible basis for a decision regarding
possible termination of pregnancy to be made
by the parents, it is essential to perform both
high-quality foetal karyotyping and a thorough
ultrasonographic examination.

Goldenhar syndrome occasionally has associated corpus callosum agenesis/dysgenesis (cf.
Goldenhar syndrome later in this chapter).

Work-up

A neuropsychological evaluation (including the
Griffiths, Leiter or WISC as appropriate plus a
test of speech and language), and a neurodevelopmental examination, including thorough
assessment of handedness and sensorimotor

coordination are usually indicated, apart from the need to perform adequate neuroimaging. An EEG should be performed in order to rule out subclinical epilepsy, document 'split brain' findings, or aid in the diagnosis of clinical seizure activity. An X-ray examination of the thorax might well be indicated, if there is a suspicion (because of a history of infantile spasms and the presence of severe mental retardation) of Aicardi syndrome.

Treatment

There is currently no specific treatment available for the various forms of corpus callosum dysgenesias, including Aicardi syndrome. Neuropsychiatric symptoms should be treated along the lines suggested for individual types of problems including epilepsy and autistictype symptoms. In the various known forms of corpus callosum dysgenesias, outcome accords with the overall level of development and symptoms exhibited in the pre-pubertal period. There is usually no progression of symptoms. However, as has been evident from the foregoing, the degree of handicap is considerable in most cases.

Hydrocephalus may be suspected because of the presence of an extremely large head (OFC may be 5 to 7 standard deviations above the age group mean). However, shunting is usually not indicated, because many such cases of 'hydrocephalus' stabilize spontaneously without causing clinical problems.

Seizures should be treated pharmacologically, but they are often very resistant to medication. In the rare case of so-called Shapiro syndrome (corpus callosum agenesis, periodic hypothermia and diaphoresis) (Shapiro, Williams & Plum, 1969), clonidine treatment may be effective (Sanfield et al., 1989).

Outcome

In the various known forms of corpus callosum dysgenesias, outcome accords with the overall level of development and symptoms exhibited in the pre-pubertal period. There is usually no progression of symptoms. However, as has been evident from the foregoing, the degree of handicap is considerable in many cases.

The outcome of corpus callosum agenesis has not been studied on a broad basis. However, it is likely to be extremely variable, ranging from excellent in the (many?) asymptomatic cases, to intermediate (socially and academically; need for special education) in some of the nonsyndromic forms, and poor in some of the named syndromes, such as Aicardi syndrome.

Angelman syndrome

Angelman syndrome, which is associated with damage to (or absence of) maternally inherited DNA material on chromosome 15q11 (at the same site as that affected in Prader–Willi syndrome), encompasses jerky movements, unprovoked laughter and varying degrees of mental retardation (hitherto mostly reported to be severe or profound).

Prevalence

To the author's knowledge, there have been no population studies of Angelman syndrome. As conceptualized today, it is bound to be rare, probably less prevalent than Prader–Willi syndrome (see below). However, as with the majority of the 'behavioural phenotypes', it is quite conceivable that current concepts of the syndrome may be too narrow, and that prevalence may be under-estimated.

Behavioural and physical phenotype

Studies supporting the notion of a particular behavioural and physical phenotype in this syndrome are beginning to appear (e.g. Clayton-Smith, 1991; Buntinx et al., 1991). So far, the evidence is too limited to suggest details in this respect, but some cautious conclusions appear to be warranted.

First of all, the typical facial features (wide mouth, prominent lower jaw and microbrachycephalia) and the jerky movements persist throughout childhood and early adolescence– adult life (Clayton-Smith, 1991).

Secondly, there are often feeding problems in the infancy period, ranging from frequent spitting to food refusal and failure to thrive. Vomiting and inadequate control of chewing and swallowing occur in some children with Angelman syndrome, but appear to abate with time in most cases.

Thirdly, there is often inappropriately little need for sleep (Zori et al., 1992).

Fourthly, walking is usually severely delayed, some never acquire this skill at all, and others, after having previously walked become nonambulant again. However, walking is usually attained by age 6 years. Those who do walk can show mild or severe ataxia.

Fifthly, difficult-to-control seizures (usually with onset between 10 and 30 months (Buntinx et al., 1991)) which are very common in early childhood, often become less severe with age. The bizarre (and typical?) EEG pattern of childhood appears to improve and more normal rhythms emerge.

Sixthly, absence of spoken language or extremely limited skills in this domain appears to be an almost invariable feature of the syndrome as conceptualized today. Nevertheless, some individuals acquire sign language skills, albeit at a rather primitive level. About 15–20% can say a few words. Most appear to have slightly better language comprehension, but caution is warranted here since no well-designed study has specifically examined this aspect yet. At least one case of Angelman syndrome and typical autism has been described so far (Steffenburg, Gillberg & Steffenburg, 1992). A few reports mention autistic-type hand-flapping stereotypies (e.g. Buntinx et al., 1991).

Seventhly, severe to profound mental retardation appears to be an invariable feature of this disorder, even though caution is warranted in accepting this statement as an absolute truth. Many behavioural phenotype syndromes (e.g. the fragile X syndrome and Prader–Willi syndrome) have originally been conceptualized as 'mental retardation syndromes'. Only several years–decades later have cases with these syndromes without mental retardation been described. Nevertheless, judging from the limited literature on Angelman syndrome, it seems clear that IQ in the 'average' Angelman case is considerably lower than in the chromosomally associated Prader–Willi syndrome. There is, in Angelman syndrome, usually a suspicion of moderately delayed mental development in the first year (or two) of life.

Eighthly, most individuals with Angelman syndrome show ocular and cutaneous hypopigmentation. Interestingly, oculocutaneous albinism can be inherited as an autosomal dominant or associated with other syndromes. It has been documented both in Prader–Willi and Angelman syndromes. Ocular hypopigmentation is consistent with a neural crest developmental abnormality. Neurocrestopathies have also been suggested to underlie neurofibromatosis and hypomelanosis of Ito.

Finally, a behavioural phenotype hallmarked by bursts of laughter, strange nighttime outbursts reminiscent of seizures (some of which probably represent epileptic phenomena), hyperactivity and impulsivity against a background of a generally happy disposition has been described by several authors. It appears that, with age, the hyperactivity subsides, giving way to more controllable behaviour. However, new problems may emerge over time. A bizarre kind of pica, with chewing of various types of objects, has been reported by some authors (Buntinx et al., 1991).

The syndrome was previously referred to as 'happy puppet syndrome', but this term is generally felt to be pejorative and should be avoided.

From the above description it should be obvious that while there are some behavioural overlapping features in Prader–Willi and Angelman syndromes, the two disorders are clearly different, in spite of the overlapping (identical?) chromosomal area affected. Genomic imprinting has been suggested to account for the fact that two different syndromes can result on the basis of chromosomal abnormality at the same site. Many (all?) cases with Prader–Willi syndrome demonstrate absence of normal paternal chromosomal material at 15q11–13. Many (all or most?) cases with Angelman syndrome demonstrate absence of normal maternal chromosomal material at 15q11–13.

Differential diagnosis

Angelman syndrome in girls may be difficult to differentiate from Rett syndrome, particularly in the first few years of life. However, most of the supportive criteria suggesting Rett syndrome (see Table 10.4) will not apply in Angelman syndrome, and a thorough check of these will usually decide the case. There are also instances of unspecific mental retardation with some, but not all, of the features of Angelman syndrome which may present diagnostic problems. However, molecular genetic diagnosis will usually help guide clinical diagnosis in such cases.

Work-up

The Angelman syndrome gene has been identified, and work-up in all suspected cases should include gene analysis. The gene defect can sometimes be visualized as a microdeletion at chromosomal analysis, but gene analysis rather than chromosomal analysis is to be preferred once the syndrome is clinically seriously considered. However, 25–40% of all Angelman patients have normal chromosomes and, even when cytogenetic studies are complemented by molecular probing, at least 20% fail to show a deletion. It merits mention in this respect that several sibling pairs with two Angelman affected individuals have not had chromosomal or molecular deletions. The EEG can be helpful in suggesting the presence of the syndrome in a child with severe–profound mental retardation. The EEG pattern is sometimes quite distinct with posterior slow wave activity with discharges facilitated by, or seen only on, passive eye closure.

CT- or MRI-scan of the brain may yield normal results (in about one-third of the cases) or show cortical atrophy, periventricular leukomalacia, dysmyelination and cerebellar hypoplasia (Zori *et al.*, 1992).

Genetic counselling

No offspring of people with Angelman syndrome have been described in the literature so far. There may be a slightly increased risk of Angelman or Prader–Willi syndromes re-occurring in a family into which one child with Angelman syndrome has been born (Fisher *et al.*, 1987), but, at the present stage, it seems that multiple incidence of the syndromes within one family is rare.

Management

There have been no studies or systematic clinical reports of management/treatment strategies in Angelman syndrome.

Outcome

A majority of the Angelman syndrome cases identified to date continue to show the same type of physical, mental and behavioural characteristics throughout childhood. Only through meticulous follow-along studies shall we learn more about the long-term outcome of this puzzling disorder.

Chronic fatigue syndrome

Chronic fatigue syndrome (also referred to as myalgic encephalomyelitis ('ME'), post-infectious neurasthenia, neurasthenia cerebralis or simply neurasthenia) comprising lethargy, a reported feeling of being overwhelmingly tired, sometimes bordering on apathy, irritability and, although not invariably, a decline in academic performance has been inconsistently noted to occur more frequently in connection with certain infectious diseases than in others. Infectious mononucleosis ('glandular fever') and coxsackie B virus (Wilson *et al.*, 1989) have been two of the most commonly reported diseases in this group. Epidemics of severe influenza have also been said to be followed by prolonged fatigue syndromes (Meijer, Zakay-Rones & Morag, 1988). However, until recently, these 'chronic fatigue syndromes', have received little attention from the scientific community, and it remains unclear to what extent they should be considered separate disorders that are linked to specific aetiological agents.

Apart from profound physical and mental fatigue, particularly after exercise, there are also commonly neuromuscular, cardiovascular and gastrointestinal symptoms.

Garralda (1992) reported two cases illustrating the potential extreme and life-threatening severity of the condition in certain children. Like other authors, she highlighted the common occurrence of physical precipitants, usually in the form of an antecedent 'flu-like' illness, and associated depressive symptomatology. She further suggested that certain features may be regarded as likely to indicate that psychopathological mechanisms are playing an important part, if not in the aetiology, possibly in the continuation of the syndrome. These factors are: *in the child:* concern (high expectations) over academic progress and a personality style characterized by obsessionality/conscientiousness, sensitivity and limited communication of emotional issues, and *in the family:* health problems (in particular fatigue and mobility symptoms) and preoccupation with illness, high academic/behavioural expectations, emotional closeness and decreased communication on emotional illness.

Prevalence

The prevalence of chronic fatigue syndrome in the general population of children is unknown, but obviously relatively common. For instance, in 7–12 year-old children attending a secondary paediatric clinic, fatigue was a major problem in 11%, even though it was the primary complaint in only 2% of all cases (Garralda & Bailey, 1990).

Work-up

It is difficult to suggest a reasonable work-up that would apply equally to all cases of chronic fatigue syndrome. It is, of course, important not to under-diagnose severe physical or psychiatric illness in young individuals, and extreme fatigue can be part of the clinical picture in a range of serious and life-threatening disorders including malignancy and endocrine disorder. Nevertheless, it is also important not to involve the young patient with chronic fatigue syndrome in too exhaustive a work-up. A screen for malignancy and severe infectious disorder in simple blood tests and a serum viral titre for the most common viruses (mononucleosis, influenza A, coxsackie B and mycoplasma) are indicated. The clinical findings should be interpreted with a view to diagnosing possible endocrine disorders such as Addison disease and hypothyroidism. The medical history should include probing into recent medications. A search for relevant family and child characteristics (see above) should be made. For a small number of children with conversion hysterical reactions (sometimes difficult to separate from chronic fatigue syndrome), sexual abuse may be the difficult, unspeakable predicament (Volkmar, Poll & Lewis, 1984; Leslie, 1988). If improvement occurs in spite of a lack of resolution of such conflicts, it would seem to argue in favour of other background factors being in operation.

Treatment

Treatment should include identification of the factors (primary viral infection, depression, over-focus on school performance, the feeling on the part of the child that returning to school and peers is an unsurmountable obstacle, over-involvement on the part of the family, etc.) which may contribute to the maintaining of symptoms over long periods of time. Talking these things over with the parents and child separately, and later together, may be very helpful in reversing the 'vicious spiral'. Separation from the family for brief inpatient management may prove necessary in some cases. Graded physiotherapy is often helpful. Antidepressant medication may be indicated. Children with chronic fatigue syndromes are an important patient group for the neuropsychiatrist. They are often in need of highly specialized care over many months, sometimes even a few years.

Outcome

Outcome is often surprisingly good, at least in the intermediate term. Most of the cases described have returned to their pre-illness level of functioning. At the height of clinical problems (one–several months after the viral illness), it may sometimes be difficult to believe that a 'cure' is really realistic. The neuropsychiatrist has an important mission in providing optimistic support during this difficult phase.

Cockayne syndrome

Cockayne syndrome is a rare autosomally recessive inherited disorder featuring leukodystrophy and leading to premature death.

Prevalence

The prevalence of Cockayne syndrome is unknown. It is undoubtedly a very rare disorder. The author has encountered two cases (familially connected) over a period of 20 years of practice, comprising more than 3000 neuropsychiatric cases.

Sex ratios

The sex ratio is likely to be equal.

Behavioural and physical phenotype

After a normal first year, growth and neurodevelopmental retardation become prominent. Occasionally, the changes do not occur until after four or five years of apparently normal development. In such cases there may be plateauing rather than regression of intellectual capacities. The presenting symptoms and diagnosis may be ADHD or DAMP. Mental retardation may be severe, moderate or mild at the time of diagnosis, but the impression is usually that of at least moderate intellectual impairment once the individual has been followed up for a few years. Skin hypersensitivity to sunlight is common and may be pronounced. Peripheral neuropathy is characteristic and nerve conduction velocity is often decreased. Cerebellar and pyramidal tract signs slowly begin to appear. Some years later (ages 4–10 years) the individuals usually have small stature, cachexic signs and large ears. Hypertension and renal failure may ensue.

Diagnosis

The diagnosis is made on the basis of the typical clinical picture in combination with the demonstration of sensitivity of cultured fibroblasts to ultraviolet light (this can also be demonstrated in amniocytes for purposes of prenatal diagnosis (Lehman, Francis & Giannelli, 1985)) and of abnormalities of the retina (pigmentary retinopathy), white matter and basal ganglia (as documented on CT scan or MRI) (Dabbagh & Swaiman, 1988). CT often discloses a considerable degree of ventricular dilatation. The CSF is usually normal.

Pathogenesis

The condition is transmitted as an autosomal recessive trait. Fibroblasts grown from individuals with Cockayne syndrome exhibit inhibition of the increased RNA synthesis which normally appears after ultraviolet irradiation (Leech et al., 1985). The pathogenesis of Cockayne syndrome is unknown.

The underlying causes of the leukodystrophy (with preservation of islands of myelin), retinal degeneration, dwarfism and skin sensitivity to light, remain to be demonstrated.

Work-up

Culture of fibroblasts and exposure to ultraviolet light and subsequent analysis of the results are only performed by a few labs at present. Such a lab should be approached and specimens sent for analysis, if the diagnosis is strongly suspected. CT and MRI should be performed, peripheral nerve cell conductance should be examined and an ophthalmologist should evaluate visual acuity and the fundi with a particular view to early detection of pigmentary retinopathy.

Treatment

There is no known treatment for Cockayne syndrome.

Outcome

Outcome is not known, but premature death often ensues. Probably, most individuals affected do not survive their thirtieth birthday and many die before that age.

De Lange syndrome (Cornelia de Lange syndrome)

The (Cornelia) de Lange syndrome is characterized by a curious face, microcepahly, mental retardation, behavioural abnormality and growth and skeletal abnormalities.

Prevalence

The prevalence of de Lange syndrome is not known. However, at least 20 cases are known to exist in children under age 18 years in Sweden. This indicates that the minimum prevalence is at least 1 in 100 000 children. Given that some cases die before age 18 years, and that other cases will remain undiagnosed, the true prevalence is likely to be considerably higher than that.

Sex ratios

The sex ratio in de Lange syndrome is reported to be equal.

Behavioural and physical phenotype

All children with de Lange syndrome reported in the literature have been mentally retarded. Most cases are profoundly mentally retarded, and it is definitely uncommon to encounter anybody with the syndrome who has a tested IQ of 50 or more.

The curious face with synophrys (the eyebrows grown together and overlapping in the midline), the low hairline on neck and forehead, long and upturned eyelashes, the depressed bridge of the nose with upturned nostrils create a typical appearance which, in itself, is usually pronounced enough to make the diagnosis clear. Moderate–severe microcephaly and over-all moderate–severe growth retardation are the rule. The arms are thin, the thumbs are proximally implanted and the thenar eminence is small. Reduction of the size of the radius and finger hypoplasia are also common features. Micrognathia is almost always present.

Behaviour problems include severe self-injurious activities (including head banging, head smashing, eye poking and hand biting), social withdrawal, full-blown autistic disorder or the triad of social, communication and behavioural/imaginative impairment/restriction combined with severe or profound mental retardation. Because motor problems are often pronounced and many individuals with the syndrome are unable to walk (and talk), it is common for the behavioural repertoire to be so limited as to preclude the development of skills elaborate enough to allow the full syndrome of autism to develop.

Diagnosis

The de Lange syndrome diagnosis is based purely on the presence of the characteristic symptoms.

Pathogenesis

The aetiology and pathogenesis of de Lange syndrome is unknown at the time of going to press with this book. Abnormalities of chromosome 3 have been reported in several cases of de Lange syndrome or, at least, in cases with a broadly similar symptomatology (Steinbach et al., 1981; McKusick, 1988a, b, c).

De Lange syndrome is believed to be inherited as an autosomal dominant, virtually all cases being new mutations. A recurrence risk of less than 5% is often quoted.

Work-up

At present, no diagnostic marker for Cornelia de Lange syndrome has been identified. Work-up should include a reasonable neuropsychological evaluation including, at least, a test of overall functioning (the Griffiths or the Vineland Social Maturity Scale; the PEP in cases with pronounced degrees of autistic behaviour). An EEG is warranted because of the high risk of seizures, some of which may be subclinical. Ophthalmological and cardiological examinations are indicated because of the high rate of ocular and cardiac problems. Hypothalamic and peripheral endocrine functions may need monitoring when there are symptoms (even mild) suggestive of Addison disease (weakness, low blood pressure, vomiting, discolouration of the skin) or other endocrine disorder.

Treatment

There is no specific treatment available for Cornelia de Lange syndrome. The autistic symptoms and self-injurious behaviours may need interventions as suggested in chapters relating to these types of problems. Restraints may be necessary in severe self-injury cases with loss of body tissue.

Outcome

Outcome is poor in many respects. Ultimate height is small, unsupported walking is often not achieved, talking is even rarer. The co-occurrence of heart disease and the variety of ocular problems also contribute to poor quality of life for many individuals with this syndrome. Mortality is increased, but there are no representative long-term follow-up studies and mean life length is not known.

Double Y syndrome (XYY)

The XYY syndrome is one of the most common chromosomal disorders. Together with Down syndrome (the most common of all major chromosomal disorders), the fragile X syndrome, XXY (Klinefelter syndrome) and XO (Turner syndrome), it accounts for as many as 1 in 300 births.

Prevalence

The prevalence of XYY syndrome is reported to be about 0.1% of the general male population.

Sex ratios

By definition, only males are affected by this syndrome.

Behavioural and physical phenotype

Boys with an extra Y-chromosome are often unusually tall but otherwise show no clear characteristic physical features. They are at increased risk of delay and other problems in language development (including dyslexia) (Ratcliffe, Butler & Jones, 1990) and prone to temper tantrums and aggressiveness. They also often show hypotonia and hyperactivity. Poor relatedness is a common feature and the risk of autism appears to be clearly increased (Hagerman, 1989). IQ is usually in the normal range, but learning disorder is relatively common and the incidence of mental retardation is possibly increased as compared with the general male population. A slightly increased tendency for aggressiveness, and features of sadism in sexual orientation in adult life, is suggested by at least one unbiased prospective study (Schiavi et al., 1988). Already in the 1960s and 1970s, Forssman suggested that individuals with XYY syndrome might be over-represented in abnormal populations with high degrees of aggressive behaviour (Forssman et al., 1975), such as in males involved in severe criminal activity. It is often stated that most individuals with XYY syndrome are indistinguishable from the normal general population of men, but the available literature on young children does not support this view.

Diagnosis

The diagnosis is made at chromosomal analysis. XYY syndrome should be suspected in children with autism, language disorders and dyslexia (particularly if associated with tall stature) and in young children with the combination of language delay and aggressive behaviour (Fig. 10.1).

Pathogenesis

The pathogenesis of XYY syndrome is unknown, in spite of the fact that the chromoso-

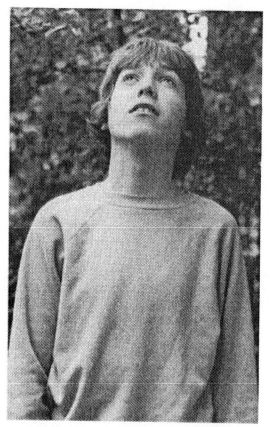

Fig. 10.1 13-year-old boy with Asperger syndrome and XYY mosaicism.

mal gonosomal aneuploidy has been known for more than 30 years. It is likely that abnormalities of testosterone metabolism or responsivity may be responsible for some of the clinical problems encountered.

Work-up

In most cases, no further work-up, apart from chromosomal analysis, is indicated.

Treatment

There is no treatment available for XYY syndrome. Parents should be informed about the risk of language disorders, dyslexia and behaviour problems. The available literature does not suggest an increased recurrence risk in future pregnancies if a mother has borne a child with XYY syndrome.

Outcome

Outcome has not been sufficiently studied in this syndrome. The only available prospective longitudinal study (Schiavi et al., 1988) suggested a high rate of sadistic sexual orientation. As regards social, academic and vocational outcome, much less is known. It is clear, however, that many individuals with XYY syndrome grow up to function well in most aspects.

Down syndrome

Down syndrome (trisomy 21, or rather triplication of 21q22.1 to 21q22.2, 'mongolism'), unlike other mental retardation syndromes, seems to be associated with a relatively low incidence of psychiatric disorder (Gillberg et al., 1986a). Down syndrome is the single most common cause of severe mental retardation, and it is not infrequently found in mild mental retardation.

Prevalence

The prevalence of Down syndrome is in the range of 1–1.2 per 1000 children born. Down syndrome accounts for about one-third of severe mental retardation and one-sixth of mental retardation of any degree of severity (Fryns et al., 1984). The prevalence is strongly related to maternal age. Thus, the rate is about 0.5–0.6 per 1000 in children born to 20 year-old mothers, around 1 per 1000 if the mother is 30 years old and almost 10% if the mother is 49 years old (Rogers & Coleman, 1992). The mortality rate in the first year was high until recently. It now appears that more than 90% of all Down syndrome infants survive the first year (and the vast majority of these will survive to adult age) (Dupont, Vaeth & Videbech, 1986).

Sex ratios

There is no clear indication that Down syndrome is in any way associated with gender.

However, just as in child psychiatry generally, it may be that the association of Down syndrome with behavioural problems may be more common in males than in females (Gillberg *et al.*, 1986a).

Behavioural and physical phenotype

There is no one behavioural or physical phenotype exclusive to, or pathognomonic of, Down syndrome. However, in a large proportion of affected individuals, it is easy to tell, both from the general physical appearance and the patterns of behaviours shown, that Down syndrome is the likely diagnosis.

It appears that additional brain damage may be common in Down syndrome, and that severe behaviour problems may be more strongly associated with this factor than with the chromosomal disorder as such. On the other hand, it is still possible, indeed quite likely, that Down syndrome *per se* predisposes to a particular personality style or behavioural phenotype.

Almost 20% of all trisomy 21 foetuses are stillborn. Furthermore, at least one in 40 spontaneous abortions contains a trisomy 21 foetus. Birthweight can be low and more than 20% of babies weighing less than 2500 g have trisomy 21.

The physical phenotype comprises neonatal (and continued) hypotonus, a typical face with outward–upward slant of the eyes, a short nose with a flat nasal bridge and white (Brushfield) spots in the central parts of the iris. There is a high incidence of cataracts and strabismus. The external auditory meatus is narrow. The fingers are short, the little finger is incurved and metacarpal bones may be missing. There may be single (rather than double) palmar creases. There are usually growth abnormalities, and most individuals with the syndrome are small, even though individual variation is considerable. Head circumference is usually small or very small.

Malformations of the atrioventricular canal and duodenal stenosis are common.

Hypotonus contributes to an increased risk of infection. This risk is increased for other reasons also, including auto-immune problems. The risk of leukaemia is much increased as compared to the general population (Krivit & Good, 1957).

Independent ambulation is usually much delayed, usually until about the age of 2–4 years.

Average IQ is below 50 (Smith & Berg, 1976; Hagberg *et al.*, 1981; Gillberg *et al.*, 1986a) and it tends to decrease with age (even when the effects of associated Alzheimer disease are partialled out). Most individuals with Down syndrome have IQs in the 20–70 range, even though, occasionally, IQ may be as high as 85.

Most children with Down syndrome have IQs under 50 and, of the 10–20% who test higher, many are cases of mosaicism (Fischler, Koch & Donnell., 1976). Such cases represent about 2–3% of all who receive a clinical diagnosis of Down syndrome. The cognitive profile in Down syndrome, in spite of a generally low level, shows considerable interindividual variation.

Epilepsy is more common than in the general population (Stafström *et al.*, 1991), even though the rate is lower than in most other mental retardation syndromes. The prevalence of infantile spasms is relatively very high (Pollack *et al.*, 1978). Hearing deficits are common, and are mostly of the conductive type. They may be made worse by chronic infections.

Hypothyroidism is a common feature and needs to be worked up and treated as appropriate for that disorder.

The very early development of children with Down syndrome is usually only slightly (if at all) retarded (Carr, 1970). Even though the stereotype of the happy, amiable and tractable personality is unsupported in many cases, and temper tantrums, irritability and stubbornness may be relatively common features in childhood, it seems clear that the majority of adolescents and young adults with Down syndrome do not have major psychiatric problems (a finding which is unusual in mental retardation generally) (Gillberg *et al.*, 1986a). However, severe problems can occur in Down syndrome, and even autism and hyperkinetic disorders have been described in a number of cases. Another subgroup of children with Down syndrome show extremely eccentric and bizarre behaviours without meeting full criteria for autistic disorder (or even an autistic-like condition). It seems that additional brain damage, or specific genetic influences on constitution, might be a pre-requisite for the development of autism in Down syndrome, and that the autistic symptoms may be unassociated with the chromosomal abnormality as such.

Diagnosis

The diagnosis of Down syndrome is based on the combined evidence of the physical phenotype and results of chromosomal analysis. Trisomy 21 is the most common chromosomal abnormality in Down syndrome, accounting for more than 90% of all cases. About 5% are due to a translocation of chromosome 21 to another chromosome, usually 14 or 21. A few per cent are composed of mosaics of normal and trisomic cells (Fischler et al., 1976). Very occasionally, only a part of chromosome 21 (including the region 21q22.1 to 21q22.2) exists in triplicate.

Interestingly, there are individuals with the physical phenotype associated with Down syndrome who do not show any currently known chromosomal abnormalities. These individuals may be intellectually normal and yet have all or most of the physical features considered typical of Down syndrome.

Pathogenesis

Trisomy 21 Down syndrome results from a mistake, called non-disjunction, when chromosomes divide. An egg or a sperm cell is created from a cell containing 46 chromosomes, which divides in half to create two germ cells, each with 23 chromosomes. In non-disjunction, the 46 chromosome cell fails to divide properly. One germ cell contains 24 and another only 22 chromosomes. At fertilization, the germ cell with only 22 chromosomes combines with a 23 chromosome cell to produce a 45 chromosome cell (a product which is rarely viable). The germ cell with 24 chromosomes when combined with a 23 chromosome germ cell (to form a 47 chromosome cell, containing one trisomy set of chromosomes) is more likely to survive. Non-disjunction occurs more often in older mothers

(see above under prevalence), and in older fathers. Recent studies suggest that there may be a paternal origin of non-disjunction in about 5% of Down syndrome cases (Antonarakis et al., 1991).

Translocations also occur that account for the clinical syndrome of Down. These always involve chromosome 21. The second involved chromosome may be chromosome 21, 14 or (uncommonly) another chromosome. The translocations may be inherited, so a check of the parents for genetic counselling is indicated.

There are also mosaicisms (cell mosaicisms or, very uncommonly, tissue mosaicisms). About 10% of all parents of children with Down syndrome are themselves mosaics. When there is no other explanation for familial Down syndrome, parental mosaicism should be considered. The affected parent may have good intelligence and few, if any, stigmata suggestive of Down syndrome.

It is still unclear how the chromosomal abnormalities encountered in the clinical Down syndrome link up with metabolic disorder to produce the specific phenotype.

Gross brain pathology is minor. Most clinicians refer to children with Down syndrome as 'brain damaged'. This would not be appropriate in many cases, in which, more accurately, there is an abnormal brain without the changes usually associated with hypoxic or other structural brain damage. The brain is small and the cerebellum particularly so. The size of the cerebrum, but not that of the cerebellum, corresponds to that of the skull (Jernigan, Bellugi & Hesselink, 1989). The first temporal gyrus is unusually small.

Microscopically there is a considerable reduction of the cells in the granular layer of the cortex in some areas and curtailment of aspinuous stellate cells (Ross, Galaburda & Kemper, 1984). The number of spines on apical dendrites are possibly reduced (Marin Padilla, 1976).

Work-up

A chromosomal analysis should be made in all neonates raising suspicion of suffering from Down syndrome. The parents should be informed about the suspicion and the reason for performing the cytogenetic assessment. Once the diagnosis is chromosomally certain, there is a need to make an in-depth work-up, including ordinary blood tests (red and white blood cells), immunological testing and evaluation of thyroid status. A cardiologist needs to make a detailed evaluation, considering the high rate of heart and large blood vessel malformations. Ophthalmologists and oto-laryngologists and audiologists should also be consulted. Some of this work-up needs to be repeated at intervals during the child's first ten years. In particular, there is a great need to monitor thyroid status and diagnose (and treat) hypothyroidism which may have insidious onset.

Treatment

There is no treatment specifically effective for Down syndrome. However, by implementing a combined medico-educational programme already at the time of diagnosis, outcome can probably be considerably improved, at least with regard to general well-being/health in childhood and adolescence (Rogers & Coleman, 1992), possibly also, although more controversial, in respect of IQ. No clearly effective treatment has yet surfaced for the Alzheimer-type changes that occur in a majority of Down syndrome individuals in adult age.

The possibility of associated hypothyroidism, hypovitaminosis and hypoimmunoglobulinaemia should be entertained at all ages and treated appropriately whenever documented. There is an increased risk of HIV and hepatitis B infection, and the threshold for performing tests to diagnose (and treat) such infections should be low.

In recent years, many studies have indicated that with early intervention programmes, mainly focusing on education of parents, parents' training of affected children and physiotherapy, much good can be achieved in Down syndrome, even though the generalizability of the results obtained in some studies has been called into question by some authors (Fields & Gibson, 1971). However, it does appear that IQ can be pushed up by 10–20 points and that motor problems associated with hypotonia can be substantially reduced. It is recommended that, since in almost all cases, the diagnosis of Down syndrome is made in the first few days of life, intensive intervention start at once. This is not the place for a detailed description of the training programme as such. The reader is referred, for instance, to Rogers and Coleman (1992). Children with Down syndrome in addition to the education programme (which, among many things, comprises a language stimulation programme) always require a continuous medical work-up because of the often associated major medical problems.

Outcome

Down syndrome is strongly associated with dementia of the Alzheimer type. Signs of early senescence, thin hair, dry and wrinkled skin, cataracts and neuropathic changes may occur as early as in the third decade (Gualtieri, 1989). Onset of seizures in a Down syndrome individual who previously did not have epilepsy may also signal change and usher in a downhill dementing development (Dalton & Crapper-McLachlan, 1986). The available evidence suggests that almost all Down syndrome individuals develop changes in brain tissue (extracellular senile, neuritic and amyloid, plaques and intracellular neurofibrillary tangles) characteristic of Alzheimer disease (Wisniewski, 1983; Iqbal & Wisniewski, 1983) already by age 40 years. Behavioural and cognitive decline may not occur until much later (Lott, 1982; Thase et al., 1984). In one study (Dalton & Crapper-McLachlan, 1986), the average age of onset of dementia symptoms was 53 years and the duration to death ranged from 3.5–10.5 years. A decline in performance on standardized neuropsychological tests is often diagnostic once the dementia is suspected (either on the basis of personality change including disinhibited behaviour, gait problems, seizure disorders or sphincteric incontinence). Serial CT scans may show temporal, frontal or widespread atrophy of brain tissue. There may also be reversible causes of deterioration, including senile depression and hypothyroidism, both of which have to be ruled out before one settles for a diagnosis of dementia of the Alzheimer type.

More than half of all Down syndrome patients in an institution showed signs of dementia in the age range of 50–59 years, and 75% had such signs at 60 years or older. Seizures developed in five out of six of those with dementia. One in five had symptoms compatible with Parkinson disease (Lai & Williams, 1989).

Duchenne muscular dystrophy

Prevalence

The prevalence of Duchenne muscular dystrophy is about 1 in 3500 male births. The prevalence in females is very much lower than this, although not precisely known (Moser, 1984; Aicardi, 1992).

Sex ratios

Duchenne muscular dystrophy is inherited from the mother as an X-linked recessive trait and affects mostly boys. Female carriers are usually asymptomatic, although in some women the disease is clinically manifest, usually in a more subtle manner than in males (Moser, 1984). The complete Duchenne phenotype has been reported in girls, some of whom have XO/XX mosaicism or structurally abnormal X chromosomes.

Behavioural and physical phenotype

The symptoms of Duchenne muscular dystrophy may be present from infancy, although rarely acknowledged until well into the child's second or third year of life. Motor milestones are severely or mildly delayed. Some degree of cognitive and social retardation appears to be common also (Sollee et al., 1985; Williams, Pleak & Hanesian, 1987), and several cases with Duchenne muscular dystrophy and autism have been reported in the literature (Komoto et al., 1984; Gillberg et al., 1991). Fitzpatrick, Barry & Garvey (1986) found a high rate of dysthymic disorder and major depression in boys with Duchenne muscular dystrophy.

Social isolation, depression and prolonged grief reactions are also commonly reported, even when DSM-III-R criteria for depressive disorders may not be met (Buchanan et al., 1979; Witte, 1985).

Wheelchair confinement is a common outcome in the pre-adolescent period, but some affected males continue to walk into the adolescent years. Progressive, symmetrical muscle weakness and atrophy run parallel with the progressive, slow loss of the ability to carry out acquired motor skills.

Diagnosis

Duchenne muscular dystrophy appears between 2 to 4 years of age with delayed motor milestones. The mutant gene has been located on the X chromosome and its protein product, dystrophin, is absent from the muscle tissue of boys with Duchenne muscular dystrophy (Hoffman, Brown & Kunkel, 1987).

Becker type dystrophy, also a heritable X-linked recessive condition, shows considerably later onset (between ages 5 and 11 years).

Once the diagnosis is suspected, genetic DNA diagnosis should be achieved.

Pathogenesis

The gene responsible for dystrophin production is located on the p-arm of the X chromosome. It is dysfunctional in Duchenne muscular dystrophy, leading to the absence of dystrophin from muscular tissue in affected boys. It is this absence that causes the muscular weakness and progressive wasting of muscular tissue, even though the exact mechanisms involved in this process are poorly understood.

It is not yet known whether dystrophin has specific effects on brain function. The retardation, depression and social interaction problems (and even autism in a few cases) seen in many cases with Duchenne muscular dystrophy suggest that there is CNS involvement in many cases. However, the mechanisms underlying this possible involvement are unknown at the time of writing this book.

Work-up

If there is delay of motor milestones, muscle weakness and suspected symmetrical muscle atrophy in a boy 2–6 years of age, Duchenne muscular dystrophy should always be suspected. Creatinephospokinase in the serum is usually raised. If the parents are known to be related, the clinical suspicion should be very strong. Genetic diagnosis at the DNA level should be accomplished.

Treatment

There is no cure for Duchenne muscular dystrophy yet. Parents, of course, are usually extremely grieved by the information about the disorder and the prediction of a downhill course. However, because the disease progresses slowly, false hope often emerges, and it is sometimes only years later, when walking becomes difficult, that grief and conflicts reappear (Carroll, 1985).

Outcome

Outcome is poor. There has been wheelchair confinement and a decreased life-span in all reported cases.

Foetal alcohol syndrome

The foetal alcohol syndrome is a common disorder with blurred boundaries both in relation to normality and other 'teratogenic' syndromes.

Prevalence

The frequency of foetal alcohol syndrome (FAS), as originally described by Lamache (1967), Lemoine, Harousseau & Borteyry (1968), and Jones et al., (1973), depends on the population under consideration. Clarren and Smith (1978) suggested that the full syndrome may be present in 1–2% of the general population, and that partial variants may be 3–5 times more common still. These figures contrast with rates of 1 in 600 for full-blown FAS and 1 in 300 for partial FAS reported by Olegård et al., (1979). Daily doses of 80 ml 'pure' alcohol (corresponding to about 700 ml of table wine) are clearly dangerous, but smaller doses should not be taken to be safe (Streissguth, Barr & Sampson, 1990). The rate of growth retardation and morphological abnormalities in young children appears to be related to the degree of use of alcohol throughout pregnancy, or during the second and third trimesters (Day et al., 1990). Even an occasional binge may be responsible for FAS in exceptional cases. Total abstinence does not appear to be necessary in order to avoid FAS developing in the offspring (Graham et al., 1988). FAS is now considered to be the leading cause of mental retardation in the western world and is found in approximately 10% of all children with mental retardation (Abel & Sokol, 1986).

Sex ratios

The sex ratio is often reported to be equal in FAS without empirical evidence being cited to support this notion. Actually, it would not be surprising if the male:female ratio was skewed, given the well-known difference in susceptibility to CNS damage between boys and girls.

Behavioural and physical phenotype

The clinical features of FAS are described in Table 10.1. A mildly–moderately retarded individual with a cheerful, slightly aloof attitude and moderate–severe degrees of hyperkinetic disorder or ADHD should always be suspected of suffering from FAS (particularly if there are associated ocular and visual abnormalities or other physical malformations). A careful history (and register search if possible) should be taken seeking to document the degree of alcohol use in pregnancy. Of all mildly mentally retarded individuals, at least 10% may suffer from FAS (Hagberg et al., 1981). If there are associated physical stigmata and growth retardation, the possibility of a FAS diagnosis should be entertained.

According to long-term follow-up (Steinhau-

Table 10.1. *The foetal alcohol syndrome (FAS): clinical features*

Domain	Symptom
General	Prenatal growth retardation (more length than weight)
	Postnatal growth retardation with considerable catch-up in the first year of life
CNS	Microcephaly[a]
	Excess neuronal migration
	Other brain malformations
	Developmental delay
	Mental retardation (mostly mild–moderate)
	Hyperkinetic disorder
	(Cheerfulness)[b]
	Occasional cases present with autistic disorder/symptoms
	Fine motor dysfunction
	Clumsiness
Facial	Microcephaly[a]
	Short palpebral fissures with epicanthal folds
	Maxillary hypoplasia with relative prognathism
	Long philtrum
	Thinning of vermillion border
	Hypoplastic upper helix
Ocular	Strabismus
	Tortuous retinal vessels
	Optic atrophy
Visceral	Congenital heart disease
	Genital abnormalities
Limbs	Limitation of elbow extension and of interphalangeal joints
	Abnormal palmar creases
Other	Hearing deficits (conductive and neurogenic)

Notes:
[a] Microcephaly can be caused both by primary growth retardation of the brain and of the skull.
[b] Cheerfulness has not been documented in the literature but is a common characteristic according to the author's clinical experience.

sen, Willms & Spohr, 1994) early childhood psychiatric problems include eating problems, sleep disorders, stereotypes, speech (and hearing) impairments and hyperactivity disorders. In school age children, particularly boys, hyperactivity tends to persist, but there are also high rates of other psychiatric problems, including depression. Those with the most pronounced dysmorphic features and those with very low IQ (<50) have the highest rate of psychiatric disorder.

Diagnosis

The diagnosis is based on the typical constellation of clinical signs and symptoms and may be further supported by the history from the mother (or relatives/friends) concerning alcohol use in pregnancy. Maturation of the EEG is delayed in alcohol-exposed infants (Ioffe & Chernick, 1988), and an EEG record from this period may aid in diagnosis.

A major problem in the diagnosis of FAS is the overlap of drugs and toxins used by mothers who also consumed large amounts of alcohol in pregnancy. Many women who abuse alcohol also abuse drugs of other kinds (including tobacco). Given this overlap, and the fact that a syndromal diagnosis of this kind is somewhat subjective, the real prevalence of mild forms of FAS is very difficult to determine.

Pathogenesis

Several types of brain malformations are common, excessive neuronal migration with leptomeningeal glioneuronal heterotopias being perhaps the most prevalent variant (Wisniewski *et al,*. 1983). Dendritic spine abnormalities appear to be common, and gross malformations such as neural tube defects, abnormal gyration and agenesis/dysgenesis of the corpus callosum have also been demonstrated in some cases (Clarren, 1979).

Work-up

A full neuropsychiatric work-up including examinations by an ophthalmologist, cardiologist, audiologist, neuropsychiatrist and neuropsychologist is always required whenever the syndrome of foetal alcohol poisoning is suspected. In addition, EEGs, CAT and MRI scans of the brain may be indicated, both in order to aid in diagnosis and to document the type and extent of damage sustained.

Treatment

There is no specific treatment for FAS. The best treatment, of course, is prevention. Reducing alcohol intake in the general population, women of child-bearing age or just pregnant women would substantially reduce the number of children born with FAS. However, this may be difficult to achieve in itself, and particularly in those women who are most at risk.

In all cases of FAS there is a need to consider the possibility that not only the intra-uterine biological but also the extra-uterine psychosocial (and biological) environment may be harmful to the child. Placement outside of the biological home (in a foster or adoptive home) might be helpful, especially if placement is achieved during the infant period (Aronsson & Hagberg, 1993).

Outcome

The outcome in FAS depends on many things, including genetic factors, the degree of brain damage sustained, the degree of intellectual handicap and behavioural disorder, associated physical disorders and the psychosocial environment during infancy and childhood (Aronsson & Hagberg, 1993). Most of the cases diagnosed in recent years have been mildly, moderately or severely mentally retarded and have shown moderate behavioural problems. These features, together with various types of malformation syndromes, imply that independent adult functioning is likely to be rare.

Fölling disease (phenylketonuria)

Fölling disease or phenylketonuria (PKU) is a disorder which can be seen as a model disorder for understanding the relationships between genes and environment, on the one hand, and mental functioning and behaviour, on the other. The disorder does not develop without a genetic defect directly or indirectly affecting several neural structures and pathways. However, it also does not develop without the contribution of an environmental stressor, in this case certain dietary constituents. It is also a perfect illustration of how the risk of specific psychiatric disorder can be screened and diagnosed and how psychiatric disorder be prevented from developing by providing a specific, rational treatment, in this case a diet.

In 1934, Fölling, a Danish physician identified excessive phenylpyruvic acid in the urine of a group of retarded patients with a musty odour to their urine. He thereby discovered PKU (Fölling, 1934). Almost 20 years later, Jervis demonstrated the inadequate functioning of phenylalanine hydroxylase in patients with PKU (Jervis, 1953). This deficiency results in failure to convert phenylalanine to tyrosine and thereby the back-up of metabolites such as phenylpyruvic acid and phenylacetic acid (the cause of the urinary odour). These metabolites flood the urine and the central nervous system (where they gradually interfere with normal nerve cell functioning causing mental deficiency and behaviour disorder).

In 1960, Dr C.E.Benda took a group of psychiatrists to a ward to see several child patients and to let them examine the children and make a diagnosis of childhood schizophrenia. Only later did he tell them that these 'schizophrenic' children were positive to PKU testing and suffered from that metabolic disease. In a paper by Friedman (1969), the publications reporting on an association of PKU with autism were reviewed, and it was concluded that there was a strong relationship between the two.

Prevalence

The mean global prevalence is about 1 in 15000 to 1 in 20000 births. However, prevalence rates tend to vary a lot. Thus, in Ireland, PKU has been reported to occur in 1 in 4000 births, whereas in Japan it is said to exist in fewer than 1 in 100 000 (Aicardi, 1992).

Sex ratios

Phenylketonuria is an autosomal recessive disorder, and the sex ratio is equal.

Behavioural and physical phenotype

Children with Fölling disease appear normal at birth, but, if untreated, soon develop signs of developmental delay, social withdrawal and inattention. Before dietary treatment, affected children were almost always mentally retarded (usually, but not always, severely so). Autistic symptoms and full-blown autism often developed months to years later. It will probably never be determined to what extent people with PKU developed autism, but from the available evidence, it appears that autistic behaviour was one of the most common associated (perhaps the most common associated) symptoms of the disorder. Hyperkinetic problems are often also encountered in untreated cases. Even some treated children have learning disabilities (Berry *et al.*, 1979) and some develop emotional and behavioural problems in adolescence and early adulthood (Levy and Waisbren, 1983).

Diagnosis

PKU is almost always impossible to detect by clinical examination of the young infant. Neonatal screening of phenylalanine levels in blood on the fourth to sixth day after birth is usually undertaken in most industrialized countries and, in itself, is virtually foolproof in identifying possible cases. However, samples can still be exchanged, lost or diagnostic results may be inadvertently ignored. This, in turn, means that all children worked up under a diagnosis of mental retardation or autism, have to be checked on again for the possibility of this diagnosis.

Pathogenesis

The lack of the enzyme phenylalanine hydroxylase (PAH) leads to a block in the conversion of phenylalanine to tyrosine, resulting in accumulation of phenylpyruvic acid, phenylactelic acid and phenylacetylamine. The gene for PAH is located on the q-arm of chromosome 12. It spans about 90 000 base pairs of DNA, has 13 exons and is decorated with a suite of highly informative DNA markers, RFLPs. PAH haplotypes are derived from a set of eight of these RFLPs. More than 50 RFLP haplotypes have now been documented at the human PAH locus (Woo, 1988). There have been reports of at least 31 different PKU mutations, and five instances of a PKU mutation, occurring more than once in history (Scriver, 1991).

The cloning of the gene (Woo *et al.*, 1983) made prenatal diagnosis possible in some families. Not all mutations have yet been found, but even when the molecular defect is not known, DNA linkage analysis can help predict which siblings may be carriers and whether or not there may be two abnormal genes in foetal tissue (Antonarakis, 1989).

The hydroxylation of phenylalanine to tyrosine requires both PAH and dihydropterine reductase and the two cofactors tetrahydrobiopterin and reduced NAD. Three different inherited phenotypes of hyperphenylalaninaemia exist: (1) classical PKU, (2) atypical PKU and (3) non-PKU hyperphenylalaninaemia (Dhondt & Farriaux, 1987). PAH activity is under 5% in (1), close to 5% in (2) and above 5% in (3). Defects in the synthesis of tetrahydrobiopterin and dihydropterine reductase are responsible for neurotransmitter dysfunction, which is universal in PKU.

The accumulation of phenylalanine and its secondary effects on brain neurochemistry, are believed to be responsible for the clinical manifestations of PKU. Classical PKU is almost always accompanied by mental retardation. Non-PKU hyperphenylalaninemia usually is not. This suggests that there might be a threshold level of phenylalanine in extracellular fluids above which irreversible brain damage occurs. If the threshold is exceeded only later in life, such as in the case of therapy discontinuation in early treated PKU patients, reversible changes appear which may affect neuropsychological function (Smith *et al.*, 1988).

High plasma phenylalanine levels in patients

with PKU lead to a reduction of amine neuro-transmitter synthesis. Secondary effects on dopamine, serotonin and norepinephrine are important. Defective neurotransmitter synthesis may be due both to a competitive inhibition of transport of large amino acids, such as tryptophan and tyrosine, into the brain across the blood–brain barrier and from the CSF back into blood, resulting in low tryptophan and tyrosine concentrations in the brain despite high levels in the CSF. The neurotransmitter dysregulation is likely to play some part in the pathogenesis of neurological and psychiatric disorder in PKU.

Abnormal myelination, reduction of myelin content and decreased brain weight are found in untreated older patients with PKU (Bauman & Kemper, 1982). Abnormal brain protein synthesis also occurs.

Work-up

The typical clinical phenotype is now almost a matter of historical interest, because the disorder is now discovered by early screening, and prevented by early diagnosis and diet treatment. However, there are still cases that are missed in the screening procedure. Also, the risk that a case might be missed increases with the new policy of discharging mothers with newborn babies after only a few days in the maternity ward. During gestation the mother's liver effectively hydroxylases phenylalanine to tyrosine. It is only after the infant is 'on its own' after birth that the rise of phenylalanine begins. If infants are screened too early (within 24–48 hours after birth), the phenylalanine test might well miss the abnormality.

The work-up that is necessary in PKU includes urine, blood and CSF sampling for determination of amino acids (including phenylalanine) and monoamines. The EEG is abnormal already after a few months in almost all untreated cases, and is reported to show increasing rates of abnormality even in early treated cases (Pietz et al., 1990). MRI may show myelin abnormalities in early treated cases (possibly due to mild hyperphenylalaninaemia which is present in spite of adequate and rigid diet therapy).

Treatment

Treatment consists of a particular diet if the diagnosis is made in infancy. A phenylalanine/protein restricted diet must be initiated shortly after birth to prevent irreversible brain damage. In individuals with persistent non-PKU hyperphenylalaninaemia, intellectual development is normal without treatment (Güttler & Lou, 1990). Discontinuation of the diet should not be tried before puberty, and even after this time, its is doubtful whether it is to be recommended (Azen et al., 1991). Subclinical deficits in patients in whom dietary restriction has been discontinued warn against the practice of early therapy discontinuation.

The effects of the diet on late treated patients is uncertain. Mental retardation cannot be prevented, but a few studies suggest that it can prevent further progress, and may even have some behavioural benefit to the child (Lowe et al., 1980).

Outcome

The outcome in PKU is variable and depends on the degree to which treatment has been implemented successfully from the start or not. Subclinical deficits in adult patients who have been treated from the first few weeks of life and, in those who discontinue therapy in adolescence, suggest that there may be negative effects of mildly elevated phenylalanine levels that may be present even with successful and rigid diet treatment.

Another severe complicating feature is the fact that a maternal PKU syndrome occurs in children born to women with PKU that was untreated in pregnancy. This syndrome consists of mental and motor retardation, growth delay, dysmorphism and congenital defects. There is clear evidence that the risk of this syndrome and the severity of its manifestations are directly correlated to the level of maternal phenylalanine during pregnancy.

Fragile X syndrome (Martin–Bell syndrome)

The fragile X syndrome constitutes a combination of physical and behavioural characteristics plus a specific fragile site on the long arm of the X chromosome (at Xq27.3). The fragile X chromosome abnormality is second only to Down syndrome in the aetiological panorama of mental retardation with IQ levels under 50. It is the most common known cause of familial mental retardation and it underlies a variety of behavioural problems (including autism and hyperactivity syndromes) (Percy *et al.*, 1990; Reiss & Freund, 1990).

Chromosomal diagnosis

After the identification of the molecular gene defect in the fragile X syndrome (Verkerk *et al.*, 1991), the diagnosis of the fragile X syndrome can now be made with a very high degree of precision. Nevertheless, at the present stage, the identification of the chromosome abnormality, usually in a chromosomal culture grown in a folic acid depleted medium, still often leads the way to molecular diagnosis. The reason for this is that children with a range of neuropsychiatric problems need to be comprehensively worked up to exclude the possibility of chromosomal abnormality generally, and not only for fragile X. Thus, a chromosomal culture is performed, and it is often via this route that the possibility of the fragile X abnormality is discovered. Physical features of the disorder in early childhood are often not striking enough to suggest the distinct syndrome of fragile X.

The problems pertaining to chromosomal diagnosis are (a) that in some cases with the fragile X syndrome, it is only possible to visualize the abnormality in a small proportion of examined cells, b) that there appear to be other, perhaps clinically insignificant, fragile sites very close to the Xq27.3 location and (c) that suspected carriers in families with clearly documented fragile X syndrome may have changes on the q-arm of the X chromosome, which, though closely located, appear to be clearly distinct from the 'true' Xq27.3 site (Butler *et al.*, 1990). It has been suggested that a diagnosis of the fragile X syndrome should be made if the fragile site at Xq27.3 is present in 4% of male cells and 2% of female cells examined. Unfortunately, this is no definite solution to all the various problems in the field, both because 2%

and 4% mean very different things depending on how many cells have actually been examined (e.g. 25 or 100) which may lead to the inclusion of false positives, and because there are definitely true fragile X syndrome cases in which it may be difficult to demonstrate even 1% of abnormal cells, leading to the risk of false negatives. Further, it seems that, with increasing age of the proband, there may be increasing problems to demonstrate the abnormality. Hopefully, these matters will be resolved now that there is a DNA marker for the syndrome. In clinical practice so far, the problems discussed necessitate a highly critical attitude on the part of the neurologist/psychiatrist and the geneticist. They also underpin the importance of repeated chromosomal cultures (sometimes more than once) in families where there is strong clinical suspicion that the syndrome might be present and negative chromosome tests or a test with 'single cell positivity'.

Genetic diagnosis

The gene defect in the fragile X syndrome involves an abnormal repetition of a CGG sequence, which normally occurs at a rate of about 20, almost at the distal end of the long arm of the X chromosome. It appears that the number of repeat CGGs is directly proportional to the increase in size of the unstable region of DNA, and, slightly more speculative at present, to the clinical presentation. Recent studies suggest that if the CGG segment is repeated six to 50–51 times, the individual is symptom free (even though unpublished data from our own centre suggests that closer to 50 there can be mild symptoms), 52 to 200 repeats can result in mild retardation and some other mild neuropsychiatric problems and risk of transmitting the severe form of the disease to offspring, and 200 to 1000 copies of the CGG region result in severe form of the disease (Verkerk *et al.*, 1991). A permutation is said to be present if there are about 52–200 CGG repeats. A full mutation is present if there are more than 200 repeats. It appears that, once the permutation has been passed through a female germ line, it will give rise to clinical disorder, at least in the male offspring. This implies that a variant of genomic imprinting is in operation in the fragile X syndrome.

After the discovery of the abnormal gene, it has been established that true cases of the fragile X syndrome may be missed if only chromosomal analysis (even in a folic acid depleted medium) is performed. This risk is particularly high if cases with a very low percentage of fragile X positive cells are discarded as clearly negative. Also, there is some risk that cases pronounced positive according to chromosomal analysis may, in fact, not have the genetic defect at all. For instance, there is both a fragile spot proximal to the fragile X q27.3 locus and one distal to it. None of these two fragile sites are associated with the clinical Martin–Bell syndrome. The proximal site is probably a 'common' fragile site with no clinical significance. The distal site probably comprises several loci, one or several of which may be associated with neuropsychiatric disorder (Wahlström, personal communication, 1994).

PCR (polymerase chain reaction) diagnosis of the abnormal (FMR–1) gene locus is now done routinely in many Clinical Genetics departments and should be used (1) when chromosomal analysis has indicated the presence of the fragile X chromosome abnormality and (2) when there is a strong clinical suspicion that the individual might suffer from the fragile X syndrome.

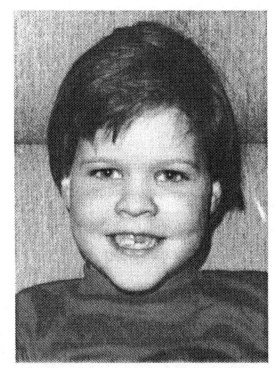

Fig. 10.2. 4-year-old girl with autism, mild mental retardation and the fragile X syndrome (low-count positivity in chromosomal culture, full mutation according to PCR-analysis).

Prevalence

Given all these reservations, it seems that the fragile X syndrome (with both the clinical features and the true chromosomal abnormality) is present in about 0.5–1 per 1000 as measured by review of mental retardation and birth records or by total screen of all retarded individuals in one area (Herbst & Miller, 1980; Hagerman, 1989). The gene defect (including full mutation and permutation cases) is bound to be more prevalent, considering that many individuals have very mild or no clinical features suggestive of the disorder.

In females, the prevalence of the chromosome abnormality may be as high as 1 per 500 (Reiss & Freund, 1990). Most affected males appear to have moderate or severe problems (even though there are 'healthy' men with the definite chromosomal abnormality), whereas most females are less severely affected (even though about one-third function in the IQ range below 70).

Sex ratios

The rate at which the genetic mutation is present in the population is likely to be marginally higher in females than in males. However, the clinical impression is different with a high number of males diagnosed with the fragile X syndrome and a considerably smaller number of females identified (Sherman, 1991). This apparent skew is caused by the more severe symptoms at the phenotypical level in males in most cases (Fig. 10.2, 10.3).

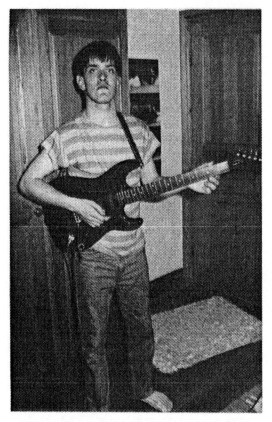

Fig. 10.3. 18-year-old young man with autism, mild mental retardation and the fragile X syndrome (low-count positivity in chromosomal culture, full mutation according to PCR-analysis).

Behavioural and physical phenotype

Many patients with the fragile X syndrome do not exhibit marked physical abnormalities of any kind, and particularly not in early childhood. Nevertheless, the clinical stereotype of the syndrome is that, in the male, there is a long face, large and prominent ears, prominent jaw and forehead, protruding lower lip, joint hypermobility (including hyperextensible finger joints), flat feet and macro-orchidism. There is obviously a disorder of connective tissue (Opitz, Westphal & Daniel, 1984), but the particulars of this are not known at the time of going to press with this book. There is also often mitral valve prolapse. Studies by Waldstein *et*

al., (1987) demonstrated abnormal elastin fibres in the skin, aorta, and cardiac valves by light microscopy in fragile X positive males. The connective tissue disorder is reminiscent of (although milder than) that seen in Marfan syndrome. (Glesby & Pyeritz (1989)) have suggested the acronym MASS phenotype to emphasize the involvement of the *m*itral valve, *a*orta, *s*keleton and *s*kin in these heritable disorders of connective tissue).

Apart from this, most physical symptoms are fairly uncharacteristic and only occasionally are they conspicuous before adolescence. It has been the present author's experience that general muscular hypotonia, protruding lower lip, hyperextensible joints and a large prepuce are the symptoms most commonly encountered in young fragile X males. In post-adolescent males it is, on the other hand, quite common to encounter the full physical phenotype even in cases who did not show much of it before puberty.

Cognitively, most males test below IQ 70, but a proportion have IQs in the normal or low normal range. The most common level of cognitive functioning seems to be 35–50. Verbal abilities are usually superior to performance and visuospatial skills. There are often relatively superior achievement results on tests reflecting verbal (particularly vocabulary) and simultaneous (gestalt) processing, and troughs in sequential (bit-by-bit) processing, short-term memory and mathematics. Most fragile X males show a decline in IQ with time (Jenssen Hagerman & Cronister Silverman, 1991). Most females with the fragile X syndrome have IQs in the low normal range, and mean IQ is significantly reduced (80–90). A subgroup of these are mildly–moderately mentally retarded (and may have autism) and many of the remaining cases present with learning disorders described as dyslexia and dyscalculia. Obligate unaffected female carriers appear to have normal IQs. There is usually no overall difference (as in the males) between verbal and performance IQ-tests. However, on the Wechsler scales there are often specific troughs on arithmetics, digit span and block design subtests. Even the obligate fragile X negative carriers show some specific neuropsychological problems reflected in tests of short-term memory. Clinical experience further suggests that they may have some abnormalities of gaze contact, poor planning and some (minor) degree of repetitive, conditionalized phrase-speech.

Psychiatrically, there is clear evidence of social dysfunction in a vast majority of male cases. Almost all male cases exhibit 'autistic' features, but only a minority exhibit the full syndrome of autism, with or without mental retardation.

The fragile X chromosome abnormality is the most common of the known causes of autism. Hyperkinetic syndromes, with and without autism, usually with many autistic features, are common as well. The cognitive test profile (see above) in the fragile X syndrome is different from that ordinarily seen in low-functioning autism, but is quite commonly encountered in high-functioning autism cases and Asperger syndrome. Several authors have described the co-occurence of Asperger syndrome and the fragile X chromosome abnormality (Hagerman, 1989).

Some of the behaviours most often encountered in the fragile X syndrome male are: gaze avoidance, tactile defensiveness and social withdrawal (age 0–2 years); gaze avoidance, avoidant greeting behaviour (turning away with head and body on greeting other people), shyness, motor stereotypies of various kinds and hyperactivity (3–4 years); echolalia, cluttering, 'nervous fidgetiness', hand flapping, stereotyped waving of things, wrist or knuckle biting, and gaze avoidance and avoidant greeting behaviour in spite of signs that there is a drive for social 'proximity' and interest in other humans (5–8 years); continuing shyness, gaze avoidance and 'nervousness' and often also a pre-occupation with certain objects or human beings in the general setting of moderate mental retardation with fast, cluttering echolalic speech (very often used in a half whispering–half 'nervously' laughing manner) (9–12 years); continuing difficulties of the same type, often aggravated by various problems associated with onset of puberty, including cross-dressing, self-injurious behaviours and clothing problems (because of large genital size) (13–20 years). Several authors have reported a cognitive stagnation, or even setback, around the time of puberty in the fragile X positive male. Hodapp et al., (1990) analysed longitudinal data from three major 'fragile X centres' and concluded that there is a significant decrease of IQ over time, with the most prominent declines occurring during the prepubertal/early pubertal period.

The same clinical picture as occurs in males is occasionally seen in affected females, but the majority of girls have less severe problems. A small percentage of all girls with the chromosome abnormality have full-blown autism, and shyness and gaze avoidance appear to be rather common phenomena even in the relatively large group with no major difficulties. Various kinds of learning problems appear to affect one-third to one-half of all fragile X positive females. These range from dyslexia to mild/moderate mental retardation. There have been occasional reports of the development of schizoaffective psychosis in some young women with the fragile X chromosome abnormality. Some of these have had relatively minor learning problems before the onset of psychosis, but have otherwise, at least outwardly, appeared to be doing well. Emotion perception and perspective-taking skills appear to be unaffected in carrier women who have normal IQ (Mazzocco, Pennington & Hagerman, 1994).

Treatment

There is no currently known specific treatment in the fragile X syndrome (Jensen-Hagerman & Cronister-Silverman, 1991).

A few authors have used stimulants to counter excessive hyperactivity (in doses recommended for children with severe hyperkinetic syndromes regardless of aetiology) and reportedly with fair or good results (Hagerman, Murphy & Wittenberger, 1988).

Folic acid (0.5–1.5 mg/kg/b.p.d.) has been used by a number of authors without consensus regarding its role having been achieved. It appears to have a mild stimulant effect which could lead to better ability to concentrate and perhaps an amelioration of hyperkinetic problems. Some reports have suggested a beneficial effect of folic acid on autistic symptoms, at least if given from the pre-school period, but no, or, in some cases, a slightly negative effect, if given after puberty (Gillberg et al., 1986a).

Genetic counselling has to be provided in all families with the syndrome. The rapidly expanding knowledge of permutations, mutations and genomic imprinting in the fragile X syndrome contributes to a situation in which more and more precise information can be shared with affected families. Molecular diagnosis is recommended for all first-degree relatives of an affected individual. Prenatal molecular diagnosis is now feasible.

Goldenhar syndrome

Prevalence

The prevalence of Goldenhar syndrome is not known. There appears to be an association between Goldenhar syndrome and autistic behaviour (Landgren, Gillberg & Strömland, 1992). Goldenhar syndrome was only identified in less than 1% of all cases with severe autistic symptoms in an autism diagnostic outpatient clinic. With an autism (classic and autistic-like conditions included) prevalence of 1 in 1000 (Wing, 1993), and assuming that not more than one in ten of all Goldenhar cases has autistic symptoms, the prevalence of Goldenhar syndrome is unlikely to be higher than 1 in 10 000 (and possibly considerably less).

Sex ratios

The sex ratio in Goldenhar syndrome is possibly equal.

Behavioural and physical phenotype

The Goldenhar syndrome, with its frequent involvement of eyes (e.g. conjunctival dermoid tumours), external ears and the vertebrae of the spinal column, shows occasional association with mild–moderate mental retardation. It is too early to decide whether there might be a more specific behavioural phenotype in this syndrome, but two female cases with a smiling face, a generally happy predisposition, slightly subnormal intelligence and many features of an autistic-like condition have been described (Landgren et al., 1992).

Diagnosis

The diagnostic criteria for Goldenhar syndrome are not yet completely clear, but it is suggested that the diagnosis be made in cases with the following features: (1) ocular abnormality including epibulbar dermoid, (2) auricular abnormality including microtia, periauricular tags or other ear anomalies and (3) vertebral abnormalities.

Pathogenesis

Most cases of Goldenhar syndrome are sporadic according to the published case report series.

Abnormalities of the development of the first and second branchial arches are involved in the pathogenesis of oculo-auriculo-vertebral syndromes. The basic aetiology is unknown, but teratogenesis has been suggested (Landgren et al 1992). Hearing loss may be conductive peripheral or due to inner ear involvement. Corpus callosum agenesis is present in some cases.

It is likely that this syndrome is multiply determined.

Work-up

The work-up depends on the degree of clinical involvement. Assessments by an ophthalmologists, oto-laryngologists and neuropsychologist are required in all cases. An MRI scan might be helpful in deciding the degree of cerebral involvement, particularly the identification of callosal dysgenesis.

Treatment

There is no specific treatment available for Goldenhar syndrome. Mental retardation and autistic symptoms should be approached in the same fashion as suggested for idiopathic cases with intellectual handicap and autism. Hearing deficits need to be carefully diagnosed and treated appropriately.

Outcome

Outcome depends on the degree of intellectual, psychiatric and hearing impairment. Limited clinical experience suggests that, if autistic symptoms are prominent in childhood, they may subside or diminish with age.

Hallervorden–Spatz Disease

Hallervorden–Spatz disease belongs (together with Huntington chorea) in the group of heredodegenerative disorders which present with predominant symptoms of involvement of the basal ganglia.

Prevalence

Hallervorden–Spatz is definitely a very rare disorder in child psychiatry and child neuropsychiatry, but, like the other heredodegenerative disorders, it often presents with behavioural and psychiatric problems, together with motor problems that may be so mild as to escape recognition (or at least diagnosis) for many years.

Sex ratios

The disorder is inherited as an autosomal recessive, and thus should have an equal sex ratio.

Behavioural and physical phenotype

Psychiatric symptoms and mental deterioration are the most common presenting features. Onset is often in infancy or early childhood, but may be in late childhood and adolescence, in which case the overall course is often slower and survival may be for 10 rather than 1–5 years (which is more common in the very early onset cases). In childhood, these symptoms may be accompanied by mild–moderate signs of motor clumsiness, including non-epileptic 'drop-attacks'. Progressive dystonia usually occurs within years after first symptoms. Choreoathetosis is present in more than half the cases. Pigmentary retinopathy occurs in about one in four patients. CT and MRI may show changes in the basal ganglia, but may also yield completely 'normal' results, even in advanced stages of the disorder.

Diagnosis

The diagnosis of Hallervorden–Spatz disease is made on the clinical presentation, sometimes supported by typical findings on CT or MRI scan (and ophthalmological examination). Occasionally, the diagnosis remains tentative until the child dies, and is only made with conviction at autopsy.

Since it is common for children with late childhood onset to present with dominating psychiatric symptoms, it is essential that the possibility of this diagnosis, and those of Huntington chorea, and other rare heredodegenerative disorders, be considered in all diagnostically obscure cases.

Pathogenesis

Hallervorden–Spatz disease is believed to be transmitted as an autosomal recessive trait.

Iron deposits (sometimes calcified) in the pallidum and substantia nigra, symmetrical destruction of these region, and 'spheroids' in the basal ganglia and cortex, are the pathophysiological hallmarks of the disorder.

Work-up

The work-up should include CT and MRI scans of the brain in order to document the typical changes (hypo- and hyperdensities in the pallidum on CT and extremely low signal from the pallidum on MRI) associated with Hallervorden–Spatz disease. The diagnosis should be suspected in children who show bizarre (schizophrenia-like, conversion-disorder-like or paranoid) psychiatric symptoms and developmental plateauing and regression. Repeated neuropsychological testing (for instance with the Griffiths in young children and the WISC-III in school-age children) may be needed to document this trend.

Treatment

There is no treatment for Hallervorden–Spatz disease, except symptomatic treatment of psychiatric and neurological symptoms.

Outcome

Outcome is very poor, and death usually occurs within one to ten years of onset of severe symptoms.

Huntington chorea

Huntington chorea usually manifests with neuropsychiatric symptoms in adult age, but childhood onset, although uncommon, is not exceptionally rare.

Prevalence

The prevalence of Huntington chorea in childhood is low but variable and highly dependent on geographic location. The rate is said to be about 1–3% of that reported in adults (Hecht, 1987). The overall prevalence of Huntington chorea in the population has been difficult to establish because of varying degrees of severity of symptoms, and variable age of onset of overt problems. An overall estimate of 0.4–0.7 per 10 000 has been considered reasonable (Gudmundsson, 1969). However, in certain areas it has been reported to occur in 56 per 10 000 cases (in a small fishing community in Scotland) (Lyon-Bolt, 1970).

Sex ratios

The sex ratio in Huntington chorea is equal.

Behavioural and physical phenotype

Commonly, the disorder begins with uncharacteristic symptoms such as attention deficits, clumsiness and learning disorder. The onset may be as early as 3 years of age. Obsessive–compulsive symptoms are usually manifest within a few years of the appearance of first symptoms. Psychosis, including schizophreniform type, has been diagnosed in adolescent onset cases that were only later shown to have Huntington chorea. Ataxia, dysarthria and personality change usually ensues. Dementia develops slowly. Seizures occur in at least half of the cases with childhood or adolescent onset (often around age 8–10 years). Rigidity and hypokinesia often progress after this.

The psychological demands on a family with a child with Huntington chorea can be enormous. First of all, the father (or mother) will be affected, and he (she) may not have been aware of this before the birth of the child. The prognosis is one in which the father (mother) may 'be given' another 13–16 years to live, the last of which will be spent in a demented state (perhaps with symptoms of schizophrenia-like disorder and paranoia), and the child may expect to live 6–8 years after the first symptoms were noted. Naturally, this places tremendous strain on all the members of the family. Such stress can contribute to further psychological and psychiatric problems.

Diagnosis

The diagnosis is made at molecular biological examination. The gene for Huntington chorea located on chromosome 4, has been cloned, and commercial kits are now available that allow the relatively simple molecular diagnosis to be made.

Pathogenesis

The pathogenetic mechanisms in Huntington chorea are not understood in spite of the fact that the gene has been cloned and that the characteristic brain changes (involving atrophy and gliosis of the frontal lobes, caudate and putamen) have been well established for decades. Genomic imprinting appears to play a role in this disorder, the severity and age of onset being affected by parental origin of the mutant gene. Although generally believed to be an autosomal dominant disorder, it has been known for a long time that if the disorder is inherited from the father, onset is likely to be earlier and the course more severe than in maternally inherited disorder. Thus, most childhood onset cases have been inherited from the father (Hecht, 1987).

Work-up

The work-up in Huntington chorea can now usually be limited to molecular genetic diagnosis of the individual and his/her family.

Treatment

There is currently no treatment available for Huntington chorea. However, the discovery of the gene defect has generated new hope for rational treatment in the foreseeable future. For obsessive–compulsive symptoms, guidelines pertaining to the treatment of OCD should be adhered to, even though muscular rigidity and hypokinesias may warrant particular attention and specific interventions.

There is a need to establish neuropsychiatric teams who can accommodate the anguish, psychiatric and physical problems faced by families with Huntington chorea. A state-of-the art genetic work-up and provision of services can only be accomplished in a centre with specific expertise in the field. Such Huntington 'follow-up centres' are often to be found in the Clinical Genetics departments, but may equally be located within the realms of a Child Neuropsychiatry service with close links to the Clinical Genetics department.

Genetic counselling needs to take account not only of recent molecular genetic findings, but also of the observations that at least 38% of gene-carrying sibs of children who have developed symptoms of Huntington chorea before the age of 10 years will themselves develop symptoms of the disorder before this age (Clarke & Bundey, 1990).

Outcome

Death usually occurs within 3 to 10 years after onset in Huntington chorea. The course from onset to death can be very variable. Some individuals show little deterioration in the first few years after onset. However, obsessive–compulsive symptoms may predominate for several years, and lead to referral to a child psychiatrist, who may not consider the possibility of a heritable disorder. Marked rigidity, hypokinesia and seizures commonly ensue. Such symptoms may also antedate the occurrence of OCD type symptoms.

Hypothyroidism

Hypothyroidism in congenital form is associated with the development of motor and mental retardation, which is irreversible if not treated during the first months of life. It may also be associated with severe psychiatric disorder, including autism.

Prevalence

Congenital hypothyroidism occurs in 1 in 3000 to 1 in 4000 births (Ilicki & Larsson, 1988). Acquired variants are considerably rarer.

Sex ratios

The sex ratio in congenital hypothyroidism is 2:1 (boys:girls).

Behavioural and physical phenotype

Untreated infants are placid and floppy and have an abnormal cry with a grunting quality. There is general pallor and dryness of the skin and an overall impression of generalized oedema in combination with lustreless hair and fontanelles and sutures that remain wide open. There may be neurological abnormalities including incoordination, ataxia and spasticity. Deafness may be present in endemic variants of hypothyroidism with goitre. The behavioural and psychiatric correlates of hypothyroidism vary, but may comprise depressive symptoms/disorder and social withdrawal including autistic behaviour (Gillberg, Gillberg, Kopp, 1992). Even with early treatment, some degree of impairment is common. Motor perception dysfunction suggestive of DAMP occurs in about 50% of all cases, gross motor clumsiness in 30%

and speech, learning and behaviour problems (mild–moderate) in about 25%, regardless of whether or not treatment was begun before the age of 10 weeks (McFaul *et al.*, 1978). Perhaps, if treatment is started within the first two weeks of life, the outcome from the neuropsychiatric point of view might be better. Heyderdahl, Kase and Lien (1991) found that the best intellectual result was obtained when serum T4 (thyroxine) levels were kept above the upper reference range during the first two years of life. It should be noted, though, that with treatment much can be achieved in the way of preventing severe retardation and physical problems.

Diagnosis

The diagnosis of congenital hypothyroidism is made by determination of the blood levels of thyroxine and thyroid stimulating hormone (TSH). There are cases that are due to developmental abnormality of the thyroid gland and others that are caused by inborn errors of metabolism. The end result is a decreased blood level of circulating thyroxine (and usually a secondarily raised level of TSH).

In most developed countries, screening for congenital hypothyroidism is accomplished by analysing the serum level of TSH, 3–5 days after birth. However, some cases of hypothyroidism may occasionally be missed in this screening, and a diagnosis of hypothyroidism needs to be considered in all cases of developmental delay.

Although acquired forms of hypothyroidism exist, the congenital variants are, by far, the most common. However, in children who slowly develop the classical symptoms of hypothyroidism (mental slowing, learning disorder, sluggishness, social withdrawal, irritability, depression, skin pallor, coarse, dry hair, hoarse voice, constipation and a constant feeling of not being warm enough), the possibility of acquired hypothyroidism has to be entertained and blood sampling for thyroid status undertaken.

Pathogenesis

Thyroid hormone is crucial for the development of the brain. In humans, foetal thyroxine is synthesized from about the 12th week of gestation. Since this hormone only partly crosses the placenta, defective synthesis will affect brain development during the second part of gestation (Fisher, 1975). Insufficient thyroxine will result in impaired RNA and protein synthesis, reduced number and size of neurons in the cortex as well as hypoplasia of axons and dendrites and deficient or retarded myelination. These abnormalities are probably directly linked to the mental, behavioural and motor problems encountered in untreated hypothyroidism. Hypothyroidism leads to a number of neurotransmitter abnormalities, the most well documented of which is hyperserotoninaemia (Gillberg & Coleman, 1992). It appears that the excessively high levels of blood serotonin encountered in infant hypothyroidism may be diminished by treatment of the underlying condition with thyroid therapy.

Work-up

In congenital hypothyroidism, TSH and thyroxine should be regularly monitored during the course of treatment. Neuropsychiatric evaluations should be made at least every 2–3 years from about age 4 years. This would be the best way of documenting and treating early onset learning and behaviour problems. Neuropsychological evaluations (the Griffiths or WPPSI scales may be used with pre-school children, the WISC-III thereafter) should be performed at a rate of about one every two years from about age 4–12 years. The WAIS-R might then be used in follow-up in late adolescence or early adulthood. It is important to document any delay or deviance in cognitive functioning as early as possible so that the effects of hypothyroidism, ineffective treatment and other disorders can be evaluated in an appropriate manner and reasonable steps taken to remedy whatever causes might underlie the problems.

Treatment

Administration of L-thyroxine is the treatment of choice. The average dose of L-thyroxine at the start of treatment is 10 to 15μg/kg of weight. Treatment with daily replacement therapy is comparatively straightforward and should not be a major burden either on the children affected or their parents.

Outcome

Treatment of thyroid insufficiency with synthetic levothyroxine can result in normal intellectual development when started before 3 months of age, and in considerably improved status when started at age 3–6 months (Klein, Meltzer & Kenny, 1972). Children treated later may have a considerably poorer outlook, and intellectual development is almost always severely compromised (Ilicki & Larsson, 1988). A cerebellar ataxic syndrome often ensues. There is now clear evidence that with onset of treatment in the first few weeks of life, overall normal functioning in early school age can be achieved (Ilicki & Larsson, 1991). However, this is not to say that there might not be some minor remaining neuropsychiatric problems. There is also evidence that those infants with low serum T4 levels (below 129 mol/L) during the first year of life, particularly if those levels are accompanied by a TSH concentration greater than 15mU/L have lower IQs than patients whose T4 levels were held constant at higher concentrations (Heyerdahl et al., 1991).

The outcome for hypothyroidism developing after infancy is much better. In such patients, in addition to mental sluggishness, withdrawal and even autistic symptoms (according to one report; Gillberg, I.C. et al., 1992), there may be muscle hypertrophy which may be associated with myotonia (which, in turn, may be the result of reduced speed of contraction and relaxation). Appropriate levothyroxine substitution usually leads to marked improvement of such symptoms, even though residual symptoms may persist.

Infection syndromes

Children may acquire permanent neuropsychiatric sequelae as a result of several different types of CNS infections. The type of psychiatric symptoms shown may be directly secondary to the CNS injury, but may also be indirectly linked to mental retardation, language disorder and hearing impairment caused by the infection. In addition, hereditary factors and socio-economic circumstances can play a part in the moulding of symptoms.

Only some of the infection syndromes that could contribute to neuropsychiatric problems in children are reviewed here. They are the infections for which a pathogenetic role has been clearly documented (CMV, herpes, mononucleosis infectiosa, rubella, and toxoplasmosis). In addition, several others, like influenza A, haemophilus influenzae and streptococcus B have been implicated in some studies, but consensus about their relevance is not as strong.

CMV infection

Infection with cytomegalovirus (CMV) in utero is a common complication which occurs in 0.2 to 2.2% of all live births (Stagno & Whitley, 1985). No more than 10% of these are symptomatic at birth and another 10% are at risk of developing neuropsychiatric symptoms within the first two years of life. A prospective study including 35 000 newborns (Peckham & Logan, 1988) found only five children (0.014% of the whole population) who had congenital CMV with clinical signs in the newborn period. Of CMV infected children 10% had CMV-related neuropsychiatric problems at age 3 years (most often sensorineural hearing loss). Most maternal infections are asymptomatic. Infection can occur either through transplacental transfer or at birth through contact with an infected cervix. It is often difficult to determine whether intra-uterine infection has occurred or not.

The most common clinical symptoms in the newborn period are hepatosplenomegaly, microcephaly and trombocytopenia (with petechiae). If there are symptoms at birth, the death rate in the first few months is high and, of those who survive, 90% will suffer severe neuropsychiatric sequelae (mental retardation, autism, epilepsy, chorioretinitis). Calcification on brain scans are suggestive of the diagnosis in infants who have negative toxoplasmosis serology. In one study, 44 children who were asymptomatic at birth, but had positive CMV titres in blood, were compared with a similar group of CMV negative controls and a random sample of normal siblings. Mean IQ was significantly lower in the CMV positive group at age 3.5 and 7 years and their rate of school failure was several times that of the comparison groups. In the CMV positive group, school failure occurred only in those who belonged to low socioeconomic classes (Hanshaw, 1976). Sensorineural hearing loss is reported to occur in 10% of those infected who do not show newborn symptoms, and it has been suggested that learning disorders, mental retardation and microcephaly in isolation may also occur (Williamson *et al.*, 1982; Hanshaw, 1976), but the evidence is conflicting. Some prospective studies have found no evidence of such late major neuropsychiatric sequelae (e.g. Pearl *et al.*, 1986).

Periventricular calcifications and cortical malformations (such as polymicrogyrias) are frequently found in CMV-infected infants. The diagnosis is suspected on the basis of clinical symptoms and these CT scan findings. If there is also excretion of CMV in urine, the diagnosis can be made with some confidence, even though it is still not proven that the neuropsychiatric symptoms and the CMV infection are causally related. Viruria may persist for many years in symptomatic and asymptomatic children alike. A low titire of complement-fixing antibodies is no guarantee that CMV is not the cause of problems in the child (Bray *et al.*, 1981).

Treatment with Geavir® (Zovir, Zovirax) or Foscavir® is effective but the brain damage which has occurred already at birth is apparently irreparable.

Herpes encephalitis

Herpes encephalitis may be contracted *in utero* (very uncommon), at the time of vaginal delivery or later in life. Caesarean section should probably be performed in all instances of maternal herpetic lesions present at the estimated onset of labour.

As in all other cases of acquired viral encephalitis, symptoms of herpes encephalitis affecting children and adolescents after the newborn period, may be diffuse and uncharac-

teristic. The first symptoms are often behavioural and memory skills are commonly affected. Low or high grade fever and malaise are also prevalent features. Acute onset loss of consciousness and convulsions (almost always focal) usually follow. Neurological and psychiatric disorders that can be referred to virtually all parts of the brain are common, but mesial, temporal and orbital regions are predominantly struck. Aphasia (followed by echolalia days to weeks later), olfactory hallucinations, social withdrawal and behavioural abnormalities (hyperkinesis, stereotypies, rage, loss of judgement) are all common. Many cases of full-blown autistic disorder and herpes encephalitis have been published (DeLong, Beau & Brown, 1981; Gillberg 1986; Gillberg, I.C., 1991; Ghaziuddin *et al.*, 1992). Several of these cases with classic autism symptoms have been children of several years of age (and one adult of 31 years). These late onset autism cases caused by herpes encephalitis provide a provocative brain model for the development of autism which suggests that autistic symptoms may not necessarily reflect developmental timing of brain development.

Unlike the diffuse slow waves characteristic of the EEG in other meningoencephalitis cases, the EEG tracing in herpes encephalitis are frequently asymmetrical and often dominated by spike foci against a background of abnormally slow activity. A low amplitude, particularly over the region of the temporal lobe, is common. The CT scan shows asymmetrical attenuation, again particularly in the temporal lobe. CSF may be normal but is usually under high pressure. An excess of lymphocytes is common, but may be as moderate as (less than) 50 cells.

An exact diagnosis is often difficult. Virus isolation from the CSF is almost always negative. Brain biopsy can provide the definitive diagnosis, but it is associated with complications and should be reserved for complicated or atypical cases. A rise of antibodies against herpes simplex virus type 1 in the CSF is significant, but it may take weeks to appear and persist for years.

According to Aicardi (1992), if the clinical

picture is consistent with herpes encephalitis, interferon alpha should be determined in the CSF and serum no less than 72 hours after initial symptoms of the disease. This is not a specific test as it is only indicative of virus replication in the CNS, but the presence of interpheron alpha in the CSF in combination with clinical symptoms concordant with herpes encephalitis is highly suggestive.

Treatment with acyclovir (cytosine arabinoside) should be started at once and, if interferon is present, continued for at least 10 days. Mortality drops radically with this treatment, but is still substantial (around 20% as compared with 70% before acyclovir was available). The addition of corticosteroids to this treatment is not recommended at present.

HIV infection and AIDS

Acquired immunodeficiency disorder (AIDS) has only recently entered the textbooks of child psychiatry (Lewis, 1991). It is a 'disease, at least moderately predictive of a defect in cell-mediated immunity, occurring in a person with no known cause for diminished resistance. Diseases diagnostic of AIDS include Kaposis's sarcoma, *Pneumocystis carinii* pneumonia and other opportunistic infections' (Institute of Medicine, 1986).

The underlying disorder in AIDS is an infection with HIV-virus. This virus infects the T-helper lymphocytes, depletes the number and alters the function of these, and indirectly compromises the function of other cells including antibody-producing B-lymphocytes. It is this process that makes the infected individual vulnerable to the opportunistic infections.

It has now been well established that AIDS is often complicated by CNS dysfunction, including a generalized form of encephalopathy characterized by progressive behavioural, motor and cognitive disturbances (Price, Inglese & Jacobs, 1991). This type of severe disorder occurs in at least two-thirds of all AIDS patients. Impaired concentration and mild memory loss are usually the presenting symptoms of this 'AIDS dementia complex'. It can occur even in the early course of systemic virus infection and may be the result of direct HIV brain infection. Neuropsychological testing may yield abnormal results very early in the course of AIDS, long before clinical signs are present (Marotta & Perry, 1989).

Most children affected with AIDS have been infected by transplacental exposure or through blood products. Sexual contact and sexual abuse are rarer, but are more likely to be involved when teenagers present with AIDS. As many as 65% percent of babies of infected mothers may develop the disease. The classic triad in this group is interstitial pneumonitis, hepatosplenomegaly and failure to thrive (Shannon & Ammann, 1985). About half of all children examined have loss of developmental milestones. Many are microcephalic and have mental retardation. According to one Italian study, the prevalence of autistic disorder may be raised in this population (Musetti *et al.*, 1993).

The clinical problems associated with AIDS are often further complicated by the fact that many children infected with the HIV-virus are psychosocially disadvantaged (Belfer, Krener & Miller, 1988).

Post-infectious measles encephalitis

Onset of post-infectious measles encephalitis is usually abrupt, of varying severity (often very severe with loss of consciousness and convulsions) and with a high mortality (around 10%). About 1 in 1000 children infected with measles develop post-infectious encephalitis (Miller, Stanton & Gibbons, 1956) on average a week after the first appearance of the rash. Many of those who survive, even those showing apparently complete recovery, develop learning disorders (including mental retardation, DAMP and dyslexia), hyperactivity and other uncharacteristic disruptive behaviour disorders.

Post-infectious mycoplasma pneumoniae encephalitis

A case of a 9 year-old girl who developed schizophreniform psychosis after contracting mycoplasma pneumoniae encephalitis has been reported in the literature (Gillberg, 1980). There were auditory hallucinations in the third person and thought blocking. A pronounced degree of lethargy, increased need for sleep and catatonic phenomena were also reported. Complete recovery occurred within 6 months.

Single cases of acute onset psychosis with confusion and hallucinations in connection with mycoplasma pneumoniae infection have also been described in 10–12 year-old boys and girls (Balassanian & Robbins, 1967; Smith & Sangster, 1972). In these cases, complete recovery occurred within weeks.

All the cases of psychosis in children and adolescents with mycoplasma pneumoniae encephalitis that have been reported to date have shown signs of a preceding episode of upper respiratory symptoms, usually comprising unproductive cough and antedating the psychotic symptoms by 2–3 weeks.

The author has also seen chronic fatigue syndrome after mycoplasma pneumoniae encephalitis and mycoplasma pneumoniae pneumonia. In such cases, it is sometimes difficult to ascertain adequately the presence of psychotic symptoms, and differential diagnosis may be difficult.

Rubella embryopathy

Rubella embryopathy is a frequent result of maternal rubella infection in pregnancy. About 80% of those mothers infected in the first 12 weeks of pregnancy, 50% of those infected in week 13–14, and 25% at the end of the second term bear children with congenital rubella. Foetal infection after this period is uncommon, but a rise occurs in the last month of pregnancy.

Severe malformations are reported to occur in all foetuses infected before the 12th week. Of those infected in the 13–16th week, deafness may be the only symptom (in about one-third of the cases originating at this point in pregnancy). Infants infected in the second term tend to show mild–moderate or severe degrees of mental retardation in combination with varying degrees of communication disorders, including autism. Intra-uterine infection of the foetus has been reported following immunizaton with

rubella vaccine, which should not be given to women of child-bearing age unless pregnancy has been ruled out.

Reduced brain weight, caused by meningeal and brain lesions in combination with inhibition of cell proliferation by the virus, is a common finding. Widespread calcification of degenerative arteries is typical. Microcephalus is a common, but not invariable, clinical feature of the syndrome.

In about 70–90% of all rubella embryopathy cases there are CNS symptoms including hypotonus, apathy and a bulging fontanelle in infancy, and overall retardation, disproportionate language delay, typical autism or autistic-type conditions in childhood (Chess, 1977; Gillberg & Coleman, 1992), and inability to lead an independent life in adulthood. Autistic symptoms occur with or without extreme sensory deficits (such as deafness or blindness). Seizures occur in a minority of patients.

Apart from CNS symptoms, congenital heart disease (patent ductus arteriosus, stenosis of pulmonary arteries and atrial or ventricular septal defects), hearing impairment and visual impairment due to cataracts, retinopathy and microphthalmus are common.

The diagnosis is made after demonstration of an elevated level of IgM (caused by a specific rubella antibody) in the child's serum at birth. Isolation of the virus in tissue culture may be possible many months after birth. Hyperserotoninaemia is common in rubella embryopathy, but the reasons for this are unclear.

Outcome is usually poor. About half the affected group is deaf or very severely hearing impaired, and a subgroup of the remainder show mild-moderate hearing impairment (Cooper & Krugman, 1967). Autism, blindness and severe mental retardation are also very common features in adult populations with rubella embryopathy. It has been reported that the autistic symptoms often subside (Chess, Korn & Fernandez, 1971), but the author's clinical experience, in this respect, does not suggest that rubella autism differs from other forms of autism.

There is no treatment available for rubella embryopathy. However, the immunization of pre-pubertal girls has become routine in developed countries and in recent years the syndrome has become rare. Nevertheless, rubella embryopathy may occur in children born to immigrant women who have arrived in developed countries from regions in which general immunization programmes do not exist, and, of course, in children born to infected mothers in the 'underdeveloped' countries. Autism in any child born to a mother who has not been immunized against rubella should always raise some suspicion that rubella embryopathy may be the underlying cause of the autistic disorder/ autistic behaviour.

Toxoplasmosis infection

Acquired toxoplasmosis is extremely rare and is said to occur only in immunodepressed patients (in whom multiple brain abscesses may signal the underlying condition of toxoplasmosis infection).

Congenital toxoplasmosis occurs particularly in cultures where meat-cooking habits allow the survival and ingestion of cysts and oocysts of the toxoplasma gondii parasite (whose usual host is the cat). It rarely gives rise to severe neuropsychiatric disorder other than severe mental retardation. Chorioretinitis may be present at birth or develop later in childhood. A few cases with autism have been described (Rutter & Bartak, 1971), but the relatively high rate of congenital toxoplasmosis and the low rate of reported autism precludes conclusions regarding a possible causal relationship.

Diagnosis is accomplished by tests measuring IgG or IgM-specific antibodies. The IgM ELISA (enzyme-linked immunosorbent assay) is considered to be the most reliable of these.

Other infections

Finally, the possible effects of pertussis (and pertussis vaccine) on the brain have been the subject of much debate over the years. Encephalopathy caused by immunization with pertussis vaccine has been estimated at 1 in 140 000 immunizations (Miller et al., 1981). However,

even these low frequencies have been contested (Shields et al., 1988). Nevertheless, most authorities believe that pertussis encephalopathy does occur, albeit extremely rarely, It is characterized by coma, status epilepticus and, sometimes, focal neurological signs 12–48 hours after administration of the vaccine (Aicardi, 1992). Cases with transient seizures or seizures that occur after 48 hours are unlikely to be complications of immunization (Menkes & Kinsbourne, 1990). However, febrile seizures may be common. Shields et al. (1988) estimated that up to 9% of all febrile seizures occurring under age 2 years might be attributable to diphtheria–pertussis–tetanus vaccine.

Some parents of children with autism attribute onset of the child's autistic symptoms to the day(s) following immunization or to the effects of the whopping cough syndrome occurring in infants under age 2 years. Because of the widespread use of immunization, and the high prevalence of pertussis in the population (and the lack of specific studies addressing the issue of autism and pertussis), little is in fact known concerning a possible relationship between the two disorders.

Pertussis encephalopathy is probably often caused mainly by hypoxia and increased venous pressure due to intense cough rather than by toxins produced by the organism (Aicardi, 1992).

Ito's hypomelanosis

Ito's hypomelanosis is also referred to as incontinentia pigmenti achromians.

Prevalence

The prevalence of Ito's hypomelanosis is not known, but judging from several clinical reports (Åkefeldt & Gillberg, 1991; Zappella, 1992a) it is possibly one of the more common neurocutaneous disorders. Zappella found 25 possible cases in a child neuropsychiatric clinic specializing in autism over a period of a few years, without specifically 'advertising'.

Sex ratios

Girls appear to be much more commonly affected than boys, but, since no population studies exist and the disorder is not known to be genetic in most cases, definite conclusions cannot be drawn as regards sex ratio in Ito's hypomelanosis.

Behavioural and physical phenotype

Ito's hypomelanosis is characterized by hypopigmented areas with a peculiar streaked or whorled appearance. The hypopigmented, sharply circumscribed spots or streaks are often unilateral or have a strong unilateral predominance and are often linearly distributed (Pascual-Castraviejo 1987; Griebel, Krägeloh-Mann & Michaelis, 1989). The skin changes (Fig. 10.4a, b) persist throughout childhood and adolescence, but tend to become less conspicuous with age. They are best seen under a Wood's lamp. CNS involvement appears to be the rule (Glover, Brett & Athreton, 1989) and may manifest with autism (Åkefeldt & Gillberg, 1991), autistic-like conditions, (Griebel, Krägeloh-Mann & Michaelis, 1989; Åkefeldt & Gillberg, 1991; Zappella, 1992a), dyslexia, mental retardation, seizures (including infantile spasms), neurological deficits, macrocephaly and microcephaly. The degree and rate of CNS symptoms seem to be correlated to the extent of the skin disorder. Hemihypertrophy has been described as well as scoliosis and malformation of the facial bones. Ocular abnormalities include corneal opacities and choroidal atrophy. There is a wide range of EEG abnormalities, including the frequent occurrence of multifocal paroxysmal features.

Diagnosis

There is no diagnostic marker, and the diagnosis has to be based on the typical set of clinical findings. Various kinds of chromosomal abnormalities have been documented in several cases, and include bizarre mosaicisms with some cell lines containing XO, others XXX and others still a completely normal karyotype (Miller & Parker, 1985; Åkefeldt & Gillberg, 1991).

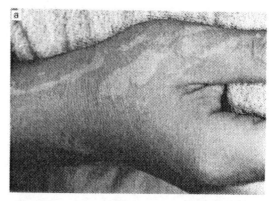

Fig. 10.4(a). Hypomelanotic areas on right hand and wrist of eight-year-old boy with hypomelanosis of Ito.

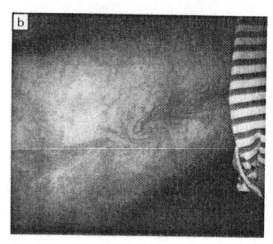

Fig. 10.4(b). Hypomelanosis of Ito: Five-year-old boy with autism, extreme hyperactivity and severe mental retardation.

Pathogenesis

The aetiology and pathogenesis of Ito's hypomelanosis is not known. The chromosomal abnormalities encountered (mosaicisms are usually found mostly in cultured fibroblasts, to a lesser extent in leukocytes; translocations have also been documented) are so varied that they fail to provide a pattern which might be used to form a theory for the development of the disorder. The disorder is usually sporadic (although familial cases have been documented, and autosomal dominant transmission has been suggested). It has been proposed that Ito's hypomelanosis is just a conglomerate of different diseases presenting with a relatively typical form of hypomelanosis.

Work-up

If Ito's hypomelanosis has been diagnosed, an EEG, a CAT scan and an MRI of the brain may be indicated. Chromosomal analysis should be performed in order to rule out additional chromosomal disorder (and to provide further indirect support for the diagnosis of Ito's hypomelanosis when unusual mosaicisms are present). An EEG may show epileptogenic discharge which could provide clues to the clinical examination of the child who may not have overt epilepsy, but may well have absence seizures not readily observable unless a prompt to search for specific symptoms has been provided by the result of the EEG examination. A CAT scan may show unilateral or bilateral hemisphere atrophy and/or areas of low attenuation in white matter (Rosemberg et al., 1984). MRI has shown neuronal heterotopias (Glover et al., 1989) and white space in between white and matter signal abnormalities (Bhushan et al., 1989). These findings are in agreement with pathological findings of Ross et al. (1982). Evaluation by an ophthalmologist and a dermatologist should be sought. An X-ray of the spine may be indicated, particularly around adolescence when scoliosis may progress at a fast rate in a few cases. Neuropsychological and neuropsychiatric evaluation should be performed as appropriate, depending on the type and degree of associated CNS symptoms.

Treatment

There is no specific treatment for Ito's hypomelanosis. Ocular and skeletal problems may have to be treated depending on the degree of involvement and functional handicaps. Autistic and other behavioural/emotional problems should be treated according to general principles for such disorders.

Outcome

Outcome is variable and tends to be associated with the degree of neuropsychiatric problems exhibited by the pre-adolescent individual with the syndrome: the more CNS symptoms the poorer the outcome. However, long-term follow-up experience with this patient group is very limited. It is also likely that a number of affected individuals never come to the attention of psychiatrists.

Joubert syndrome

Joubert syndrome is an autosomal recessive disorder characterized by partial or complete agenesis of the cerebellar vermis and episodic tachypnoea alternating with prolonged apnoea (Joubert et al., 1969).

Prevalence

The Joubert syndrome is very rare, but no accurate population prevalence figures are available.

Sex ratios

The syndrome is probably equally common in the two sexes.

Behavioural and physical phenotype

Episodic tachypnoea alternating with prolonged apnoea are the clinical hallmarks of the syndrome. Mental retardation (usually severe or profound), ataxia, abnormal eye movements, tongue protrusion and hypotonia are standard features. Two individuals with Joubert syndrome have been described with pronounced autistic behaviour, at least one of whom met full criteria for DSM-III-R autistic disorder (Holroyd, Reiss & Bryan, 1991). These two individuals had exceptionally high IQs (full-scale IQ 64 and 85, respectively). The report of concurrence of Joubert syndrome and autistic disorder is particularly interesting, given that partial or complete agenesis of the cerebellar vermis is part of the diagnosis of Joubert syndrome, and it has been described to occur in autism as well (Courchesne et al., 1988).

Diagnosis

The diagnosis is made on the basis of clinical symptoms as described plus the documentation of cerebellar vermis agenesis (partial or complete).

Pathogenesis

The symptoms of Joubert syndrome are probably caused by the agenesis of the cerebellar vermis, which, in turn, is caused by an autosomal recessive hereditary disorder.

Work-up

The work-up required is limited. It should always include an IQ-test and a baseline evaluation by a child neuropsychiatrist. In case there is associated autistic symptomatology, further neuropsychological, psychiatric and educational work-up may be necessary along lines appropriate for the syndrome of autism.

Treatment

There is no specific treatment available for Joubert syndrome.

Outcome

Outcome in Joubert syndrome is unknown. However, because of the common association with severe and profound levels of mental retardation, the psychosocial and academic outcome in adult age must be poor in most cases.

Kleine–Levin syndrome

Originally described in the 1930s, the Kleine–Levin syndrome has received attention in paediatrics and child psychiatry only in recent years.

Prevalence

The Kleine–Levin syndrome occurs mostly in adolescent boys, but female cases have been reported occasionally (Lishman, 1978). The population prevalence of Kleine–Levin syndrome is unknown, but it is clearly more prevalent than suggested by the fact that, for many years, it was not mentioned at all in the child and adolescent psychiatric literature. The author has personally examined six cases over the last five-year period.

Diagnosis and clinical picture

The syndrome usually presents with greatly increased need for sleep and a tendency for the affected adolescent to eat any food within sight/reach during the few waking hours of the day. There is usually little or no mention of increased hunger by the person him/herself. There is also a variety of emotional/behaviour/neuropsychiatric problems, often coloured by intense irritability, and occasionally amounting to severe aggression. The behavioural problems sometimes antedate the appearance of hypersomnia and hyperphagia by a few days. The symptom constellation often appears abruptly and is present for a few days to a few weeks whereafter symptoms subside in an otherwise perfectly healthy adolescent boy, and things go back to normal again. Weeks to months later, a new episode occurs and follows a similar pattern, albeit quite often of more limited duration. New episodes can appear for a period of one–several years. However, gradually relapses tend to occur less often and the episodes become shorter and shorter.

The onset of problems may be so abrupt as to suggest encephalitis or psychosis. Memory loss is often partial, but may be complete for the first few days of an episode.

Pathogenesis

Hypothalamic dysfunction has been proposed (Lishman, 1978; Gillberg, 1987) to account for the symptomatology because (a) the appetite and sleep symptoms implicate hypothalamic systems, (b) the syndrome occurs mostly in the teenage period, (c) it affects mostly boys and its episodic nature could be seen as a counterpart to variable behaviour in connection with onset of menarche in girls and (d) some EEG findings are compatible with hypothalamic dysfunction.

Work-up

The work-up should include a neuropsychiatric assessment (but not necessarily a major neuropsychiatric evaluation), including a neuropsychological test (such as the WISC-III or the WAIS-R), which should be performed in the first symptom-free interval. If the history and symptoms are typical, there is no need for further work-up, but in case of doubt, neurological and laboratory work-up to exclude encephalitis and other neurological disorders, brain tumour and metabolic problems may be essential. A urine and/or blood screen for narcotic/drug substances might also be appropriate in some cases.

Treatment

Treatment need often consist only of assessment and a proper diagnosis. In severe cases, negatively affecting school attendance over long periods, a trial of stimulants (e. g. D-amphetamine 5–15 mg × 2–3 given at 3–4 hour intervals) might be indicated (Lishman, 1978). Lithium (in doses consistent with prophylactic treatment for bipolar disorder, i.e. doses leading to serum concentrations of 0.4–0.7 mE/l) has also been advocated by some authors, but is probably best reserved for those very rare extremely severe cases with frequent long episodes of hypersomnia and short spells of normal functioning in-between. In most cases, however, information given to the affected child/teenager, his/her parents and teachers is adequate. Nevertheless, there is sometimes a need to repeat at least one school grade. This is because the diagnosis is rarely made in the very early stages of the disorder, and several untreated episodes may have led to poor school attendance for many months before appropriate treatment can be started.

Follow-up should be continued into early adulthood to make certain that the episodes subside and that there are no residual neuropsychiatric symptoms. A repeated neuropsychological test (such as the WAIS-R) should be performed a few/several years after initial diagnosis and work-up.

Outcome

Long-term outcome is reported to be good (even though, as has already been mentioned, a year (or two) of school work could have been wasted), and most cases are reported to do well by early adult life. However, a few reports have questioned the consistently good outcome described in most of the early literature. There is a need for longitudinal follow-up studies of Kleine–Levin syndrome cases.

The behaviour problems encountered are extremely variable and often associated with some degree of somnolence and clouded consciousness. All sorts of psychiatric diagnosis have been discussed or assigned before a correct diagnosis is established. These may range from 'depression' (or 'manic-depression' because of the episodic character of the disorder) to 'schizophrenia' and 'drug abuse'. Encephalitis is commonly suspected, if the family seeks help during the first episode. Episodic severe aggression may rarely be the major presenting problem.

The episodic nature of the disorder might not be evident until three or more episodes have occurred. There is also commonly partial or total amnesia for the episodes.

Klinefelter syndrome (XXY)

Prevalence

Klinefelter syndrome affects about 0.1–0.15% of all live-born males.

Sex ratios

Klinefelter syndrome, by definition, can only occur in males.

Behavioural and physical phenotype

Boys with an extra X chromosome usually have a relatively low verbal IQ even though full-scale

IQ is often in the normal (or slightly subnormal range). They are often described as clumsy, and show many of the problems typical of children with DAMP (sometimes with a tendency towards hypoactivity). These problems may be enhanced by an unusual body-build/neuromotor performance. From middle childhood their legs tend to be long and arm span may exceed height. Penis and testicles are small or small normal. The testicles tend to be softer than normal. Many develop breast enlargement and the incidence of breast cancer is increased as compared with normal males.

The boys are often described as timid and with poor self-confidence. They have mild–moderate social interaction problems. Language disorders (first showing as language delay) and dysarticulation are common. A small number of cases with Klinefelter syndrome have been described who have autism.

One prospective study suggests that, in adult life, they may be less sexually active and more submissive in sexual orientation than other men (Schiavi et al., 1988).

Diagnosis

The diagnosis is generally not clinically suspected (and therefore altogether missed) in the pre-adolescent period, unless chromosomal analysis is performed in all children with typical problems.

The diagnosis of Klinefelter syndrome is made at chromosomal analysis. The typical karyotype is 47, XXY. Mosaicisms are not uncommon. Children with social interaction problems and a 47, XXY (low count) mosaicism have been described (Gillberg & Wahlström, 1985).

Pathogenesis

The pathogenesis in Klinefelter syndrome is not known, although, of course, hormonal changes are likely to result from the chromosomal abnormality, and these changes, in turn, could cause the physical and behavioural abnormalities.

Work-up

The work-up of Klinefelter syndrome males, other than the chromosomal examination and the possible need to repeat this, should include a physical and neurodevelopmental examination, neuropsychiatric assessment, neuropsychological work-up (including one of the Wechsler scales) and any other examination that is deemed clinically relevant depending on the type of symptoms shown by the individual patient.

Treatment

There is currently no specific treatment available for males with Klinefelter syndrome.

The old notion that 'these cases are probably best left to themselves, and a diagnosis may only be more upsetting than helpful' is probably inadequate. Instead, individuals with Klinefelter syndrome and their families may need careful counselling for many years, albeit at relatively long intervals, often well into the Klinefelter individual's adult age.

Outcome

The diagnosis of XXY syndrome implies later infertility, and counselling will be needed for this.

Krabbe disease

Krabbe disease (or Krabbe leukodystrophy) is not usually a diagnostic concern for the clinical child neuropsychiatrist, considering that most cases present with overt neurological symptoms in the first year of life and that few, if any, survive their fourth birthday. Nevertheless, it is included here, because occasionally, cases with juvenile onset may cause problems as regards differential diagnosis. The underlying neurometabolic disorder is a defect in the production of cerebroside-beta-galactosidase, which, in turn, leads to the accumulation of ?, a substance toxic to nerve cells, and consequently to neuronal death, major neurological disorder, developmental stagnation, regression and death.

Lesch–Nyhan syndrome

Lesch–Nyhan syndrome (Lesch & Nyhan, 1964; Nyhan *et al.*, 1969) is possibly the first disorder described in the literature which was believed to present with a particular *behavioural* phenotype.

Prevalence

The prevalence of Lesch–Nyhan syndrome is not known. However, the full-blown clinical picture is almost definitely rare, considering that, even in highly specialized neuropsychiatric/neurological clinics, only a few cases per thousand are seen.

Sex ratios

Lesch–Nyhan syndrome is inherited as an X-linked recessive disorder; only males are affected and females are carriers.

Behavioural and physical phenotype

Children with Lesch–Nyhan syndrome usually exhibit the combination of severe self-mutilation (mostly involving biting of own body, particularly lips and fingers) and choreoathetoid movements. Many (though not all) are moderately to severely mentally retarded. Some are friendly and cheerful (in spite of the self-mutilation which may take on grotesque proportions), but others demonstrate severely aggressive behaviour. Many show both physical and verbal aggression against others, and coprolalia, reminiscent of Tourette syndrome is common (Anderson & Ernst, 1994). A very common behaviour is throwing either an arm, a leg or the head out at doorways in order to inflict self-injury. Biting and head snapping directed at other people are also very common. A subgroup has classical symptoms of autism (Nyhan *et al.*, 1969; Gillberg & Coleman, 1992). The majority of the patients have a particularly severe form of self-mutilation involving biting of the lower lip. About half the children have seizures. In adolescence, haematuria, renal calculi and renal failure often develop. Gouty arthritis and urate tophi can also be observed.

Diagnosis

The diagnosis of Lesch–Nyhan syndrome should be suspected on the basis of the presence of the particular phenotype. It is confirmed by the demonstration of a particular inherited biochemical defect. The purine salvage enzyme, hypoxanthine–guanine–phosphoribosyl transferase (HGPRT) is deficient and this results in massive overproduction of uric acid (Wilson, Young & Kelley, 1983).

Pathogenesis

The HPRT gene has been mapped to the distal portion of the X chromosome (Becker *et al.*, 1979). The activity of the enzyme HGPRT is markedly reduced or absent (Seegmiller, Rosenbloom & Kelley, 1967) in Lesch–Nyhan syndrome. In normal human beings, HGPRT activity is highest in brain tissue. In the brain, the region containing the greatest activity is the basal ganglia. So far, post-mortem analyses of Lesch–Nyhan cases have revealed no specific neuropathological changes. Castells *et al.* (1979) and Silverstein *et al.* (1985) reported a decrease in dopamine and serotonin metabolites in cerebrospinal fluid. Although the discovery of the specific biochemical abnormality of the Lesch–Nyhan syndrome and the association of the syndrome with severe self-mutilating behaviours led to optimism of finding a rational pharmacological treatment, not only for self-injury in this particular syndrome, but perhaps more generally, so far, no clear-cut progress has been made. Further, it is still quite unclear just which are the pathways from the biochemical abnormality to brain functions to behaviour in the Lesch–Nyhan syndrome.

Work-up

A blood test for the HGPRT enzyme is the basis for the work-up. A uric acid clearance study should also be performed in order to establish if kidney function is intact and if the abnormality is metabolic rather than renal. The work-up should also include an evaluation of behavioural problems, including a detailed account of the self-injurious behaviours. A neurologist should evaluate the motor/movement disorder. Behavioural interventions similar to those employed in autism might be worthwhile and an appropriate assessment of factors contributing to elicitation/maintenance of abnormal behaviours should be performed.

Treatment

There is no known treatment for Lesch–Nyhan syndrome. However, it is generally recommended that interventions aimed at lowering the blood level of uric acid be used. This could include the administration of allopurinol and the introduction of low-purine diets (Hooft, Van Nevel & De Schaepdryver, 1968; Coleman, 1989). Physical restraints are usually required to prevent some forms of self-mutilation. Behaviour modification (particularly through negative reinforcement) is of limited efficacy. Of all the various medications tried in this devastating disorder, benzodiazepines tend to have the highest rate of success.

Outcome

Outcome in the Lesch–Nyhan syndrome is poor at the present time. The neurological symptoms tend to progress over the years. The self-injury can be so bad as to necessitate the extraction of all teeth, the fixation of arms and hands to the body and plastic surgery to repair the sometimes extensive damage accomplished by constant biting and hitting. Life expectancy is much lowered compared to the general population and to mentally retarded populations.

Lowe syndrome

Lowe syndrome, or oculocerebrorenal dystrophy, is a syndrome which has been poorly outlined with regard to behavioural characteristics. Nevertheless, there are often learning disorders (usually severe) and disruptive behaviour problems, and so a brief presentation is included here.

Prevalence

The prevalence of Lowe syndrome is unknown. A recent, very rough, estimate was reported at 1 in 200 000 live births (Charnas & Gahl, 1991).

Sex ratios

The syndrome is reported to occur in males mostly and is believed to be inherited in a sex-linked partially dominant fashion. At least 15 females with the syndrome have been described in the literature, but only five of these meet rigid diagnostic criteria, and only one of these five has been shown to have a normal (unbanded) 46 XX karyotype.

Behavioural and physical phenotype

The physical phenotype is characterized by cataracts or scattered opacities of the lens, glaucoma, organic aciduria, aminoaciduria and diminished renal production of ammonia. The eyes are often deep-set, there may be frontal 'bossing' and cryptorchidism. Growth retardation is common (Charnas & Gahl, 1991). Hypotonia and hypo/areflexia appear towards the end of the first year. Hyperkinetic syndromes often emerge around this age, and developmental delay becomes obvious. The most frequently described behaviours in school-age children are self-injury, consisting of scratching, biting, or hand and head banging, episodic dyscontrol, oculodigital phenomena (with hands placed between eyes and light source where they are rapidly and stereotypically moved) and resistance to change. Aggressive behaviour towards objects and people occur in about one-third of individuals diagnosed with Lowe syndrome (Lowe Syndrome Association Survey, 1989). Febrile episodes are common. Metabolic acidosis and rickets are frequent, but not invariable, features of the disorder. Seizures, including staring spells, infantile spasms and generalized tonic-clonic seizures occur in one-third of patients (Charnas 1989).

Diagnosis

The diagnosis is made on the basis of the typical combination of 'oculocerebrorenal' symptoms, i.e. congenital cataracts, mental retardation and generalized amino aciduria. A small number of individuals with low normal IQ exists (Charnas & Gahl, 1991).

Pathogenesis

The pathogenetic mechanisms are not understood so far. The disorder is believed to be inherited in a (parial) dominant sex-linked fashion. The chromosomal location is believed to be Xq24–26 (Silver, Lewis & Nussbaum, 1987). Female carriers are usually healthy except that they may have lenticular opacities.

Work-up

Ophthalmological examination, neuropsychological work-up (including an age-appropriate IQ test) and neuropsychiatric evaluation (with a particular view to diagnosing possible severe hyperactivity) and continuous follow-up of renal function are the basic requirements in the work-up of young patients with Lowe syndrome.

Genetic counselling is still difficult, but when the mother of a patient or another female in the family has typical lens opacities, it is relatively straightforward: each male foetus of the affected woman has a 50% risk of being affected, and each female foetus has a 50% chance of being a carrier.

Treatment

No specific treatment is available, and large doses of vitamin D have been ineffectual in the treatment of rickets. However, with the addition of calcium and sodium supplements, better results have been obtained with this regime. A more detailed account of treatment in this syndrome can be found in Charnas and Gahl (1991) .

Outcome

Severe mental retardation is common. Outcome in the longer-term perspective has been incompletely studied.

Marfan syndrome

Abraham Lincoln is the most famous individual who is believed to have suffered from Marfan syndrome (Randall, 1990). Marfan syndrome is well known in most branches of medicine because it presents with a number of symptoms and signs that concern a wide variety of different specialists, such as ophthalmologists, cardiologists and orthopaedic surgeons, quite apart from psychiatrists (McKusick, 1972).

Prevalence

The prevalence of Marfan syndrome is unknown, but may be relatively high given the common observation of individuals with long arms and legs and 'spider-like' fingers and toes.

Sex ratios

The sex ratio in Marfan syndrome is probably equal.

Behavioural and physical phenotype

There is no particular behavioural phenotype in Marfan syndrome. The physical hallmarks of the syndrome are usually characteristic, though. The long bones are strikingly long and the fingers are unusually thin and elongated giving the appearance of 'spider fingers'. There may be abnormalities of the vertebrae (scoliosis or kyphosis), cardiac anomalies (mitral valve deformities, cardiac hypertrophy), aortic cystic medianecrosis, aortic aneurysm (sometimes dissecting), abnormal location of the lungs and intracerebral aneurysms. There are often characteristic abnormalities of the lens (most often subluxation). Recently, poliosis (a white forelock) was described in Marfan syndrome (Herman et al., 1991), indicating that this phenomenon may not be as typical of tuberous sclerosis (Bourneville disease) as previously believed. Striae distensae are also common dermatological phenomena encountered in Marfan syndrome.

Intelligence is usually normal, and, indeed sometimes, superior. Single cases of autism, obsessive–compulsive disorder, and panic disorder with Marfan syndrome have been examined by the author, but it is not possible to suggest that these would be syndromes that are associated with Marfan syndrome at a rate over and above that expected by chance alone.

Diagnosis

The diagnosis is made on the basis of presence of the characteristic physical features: arachnodactyly (the abnormal length of the extremities, particularly the fingers and toes), luxation of the lens and other malformations (of the heart and large blood vessels). A similar phenotype with arachnodactyly and extopia lentis is sometimes associated with homocystinuria (which is inherited as an autosomal recessive), suggesting that a screen for aminoacidopathies would be appropriate in all cases suspected of suffering from Marfan syndrome.

Pathogenesis

Marfan syndrome is believed to be inherited as an autosomal dominant trait. Sporadic cases that are probably the result of new mutations also exist. It is possible that subclinical Marfan syndrome cases may exist in which only the arachnodactyly is impressive. The disorder is considered to represent a general 'mesodermal dystrophy'. The pathogenetic chain of events in Marfan syndrome is not known. Involvement of chromosome 15 (the fibrillin gene) has been suggested by a number of studies. There is a disorder of elastin and other connective tissues which accounts for some of the skeletal and angiodysplastic findings.

Work-up

The work-up required includes assessment by a cardiologist, ophthalmological examination, an X-ray examination of the vertebral column, blood and urine aminoacidograms and a test of kidney function.

Treatment

There is no specific treatment for Marfan syndrome. However, cardiac, vascular and skeletal abnormalities should be treated according to guidelines for such disorders. It has been suggested that beta-blockers may help arrest progressive dilatation of the aorta (Tahernia, 1993).

Outcome

Outcome depends on the degree of vascular involvement, in the brain, the heart and kidneys. Cardiac symptoms may begin as early as in the fifth year of life. In adolescence and adulthood, there may be left ventricular failure with or without angina pectoris. Respiratory problems are relatively common. With low-grade abnormalities in these organs, the syndrome is likely to be associated with normal longevity, but prospective follow-up studies are lacking and knowledge in this area is patchy.

Marker chromosome (15) syndrome (partial tetrasomy 15)

This syndrome (Fig. 10.5) has only recently been suggested to constitute a relatively homogeneous entity (Gillberg et al., 1991; Blennow et al., 1994), but it has been described by many different authors over the last 10 years (Maraschio et al., 1981; Buckton et al., 1985; Ghaziuddin et al., 1993; Baker et al., 1994; Bundey et al., 1994).

Prevalence

The prevalence of this chromosomal syndrome is unknown. However, it is almost definitely rare, since it has not been described in large series of patients who have undergone chromosomal examination. It appears that one hallmark of the clinical syndrome may be autism (Gillberg et al., 1991). In the only published

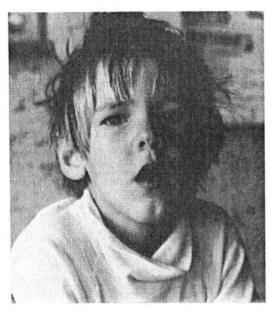

Fig. 10.5. Boy with marker chromosome 15 (partial tetrasomy 15) and autism.

systematic population-based study of chromosomes in children with autism, not a single case was identified (Gillberg & Wahlström 1985), indicating that the prevalence may be less than 1 in 100 000 children born.

Sex ratios

The sex ratio of marker chromosome 15 syndrome (partial tetrasomy 15) has not been specifically examined. Most published cases have been male. However, the publications of typical female cases by Ghaziuddin *et al.* (1993) and by Baker *et al.* (1994) show that it is not confined to males. Several of the males described by Gillberg *et al.* (1991) showed episodic hyperventilation, but this was not noted in the girl described by Ghaziuddin *et al.* (1993). This suggests the possibility that there may be symptomatic differences accounted for by the sex of the proband.

Behavioural and physical phenotype

The typical behavioural and physical phenotype is described in Table 10.2.

Table 10.2. *The clinical features of marker chromosme 15 syndrome (partial tetrasomy 15) as described by Gillberg et al.,* (1991)

Clinical feature
Autistic features usually amounting to full-blown autism
Moderate to profound degrees of mental retardation
Epilepsy
Hypotonus
Motor restlessness and hyperactivity
Muteness or extreme echolalia
Hand flapping and hand patting/hand wringing
Kyphosis/scoliosis
Esotropia
Facial nerve cell palsies
General growth retardation
Epicanthal folds
(Big protruding ears)[a]
(High-arched palate)[a]
(Episodic hyperventilation)[a]
(Hypertelorism)[a]

Note: [a] *described specifically only by Gillberg et al.* (1991)

There is usually developmental delay already in the first six months of life, although occasionally this may not be clearly noted until the second, or even third, year of life. Social interaction is typically impaired and there may be marked unawareness of the existence or feelings of other people. Stereotyped motor movements are present from early on. Hand flapping, as typically seen in autism, and body patting, as often encountered in Rett syndrome, are the rule. Delayed language development and muteness are the most common types of abnormality in the communication domain. A subgroup develops echolalic speech around age 3–4 years. One of the boys seen in our centre was able to sing well (including with words), but otherwise had very poor language skills. Motor activity is often very high.

There is often retarded physical growth and

Kr. 15.   Mar. 15

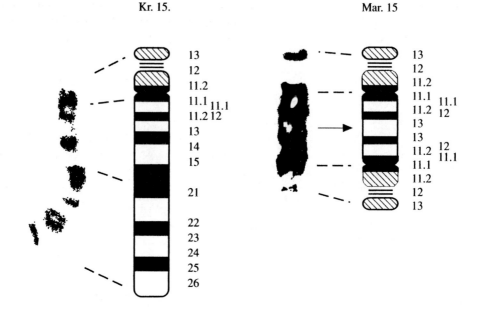

Fig. 10.6. Marker chromosome 15 (partial tetrasomy 15).

some of the cases seen in our centre (and the girl reported by Ghaziuddin *et al.*, 1993) have been exceptionally short with small hands and feet. Hypotonia is often present. Epilepsy (juvenile myoclonic in the Gillberg *et al.* series, infantile seizures in the Ghaziuddin *et al.* girl) has been a common finding. Other physical hallmarks of the syndrome include epicanthal folds and scoliosis/kyphosis.

Gillberg *et al.* (1991) suggested some similarities between this disorder and that of Rett syndrome. The growth retardation, occurrence of epilepsy after infancy, episodic hyperventilation and intermittent hand-clapping and hand-wringing are all reminiscent of the same types of symptoms seen in females with Rett syndrome.

Diagnosis

The diagnosis is made after chromosomal culture, which should be undertaken on the basis of the clinical suspicion that the child might have the syndrome. Tetrasomy of a part of chromosome 15 appears as a separate marker chromosome (Fig. 10.6.). The karyotype is 47

XY or XX + inv dup (15)(p13q12). It seems that the chromosomal material involved may have been inherited by the mother, but it is too early for definite conclusions to be drawn in this respect.

Pathogenesis

It is not known how the genetic abnormality contributes to the development of the characteristic behavioural and physical phenotype. The possibility that the parental origin of the chromosomal material may be important (at least in males, Martinsson *et al.*, 1994) should be further researched in view of the clinical implications of specific differential parental genetic effects on the expressed phenotype in other syndromes (most notably the fragile X, Prader–Willi and Angelman syndromes). Our group recently examined a male with the typical physical and behavioural phenotype who was marker X chromosome negative on first cytogenetic analysis. Because the phenotype was so strikingly similar to the marker chromosome cases described in the literature, the cytogenetic analysis was extended, and it was established that partial tetrasomy of chromosome 15 q11–13 was present in this case also, even though the material did not occur as an extra marker chromosome but as inserted extra material on chromosome 21. The affected boy's father had the same chromosomal abnormality, functioned in the normal range of intelligence, but was psychiatrically disturbed with several features of Asperger syndrome. The father had inherited the extra chromosomal material from his mother, suggesting, again, that genomic imprinting may be operating in this syndrome.

Work-up

The work-up, apart from chromosomal culture, should include a detailed family history, and, depending on availability, a further molecular biological work-up to determine the parental origin of the 'extra' chromosome material. A clinical autism and mental retardation screen should include appropriate tests for these diagnoses (see the chapters on autism and mental retardation). The medical work-up can be relatively limited, and should focus on possible epilepsy and spinal deformities.

Treatment

There is no known treatment for marker chromosome 15 syndrome. Intervention strategies as suggested for autism may be appropriate if the autistic symptomatology is prominent. The author has some positive preliminary experience with fenfluramine in this group of patients (1 mg/kg/day divided in two doses). Valproic acid appears to be the best antiepileptic drug regime in this disorder.

Outcome

Outcome is not known in the longer term. In the ten-year perspective through adolescence and early adult life it appears to be similar to that in moderately mentally retarded individuals with moderately severe autism without the marker chromosome. The onset of juvenile myoclonic seizures in the 8–10 year-old age range could be typical of the males. Although initially often frequent and severe, the seizure disorder tends to become less dramatic with age.

Moebius syndrome

Moebius syndrome was first described by Moebius in 1888. Its peculiar symptoms derive from bilateral congenital facial nerve palsies. The underlying aetiology may differ from one case to another, and it is not clear that it constitutes a homogeneous syndrome from the neurobiological point of view.

Prevalence

The prevalence of Moebius syndrome is not known, but complete and incomplete cases (for instance, with severe congenital unilateral facial nerve palsy in combination with mild–moderate congenital unilateral facial nerve palsy) are common enough to warrant consideration of a diagnosis of Moebius syndrome several times every year in a medium-sized paediatric or child neuropsychiatric clinic.

Sex ratios

There are no clear clues as to the typical sex ratio in Moebius syndrome, but it appears that boys may be slightly more often affected than girls. There is a higher male:female ratio in those Moebius syndrome cases that exhibit severe neuropsychiatric associated disorders (Gillberg & Steffenburg, 1989).

Behavioural and physical phenotype

The typical facial appearance of many cases with Moebius syndrome is often striking. In addition to the typical mask-like facies there is also often bilateral internal strabismus due to the involvement of both abducens nerves. There may, or may not, be associated abnormalities of limbs, pectoral muscles and/or visceral organs.

The behavioural phenotype is variable. According to one study (Gillberg & Steffenburg, 1987), as many as one-third of the cases may show autistic symptoms or even full-blown autism. Social competence may be both under- and overvalued depending on the point of view of the observer: while it is true that a child with congenital bilateral facial nerve palsy will not be able to exhibit the range of facial responses to underlying emotions, it is equally clear that social incompetence may be falsely attributed to the presence of the neurological symptoms.

Diagnosis

The diagnosis of Moebius syndrome depends on the demonstration of congenital (clear-cut or suspected) bilateral (usually equally pronounced) facial nerve palsy and is supported if such palsy is accompanied by signs and symptoms of involvement of other brainstem nuclei (especially the nerve cell nuclei of nervus trochlearis and nervus abducens) and of peripheral limb abnormalities (including abnormalities of fingers and toes) and pectoral muscle and visceral malformation (Towfighi et al., 1979).

Pathogenesis

The pathogenesis of Moebius syndrome is likely to be multiple. A few cases may be caused by congenital aplasia of muscles or by other muscular disorders (Hanson & Rowland, 1971). Certain cases could be caused by specific absence of brainstem nuclei (Towfighi et al., 1979), but the majority are likely to be the result of brainstem damage which, in turn, may be caused by ischaemia (with resultant calcification of the facial nuclei (Govaert et al., 1989)). Moebius syndrome (and other regional facial/neck abnormalities, such as the Klippel–Feil syndrome) may be associated with disrupted blood supply in the region covered by the subclavian artery (Bavinck & Weaver, 1986).

A limited number of familial cases of Moebius syndrome has been described in the literature (Garcia-Erro et al., 1989), but the evidence to date suggests that the majority appears to be caused by non-genetic factors.

Work-up

The work-up indicated in cases suspected of suffering from Moebius syndrome should include a screen for autism, an age-appropriate IQ-test, a CT- or MRI-scan to exclude space-occupying lesions which could contribute to the effects on cranial nerves and audiological plus auditory brainstem response examination to document brainstem neurophysiological dysfunction and/or hearing deficits. Ophthalmological evaluation is also mandatory to detect visual and visuomotor deficits.

Treatment

There is no known treatment for Moebius syndrome. Various kinds of intervention aimed at reducing the negative effects of facial paralysis (ocular, oculomotor, specific training of chewing and masticating) and any associated limb, skeletal or muscular problems as well as of disturbed behaviour may be indicated.

Outcome

No long-term outcome study of cases with Moebius syndrome has been published which means that to a considerable extent outcome is unknown. Nevertheless, many cases with the syndrome have been followed to adult life, and the evidence suggests that there is little change in overall functioning. However, in cases with severe autistic symptoms, outcome may be better predicted on the basis of this type of symptoms than from what is known about the physical disorder in itself.

Neurofibromatosis (von Recklinghausen disease)

Like tuberous sclerosis and Ito's hypomelanosis, von Recklinghausen disease, or neurofibromatosis, is classified as a phakomatosis, i.e. a group of disorders characterized by their dysplastic nature and proclivity to tumour formation in the CNS, skin and viscera.

Prevalence

Neurofibromatosis is reported to occur in at least 1 of every 3000 people (Crowe, Schull & Neil, 1956; Riccardi & Eichner, 1986). The clinical expression of the disorder is highly variable, and, in consequence, prevalence estimates are difficult to interpret. Mild forms of the disorder are almost definitely considerably more common than the prevalence rates in the literature suggest.

There are at least two subtypes of neurofibromatosis, type 1 (NF–1) and type 2 (NF–2). NF–1 is by far the most common. Its prevalence has been estimated at 1 in every 3500 people (Riccardi & Eichner, 1986).

Pathogenesis

NF–1 is caused by a gene defect on the long arm of chromosome 17 (the q11.2 area). The gene is large, comprising 2–3000 kb in length and encoding a protein of at least 2485 amino acids (Cawthon *et al.* 1990). Direct DNA diagnosis is now available.

A variety of types of mutational events can lead to the expression of the NF–1 phenotype, including chromosome translocations, insertions, deletions and point mutations (Riccardi, 1991*a*, *b*, *c*, 1993).

NF–2 patients appear to have a gene locus on chromosome 22 (Rouleau, Wertelecki & Haines, 1987), but, so far, direct DNA diagnosis is not available.

Behavioural and physical phenotype

In NF–1, the cutaneous changes include *café au lait* spots (at least six with a diameter of more than 15 mm if the presence of such skin changes alone are taken as evidence of the disorder), molluscum fibromas, hypopigmented spots (best seen with a Wood's lamp) and diffuse areas of pigmentation (one or several of these skin signs may be present in the individual patient). Although there may be hyperpigmented patches visible already at birth, they often appear later during the first decade, and the degree of pigmentation usually increases by adolescence leading to their recognition only at that age or later in many cases. Neurofibromata are often present, and optic gliomas are diagnosed occasionally. Axillary or inguinal freckling is a useful diagnostic aid. Lisch nodules (tiny melanocyte-containing hamartomas pro-jecting from the surface of the iris) appear to be of diagnostic value in differentiating the type 1 neurofibromatosis (Lubs *et al.*, 1991).

In NF–2, the cardinal feature is the development of bilateral acoustic neuromas in 96% of the cases. The number of *café-au-lait* spots are generally fewer than in NF–1 (Huson & Thrush, 1985).

There does not appear to be a consistent behavioural phenotype in any of the variants of NF. In all probability, many individuals with NF are completely free of psychiatric disorder, major behavioural or emotional problems. Nevertheless, autism has been described in some cases (Gillberg, 1992). Also, in populations of young people with autism, neurofibromatosis has been suggested to be relatively common, occurring in as many as 4–8% of all autism cases (Gillberg & Forsell, 1984). Deficits in attention, motor control and perception may be quite common in NF (Samuelsson, 1981). The present author has examined a number of young people with NF who showed severe DAMP (see Chapter 8), some of whom also had autistic features.

Outcome

Outcome in NF is highly variable, ranging from no or little psychosocial handicap to severe autism, mental retardation and disfiguring skin and bone changes. There is currently no better way of making a reasonable prognosis than to compile the clinical signs in childhood, and to expect the most severely affected cases at that point in time to be those with the poorest outcome. Nevertheless, some with negative odds in childhood have relatively good outcomes, whereas a subgroup of those with no, or very few, signs develop some rather devastating skin and skeletal problems later, so that there is no good guideline for the individual case.

Noonan syndrome

Jacqueline Noonan, in 1968, described a syndrome of hypertelorism, Turner syndrome phenotype and associated congenital heart disease (Noonan, 1968). Some years later, Jones,

Turner & Ferguson-Smith (1966), and Kaplan, Opitz & Gosset (1968) reviewed the literature on Turner syndrome phenotype and named the 'new' syndrome Noonan syndrome. Not much is yet known about the prevalence, genetics or specificity of this syndrome.

Noonan syndrome, so far, has been presumed to be possibly overrepresented in the male sex, but there is actually no good empirical support for the notion of Noonan syndrome as a 'male' variant of Turner syndrome in the female.

The most striking characteristics of Noonan syndrome are the typical face and short stature, similar to those observed in Turner syndrome, in combination with a normal karyotype on cytogenetic examination.

The following features have been reported in more than 75% of cases: short stature, pterygium colli, low-set ears, low nuchal hairline, high-arched palate, cubitus valgus, cryptorchism and various cardiovascular anomalies. Somewhat less common features (25–50% of reported cases) include: micrognathia, hypertelorism, epicanthus, antimongoloid slant of the palpebral fissures, ptosis, short neck, scutiform thorax, pulmonary stenosis and mental retardation.

Recent reports suggest that, just as in Turner syndrome, congenital peripheral hearing loss may be common in Noonan syndrome (Heller, 1965; Cremers & van der Burgt, 1992). This could be due to ossicular chain anomalies which may be successfully surgically corrected with restoration of hearing (Cremers & van der Burgt, 1992).

It is unclear to what extent the behavioural phenotype of Noonan syndrome overlaps with that of Turner syndrome.

Prader–Willi syndrome

Prader–Willi syndrome has attracted particular interest in the last decade both because of its peculiar behavioural phenotype (often more typical and suggestive of the diagnosis than the physical syndrome) and the fact that its genetics has cast new light on genetic mechanisms,

including genomic imprinting, that have previously been elusive to clinicians and researchers alike.

Prevalence

The prevalence of 'classic' Prader–Willi syndrome appears to be in the range of 1 per 10000 to 1 per 13000 children and young adults, depending on the exact criteria used for defining the syndrome and the type of screening method used. However, a population-based study in Sweden (Åkefeldt, Gillberg & Larsson, 1991) suggested that Prader–Willi syndrome might be considerably more common than previously believed, particularly if IQ under 70 is not considered a necessary defining feature. If, when diagnosing Prader–Willi syndrome, a learning disorder is allowed to substitute for clear-cut mental retardation as a diagnostic criterion, the syndrome is likely to be several times more common than previously suspected. The identification of the gene defect has now provided the theoretical tool for determining the true prevalence of Prader–Willi syndrome in the general population. Nevertheless, this should not be taken to imply that there is necessarily only one variant of Prader–Willi syndrome. There may be Prader–Willi syndrome with DNA abnormalities on chromosome 15q11q13 and there may, theoretically at least, be other cases with the full clinical syndrome but without this particular DNA abnormality. Also, the discovery that the typical gene abnormality may be present in the absence of classical signs of the syndrome (at least in young infants) could imply that the link between Prader–Willi syndrome and a particular gene defect may not be as straightforward as currently believed.

Sex ratios

The male:female ratio in Prader–Willi syndrome is probably equal according to the clinical and epidemiological studies that have been published to date.

Behavioural and physical phenotype

The common symptoms encountered in Prader–Willi syndrome are neonatal hypotonia, early feeding problems, overeating, obesity, short stature, small hands and feet, scoliosis, learning problems (but not, as previously believed, necessarily mental retardation) and a peculiar behavioural phenotype. Distinctive dysmorphic facial features (narrow bifrontal diameter, almond-shaped palpebral fissures and a thin down-turned upper lip) are often present but rarely conspicuous in the youngest age group. Hypogonadism is also a salient feature of the syndrome, but it is not always easily observable in very young children. The diagnosis of Prader–Willi syndrome may be delayed for many years, even into adulthood, and the delay is often caused by the failure on the part of clinicians to recognize that symptoms may not be as striking in childhood as they are later in life. Hypogonadism may be particularly difficult to diagnose in infants, and especially in female infants. In pre-school boys, penile size is often judged to be normal, but there may be scrotal hypoplasia or cryptorchidism.

About one in five of children with Prader–Willi syndrome are born in breech presentation.

The head size in the infant period is often relatively large, but only occasionally is true macrocephalus present. Most Prader–Willi syndrome infants are reported to have abnormalities of the quality of cry, and are described as having a weak, stridorous, high pitched, 'not sustained' or 'squeaky' cry (Aughton & Cassidy, 1990).

Diagnosis

Recent studies have shown that mental retardation is not an invariable feature (Clarke, Waters & Corbett, 1989) of Prader–Willi syndromes, and that there are cases with microdeletions at 15q11 with all the characteristics of the syndrome except mental retardation and short stature and small hands and feet. It now seems likely that Prader–Willi syndrome as originally described may be only part of a wider pheno-

Table 10.3. *Diagnostic criteria for Prader–Willi syndrome according to Åkefeldt et al. (1991)*

Necessary criteria
Severe hypotonia in neonatal period
Hypogonadism/delayed sexual development
Major weight problems (overweight)
Learning disorder

Supportive criteria
Deletion of chromosome 15/characteristic genetic (DNA) abnormality
Short stature
Typical dysmorphic features
Typical personality traits
Scoliosis
Skin-picking

---

type involving a particular behavioural profile with onset in the first year of life.

Diagnostic criteria for Prader–Willi syndrome are detailed in Table 10.3. A distinction has been made between necessary and supportive criteria. These criteria were used in the only population-based study of Prader–Willi syndrome published to date (Åkefeldt *et al.*, 1991).

As the child in the second or third year of life begins to grow fat, many parents often apply for help. By this time, there is often the description of a docile, still and kind child, who will, nevertheless, be irritable at times and who occasionally throws exceptionally severe temper tantrums (during which furniture and whole parts of apartments may be smashed to pieces). The tantrums are usually immediately followed by the 'baseline' hypoactivity and remorse.

The majority of children with Prader–Willi syndrome exhibit the strange habit of picking their skin, inflicting wounds, bruises and scratches. A few extract nails, tear at their hair, bite their lower lip or bang their head.

Most children with the syndrome will go for food like a bulimia patient during exacerbation. They eat and eat and just will not stop. They will go to any difficulty in order to be able to get access to the food in the fridge, freezer or pantry. Almost all parents have had to install lock mechanisms of varying degree of ingenuity in order to limit the amount of food otherwise bolted by the child. Even in scientific investigations, their inability to stop eating (in an experimental setting) has been amply demonstrated.

It now appears that there may be very mild forms of this disorder also. There may be relatively wide clinical variation across cases (see above in prevalence section). Many children may not have a severe learning disorder. The particular learning disorder variant termed 'hyperlexia' (see the chapter on dyslexia) is sometimes present in Prader–Willi syndrome (Burd & Kerbeshian, 1989).

In summary, 'extremely fat and hungry' children who show features of the behavioural phenotype described in the foregoing should be seriously considered for a diagnosis of Prader–Willi syndrome.

Hypothalamic dysfunction in Prader–Willi syndrome has long been suspected because of the combination of overeating–obesity, hypogonadism and short stature. However, it is only recently that clear evidence for hypothalamic hypofunction has been presented. Costeff *et al.* (1990) found low plasma growth hormone levels (but normal TSH) in short children with Prader–Willi syndrome, and suggested that these low levels were not an artefact of obesity.

Pathogenesis

Prader–Willi syndrome (or Prader–Labhart–Willi syndrome) is believed to be caused by an absence of paternal DNA at the chromosome 15q11q13 location. Angelman syndrome also exhibits a chromosomal abnormality at this location in some cases. Genomic imprinting of the chromosome 15q11–12 region has been suggested to account for the fact that two fairly distinct syndromes can arise on the basis of abnormality in the same chromosome segment. Absence of normal *paternal* DNA according to this hypothesis leads to Prader–Willi syndrome and absence of normal *maternal* DNA to Angelman syndrome. There are also cases with atypical hypotonia in the infancy period, but without the full-blown syndrome of Prader–Willi syndrome, who demonstrate the same type of chromosome abnormality as do patients

with the full syndrome (Holm *et al.*, 1993). Follow-up studies will reveal whether these cases eventually develop more symptoms of Prader–Willi syndrome or not.

Almost all cases of Prader–Willi syndrome (and of Angelman syndrome) are sporadic, but occasional families exist with translocation/inversion containing individuals with Angelman syndrome (with a maternally derived unbalanced translocation) and other individuals with Prader–Willi syndrome (with the same unbalanced translocation but of paternal derivation) (Hultén *et al.*, 1991).

It appears that about 20% of all cases of unequivocal Prader–Willi syndrome result from inheritance of both copies of chromosome 15 from the mother (so-called maternal uniparental disomy) and that the remaining cases are due to 'chromosomal' (detectable at chromosomal culture) or 'molecular' (detectable only at DNA analysis) deletions (Masscari *et al.*, 1992). Maternal uniparental disomy may be associated with advanced maternal age. There are also cases with some (and possibly without) atypical Prader–Willi symptoms, but with the overall behavioural/physical phenotype suggestive of the syndrome, who do not demonstrate any detectable DNA abnormalities, structural or associated with genomic imprinting. Whether or not these are to be regarded as true cases remains open to speculation at the present stage.

Intervention and treatment

Parents need to be informed about the nature of their child's condition. Oral and written information is essential in all cases. The parents have often been blamed by doctors, dieticians and psychologists (and by themselves) for the child's extreme obesity. The associated behavioural problems have often led to referral to a child psychiatric service. Without a proper diagnosis at the syndrome level, there is obviously a great risk that counselling may come to focus on child rearing practices with an underlying implication that disturbances in this area might be at the root of all the child's problems. Informing the parents about the almost identical behaviour problems encountered in other children with Prader–Willi syndrome, often has very positive psychological consequences. For the family to belong to a national (or local) Prader–Willi Society is almost always valuable.

The parents may need to be advised (although most have already found out for themselves) about locking fridges and various other cupboards, etc. With a very strict attitude on the part of parents and staff at school, it is sometimes feasible to make the child lose weight and even to achieve normal weight. However, retaining this strict attitude is by no means easy and, at the present stage, the family that cannot cope with all the restrictions is not to be blamed.

Once the behaviour problems are seen for what they are (i.e. part of the syndrome as such), some of the major conflicts in the family may be kept at a more reasonable level without blaming or self-blaming. Nevertheless, temper tantrums will often continue to cause great concern.

Various diets and drug treatments (including fenfluramine to reduce weight) have been tried in Prader–Willi syndrome, but the long-term effects, if any, remain to be demonstrated. Fenfluramine might be useful in short-term treatment, e.g. during periods when exposure to great amounts of food cannot be avoided and aggressive behaviour may be particularly difficult to control or contain (Selikowitz *et al.*, 1990).

Outcome

Prader–Willi syndrome usually leads to considerable handicap in adult life. It is not clear how serious or frequent are the problems faced by young (or older) adults with the syndrome. This is because no controlled population-based follow-up studies have been performed, to date. However, clinical experience suggests that individuals diagnosed in specialized clinics have considerable problems both in academic, psychosocial and physical domains.

Rett syndrome

Rett syndrome is one of the most common causes of severe mental retardation in young girls, second only to Down syndrome and, possibly, the fragile X syndrome in frequency in severely mentally retarded female populations (Hagberg, 1993). Various types of behavioural problems (including autistic symptoms, stereotypies and bruxism) are common, although not invariable features of the disorder. Many cases of Rett syndrome have previously been diagnosed as suffering from autism or 'childhood psychosis' (Witt-Engerström & Gillberg, 1987).

Prevalence

The prevalence of classical Rett syndrome has been estimated at at least 1 in 10 000 girls in Sweden (Hagberg, 1993). This figure is possibly an underestimate given that the epidemiological figure has been calculated from studies performed on children seen in certain clinics rather than from general population data. Nevertheless, the prevalence rate is likely to be close to population rates, considering that as severe a disorder as Rett syndrome would not likely be missed completely in Swedish health services. However, it is possible that some cases could have been obscured by being diagnosed as 'autistic' or 'psychotic'. Also, the recent acceptance that Rett syndrome variants also exist (Hagberg & Gillberg, 1993) has made it more difficult to decide where the boundaries of the syndrome are, and thus what the true prevalence might be.

Sex ratios

At the time of the production of this book, no unequivocal case of male Rett syndrome has been published or reported in other ways. The general consensus is that Rett syndrome is probably a disorder which occurs only in females. Nevertheless, a number of males with phenotypes strikingly similar to those observed in classical female cases have been reported (Hagberg & Gillberg, 1993), and it is yet too early to say with certainty that male Rett syndrome does not exist.

Behavioural and physical phenotype

Most girls with Rett syndrome show normal or almost normal development up to the age of

6–16 months. However, some authors (Kerr, 1993) have long maintained that Rett syndrome girls may not be quite normal from birth. They are often reported by their parents to have been, not just 'good', but 'very, *very* good'. At age 6–16 months, many then stagnate or rapidly begin to lose skills (social smile, interaction and some language skills might be lost). Some, but not all, of these become aloof, emotionally detached and are described as 'autistic'. Others slowly develop an emotionally stunted style of social interaction which may eventually also be described as autistic. A few seem almost toxically affected with attacks of rage, anxiety, confusion and chaotic hyperactivity. If there is an autistic or autistic-like phase, this may last from a month to several years. Usually by school age, or at least by puberty, the autistic aloneness begins to subside. The available evidence shows that the same type of development applies in most people with autism almost regardless of underlying cause.

With age, communicative intent becomes more pronounced. Many girls with Rett syndrome use their eyes for pointing to things that they want or which are otherwise of interest to them.

Girls with Rett syndrome show a variety of hand stereotypies, most of which involve 'midline procedures', i.e. both hands are 'washed' or clapped in the midline or used to slap the forehead or neck in the midline. At an early stage some may show more typical 'autism-type' hand flapping stereotypies. There are also hand stereotypies with hands apart.

Some girls are reported to laugh in the middle of the night. This occurs in a number of neuro-metabolic/neurological disorders affecting the brain (e.g. the Sanfilippo variant of mucopolysaccharidosis) and in many autism cases without Rett syndrome.

Bruxism and hyperventilation are common features in Rett syndrome and are sometimes interpreted as signs of extreme anxiety, a notion for which there is generally no empirical support. Nevertheless, it is clear that, in the regression stage (the so-called stage II, see below), many young children with Rett syndrome are very severely disturbed, autistic and appear to

be frightened or possibly even in pain. Bruxism is usually of a very particular type and reported to sound like the slow uncorking of a bottle of wine (Hagberg, 1993). Hyperventilation with bloating, swallowing of air and distension of the stomach is very common. There are also attacks of apnoea, sometimes following directly after bouts of hyperventilation, more rarely occurring without such antecedents. Episodes of hyperventilation alternating with apnoeic episodes and stereotypic hand movements also occur, but these behavioural phenomena have not been shown to correlate consistently with paroxysmal EEG events.

Rett syndrome variants

It is now clear that there exist a number of variants of Rett syndrome (Fig. 10.7, 10.8).

Infantile onset of seizures may blur the clinical picture in otherwise classical Rett syndrome cases. There are obvious congenital variants as well as 'late regression variants'. The most commonly described variant of Rett syndrome is the so called 'forme fruste' (Hagberg & Rasmussen 1986), in which the course is slower, the original diagnosis is often one of 'uncomplicated' severe mental retardation, and yet the clinical picture at adolescence usually indisputably favouring a diagnosis of Rett syndrome. Variants with preserved speech have also been described (Zappella, 1992*b*). The considerable variability in monozygotic twins supports a concept of a variable behavioural and physical phenotype.

Diagnosis

The diagnostic criteria of Rett syndrome are detailed in Table 10.4. Many girls with Rett syndrome in the early stages of the disorder show many autistic features without demonstrating clear-cut major neurological signs of any other kind. Therefore, it is common to make an autism diagnosis in the under 2–3 year-old age group. Occasionally one comes across a child with Rett syndrome with an unusually slow course. In such cases, the diagnosis of

Forme fruste RS variants
several different types

Rett syndrome
classical 'core'

Late
regression
RS

Preserved
speech
RS

Early
seizure
onset
RS

Congenital
onset
RS

?
Male
RS

Fig. 10.7.

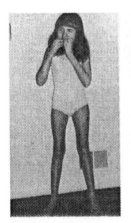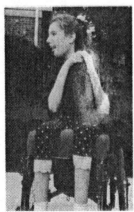

Fig. 10.8. Two teenage girls with Rett syndrome who followed different clinical courses. (*left:* Stage III (ambulatory), *right:* Stage IV-B (non-ambulatory).

'pure autism' with severe/moderate mental retardation can be retained for many years.

Stunting of head (and general) growth, occurrence of epilepsy, development of scoliosis and progressive loss of lower limb motor functions are common features.

Perhaps the most typical features of Rett syndrome are the abrupt or gradual decline in the use of acquired hand skills, generalized dyspraxia, and the delay (sometimes for minutes) in response to stimuli and prompts from the environment.

Hagberg (1993) has suggested diagnostic criteria for Rett syndrome variants (forme fruste, forme fruste allied and other variants) (see Table 10.5). The Rett syndrome variants are further discussed in the section on differential diagnosis.

Table 10.4. *Diagnostic criteria for classical Rett syndrome according to Trevathan et al.* (Rett Syndrome Diagnostic Criteria Work Group 1988)

Necessary criteria[a]
Apparently normal prenatal and perinatal period
Apparently normal psychomotor development through the first 6 months[b]
Normal head circumference at birth
Deceleration of head growth between ages 5 months and 4 years
Loss of acquired purposeful hand skills between ages 6 and 30 months, temporally associated with
    communication dysfunction and social withdrawal
Development of severely impaired expressive and receptive language, and presence of apparent severe
    psychomotor retardation
Stereotypic hand movements such as hand wringing/squeezing, clapping/tapping, mouthing and
    'washing"/rubbing automatisms appearing after purposeful hand skills are lost
Appearance of gait apraxia and truncal apraxia/ataxia between ages 1 and 4 years
Diagnosis tentative until 2 to 5 years of age

Supportive criteria
Breathing dysfunction
    Periodic apnea during wakefulness
    Intermittent hyperventilation
    Breath-holding spells
    Forced expulsion of air of saliva
EEG abnormalities
    Slow waking background and intermittent rhythmical slowing (3-5–Hz)
    Epileptiform discharges, with or without clinical seizures
Seizures
Spasticity, often with associated development of muscle wasting and dystonia
Peripheral vasomotor disturbances
Scoliosis
Growth retardation
Hypotrophic small feet

Exclusion criteria[a]
Evidence of intra-uterine growth retardation
Organomegaly or other signs of storage disease
Retinopathy or optic atrophy
Microcephaly at birth
Evidence of perinatally acquired brain damage
Existence of identifiable metabolic or other progressive neurological disorder
Acquired neurological disorders resulting from severe infections or head trauma

Notes:
[a] Modified from Hagberg *et al.* 1985
[b] Development may appear to be normal for up to 18 months

Table 10.5. *Diagnostic criteria for Rett syndrome variants according to Hagberg, 1993*

Group I (Clear, though not classical Rett syndrome). A female at least 10 years of age with mental retardation of unexplained origin, meeting at least three of the following six main criteria:

Loss of (partial or subtotal) acquired fine finger skills in late infancy/early childhood
Loss of aquired single words/phrases/nyanced babble
Rett syndrome type hand stereotypies, hand together or apart
Early onset communication disorder
Deceleration of head growth of 2SD or more (even when still within normal limits)
The characteristic Rett syndrome disease profile: a regression period (stage II) followed by amelioration in social and communication areas (stage III) despite continous slow neuromotor regression through school age and adolescence

and, in addition at least 5 of the following 11 supporting criteria:

Breathing irregularities (hyperventilation and/or breath-holding)
Bloating/marked air swallowing
Gait dyspraxia
Characteristic teeth grinding
Neurogenic scoliosis (long curve of neurogenic type) or high kyphosis (ambulant girls)
Gradual appearance of lower limb neurological signs
Small blue/cold impaired feet, autonomic/trophic dysfunction
Insidious development of EEG sleep pattern characteristic of Rett syndrome
Unmotivated sudden laughing/screaming spells
Impaired/delayed nociception
Eye pointing characteristic of Rett syndrome

Group II (Probable Rett syndrome). An adult woman with mental retardation of unexplained origin, where only incomplete data are recorded/available, meeting all the following four criteria:
Hand dyspraxia/apraxia which cannot be accounted for in other ways and which stands out against development in other areas
Rett syndrome type hand stereotypies or locked, distorted position of the hands which can be characteristic of Rett syndrome
Discrepancy between progressive neuro-impairments (particularly distal lower limb dystonia, lower neuron dysfunction) and slowly stabilizing/improving communication abilities
Communication dominated by the eye pointing, characteristic of Rett syndrome

and, in addition, at least 4 of the first 9 RS supporting characteristics given under group I.

Specify: congenital, infant onset (0–1 year) early childhood onset (1–3 years) late childhood regression (4–10 years)
seizure onset
preserved speech

Pathogenesis

The brain in Rett syndrome is much smaller than normal, the average weight being around 850 g (Armstrong, 1992). There appear to be poor development of dendrites, dense cell packing and small cells (Bauman, 1992; Armstrong, 1992), all compatible with an arrest in brain development beginning around age 1–3 months postnatally. It is currently believed that Rett syndrome is a genetic disorder of neurodevelopment rather than a truly and inevitably progressive neurodegenerative brain disorder. Hagberg (1992) suggested the term 'neuronal disconnection failure' for the type of neural abnormality typical of Rett syndrome.

A number of familial cases have been described (siblings concordant for Rett syndrome, monozygotic concordant twins, a monozygotic discordant twin pair, a dizygotic concordant twin pair, an aunt and a niece concordant for Rett syndrome, a mother and daughter who both have Rett syndrome). Attempts have been made to fit these cases into one genetic model, so far without complete success. A two-step mutation involving a mutant gene on the X-chromosome and lethality in the male is still the most espoused theory for genetic transmission of Rett syndrome (Clarke, 1993). Nevertheless, transmission through males (as has been observed in a large genealogical Swedish study, Åkesson *et al.*, 1992) presents a problem for this model. Bühler (Bühler, Malik & Alkan, 1990) has suggested an autosomal locus interacting with X-linked inheritance.

Recently, a number of extended families have been observed in which maternally related first cousins have classical Rett syndrome, autism with ataxia and severe mental retardation with autism (Gillberg, Ehlers & Wahlström, 1990) or classical Rett syndrome and other variants of Rett syndrome (Anvret *et al.*, 1990) or classical Rett syndrome, autism, Asperger syndrome and anorexia nervosa (Gillberg, Råstam & Gillberg, 1994). These observations suggest that what is inherited in Rett syndrome may not be the classical phenotype, but some other symptom/sign of neuroimpairment which, depending on other associated factors, may present in slightly or even very different ways.

Work-up

There is still no unique diagnostic marker for Rett syndrome. Thus, the diagnosis rests on the description of the typical core symptoms and supportive findings. The work-up required depends on the degree of certainty of the clinical diagnosis made, the age of the individual affected, and the type of most prominent symptoms encountered.

Rett syndrome can be confused with a number of other conditions, particularly in young girls. Thus, mucopolysaccharidoses may mimic the clinical picture of Rett syndrome almost to perfection. In infantile spasms, with or without tuberous sclerosis, the symptoms can be almost identical. The differential diagnosis is rendered even more difficult in such cases because Rett syndrome and infantile spasms can occur together (see below under Rett variants). Thus, before a final diagnosis of Rett syndrome is made in a young girl, an extensive medical, neurophysiological and metabolic work-up will almost always have been done before. This may involve screening for aminoacidopathies, organic acidopathies, poly- and oligosaccharides, EEG and CAT-scan examination and chromosomal analysis.

The EEG can often be helpful in early differential diagnosis in Rett syndrome. During stage I there is usually no changes or slight general slowing. During stage II, focal spikes in central, often centroparietal (parasagittal) leads are common (Niedermeyer & Naidu, 1990). The spikes are most consistently seen in sleep. Although characteristic of stage II, spikes sometimes persist into stage III. This clinically rather uneventful stage is sometimes accompanied by some rather typical changes, particularly during sleep. First, there may be intermittent bursts of irregular delta waves, appearing against a rather flat background. Discrete theta episodes can be seen in drowsiness. The intermittent pattern of bursts is similar to that seen in subacute sclerosing panencephalitis. Epileptic discharge phenomena are common EEG findings in stage IV, in spite of the fact that overt epileptic seizures are uncommon.

SPECT studies (e.g. Uvebrant *et al.*, 1993) have shown hypoperfusion in the midbrain, brainstem and frontal areas. Whether these pathologies have developed in parallel in different brain localities, or represent one dysfunction leading to the other two remains to be resolved.

The work-up required once the diagnosis has been established should be guided more by the type of main problem shown by the patient, than by any one overall guideline for the whole group.

Outcome

Rett syndrome is divided into four developmental stages according to prevailing symptoms and course of the disorder (Witt-Engerström, 1993). In *stage I (infancy)* there may be subtle signs of the child being 'too good' (Kerr, Montague & Stephenson, 1987). Dissociation of motor development and delay in equilibrium control is often apparent by age 10 months. In *stage II (regression)* early development is reversed (around age 11–25 months) and movement and behaviour become increasingly dyscoordinated. The girls often appear withdrawn and even frightened. There is often an impression of 'toxaemia', and the regressive phenomena may take on a fulminating course. At about age 2.5 years (20–50 months) *stage III (established syndrome/pseudostationary period)* emerges with some beginning signs of renewed sociability and a decrease in 'toxic' symptoms. Hand dyspraxia and stereotypic movements are prominent. Some girls/women with Rett syndrome develop more symptoms of lower limb involvement years to decades later and enter into *stage IV (late motor deterioration)*. They may then become completely non-ambulant and wheelchair dependent.

Epilepsy was once believed to be almost universal in Rett syndrome, but is now believed to occur in perhaps no more than half of all cases. Vacant staring spells, which are very often encountered, do not necessarily represent true epileptic phenomena.

Scoliosis is extremely common, and should be monitored and treated early (Budden, 1993).

Outcome in Rett syndrome was once believed to be extremely poor with a gradually downhill course and premature death. Follow-up of larger groups of cases, and the identification of classical Rett syndrome in middle-aged women, have contributed to a better understanding of the prognosis. It is now clear that plateauing usually occurs in Rett syndrome, and that further major loss of function rarely occurs after adolescence, even though (secondary?) progressive loss of function and increased posturing in the lower limbs may be seen. Communicative function often improves in stage IV.

Diagnosis

The diagnosis of Rett syndrome is based on a set of necessary and supportive criteria (Table 10.4). As has been repeatedly pointed out, it now appears that these criteria for diagnosing classical Rett syndrome may be overly restrictive and artificially narrow. In research, it is still necessary to apply these criteria with rigour (until a possible biological marker for the syndrome is found). In clinical practice, there may be many cases meeting almost all (though not full) criteria for Rett syndrome. Such cases should be acknowledged as possible Rett syndrome (Table 10.5).

Psychiatric/behavioural aspects

There are a number of important neuropsychiatric aspects and behavioural phenomena that need to be taken into account when planning a good intervention programme in Rett syndrome. The autistic symptoms shown by young girls with this disorder often lead to a diagnosis of autism. However, the behavioural treatment approach advocated in autism may not be quite appropriate for the type of autistic problems shown by Rett syndrome girls. Rather than resisting change (a typical symptom of autism), girls with Rett syndrome tend to be withdrawn, socially dyspractic and lacking initiative while in stage II. Communication through gaze should be tried, since it appears that visuospatial pathways may be relatively spared (Uvebrant *et al.*, 1993). Constant training of motor function, equilibrium and communication skills may help preserve some functions through stage II into stages III and IV.

It is important to remember that most, though not all (Gillberg 1989), girls with Rett syndrome grow out of the most severe forms of autistic withdrawal once they are in stage III and may, instead, become relatively very communicative, smiling and pointing with their eyes.

Differential diagnosis/Rett variants

A number of cases show symptoms in the borderland of Rett syndrome and autism (Gillberg, 1989; Hagberg & Gillberg, 1993).

Among these are the so-called 'forme fruste variants' (Hagberg & Rasmussen, 1986). These borderland cases all show many of the features of Rett syndrome, albeit to a milder degree (at least initially), but they do not fulfil all the classical criteria. The course is more protracted and a definite diagnosis usually cannot be made until after age (10–) 13 years. The regression often occurs later (at 12–36 months of age), and its onset is more insidious. These girls also usually meet most, or all, of the criteria for autistic disorder (or infantile autism). Some girls show all the classical symptoms of autism, but only after a prolonged premorbid or stage I period of the disorder.

Early onset epilepsy can distort the clinical picture of Rett syndrome to the extent that the true nature of the major 'underlying' disorder may not be realized for many years, if at all.

Congenital variants have been described in which all the diagnostic criteria, except normal psychomotor development during the first months of life, are met (Rolando, 1985; Nomura, Segawa & Hasegawa, 1985; Goutières & Aicardi, 1987; Lin et al., 1991). Such cases have been described in families containing at least one case of classical Rett syndrome, making it likely that the atypical congenital variant is, in fact, a case of 'true' Rett syndrome.

Other familial cases have been described in which one girl had classical Rett syndrome, a maternal first cousin had classical autism later developing into more Rettoid symptomatology, and another maternal first cousin had autism with severe mental retardation (Gillberg et al., 1990).

Zappella (1992b, 1994) has described a number of girls with autism, developmental arrest, hand-washing stereotypies and other Rett syndrome suspected symptoms in the presence of some preserved (in some cases even elaborate) speech. The present author and Professor Bengt Hagberg have seen several such cases also. A few cases of boys with these borderline conditions have been described in the literature.

However, most authors agree that, to date, no undisputable male cases of Rett syndrome have been described (Hagberg & Gillberg, 1993). Rett-like symptomatology also occurs in conjunction with other neurological disorders such as infantile neuronal ceroid lipofuscinosis (Hagberg, 1989), Moebius syndrome (Gillberg, 1989) and mucopolysaccharidosis. The different types of Rett variants and their distribution in relation to the 'nuclear' or 'classical' form of Rett syndrome have already been outlined in Fig. 10.7 and Table 10.5.

Treatment/management

There is no cure or rational treatment for Rett syndrome at present. Nevertheless, a lot of good things can be accomplished through state-of-the art medical treatment and education.

In the management of the behavioural/psychiatric problems encountered in Rett syndrome it is essential for the clinician to be aware of the natural course of the disorder so that symptoms such as autism and night laughter are not inappropriately interpreted as signalling specific psychological or interactional problems. The degree of language comprehension, and production, is extremely low in Rett syndrome. Communication should be achieved by other means such as through eye gaze and manual prompting. Some degree of hand function can often be maintained if both hands are trained separately for long periods of time every day.

Pharmacologically, some worthwhile results with bromocriptin (20 mg/kg/day b.p.d.) have been reported (Zappella, 1990a), but confirmatory double-blind, placebo-controlled studies are needed before this drug can be recommended. Naltrexone has also been tried, but with conflicting results (Percy et al., 1994).

Outcome

The ultimate course of Rett syndrome is only partly known. It seems clear that the vast majority become extremely mentally and/or neurologically handicapped and remain dependent on other people for virtually all matters in every day life. Epilepsy, constipation, scoliosis, progressive motor (and vasomotor) control problems complicate the clinical picture in a majority of cases. The psychiatric/behavioural problems can be frustrating through childhood, and sometimes adolescence, but usually cause less concern in the adult age group.

It appears that many of the characteristic symptoms of Rett syndrome in childhood are no longer as clearly evident in later life. The author knows about a 50 year-old woman with a classic Rett syndrome history, who gave up clapping and wringing her hands (in the midline) around age 30 years. As a child she had been extremely aloof, but after about age 15 years, she seemed to become more and more interested in social interaction. Her clinical profile at age 50 years was characteristic of sociable severely mentally retarded people.

Concluding comments

Thinking about the possibility of a diagnosis of Rett syndrome is essential in all very young girls presenting with autistic symptoms. In one study, 80% of all Rett syndrome girls were first suspected of suffering from autism or autistic features (Witt-Engerström & Gillberg, 1987) and, on the basis of available prevalence estimates for Rett syndrome, it was concluded that, of all girls presenting in the first few years of life with autistic symptoms, 1/3–1/2 will eventually turn out to have Rett syndrome.

Sanfilippo syndrome and other mucopolysaccharidoses

The mucopolysaccharidoses are severe neurometabolic disorders, invariably leading to nerve cell death and premature death. They are caused by inborn errors of metabolism due to deficiencies of lysosomal glucosidase or sulphatase, which lead to the accumulation of mucopolysaccharides or glycosaminoglycans in the lysosomes. The enzymes that are deficient vary from one disease subgroup to another, and may even vary within the subgroups. For instance, in Sanfilippo disease, there are at least four different types of enzyme disorders, even though the urine final product (heparan sulphate) is the same.

Prevalence

The prevalence of the whole group of these disorders is not known. However, for some of them, like Hurler disease, prevalence data are available, and are in the range of 1 per 100 000 births.

Sex ratios

The sex ratio, except in Hunter disease is reported to be equal.

Behavioural and physical phenotype

There is no characteristic phenotype, although Sanfilippo disease often presents with marked behavioural problems including hyperactivity, self-mutilation and autistic features, often after a period of seemingly normal development. There is then usually progressive mental and neurological deterioration. The physical characteristics, at first, may be minor, although hypergenitalism and some degree of overall coarseness is the rule. In Hunter disease, osseuos anomalies including kyphoscoliosis and dwarfism are common, but neurological and psychiatric impairment much less frequent. In Hurler disease, there is usually a combination of severe osseous anomalies and severe CNS involvement.

Diagnosis

The diagnosis is usually suspected on the basis of any combination of two of the following: (1) increasing degree of coarse physical features, (2) dwarfism, (3) behavioural disturbance characterized by unmalleability, autistic features, aggressiveness, hyperactivity and self-mutilation and (4) progressive neurological and mental impairment. Urine and blood work-up are essential in order to identify the specific biochemical markers associated with Sanfilippo and other mucopolysaccharidosis syndromes (McKusick, 1972; Aicardi, 1992). Differential diagnostic problems may arise in relation to the so-called DDD – or CDG –

syndrome (disialotransferrin deficiency disorder – or carbohydrate deficiency glycoprotein disorder) (Kristiansson *et al.*, 1989), a glycoprotein metabolism disorder also characterized by mental and behavioural deterioration and progressive kyphosis.

Pathogenesis

Most of the mucopolysaccharidoses are inherited as autosomal recessive traits. Hunter disease is an exception and is X-linked recessive. The various enzyme deficiencies have been fairly well established, and cause storage of substances that lead to progressive nerve cell death. The way in which CNS destruction develops is poorly understood, however. There is clinical (and theoretical) overlap with disorders of glycoprotein metabolism.

Work-up

Urine screening for excretion of mucopolysaccharides should be routine in all young people with progressive regression and in those with escalating autistic and disruptive behavioural symptoms.

Treatment

Hurler disease can be treated with some success (Whitley *et al.*, 1986): enzyme replacement therapy by bone marrow transplant is recommended. In most other variants of the mucopolysaccharidoses, no rational treatment is available at the time of going to press with this book.

Outcome

Outcome is poor, perhaps particularly in Hurler disease and Sanfilippo disease. In these syndromes, death usually supervenes before age 20 years.

Schilder disease

The combination of so-called sudanophilic degeneration of the central nervous system and adrenal medullar failure is often referred to as Schilder disease or Schilder syndrome. This is not a single disease entity but represents a variety of 'cerebral sclerosis' conditions, some of which are sporadic and others hereditary. Sex-linked recessive, autosomal recessive and autosomal dominant forms have been described.

Schilder syndrome shows variable clinical onset age depending on which variant of the disorder is inferred. Nevertheless, the majority of cases show progressive symptoms and signs of a brain disorder before age 8 years. To confirm the diagnosis, brain biopsy (or autopsy) is necessary.

The neuropsychiatric profile is related to signs and symptoms of progressive dementia. Aggressive outbursts and autistic-type behaviour has been encountered in one case of hereditary (autosomal dominant) Schilder syndrome.

Sex chromosome aneuploidies

It now seems that most cases of sex chromosome aneuploidies (which occur in about 0.3% of all live births) have an increased risk of problems which can lead to a high rate of psychiatric disorders. Conversely, sex chromosome aneuploidies are relatively common in child psychiatric clinic attenders. In one study (Crandall, Carrel & Sparkes, 1972), 1.6% of children referred to a child psychiatry clinic had sex chromosome aneuploidies.

For further details, see the various identified syndromes (Double Y, Klinefelter, Triplo X and Turner syndromes).

Sotos syndrome

This syndrome, described by Sotos in 1952, is now variously referred to as cerebral gigantism or Sotos syndrome. Its aetiology is unknown and the prevalence has not been studied in detail. There are typical gargoyle features in early childhood, but puberty onset is often early, and so ultimate height does not usually take on gigantic proportions.

Dodge, Holmes & Sotos (1983) characterized Sotos syndrome in the following way: the children are large at birth and show excessive growth in the first four years, they have macrocrania, a high forehead, frontal bossing, a prominent jaw, hypertelorism, antimongoloid slanting of the palpebral fissures and a high arched palate. The profile of the head is 'triangulated' with a tendency for the projection of the lower jaw backwards to be identical with the posterior limit of the occipital part of the skull. Bone age is usually advanced in prepubertal children. Hands and feet are described as large. Affected patients often resemble each other more than they do other members of their families. A number of cases associated with hyper- and hypothyroidism have been described in the literature. The occasional occurrence of tumours (including neurofibromatosis) in Sotos syndrome has been taken to reflect a general growth disorder.

Sotos syndrome often appears to be sporadic, but it is quite clear that familial–hereditary cases are not uncommon. It has been suggested that an autosomal dominant mode of inheritance might be present in such cases. Parents are perhaps slightly older than average, but data in this respect is scarce.

Early teething, delay in beginning to walk and speak and some degree of intellectual retardation are common early manifestations, apart from the physical characteristics described above.

The neuropsychiatric profile in Sotos syndrome is only partly known. About 80% of patients are believed to be mentally retarded, but, as in many other behavioural phenotype syndromes, this may be an over-estimate based on studies of atypical institutionalized groups. There is often a large discrepancy between verbal and performance IQ, the latter being considerably lower as a result of severe perceptual problems in many cases. Nevertheless, spoken language is often deficient with a marked tendency for echolalia, slurred speech and slow articulation ('oral apraxia'). According to a recent study by Rutter and Cole (1991) behavioural problems, attention deficits and mild cognitive dysfunction are common

features. About two-thirds of cases were reported to have IQ-levels in the 50–70 range and the majority of the remainder in the 70–90 range.

Zappella (1990b) recently described autistic symptoms and even full-blown autistic disorder in 5 out of 12 examined cases with Sotos syndrome and associated mental retardation. One further case, the only girl in the series showed excessive degrees of insistence on sameness. Four further boys were hyperactive. Morrow, Whitman & Accardo (1990) have also described autism in connection with Sotos syndrome.

Spielmeyer–Vogt disease

Spielmeyer–Vogt disease is one of the syndromes leading to early onset visual problems (followed by complete blindness/'amaurosis'), followed (occasionally preceded) by mental and neurological motor symptoms.

The onset of this disorder (or 'juvenile neuronal ceroid lipofuscinosis') is usually around age 5–7 years. Behavioural problems of various kinds (including withdrawal, panic attacks and hyperactivity) are very often the presenting symptoms (Armstrong, Koppang & Rider, 1982). Dysarthria is often the next problem to develop, and it may be many months or years before the typical progressive visual deterioration occurs. Macular degeneration with pigment accumulations occur from about age 10–12 years. Slow waves or a low amplitude are common findings on the EEG. Mild/moderate atrophy may be present on neuroimaging and extensive calcification may be a characteristic finding on CT scanning.

Death, with current methods of intervention, occurs between 16 and 35 years of age.

Thalidomide syndrome

Thalidomide was introduced as a tranquillizer in the 1950s. It was in widespread use for a short time until it became known that the drug could have teratogenic effects. More about this specific syndrome is reported in Chapter 3. The recent description of autism in thalidomide embryopathy (Strömland *et al.*, 1994) makes it mandatory to screen for possible teratogenic influences in autistic disorder (and autistic-like conditions with varying degrees of mental retardation).

Triplo X syndrome (XXX, 'super female syndrome')

Girls with this syndrome constitute 0.1% of all live-born females. They are at much increased risk of language disorder, learning disorder (with a need for special education in most cases and IQs in the low normal range), shyness, immaturity and conduct problems of various kinds (Linden *et al.*, 1988). They are tall and poorly coordinated as regards motor movements. This, in connection with their odd behaviour and conduct problems, leads to a much increased risk of referral for institution treatment of different kinds.

Tuberous sclerosis (Bourneville disease)

Tuberous sclerosis (epiloia, Bourneville disease) is inherited as an autosomal dominant with variable penetrance. The rate of new mutations is said to be high (58–68% according to Fleury *et al.*, 1980 and Hunt & Lindenbaum 1984), but the evidence for this is not unequivocal, since no population studies dealing specifically with this issue have been published. There is some evidence for familial transmission in at least 50% of all cases with early childhood severe symptoms (Ahlsén *et al.*, 1994).

Prevalence

Several population studies suggest that the prevalence of tuberous sclerosis in children and adolescents is in the range of 1/12000–1/6800 (Hunt & Shepherd, 1993; Ahlsén *et al.*, 1994). The highest rate reported to date comes from a Swedish population study. In that study, the 11–15 year-olds had the highest prevalence of diagnosed early 'onset' (symptoms before 5

years of age) tuberous sclerosis. The true number of cases is likely to be considerably higher than 1/6800, given the well-established fact that many tuberous sclerosis cases exhibit few symptoms and may go unrecognized for many years, sometimes throughout life.

Sex ratios

The sex ratio in cases with early symptoms is probably equal (Ahlsén *et al.*, 1994). The results of some studies might suggest a higher rate in males than in females (e.g. Shepherd *et al.*, 1991), but this could be an artefact of very small numbers of cases.

Diagnosis

Gomez (1988) has suggested definitive and suggestive criteria for the diagnosis of tuberous sclerosis (Table 10.6). It is anticipated that the gene(s) for tuberous sclerosis will be mapped in the next few years, and it is likely that, just as in the case of neurofibromatosis, a clearer distinction between various types of tuberous sclerosis will then be possible.

Aetiology, pathogenetic factors and pathology

The aetiology of tuberous sclerosis is unknown at the production of this book. However, linkage has been obtained in some families to chromosome 9q34 (Fryer *et al.*, 1987; Connor, 1990), and in others to chromosome 16 (Webb *et al.*, 1993). Chromosome 11 has also been implicated, but this location is currently not being pursued with the same intensity as the other two. All three gene sites are adjacent to genes regulating dopamine turnover/function, which is of theoretical interest, considering that so many tuberous sclerosis patients have autistic symptoms. The general hypothesis at the time of writing this book is that a faulty protein is the result of the gene defect, and that the protein produces disordered cell differentiation and migration in early tissue development, resulting in abnormal tissue growths in many body organs. The brain, skin, kidney and heart are the organs most notably affected. The varia-

Table 10.6. *Diagnostic criteria for tuberous sclerosis according to Gomez*

Criterion
Definitive diagnosis if any one of the following:
Subependymal glial nodules
Cortical tubers
Giant cell astrocytomas
Retinal hamartomata
Facial angiofibromas (adenoma sebaceum)
Ungual fibroma
Forehead/scalp fibrous plaques
Multiple renal angiomyolipomas
Presumptive diagnosis if any two of the following:
Infantile spasms
Myoclonic tonic or atonic seizures
Hypomelanotic macules
Shagreen patches
Peripapillary retinal hamartoma undistinguishable from Drusen
Gingival fibromas
Dental enamel pits
Multiple renal tumours
Renal cysts
Cardiac rhabdomyoma
Pulmonary lymphangiomatosis
Radiographic 'honeycomb' lungs
Wedge-shaped cortical-subcortical calcification
Multiple subcortical hypomyelinated lesions
Immediate relative with TS

bility of expression in tuberous sclerosis is enormous both as regards the position and number of lesions. This, in turn, produces wide variation in respect of associated physical and behavioural problems.

It is quite possible that tuberous sclerosis, just like neurofibromatosis, may represent a complex of disorders rather than one disease entity.

Cortical tubers, subependymal nodules and giant cell tumours are the characteristic brain lesions found in tuberous sclerosis. The tubers are hard nodules of variable size which have a structure of areas of disordered stellate neurons and areas of astrocytes which are distinct from one another. There is reduction of the number of neurons, which are replaced by bizarre-shaped giant cells (Trombley & Mirra, 1981;

Steffanson, Wollman & Huttenlocher, 1988). The tubers may become calcified. Large abnormal heterotopic neurons extend beneath the tubers all the way to the ventricular walls. The subependymal nodules are usually located in, or next to, the caudate nucleus and thalamus, mostly on the outer walls of the frontal horn and body, and resemble wax that has dripped down the side of a candle on the lining of the ventricular walls. The cells making up the subependymal nodules are thought to be of astrocytic origin. The giant cell astrocytomas are not as common as the other two abnormalities and are located to the region of the Monro foramina. Unlike the other tumours, they may grow to become large, but only very rarely do they turn malignant. All these brain tumours can contribute to socially impaired behaviour, overactivity, epilepsy and mental retardation.

In addition to the brain lesions there are often visceral tumours, such as rhabdomyomas of the heart (occurring in 40 to 50% of all tuberous sclerosis cases). Renal lesions may consist of angiomyolipomas (which in some patients may be the only sign that the patient is suffering from tuberous sclerosis) and renal cysts (Robbins & Bernstein, 1988). In the fundi of the eyes, retinal hamartomas (phakomas) are astrocytic and usually benign tumours that may calcify (Gomez, 1988). These hamartomas are round or oval in shape and often take on a typical mulberry appearance. They may be difficult to differentiate from so-called 'Drusen'. Cataracts and iris colobomas are also occasionally encountered in tuberous sclerosis.

The cutaneous problems include hypomelanosis (usually in patches, ash-leaf spots or minimal macules the size of grains of rice, or affecting the scalp and resulting in depigmented hair; the most common cutaneous signs of tuberous sclerosis according to Hunt (1983) and probably present from birth but often not recognized until much later), facial angiofibromas (the characteristic red papular lesions that are considered by many to be the typical hallmark of the disorder, but which are present in less than two-thirds of cases and which make their appearance at any time from 3 to 15 years of age), fibrous plaques on the forehead or scalp, periungual fibromas (usually not present until pre-adolescence (Ahlsén et al., 1994)) and shagreen patches (consisting of slightly elevated plaques of epidermis with an almost granular surface and usually, but not always, a (slight) yellowish–brown discolouration which appear only after a few years of life).

Behavioural phenotype in tuberous sclerosis

The triad of mental retardation, epilepsy and adenoma sebaceum/facial angiofibroma (the typical skin rash which appears in many severely affected cases at least before adolescence) is considered diagnostic. In recent years it has been discovered that most patients with tuberous sclerosis presenting with major symptoms before age 2–5 years have autism or autistic features with severe hyperactivity (Hunt & Dennis, 1987; Gillberg, Gillberg & Ahlsén, 1994a). The triad of mental retardation, epilepsy and autism has since emerged as a clinical warning that the underlying cause might be tuberous sclerosis. It is of considerable interest that, long before Kanner described the condition of 'early infantile autism' (Kanner 1943), Critchley and Earl (1932) described its classic symptoms in a child with tuberous sclerosis.

Epilepsy is a very common feature of early symptomatic tuberous sclerosis. All kinds of seizures may occur, but it appears that, at least in childhood, infantile spasms and complex partial seizures may be particularly common (Hunt & Shepherd, 1993; Ahlsén et al., 1994). These types of seizures, in turn, are often associated with autistic and hyperactive symptomatology. However, some cases with seizures of these types do not develop autistic behaviour and a few individuals with autistic behaviour, in tuberous sclerosis have not shown seizure activity either clinically or according to EEG examination.

At least 40% of all children with tuberous sclerosis diagnosed before age 5 years have autism or autistic-like conditions (Hunt & Shepherd, 1993; Gillberg I.C. et al., 1994a). In the remaining cases, autistic features (including Asperger syndrome) and hyperactivity are common. Transient problems compatible with a diagnosis of elective mutism have also been described (Gillberg I.C. et al., 1994a). There is a very high rate of sleep problems in tuberous sclerosis regardless of whether the 'main' behavioural diagnosis is autism, autistic-like condition, autistic features or hyperkinetic disorder.

Children with autism in association with tuberous sclerosis are often severely aloof, exhibit a staring, empty gaze and generally have major behaviour problems (including uncontrollable hyperactivity) which can be extremely difficult to manage. Mental retardation is often severe. However, autism can appear in tuberous sclerosis even when mental retardation is not present.

The high prevalence of autism in tuberous sclerosis means that tuberous sclerosis is a common associated disorder in autism. It has been estimated that tuberous sclerosis accounts for 5–8% of all autism cases in the general population (Hunt & Shepherd, 1993; Gillberg, I.C. et al., 1994a).

The reason for the link between tuberous sclerosis and autism/hyperactivity remains obscure. In tuberous sclerosis there are often widespread brain problems. The brain areas around the ventricles are often affected already at an early stage. Changes here could account for the common co-occurrence of tuberous sclerosis, infantile spasms, complex partial seizures and autism. It appears that there may be two or more forms of tuberous sclerosis (possibly linked to, at least, chromosome 9 (Fryer et al., 1987) and chromosome 16 (Kandt et al., 1992) (possibly also chromosome 11 (Smith et al., 1988)). The possibility of a gene defect close to loci for enzymes which are important in dopamine metabolism and dopamine receptor function has led to increased interest in the hypothesis that underlying the connection between autism and tuberous sclerosis may be a genomic change involving both the 'pure' tuberous sclerosis gene and dopamine genes (which might be involved in the pathogenesis of autism).

Autism and hyperactivity in tuberous sclerosis are not invariably connected with epilepsy, even though the vast majority of those who

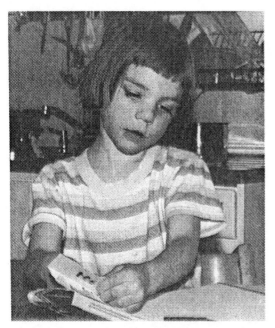

Fig. 10.9. Four-year-old girl with autism, epilepsy, near-normal intelligence and tuberous sclerosis.

have autism/hyperactivity also have early onset seizures (and mental retardation). Epilepsy, in turn, is often hard to treat. Unfortunately, both autism and hyperactivity, under such circumstances, may be difficult to treat (Fig. 10.9).

Work-up

Any child suspected of suffering from tuberous sclerosis (for instance, on the basis of the combination of severe mental retardation, epilepsy and autism) should receive a full work-up including an MRI *and* a CT (the risk that a child has tuberous sclerosis is minimal if both MRI and CT are normal (Gomez, 1988); MRI shows high signal areas in T2–weighted spin-echo sequences and usually depicts the cortical and subcortical tubers with considerable specificity and sometimes reveals cerebellar lesions as well; CT is better at demonstrating the calcified lesions), an EEG (to clarify the type of epilepsy associated with tuberous sclerosis), an ECG (which may demonstrate the typical syndrome of Wolff–Parkinson–White possibly mirroring

underlying cardiac rhabdomyomas) skin examination under Wood's light, renal ultrasound, and evaluations/assessments by a cardiologist and an ophthalmologist.

Treatment

There is no specific treatment for tuberous sclerosis, but many of the manifestations of the disorder are amenable to treatment. Anticonvulsants should be given for seizures, although it is essential to recognize that seizure control is often not possible to achieve. If infantile spasms are present in a very young child with tuberous sclerosis, corticotropin or steroid treatment may be indicated. Brain tumours may be removed surgically, and there is good evidence from individual case reports that such therapy can lead both to the reduction of seizures and autistic symptoms (Urebrant *et al.*, 1993). Facial angiofibromas should be treated with plastic surgery as indicated by disfigurement, psychological problems or (occasionally) obstruction of the eyes or nose.

Genetic counselling

Genetic counselling is an integral part of intervention in tuberous sclerosis. A thorough history and examination of both parents are essential. A cautiously positive attitude concerning recurrence risks may be appropriate when there is no abnormality (including skin problems) suggestive of tuberous sclerosis in the parents or the extended family, and there is no history of epilepsy, mental retardation, autism or kidney disease suggestive of tuberous sclerosis in the immediate family. However, it is often very difficult to determine with any degree of accuracy that tuberous sclerosis does not run in the family, and most genetic counselling in this field needs to be done with considerable reservations: it is not clear to what extent tuberous sclerosis is the result of spontaneous mutations. Nevertheless, if there are no clear signs of a hereditary variant, the following figures may be useful in clinical practice. Even if one of the parents does have tuberous sclerosis, the risk that the offspring may have the disorder is 1 in

2. Most people with tuberous sclerosis are likely to be mildly affected. It is likely that only about 1 in 5 has a severe form of tuberous sclerosis. Of these, not all have severely debilitating symptoms such as autism and severe mental retardation. Thus, it would be safe to say that, even when there is a family history, the risk that the next child will be affected by very severe symptoms of tuberous sclerosis is probably less than 1 in 10. In cases where there is no family history and no physical signs of the disorder in the parents, the risk will be considerably lower than this. However, it would be unethical to make too little of the risks of having a child with tuberous sclerosis faced by parents who have already had a child with the disorder.

Outcome

Outcome in tuberous sclerosis depends on the degree of involvement of the brain and other visceral organs. Clearly, even though there have been no specific empirical studies in the field, the majority of all individuals affected with tuberous sclerosis lead long productive lives. Only in cases with early symptomatic tuberous sclerosis (e.g. with severe symptoms of the disorder showing already under age 4 years) is outcome likely to be restricted. The risk that the individual might die from prolonged seizures or renal failure is considerable. The author has seen several such cases terminating in death under age 30 years.

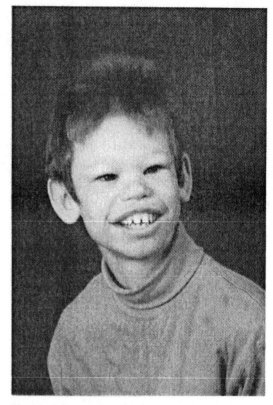

Fig. 10.10. Boy with Williams syndrome.

external and internal genitalia. Nevertheless, it seems that many marry and lead well-adjusted lives in adult age.

Turner syndrome (X0)

Girls with this syndrome have a low rate of psychiatric disorder. IQ is usually normal, but performance IQ shows a downward shift. Visuospatial skills are often particularly poor, and this tends to affect mathematics skills. An association of X0 syndrome with anorexia nervosa (particularly X0 mosaicism) has been suggested, but a recent systematic chromosome study including a population sample did not yield support for this (Råstam, Gillberg & Wahlström, 1991). After adolescence, these cases are of short stature and have infantile

Williams syndrome

A constellation of symptoms consisting of infancy feeding problems, transient hypercalcuria, a specific abnormality of the face, facial skeleton and skull (referred to as elfin face), unusual sacral creases and variable stenosis of big blood vessels (particularly the aorta) is now often referred to as Williams syndrome (see Fig. 10.10). It is important to make note of the fact that so-called specific facial abnormalities (including a long, smooth philtrum, full lips, wide mouth, full cheeks, long neck, short upturned nose and flat malar eminences plus, often, microcephalus) are not invariably so conspicuous as to arouse suspicion of the disorder, particularly in the younger age group. Quite often it takes until the age of 4–6 years before the full syndromal character of the disorder is recognized.

In the following, we shall be dealing mostly with the emotional and behavioural problems invariably encountered in this syndrome.

Prevalence

The prevalence of Williams syndrome is unknown. Estimates have ranged from 1 in 20000 to 1 in 50000, but no population studies have been published and hence no conclusions can be drawn. According to the author's experience it is almost definitely more common than suggested by previous writings. At least 100 childhood cases are currently known in Sweden. This is similar to Rett syndrome (girls) and tuberous sclerosis (boys and girls), conditions which, in regional Swedish population studies have been shown to have a prevalence of at least 1 in 10000 in school-age children. Clinical experience also suggests that many cases with Williams syndrome go unrecognized for many years, perhaps into adulthood.

Sex ratios

The male:female ratio is believed to be equal, but, in this respect too, conclusions have to be tentative.

Behavioural and physical phenotype

In studies by Udwin, Yule & Martin, (1987), Dilts, Morris & Leonard (1990) and Udwin (1990), a possibly rather specific behavioural phenotype has been identified in Williams syndrome. In the first two years of life there is often a considerable problem over feeding and the child may seem fussy and could have a sleep problem. Later on, overall development will be noted to be slow. Some children with Williams syndrome show autistic type behaviour up to about age 5 years (Reiss et al., 1985; Gillberg & Rasmussen, 1994). A few of these fulfil criteria for autistic disorder/infantile autism and have been identified in population screening samples of young children with autism (Gillberg et al., 1991). However, some of those with autistic behaviour in early childhood later show less social and communication impairments. A small number of cases with Williams syndrome continue to exhibit symptoms compatible with full diagnostic criteria for autistic disorder. Reiss et al. (1985) proposed that serotonergic dysfunction (as implicated by higher than normal blood serotonin levels in two cases) might be the underlying 'autismogenic' factor in Williams syndrome cases showing high degrees of autistic behaviour. However, in the four Williams syndrome-autism cases reported by Gillberg and Rasmussen (1994), CSF–5–HIAA was raised only in three. In contrast, there was evidence of dopamine dysfunction in all four.

By age 6 years, the typical Williams syndrome behavioural/emotional profile is usually present. The intellectual level is then usually in the mildly–moderately retarded range, but a few cases have severe–profound mental retardation and even fewer have low normal levels of intelligence. Superficial language capacities are usually relatively good, and the most typifying feature is the way the Williams syndrome person will approach other people to make superficial conversation in a seemingly happy-go-lucky manner. Questions may be asked in a highly repetitive manner, but with a social amiability such that most people will not, at first, feel pestered by the monotony of them. Underneath this superficial sociability is usually an anxious obsession and preoccupation with certain ideas and also an emotional problem bordering on a chronic anxiety state. A 'cocktail party syndrome' has been invoked, but only about one-third of school-age children with Williams syndrome show many of the salient features of cocktail party speech (Udwin & Yule, 1990).

Hyperacusis and over-reaction to vestibular stimuli have been noted by many authors (including Dilts et al., 1990).

There are generally rather severe problems with visual perception, but these may be effectively obscured by the talkativeness. Eventually, however, the learning problem becomes more and more obvious. Reading skills may be considerably less impaired than mathematics. It is of interest that facial recognition, in spite of the visual perception problems, seems to be unaffected in Williams syndrome (Bellugi *et al.*, 1990).

The following characteristic behavioural phenotype has been suggested by Dilts *et al.* (1990): (1) multiple developmental motor disabilities affecting strength, balance, coordination and motor planning, (2) sensory integration dysfunction (hyperreactivity to sound ('hyperacusis') and hypersensitivity to vestibular input), (3) hyperreactivity in the fields of emotion (perseverative worrying and sensitivity), activity (ADHD), sociability (impulsive social seeking, over-enthusiasm, over-talkativeness and problems making and keeping friends), (4) delayed expressive and receptive language skills with simultaneous age-appropriate grammar and articulation, (5) better reading than mathematics ability and (6) cognitive dysfunction ranging from learning disability to mental retardation.

Diagnosis

The diagnosis of Williams syndrome is clinical and depends on the demonstration of the peculiar 'elfin face' and a number of additional features, including supravalvular aortic stenosis and typical behavioural/emotional problems (see Table 10.7). With the recent demonstration of a mutant elastin gene on chromosome 7, it is possible that genetic molecular genetic diagnosis may soon become routine.

Work-up

The work-up in the young child with Williams syndrome needs to be slightly different than in adults presenting with a possible diagnosis.

Pathogenesis

Now that the mutant elastin gene has been located on chromosome 7 and linked to the

Table 10.7. *Behavioural and emotional problems in Williams syndrome (modified from Udwin, 1990)*.

Feature	% children	% adults
Solitary	84	71
Worried	71	88
Irritable	68	67
Over-friendly with strangers	64	73
Fearful	64	73
Temper tantrums	61	47
Disobedient	59	34
Eating difficulties	57	45
Obsessive/preoccupations	52	82
Incessant chatter	48	58
Destructive	48	25
Fights	48	20
Excessive use of social phrases/ clichés	46	51
Sleeping difficulties	46	40
Complains of aches and pains	39	67
Fussy	39	40
Fear of heights and uneven surfaces	25	33
Cannot manage money	–	94
Cannot settle	–	77
Restless	–	71

appearance of supravalvular aortic stenosis in Williams syndrome (Ewart *et al.*, 1993), it is possible that there may soon be a simple genetic test for all cases of Williams syndrome. However, at this point in time, the aetiology of Williams syndrome is still unknown. The syndrome has been described in several sets of concordant monozygotic twins (e.g. Murphy *et al.*, 1990), but so far not in dizygotic twins. This has been taken as supporting a genetic basis for the disorder. However, in the absence of studies on representative twin samples, and a definite genetic marker in the field, no conclusions are warranted.

Hypercalcaemia is a common, but probably not invariable, feature of the disorder in the first few years of life. It can often not be demonstrated later in childhood. It has been proposed to be the cause of many of the symptoms encountered in Williams syndrome (supraval-vular aortic stenosis or calcification of large vessels including aorta and pulmonary and renal arteries, facial abnormalities, etc.). Even if hypercalcaemia were present in all cases, it is unlikely that it is the cause or involved in the basic pathogenetic chain of events in Williams syndrome. Calciotonin deficiency is present in many cases and is probably responsible for or associated with the hypercalcaemia (Jones, 1990). A gene on chromosome 11 is alternatively processed to produce calciotonin and a 'calciotonin-gene-related peptide'. This peptide has established biological effects in the central nervous system, the cardiovascular system and the gastrointestinal system, all of which are implicated in most Williams syndrome cases. It has been hypothesized (Jones, 1990) that it is the possible shift from calciotonin to calciotonin-gene-related peptide production which accounts for the behavioural and physical phenotype characteristic of Williams syndrome, but, at present, this remains speculative.

Treatment

It is essential to provide parents with up-to-date information concerning the typical psychological problems shown by most, if not all, children with the syndrome. This will go a long way in alleviating feelings of guilt and concern that parents may have contributed to the development of a particular behavioural style. Sleep and anxiety problems may sometimes, at least for short periods of time, have to be dealt with by pharmacological treatment. One must take care not to over-use the benzodiazepines (which can cause aggressive behaviour and (rarely) addiction problems). A trial of clomipramine (10–75 mg in the under 12 year olds, 25–150 mg in the teenage period) is sometimes helpful. Educational measures of various kinds (including instructing the child/teenager that you cannot approach strangers in the street and immediately ask them a lot of questions) are often required. Placement in a classroom for the mentally retarded is often necessary. Whether this is done or not, it is essential to inform the teacher about all the behavioural/emotional

aspects of Williams syndrome. Usually, this is not done, even in cases where the teachers are informed in some detail about the physical characteristics of the child. Information to teachers about psychological matters related to Williams syndrome will often make life for the child, family and teacher much easier to cope with.

Outcome

Udwin's studies of adults with Williams syndrome have demonstrated that many of the behavioural and emotional problems persist throughout childhood and adolescence into adult life. The table outlines the frequency of various problems shown by children and adults with Williams syndrome (Table 10.7).

Wilson's disease

Wilson's disease is a genetic disorder, affecting the CNS and associated with liver cirrhosis. It is often referred to as hepatolenticular degeneration, and it is related to a derangement of copper metabolism. High levels of liver copper and grey matter accumulation of copper in the brain are usually found.

Prevalence

The prevalence of homozygous Wilson's disease is reported to be about 1 in 100 000 (Aicardi, 1992), but the epidemiology of the disorder has not been studied in enough depth to decide whether this is an accurate clinical guess or not.

Sex ratios

The sex ratio in Wilson's disease is reported to be equal.

Pathogenesis

Wilson disease is inherited as an autosomal recessive trait.

In the normal liver, copper is incorporated

into newly synthesized ceruloplasmin, a protein used for the transportation of copper to the rest of the body. More than 95% of copper is normally incorporated into ceruloplasmin, and the concentration of this protein in plasma is 300–400 mg/l. Plasma levels are elevated in pregnancy, liver cirrhosis and other disorders with high circulating oestrogen, malignant disease and hyperthyroidism. The vast majority of patients with Wilson disease have markedly lowered levels of plasma ceruloplasmin, but a minority do not. There is also a variant of familial ceruloplasmin deficiency, which is asymptomatic or presents only with retinal degeneration and blepharospasms (Miyajima et al., 1987).

It appears that a defect in the cells of the liver prevents the incorporation of copper into ceruloplasmin and this, in turn, results in the accumulation of copper in the liver, damage to hepatocytes and their mitochondria and peroxisomes. With time, copper leaks from the liver and is taken up by tissues, the brain in particular, with resulting secondary damage.

The liver shows focal necrosis and secondary cirrhosis. In the basal ganglia there is spongy degeneration, loss of neurons and large numbers of big astrocytes (Alzheimer type II glia). The frontal lobes are involved in a similar way, but other parts of the brain are relatively spared.

Copper is deposited in clumps close to the endothelial surface of the Descemet membrane, which is responsible for the Kayser–Fleischer ring.

The gene for Wilson disease has been mapped to chromosome 13.

Behavioural and physical phenotype

There are roughly three modes of clinical presentation of Wilson disease: (1) hepatic manifestations at age 3–5 years in one-third, (2) neurological manifestations after age 8–10 years in one-third and (3) a mixture of hepatic, cerebral and blood symptoms (including acute or intermittent haemolytic anemia) in the remaining third.

There is no specific behavioural phenotype

suggestive of Wilson disease. Facio-linguo-pharyngeal involvement, causing a mask-like appearance, dysarthria and dysphagia, is common in childhood and adolescent onset cases of type (2) and (3). Tremor may be Parkinsonian or flapping. The course is usually slowly progressive, but may be acute. In the late stages, muscular rigidity is pronounced and generalized, dyskinesias take on bizarre forms and the patient may be neurologically severely incapacitated.

Psychiatric symptoms are often the only, or most prominent feature of Wilson disease for many years (Medalia, Isaacs, Glaberman & Scheinberg, 1988). Schizophrenia-like disorders, autistic symptoms and the clinical picture of Asperger syndrome (unpublished, personal observations) may all be presenting features. Most patients (perhaps all) with psychiatric and neurological manifestations of the disease will turn out to have a Kayser–Fleischer ring. Alcoholism is believed to be a common indirect complication, due to the knowledge that alcohol decreases the tremors usually associated with Wilson disease.

Diagnosis

The diagnosis of Wilson disease is still based on clinical findings. The possibility of a diagnosis of Wilson disease must always be considered in child and adolescent neuropsychiatry. Any child or adolescent with mild, moderate or severe neuropsychiatric problems (including deterioration, social and academic dysfunction) should be examined with a view to excluding or diagnosing this, potentially treatable, disorder.

Work-up

The Kayser–Fleischer ring is probably always present in cases with neurological/psychiatric symptoms. It can often be seen with the naked eye, but slit-lamp examination may be required, which, among many other factors, argues for a high rate of referral of young neuropsychiatric patients to ophthalmologists. CT and MRI scans will reveal symmetrical areas of hypodensity in the thalamus and basal ganglia (Takano *et al.*, 1983; Lukes *et al.*, 1983) in about half of the cases with neurological symptoms. These abnormalities may decrease or disappear altogether after appropriate treatment. Serum ceruloplasmin is usually low (< 100 mg/l) as is serum copper (< 7.8 μmol/l corresponding to < 50 μg/dl). Low ceruloplasmin unaccompanied by any clinical abnormality may indicate a heterozygous state. Liver biopsy and determination of liver copper may be required to make a final diagnosis.

Treatment

D-penicillamine (0.5–0.75 g/day for children under 10 years, 1.0 g/day for older patients) is the treatment of choice in Wilson disease. It is given orally in divided doses. Pyridoxine (25 mg/day) should be added because of the antivitamin effect of penicillamine. Side effects are common (e.g. fever, nephrotic syndrome, pyridoxine deficiency, thrombocytopenia). Steroids may be needed to overcome these. Tetrahydromolybdate is a theoretically interesting drug which has shown some promising preliminary results (Brewer *et al.*, 1991).

Outcome

Approximately 50% of those with neurological/psychiatric manifestations become asymptomatic. Those with purely hepatic forms usually do very well after treatment. The subgroup with mixed problems have intermediate outcomes (Aicardi, 1992).

There is a group of (clinically, genetically or metabolically) related disorders with some features of Wilson disease but with a different or less pronounced disturbance in copper metabolism. The status of this group *vis à vis* 'pure' Wilson disease remains to be determined.

Other named or aetiologically distinct syndromes

Many other named syndromes can present with psychiatric problems or a combination of psychiatric problems, signs of involvement of internal organs such as the spleen and liver, and clear-cut neurological abnormality. In this group are included *Coffin–Lowry syndrome*, *Gaucher disease*, and *Salla disease* to mention but a few. It has not been established, or suggested, that these syndromes have a specific behavioural phenotype. Coffin–Lowry syndrome has been reported to be associated with a 'happy temperament' (Arena & Lubs, 1991), and also with autism (Bryson, Clark & Smith, 1988). Nevertheless, the study of the psychiatric symptoms that are common in these syndromes is only just beginning, and it is too early to conclude that they too might not constitute clearly delineated behavioural phenotype syndromes.

There are also a number of syndromes named after aetiology/pathogenetic factors rather than after their discoverers. Included in this group is non-ketotic hyperglycinaemia, acute intermittent porphyria and other inherited disorders of porphyrin metabolism and metachromatic leukodystrophy.

Non-ketotic hyperglycinaemia (Deutsch, Weizmann & Weizman, 1991), which, like some other metabolic disorders, may present with 'pure' neuropsychiatric problems such as attention deficits, motor control problems, language delay and mental retardation. The diagnosis is based on a finding of a CSF-to-plasma glycine ratio of > 0.03. Mitochondrial disease (including syndromes that give rise to high level of blood and CSF lactate) is also known to cause neuropsychiatric disorders. Dietary treatment may be appropriate in these syndromes.

Acute intermittent porphyria (Becker & Kramer, 1977) *and other inherited disorders of porphyrin metabolism* are rare in childhood. Occasionally, such disorders present with psychiatric symptoms, including schizophreniform psychosis. The author has examined one case of acute intermittent porphyria with classic autism, the symptoms of which were first precipitated by the administration of a drug. Exacerbations in the neuropsychiatric symptom profile occurred with changes in the metabolic state of this 6 year-old boy. Polyneuropathy can involve both the upper and lower limbs, and intermittent abdominal pains are reported to be as common as in adult patients. Seizure disorders may be more frequent in children than in adults (Houston *et al.*, 1977).

Metachromatic leukodystrophy (a rare inherited disorder) with childhood or adolescent onset seems to be strongly associated with psychosis comprising complex auditory hallucinations and bizarre delusions. In a review of 129 case reports of metachromatic leukodystrophy, 53% presented with psychosis, a considerably higher rate than in almost all other primary neurological disorders (Hyde, Ziegler & Weinberger, 1992).

It is likely that the next decade will witness important developments in this field.

References

Abel, E.L., Sokol, R.J. (1986). Fetal alcohol syndrome is now leading cause of mental retardation. *Lancet*, **ii**, 1222.

Ahlsén, G., Gillberg, I.C., Lindblom, R., Gillberg, C. (1994). Tuberous sclerosis in Western Sweden. A population study of cases with early childhood onset. *Archives of Neurology*, **51**, 76–81.

Aicardi, J. (Ed.) (1992). *Diseases of the Nervous System in Childhood. Clinics in Developmental Medicine, No. 115/118*. London: MacKeith Press.

Aicardi, J., Chevrie, J.J., Baraton, J. (1987). Agenesis of the corpus callosum. *In* Vinken, P.J., Bruyn, G.W.,Klawans, H.L. (Eds.). *Handbook of Clinical Neurology, Revised Series Vol. 6: Brain Malformation*. Amsterdam: North Holland.

Åkefeldt, A., Gillberg, C. (1991). Hypomelanosis of Ito in three cases with autism and autistic-like conditions. *Developmental Medicine and Child Neurology*, **33**, 737–43.

Åkefeldt, A., Gillberg, C., Larsson, C. (1991). Prader–Willi syndrome in a Swedish rural county: epidemiological aspects. *Developmental Medicine and Child Neurology*, **33**, 715–21.

Åkesson, H.0., Hagberg, B., Wahlström, J., Engerström, I.W. (1992). Rett syndrome: a search for gene sources. *American Journal of Medical Genetics*, **42**, 104–8.

Anderson, L.T., Ernst, M. (1994). Self-injury in Lesch–Nyhan disease. *Journal of Autism and Developmental Disorders*, **24**, 67–81.

Antonarakis, S.E. (1989). Diagnosis of genetic disorders at the DNA level. *New England Journal of Medicine*, **320**, 153–63.

Antonarakis, S.E., and the Down syndrome Collaborative Group. (1991). Parental origin of the extrachromosome in trisomy 21 as indicated by analysis of DNA polymorphisms. *New England Journal of Medicine*, **324**, 872–6.

Anvret, M., Wahlström, J., Skogsberg, P. & Hagberg, B. (1990). Segregation analysis of the X-chromosome in a family with Rett syndrome in two generations. *American Journal of Medical Genetics*, **37**, 31–5.

Arena, J.F., Lubs, H.A. (1991). Computerized approach to X-linked mental retardation syndromes. *American Journal of Medical Genetics*, **38**, 190–9.

Armstrong, D.D. (1992). The neuropathology of the Rett syndrome. *Brain and Development*, **14**, Suppl:S89–98.

Armstrong, D., Koppang, N. & Rider, J.A. (Eds.) (1982). *Ceroid-lipofuscinosis (Batten's Disease)*. Amsterdam: Elsevier.

Aronsson, M., Hagberg, B. (1993). Hur har det gått för de alkoholskadade barnen? *Läkartidningen*, **90**, 2214–19 (In Swedish.)

Aughton, D.J., Cassidy, S.B. (1990). Physical features of Prader–Willi syndrome in neonates: Comment in: *Am J Dis Child* 1992 Feb;146(2):151–2. *American Journal of Diseases in Childhood*, **144**, 1251–4.

Azen, C.G., Koch, R., Gross-Friedman, E., Berlow, S., Coldwell, J., Krause, W., Matalon, R., McCabe, E., O'Flynn, M., Peterson, R., *et al.* (1991). Intellectual development in 12–year-old children treated for phenylketonuria. *American Journal of Diseases of Children*, **145**, 35–9.

Baker, P., Piven, J., Schwartz, S., Patil, S. (1994). Duplication of chromosome 15q 11–13 in two individuals with autistic disorder. *Journal of Autism and Developmental Disorders*, **24**, 529–35.

Balassanian, N., Robbins, F.C. (1967). Mycoplasma pneumoniae infection in females. *New England Journal of Medicine*, **277**, 719–25.

Bauman, M. (1992). Neuroanatomical observations in autism. What's wrong with the brain? Paper given at the meeting on Prevention of Autism. Welshpool, November.

Bauman, M.L., Kemper, T.L. (1982). Morphologic and histoanatomic observations of the brain in untreated human phenylketonuria. *Acta Neuropathologica*, **58**, 55–63.

Bavinck, J.N.B., Weaver, D.D. (1986). Subclavian artery supply disruption sequence: hypothesis of a vascular etiology for Poland, Klippel–Feil and Möbius anomalies. *American Journal of Medical Genetics*, **23**, 903–18.

Becker, D.M., Kramer, S. (1977). The neurological manifestations of porphyria: a review. *Medicine*, **56**, 411–23.

Belfer, M.L., Krener, P.K., Miller, F.B. (1988). AIDS in children and adolescents. *Journal of the American Academy of Child and Adolescent Psychiatry*, **27**, 147–51.

Bellugi, L., Bihrle, A., Jernigan, T., Trauner, D., Doherty, S. (1990). Neuropsychological, neurological and neuroanatomical profile of Williams syndrome. *American Journal of Medical Genetics*, **Suppl. 6**, S115–25.

Berry, H.K., O'Grady, D.J., Perlmutter, L.J., Bofinger, M.K. (1979). Intellectual development and academic achievement of children treated early for phenylketonuria. *Developmental Medicine and Child Neurology*, **21**, 311–20.

Bhushan, V., Gupta, R.R., Weinreb, J., Kairam, R. (1989). Unusual brain MRI findings in a patient with hypomelanosis of Ito. *Pediatric Radiology*, **20**, 104–6.

Blennow, E., Bröndum-Nielsen, K., Telenius, H., Carter, N.P., Kristoffersson, U., Holmberg, E., Gillberg, C., Nordenskjöld, M. (1994). Characterization of 49 cases with extra structurally abnormal chromosomes by fluorescence *in situ* hybridization. *Submitted*,

Blum, A., André, M., Broullé, P., Husson, S., Leheup, B. (1990). Prenatal echographic diagnosis of corpus callosum agenesis: The Nancy experience 1982–1989. *Genetic Counseling*, **38**, 115–26.

Bray, P.F., Bale, J.F., Anderson, R.E., Kern, E.R. (1981). Progressive neurological disease associated with chronic cytomegalovirus infection. *Annals of Neurology*, **9**, 499–502.

Brewer, G.J., Dick, R.D., Yuzbasiyan-Gurkin, V., Tankanow, R., Young, A.B., Kluin, K.J. (1991). Initial therapy of patients with Wilson's disease with tetrathiomolybdate. *Archives of Neurology*, **48**, 42–7.

Bryson, S.E., Clark, B.S., Smith, I.M. (1988). First report of a Canadian epidemiological study of autistic syndromes. *Journal of Child Psychology and Psychiatry*, **29**, 433–45.

Buchanan, D.C., LaBarbera, D.J., Roelofs, R., Olsen, W. (1979). Reactions of families to children with Duchenne muscular dystrophy. *General Hospital Psychiatry*, **1**, 262.

Buckton, K.E., Spowart, G., Newton, M.S., Evans, H.J. (1985). Forty four probands with an additional 'marker' chromosome. *Human Genetics*, **69**, 353–70.

Budden, S. (1993). Medical and general management of RS girls. Medical World Congress on Rett Syndrome. Antwerp, Belgium, 8–10 October.

Bundey, S., Hardy, C., Vickers, S., Kilpatrick, M.W., Corbett, J.A. (1994). Duplication of the 15q 11–13 region in a patient with autism, epilepsy and ataxia. *Developmental Medicine and Child Neurology*, **36**, 736–72.

Buntinx, I.M., Willems, P.J., Mangelschots, K.J., Kennekam, R.C., Brouwer, O.F., Beuten, J., Dumon, J.E. (1991). Clinical evaluation of the Angelman syndrome in Belgium and the Netherlands. International NATO-supported Advanced Research Workshop on Prader–Willi Syndrome and Other Chromosome 15q Deletion Disorders. Norwijkerhout, the Netherlands.

Burd, L., Kerbeshian, J. (1989). Hyperlexia in Prader–Willi syndrome. *The Lancet*, **ii**, 983–4.

Butler, M.G., Allen, A., Haynes, J.L., Clark, S.J. (1990). Chromosome lesions which could be interpreted as 'fragile sites' on the distal end of Xq. *American Journal of Medical Genetics*, **37**, 250–3.

Bühler, E.M., Malik, N.J., Alkan, M. (1990). Another model for the inheritance of Rett syndrome. *American Journal of Medical Genetics*, **36**, 126–31.

Carr, J. (1970). Mental and motor development in young mongol children. *Journal of Mental Deficiency Research*, **14**, 205–20.

Carroll, J.E. (1985). Diagnosis and management of Duchenne muscular dystrophy. *Pediatric Research*, **6**, 195.

Castells, S., Chakrabarti, C., Winsberg, B.G., Hurwic, M., Perel, J.M., Nyhan, W.L. (1979). Effects of L-5-hydroxytryptophan on monoamine and amino acids turnover in the Lesch–Nyhan syndrome. *Journal of Autism and Developmental Disorders*, **9**, 95–103.

Cawthon, R.M., Weiss, R., Xu, G.F., Viskochil, D., Culver, M., Stevens, J., Robertson, M., Dunn, D., Gesteland, R., O'Connell, P., *et al.* (1990*b*). A major segment of the neurofibromatosis type 1 gene: cDNA sequence, genomic structure, and point mutations: published erratum appears in *Cell* 1990 Aug 10;62(3):following 608: *Cell*, **62**, 193–201.

Charnas, L. (1989). Seizures in the oculocerebrorenal syndrome of Lowe. *Neurology*, **39 (suppl)**, 216.

Charnas, R., Gahl, W.A. (1991). The oculocerebrorenal syndrome of Lowe. *Advances in Pediatrics*, **38**, 75–107.

Chess, S. (1977). Follow-up report on autism in

congenital rubella. *Journal of Autism and Childhood Schizophrenia*, **7**, 68–81.

Chess, S., Korn, S.J., Fernandez, P.B. (1971). *Psychiatric Disorders of Children with Congenital Rubella*. New York: Brunner/Mazel.

Chevrie, J.J., Aicardi, J. (1986). The Aicardi syndrome. *In* Pedley, T.A.,Meldrum, B.S. (Eds.). *Recent Advances in Epilepsy*. Edinburgh: Churchill Livingstone.

Clarke, A. (1993). Metabolic and molecular genetic studies on familial cases of RS. Medical World Congress on Rett Syndrome. Antwerp, Belgium 7–10 October.

Clarke, D.J., Bundey, S. (1990). Very early onset Huntington's disease: genetic mechanism and risk to siblings. *Clinical Genetics*, **38**, 180–6.

Clarke, D.J., Waters, J., Corbett, J.A. (1989). Adults with Prader–Willi syndrome: Abnormalities of sleep and behaviour. *Journal of the Royal Society of Medicine*, **82**, 21–4.

Clarren, S.K. (1979). Neural tube defects and fetal alcohol syndrome (letter). *Journal of Pediatrics*, **95**, 328.

Clarren, S.K., Smith, D.W. (1978). The fetal alcohol syndrome. *New England Journal of Medicine*, **298**, 1063–7.

Clayton-Smith, J. (1991). Angelman syndrome in the adolescent and young adult. International NATO-supported Advanced Research Workshop on Prader–Willi Syndrome and Other Chromosome 15q Deletion Disorders. Nordwijkerhout, the Netherlands.

Coleman, M. (1989). Autism: Non-drug biological treatments. *In* Gillberg, C. (Ed.) *Diagnosis and Treatment of Autism*. New York: Plenum Press.

Connor, J.M. (1990). Epidemiology and genetic approaches in tuberous sclerosis. *In* Ishibashi, Y.,Hori, Y. (Eds.). *Tuberous Sclerosis and Neurofibromatosis: Epidemiology, Pathophysiology, Biology and Management*. Amsterdam: Elsevier Science Publishers.

Cooper, L.Z., Krugman, S. (1967). Clinical manifestations of postnatal and congenital rubella. *Archives of Ophthalmology*, **77**, 434–9.

Costeff, H., Holm, V.A., Ruvalcaba, R., Shaver, J. (1990). Growth hormone secretion in Prader–Willi syndrome. *Acta Paediatrica Scandinavica*, **79**, 1059–62.

Courchesne, E., Yeung-Courchesne, R., Press, G.A., Hesselink, J.R., Jernigan, T.L. (1988). Hypoplasia of cerebellar vermal lobules VI and VII in autism. *New England Journal of Medicine*, **318**, 1349–54.

Crandall, B.F., Carrel, R.E., Sparkes, R.S. (1972).

Chromosome findings in 700 children referred to a psychiatric clinic. *Journal of Pediatrcs*, **80**, 62–8.

Cremers, C.W., van der Burgt, C.J. (1992). Hearing loss in Noonan syndrome. *International Journal of Pediatrics and Otorhinolaryngology*, **23**, 81–4.

Critchley, M., Earl, C.J.C. (1932). Tuberose sclerose and allied conditions. *Brain*, **55**, 311–46.

Crowe, F.W., Schull, W.J., Neil, J.W. (1956). *Pathological and Genetic Study of Multiple Neurofibromatosis*. Springfield, Ill: Thomas.

Dabbagh, O., Swaiman, K.F. (1988). Cockayne syndrome: MRI correlates of hypomyelination. *Pediatric Neurology*, **4**, 113–6.

Dalton, A.J., Crapper-McLachlan, D.R. (1986). Clinical expression of Alzheimer's disease in Down's syndrome. *Psychiatric Clinics of North America*, **9**, 659–70.

Day, N.L., Richardson, G., Robles, N., Sambamoorthy, J., Taylor, P., Scher, M., Stoffer, D., Jaspese, D., Cornelius, M. (1990). Effect of prenatal alcohol exposure on growth and morphology of offspring at 8 months of age. *Pediatrics*, **85**, 748–52.

DeLong, G.R., Beau, S.C., Brown, F.R. (1981). Acquired reversible autistic syndrome in acute encephalopathic illness in children. *Archives of Neurology*, **38**, 191–4.

Deutsch, S.I., Weizman, A., Weizman, R. (1991). *Application of Basic Neuroscience to Child Psychiatry*. New York and London: Plenum Medical Book Company.

Dhondt, J.L., Farriaux, J.P. (1987). Atypical cases of phenylketonuria. *European Journal of Pediatrics*, **146 (Suppl.)**, A38–43.

Dilts, C.V., Morris, C.A., Leonard, C.O. (1990). Hypothesis for development of a behavioral phenotype in Williams syndrome. *American Journal of Medical Genetics*, **6**, 126–31.

Dodge, P.R., Holmes, S.J., Sotos, J.F. (1983). Cerebral gigantism. *Developmental Medicine and Child Neurology*, **25**, 248–52.

Dupont, A., Vaeth, M., Videbech, P. (1986). Mortality and life expectancy of Down's syndrome in Denmark. *Journal of Mental Deficiency Research*, **30**, 111–20.

Ewart, A., Morris, C.A., Atkinson, D., Jin, W., Sternes, K., Spallone, P., Stock, A.D., Leppert, M., Keating, M.T. (1993). Hemizygosity at the elastin locus in a developmental disorder, Williams Syndrome. *Nature Genetics*, **5**, 11–6.

Fields, D.L. & Gibson, D. (1971). Forecasting mental growth for at-home mongols (Down's syndrome). *Journal of Mental Deficiency Research*, **15**, 163–8.

Fischler, K., Koch, R. & Donnell, G.N. (1976). Comparison of mental development in individuals with mosaic and trisomy 21 Down's syndrome. *Pediatrics*, **58**, 744–8.

Fisher, D.A. (1975). Thyroid function in the fetus. *In* Fisher, D.A.,Burrow, G.N. (Eds.). *Perinatal Thyroid Physiology and Disease.* New York: Raven Press.

Fisher, J.A., Burn, J., Alexander, F.N., Gardner-Medwin, D. (1987). Angelman (happy puppet) syndrome in a girl and her brother. *Journal of Medical Genetics*, **24**, 294–8.

Fitzpatrick, Barry, G., Garvey, C. (1986). Psychiatric disorder among boys with Duchenne muscular dystrophy. *Developmental Medicine and Child Neurology*, **28**, 589.

Fleury, P., De Groot, W.P., Delleman, J.W., Verbeeten, B., Franken-Molen-Witziezwicz, I.M. (1980). Tuberous sclerosis: the incidence of sporadic cases versus familial cases. *Brain and Development*, **2**, 107–17.

Forssman, H., Wahlström, J., Wallin, L., Åkesson, H.-O. (1975). Males with double Y-chromosomes. Reports from the Psychiatric Research Centre, St Jörgen's Hospital, Göteborg, Sweden.

Friedman, E. (1969). The autistic syndrome and phenylketonuria. *Schizophrenia*, **1**, 249–61.

Fryer, A.E., Chalmers, A., Connor, J.M., Fraser, I., Povey, S., Yates, A.D., Yates, J.R.W., Osborne, J.P. (1987). Evidence that the gene for tuberous sclerosis is on chromosome 9. *Lancet*, **i**, 659–61.

Fryns, J.P., Kleczkowska, A., Kubie:n, E., Van den Berghe, H. (1984). Cytogenetic findings in moderate and severe mental retardation. A study of an institutionalized population of 1991 patients. *Acta Paediatrica Scandinavica Suppl*, **313**, 1–23.

Fölling, A. (1934). Über Ausschiedung von Phenylbenztraubensaure in den Haarn als Stoffwechselanomalie in Verbinduning mit Imbessillität. *Hoppe Seüöers Zeitschrift für Physiologie und Chemie*, **227**, 169.

Garcia-Erro, M.I., Correale, J., Arberas, C., Sanz, O.P., Muchnik, S., Sica, R.E.P. (1989). Familial congenital facial diplegia: electrophysiologic and genetic studies. *Pediatric Neurology*, **5**, 262–4.

Garralda, M.E. (1992). Severe chronic fatigue syndrome in childhood: a discussion of psychopathological mechanisms. *European Child & Adolescent Psychiatry*, **1**, 111–18.

Garralda, M.E., Bailey, D. (1990). Paediatrician identification of psychological factors associated with general paediatric consultations. *Journal of Psychosomatic Research*, **34**, 303–12.

Ghaziuddin, M., Tsai, L.Y., Eilers, L., Ghaziuddin, N. (1992). Brief report: autism and herpes simplex encephalitis. *Journal of Autism and Developmental Disorders*, **22**, 107–13.

Ghaziuddin, M., Sheldon, S., Tsai, L.Y., Alessi, N. (1993). Abnormalities of chromosome 18 in a girl with mental retardation and autistic disorder. *Journal of Intellectual Disability Research*, **37**, 313–17.

Gillberg, C. (1980). Schizophreniform psychosis in a case of mycoplasma pneumoniae encephalitis. *Journal of Autism and Developmental Disorders*, **10**, 153–8.

Gillberg, C. (1986). Brief report: Onset at age 14 of a typical autistic syndrome. A case report of a girl with herpes simplex encephalitis. *Journal of Autism and Developmental Disorders*, **16**, 369–75.

Gillberg, C. (1987). Kleine–Levin syndrome: unrecognized diagnosis in adolescent psychiatry. *Journal of the American Academy of Child and Adolescent Psychiatry*, **26**, 793–4.

Gillberg, C. (1989). The borderland of autism and Rett syndrome: five case histories to highlight diagnostic difficulties. *Journal of Autism and Developmental Disorders*, **19**, 545–59.

Gillberg, C. (1992). Subgroups in autism: are there behavioural phenotypes typical of underlying medical conditions? *Journal of Intellectual Disability Research*, **36**, 201–4.

Gillberg, C., Coleman, M. (1992). *The Biology of the Autistic Syndromes.* 2nd edition. London, New York: MacKeith Press, Cambridge University Press.

Gillberg, C., Forsell, C. (1984). Childhood psychosis and neurofibromatosis – more than a coincidence? *Journal of Autism and Developmental Disorders*, **14**, 1–8.

Gillberg, C., Coleman, M. (1994). Autism and possibly related medical disorders. A review of the pertinent literature. *Journal of Child Psychology and Psychiatry*, submitted.

Gillberg, C., Rasmussen, P. (1994). Four case histories and a literature review of Williams syndrome and autistic behavior. *Journal of Autism and Developmental Disorders*, **24**, 381–93.

Gillberg, C., Steffenburg, S. (1987). Outcome and prognostic factors in infantile autism and similar conditions: a population-based study of 46 cases followed through puberty. *Journal of Autism and Developmental Disorders*, **17**, 273–87.

Gillberg, C., Steffenburg, S. (1989). Autistic behaviour in Moebius syndrome. *Acta Paediatrica Scandinavica*, **78**, 314–16.

Gillberg, C., Wahlström, J. (1985). Chromosome abnormalities in infantile autism and other childhood psychoses: a population study of 66 cases. *Developmental Medicine and Child Neurology*, **27**, 293–304.

Gillberg, C., Persson, E., Grufman , M., Themnér, U. (1986*a*). Psychiatric disorders in mildly and severely mentally retarded urban children and adolescents: epidemiological aspects. *British Journal of Psychiatry*, **149**, 68–74.

Gillberg, C., Wahlström, J., Johansson, R., Törnblom, M., Albertsson-Wikland, K. (1986*b*). Folic acid as an adjunct in the treatment of children with the autism fragile-X syndrome (AFRAX). *Developmental Medicine and Child Neurology*, **28**, 624–7.

Gillberg, C., Ehlers, S., Wahlstrom, J. (1990). The syndromes described by Kanner and Rett-Hagberg: overlap in an extended family. *Developmental Medicine and Child Neurology*, **32**, 258–61.

Gillberg, C., Steffenburg, S., Wahlström, J., Gillberg, I.C., Sjöstedt, A., Martinsson, T., Liedgren, S., Eeg-Olofsson, O. (1991). Autism associated with marker chromosome. *Journal of the American Academy of Child and Adolescent Psychiatry*, **30**, 489–94.

Gillberg, I.C. (1991). Autistic syndrome with onset at age 31 years. Herpes encephalitis as one possible model for childhood autism. *Developmental Medicine and Child Neurology*, **33**, 920–4.

Gillberg, I.C., Gillberg, C., Kopp, S. (1992). Hypothyroidism and autism spectrum disorders. *Journal of Child Psychology and Psychiatry*, **33**, 531–42.

Gillberg, I.C., Gillberg, C., Ahlsén, G. (1994*a*). Autistic behaviour and attention deficits in tuberous sclerosis. A population-based study. *Developmental Medicine and Child Neurology*, **36**, 50–6.

Gillberg, I.C., Råstam, M., Gillberg, C. (1997). Anorexia nervosa 6 years after onset. Part I. Personality disorders. *Comprehensive Psychiatry*, In press.

Glesby, M.J., Pyeritz, R.E. (1989). Association of mitral valve prolapse and systemic abnormalities of connective tissue. A phenotypic continuum: see comments: Comment in: *JAMA* 1989. Dec 8;262(22):3132. *JAMA*, **262**, 523–8.

Glover, M.T., Brett, E.M., Athreton, D.J. (1989). Hypomelanosis of Ito: spectrum of the disease. *Journal of Pediatrics*, **115**, 75–80.

Gomez, M.R. (1988). *Tuberous Sclerosis*. New York: Raven Press.

Gordon, C.T., Krasnewich, D., White B., Lenane, M., Rapoport, J.L. (1994). Brief report: translocation involving chromosomes 1 and 7 in childhood-onset schizophrenia. *Journal of Autism and Developmental Disorders*, **24**, 537–45.

Goutières, F., Aicardi, J. (1987). New experience with Rett syndrome in France: the problem of atypical cases. *Brain and Development*, **9**, 502–5.

Govaert, P., Vanhaesebrouck, P., De Praeter, C., Fränkel, U., Leroy, J. (1989). Moebius sequence and prenatal brainstem ischemia. *Pediatrics*, **84**, 570–3.

Graham, J.M., Hanson, J.W., Darby, A.L., Barr, H.M., Streissguth, A.P. (1988). Independent dysmorphology evaluations at birth and 4 years of age for children exposed to varying amounts of alcohol *in utero*. *Pediatrics*, **81**, 772–8.

Griebel, V., Krägeloh-Mann, I., Michaelis, R. (1989). Hypomelanosis of Ito – report of four cases and survey of the literature. *Neuropediatrics*, **20**, 234–7.

Gualtieri, C.T. (1989). The differential diagnosis of self-injurious behavior in mentally retarded people. *Psychopharmacological Bulletin*, **25**, 358–63.

Gudmundsson, K.R. (1969). Prevalence and occurrence of some rare neurological dieases in Iceland. *Acta Neurologica Scandinavica*, **45**, 114–18.

Güttler, F., Lou, H. (1990). Phenylketonuria and hyperphenylalaninemia. *In* Fernandes, J., Saudubray, J.M.,Tada, K. (Eds.). *Inborn Metabolic Diseases, Diagnosis and Treatment*. Berlin: Springer Verlag.

Hagberg, B. (1989). Rett syndrome: clinical pecularities, diagnostic approach and possible cause. *Pediatric Neurology*, **5**, 75–83.

Hagberg, B. (1992). The Rett syndrome: an introductory overview 1990. *Brain and Development*, **Suppl**, S5–8.

Hagberg, B. (Ed.) (1993). *Rett Syndrome – Clinical & Biological Aspects*. London: Mac Keith Press.

Hagberg, B., Gillberg, C. (1993). Rett variants – Rettoid phenotypes. *In* Hagberg, B. (Ed.) *Rett Syndrome – Clinical & Biological Aspects*. London: Mac Keith Press.

Hagberg, B., Rasmussen, P. (1986). 'Forme fruste' of Rett syndrome – a case report. *American Journal of Medical Genetics*, **24: suppl. 1**, 175–81.

Hagberg, B., Hagberg, G., Lewerth, A., Lindberg, U. (1981). Mild mental retardation in Swedish school children. I. Prevalence. *Acta Paediatrica Scandinavia*, **70**, 441–4.

Hagberg, B., Goutiéres, F., Hanefeld, R., Rett, A., Wilson, J. (1985). Rett syndrome: criteria for excursion and inclusion. *Brain and Development*, **7**, 372–3.

Hagerman, R.J. (1989). Chromosomes, genes and autism. *In* Gillberg, C. (Ed.) *Diagnosis and Treatment of Autism*. New York: Plenum Press.

Hagerman, R.J., Murphy, M.A., Wittenberger, M.D. (1988). A controlled trial of stimulant medication in children with the fragile X syndrome. *American Journal of Medical Genetics*, **30**, 377–92.

Hagerman, R.J., Amiri, K., Cronister, A. (1991). Fragile X checklist. *American Journal of Medical Genetics*, **38**, 283–7.

Hamano, S.I., Yagishita, S., Kawakami, M., Ito, F., Maekawa, K. (1989). Aicardi syndrome: postmortem findings. *Pediatric Neurology*, **5**, 259–61.

Hanshaw, J.B. (1976). Cytomegalovirus. *In* Remington, J.S.,Klein, J.O. (Eds.). *Infectious Diseases of the Fetus and Newborn Infant*. Philadelphia: W.B. Saunders.

Hanson, P.A., Rowland, L.P. (1971). Möbius syndrome and facioscapulohumeral muscular dystrophy. *Archives of Neurology*, **34**, 31–9.

Hecht, F. (1987). Advances in medical genetics: Huntington disease. *Pediatric Review*, **9**, 13–14.

Heller, R.H. (1965). The Turner phenotype in the male. *Journal of Pediatrics*, **66**, 48–63.

Herbst, D.S., Miller, J.R. (1980). Nonspecific X-linked mental retardation II: the frequency in British Columbia. *American Journal of Medical Genetics*, **7**, 461–9.

Herman, K.L., Salman, K., Rose, L.I. (1991). White forelock in Marfan's syndrome: an unusual association, with review of the literature. *Cutis*, **48**, 82–4.

Heyerdahl, S., Kase, B.F., Lie, S.O. (1991). Intellectual development in children with congenital hypothyroidism in relation to recommended thyroxine treatment. *Journal of Pediatrics*, **118**, 850–7.

Hodapp, R.M., Dykens, E.M., Hagerman, R.J., Schreiner, R., Leckman, J.F. (1990). Developmental implications of changing trajectories of IQ in males with fragile X syndrome. *Journal of the American Academy of Child and Adolescent Psychiatry*, **29**, 214–19.

Hoffman, E.P., Brown, R.H., Kunkel, L.M. (1987). Dystrophin: the protein product of the Duchenne muscular dystrophy locus. *Cell*, **51**, 919.

Holm, V.A., Cassidy, S.B., Butler, M.G., Hanchett, J.M., Greenswag, L.R., Whitman, B.Y.,

Greenberg, F. (1993). Prader–Willi syndrome: consensus diagnostic criteria. *Pediatrics*, **91**, 398–402.

Holroyd, S., Reiss, A.L., Bryan, R.N. (1991). Autistic features in Joubert syndrome: A genetic disorder with agenesis of the cerebellar vermis. *Biological Psychiatry*, **29**, 287–94.

Hooft, C., Van Nevel, C., De Schaepdryver, A.F. (1968). Hyperuricosuric encephalopathy without hyperuricaemia. *Archives of Diseases in Childhood*, **43**, 734–7.

Houston, A.B., Brodie, M.J., Moore, M.R., Stephenson, J.B.P. (1977). Hereditary coproporhyria and epilepsy. *Archives of Disease in Childhood*, **52**, 646–50.

Hultén, M., Armstrong, S., Challinor, P., Gould, G., Hardy, G., Leedham, P., Lee, T., McKeown, C. (1991). Genomic imprinting in an Angelman and Prader–Willi translocation family. *The Lancet*, **338**, 638–9.

Hunt, A. (1983). Tuberous sclerosis: a survey of 97 cases. *Developmental Medicine and Child Neurology*, **25**, 346–57.

Hunt, A., Dennis, J. (1987). Psychiatric disorder among children with tuberous sclerosis. *Developmental Medicine and Child Neurology*, **29**, 190–8.

Hunt, A., Lindenbaum, R.H. (1984). Tuberous sclerosis: A new estimate of prevalence within the Oxford region. *Journal of Medical Genetics*, **21**, 272–7.

Hunt, A., Shepherd, C. (1993). A prevalence study of autism in tuberous sclerosis. *Journal of Autism and Developmental Disorders*, **23**, 323–39.

Huson, S.M., Thrush, D.C. (1985). Central neurofibromatosis. *Quarterly Journal of Medicine*, **55**, 213–24.

Hyde, T.M., Ziegler, J.C., Weinberger, D.R. (1992). Psychiatric disturbances in metachromatic leukodystrophy. Insights into the neurobiology of psychosis: Comment in: *Arch Neurol* 1993 Feb;50(2):131. *Archives of Neurology*, **49**, 401–6.

Hynd, G.W., Semrud-Clikeman, M., Lorys, A.R., Novey, E.S., Eiopulos, D., Lyytinen, H. (1991). Corpus calossum morphology in attention deficit-hyperactivity disorder: morphometric analysis of MRI. *Journal of Learning Disabilities*, **27**, 141–6.

Ilicki, A., Larsson, A. (1988). Psychomotor development of children with congenital hypothyroidism diagnosed by neonatal screening. *Acta Paediatrica Scandinavica*, **77**, 142–7.

Ilicki, A., Larsson, A. (1991). Screening for congenital hypothyroidism results in early treatment and good psychomotor development.

Läkartidingen, **88**, 2062–4 (in Swedish).

Institute of Medicine, National Academy of Sciences (1986). *Confronting AIDS: Directions for Public Health, Health Care, and Research.* Washington: National Academy Press.

Ioffe, S., Chernick, V. (1988). Development of the EEG between 30 and 40 weeks gestation in normal and alcohol-exposed infants. *Developmental Medicine and Child Neurology*, **30**, 797–807.

Iqbal, K., Wisniewski, H.M. (1983). Neurofibrillay tangles. *In* Reisberg, B. (Ed). *Alzheimer's Disease.* New York: Free Press.

Jeeves, M.A., Temple, C.M. (1987). A further study of language function in callosal agenesis. *Brain and Language*, **32**, 325–35.

Jellinger, K., Gross, N., Kaltenbäck, E., Grisold, W. (1981). Holoprosencephaly and agenesis corpus callosum. Frequency of associated malformations. *Acta Neuropathologica*, **55**, 1–10.

Jenssen Hagerman, R.J. & Cronister Silverman, A. (1991). *Fragile X Syndrome. Diagnosis, Treatment, and Research.* Baltimore and London: The Johns Hopkins University Press.

Jeret, J.S., Serur, D., Wisniewski, K., Fish, C. (1985–1986). Frequency of agenesis of the corpus callosum in the developmentally disabled population as determined by computerized tomography. *Pediatric Neuroscience*, **12**, 101–3.

Jeret, J.S., Serur, D., Wisniewski, K., Fish, C., Lubin, R. (1987). Clinicopathological findings associated with agenesis of the corpus callosum. *Brain and Development*, **9**, 225–64.

Jernigan, T., Bellugi, U., Hesselink, J. (1989). Structural differences on magnetic resonance imaging between Williams and Down syndrome. *Neurology*, **39**, 277.

Jervis, G.A. (1953). Phenylpyruvic oligiphrenia deficiency of phenylalanine-oxidizing system. *Proceedings of the Society for Expereimental Biology and Medicine*, **82**, 514–15.

Jones, H.W., Turner, H.H., Ferguson-Smith, M.A. (1966). Turner's syndrome and phenotype. *Lancet*, **i**, 1155.

Jones, K., Smith, D.W., Ulleland, C., Streissguth, A.P. (1973). Pattern of malformations in offspring of chronic alcoholic mothers. *Lancet*, **i**, 1267–71.

Jones, K.L. (1990). Williams syndrome: an historical perspective of its evolution, natural history and etiology. *American Journal of Medical Genetic*, **Suppl. 6**, S89–96.

Joubert, M., Eisenring, J.J., Robb, J.P., Andermann, F. (1969). Familial agenesis of the cerebellar vermis. A syndrome of episodic hypernea, abnormal eye movements, ataxia and retardation. *Neurology*, **19**, 813–25.

Kandt, R.S., Haines, J.L., Smith, M., Northup, H., Gardner, R.J.M., Short, M.P., Dumars, K., Roach, E.S., Steingold, S., Wall, S., Blanton, S.H., Flodman, P., Kwiatkowski, D.J., Jewell, J.L., Roses, A.D., Pericak-Vance, M.A. (1992). Linkage of an important gene locus for tuberous sclerosis to a chromosome 16 marker for polycystic kidney disease. *Nature Genetics*, **2**, 37–41.

Kanner, L. (1943). Autistic disturbances of affective contact. *Nervous Child*, **2**, 217–50.

Kaplan, M.S., Opitz, J.M., Gosset, F.R. (1968). Noonan's syndrome. A case with elevated serum alkaline phosphatase levels and malignant schwannoma of the left forearm. *American Journal of Diseases in Childhood*, **116**, 359–66.

Kerr, A.M., Montague, J., Stephenson, J.B. (1987). The hands, and the mind, pre- and post-regression, in Rett syndrome. *Brain and Development*, **9**, 487–90.

Kerr, A. (1993). (8–10 October) The first five years in Rett syndrome. Paper given at the World Congress on Rett Syndrome. Antwerp, Belgium.

Klein, A.H., Meltzer, S., Kenny, F.M. (1972). Improved prognosis in congenital hypothyroidism treated before three months. *Journal of Pediatrics*, **81**, 912–15.

Klingensmith, W.C., Cioffi-Ragan, D.T. (1986). Schizencephaly: diagnosis and progression in utero. *Radiology*, **159**, 617–18.

Komoto, J., Udsui, S., Otsuki, S., Terao, A. (1984). Infantile autism and Duchenne muscular dystrophy. *Journal of Autism and Developmental Disorders*, **14**, 191–5.

Kristiansson, B., Andersson, M., Tonnby, B., Hagberg, B. (1989). Disialotransferrin developmental deficiency syndrome. *Archives of Disease in Childhood*, **64**, 71–6.

Krivit, W., Good, R.A. (1957). Simultaneous occurrence of mongolism and leukemia. *American Journal of Diseases of Children*, **94**, 289.

Lai, F., Williams, R.S. (1989). A prospective study of Alzheimer disease in Down syndrome. *Archives of Neurology*, **46**, 849–53.

Lamache, M.A. (1967). Communications: Réflections sur la déscendance des alcooliques. *Bull Acad Nat Médicine*, **151**, 517–21.

Landgren, M., Gillberg, C., Strömland, K. (1992). Goldenhar syndrome and autistic behaviour. *Developmental Medicine and Child Neurology*, **34**, 999–1005.

Leech, R.W., Brumback, R.A., Miller, R.H.,

Otsuka, F., Tarone, R.E., Robbins, J.H. (1985). Cockayne syndrome: clinicopathologic and tissue culture studies of affected siblings. *Journal of Neuropathology and Experimental Neurology*, **44**, 507–19.

Lehman, A.R., Francis, A.J., Giannelli, F. (1985). Prenatal diagnosis of Cockayne's syndrome. *Lancet*, **i**, 486–8.

Lemoine, P., Harousseau, H., Borteyry, J. (1968). Les enfants de parents alcooliques: anomalies observées. *Ouest Médicale*, **25**, 476–82.

Lesch, M., Nyhan, W.L. (1964). A familial disorder of uric acid metabolism and central nervous system function. *American Journal of Medicine*, **36**, 561–70.

Leslie, S.A. (1988). Diagnosis and treatment of hysterical conversion reactions. *Archives of Disease in Childhood*, **63**, 506–11.

Lewis, M. (Ed.) (1991). *Child and Adolescent Psychiatry. A Comprehensive Textbook*. Baltimore, Maryland: Williams & Wilkins.

Levy, H.L., Waisbren, S.E. (1983). Effects of untreated maternal phenylketonuria and hyperphenylalaninemia on the fetus. *New England Journal of Medicine*, **309**, 1269–74.

Lin, M.Y., Wang, P.J., Lin, L.H., Shen, Y.Z. (1991). The Rett and Rett-like syndromes: a broad concept. *Brain and Development*, **13**, 228–31.

Linden, M.G., Bender, G.G., Harmon, R.J., Mrazek, D.A., Robinson, A. (1988). 47XXX: what is the prognosis? *Pediatrics*, **82**, 619–30.

Lishman, W.A. (1978). *Organic Psychiatry. The Psychological Consequences of Cerebral Disorder*. Oxford: Blackwell Scientific Publications.

Lott, I.T. (1982). Down's syndrome, aging, and Alzheimer's disease: a clinical review. *Annals of the New York Academy of Sciences*, **396**, 15–27.

Lowe Syndrome Association (1989). *Lowe Syndrome Association Comprehensive Survey: Preliminary results on Behavior*. West Lafayette, Indiana: The Association.

Lowe, T.L., Tanaka, K., Seashore, M.R., Young, J.G., Cohen, D.J. (1980). Detection of phenylketonuria in autistic and psychotic children. *Journal of the American Medical Association*, **20**, 104–11.

Lubs, M.L., Bauer, M.S., Formas, M.E., Djokic, B. (1991). Lisch nodules in neurofibromatosis type q. *New England Journal of Medicine*, **324**, 1264–6.

Lukes, S.A., Aminoff, M.J., Crooks, L., Kaufman, L., Mills, C., Newton, T. (1983). Nuclear magnetic resonance imaging in movement disorders. *Annals of Neurology*, **13**, 690–1.

Lyon-Bolt, J.M. (1970). Huntington's chorea in the West of Scotland. *British Journal of Psychiatry*, **116**, 259–70.

McFaul, R., Dorner, S., Brett, E.M., Grant, D.B. (1978). Neurological abnormalities in patients treated for hypothyroidism from early life. *Archives of Disease in Childhood*, **53**, 611–19.

McKusick, V.A. (1972). *Heritable Disorders of Connective Tissue*. Saint Louis: C.V. Mosby.

McKusick, V.A. (1988a). The morbid anatomy of the human genome: a review of gene mapping in clinical medicine. 4. *Medicine (Baltimore)*, **67**, 1–19.

McKusick, V.A. (1988b). The new genetics and clinical medicine: a summing up. *Hosp Pract*, **23**, 177–183, 186, 191.

McKusick, V.A. (1988c). *Mendelian Inheritance in Man. Catalogs of Autosomal Dominant, Autosomal Recessive and X-linked Phenotypes*. Baltimore: Johns Hopkins Press.

Maraschio, P., Zuffardi, O., Bernardi, F., Bozzola, M., De Paoli, C., Fonatsch, C., Flatz, S.D., Ghersini, L., Gimelli, G., Loi, M., Lorini, R., Peretti, D., Poloni, L., Tonetti, D., Vanni, R., Zamboni, G. (1981). Preferential maternal derivation in inv dup(15): analysis of eight new cases. *Human Genetics*, **57**, 345–50.

Marin Padilla, M. (1976). Pyramidal cell abnormalities in the motor cortex of a child with Down's syndrome. A Golgi study. *Journal of Comparative Neurology*, **167**, 63–81.

Marotta, R., Perry, S. (1989). Early neuropsychological dysfunction caused by human immunodeficiency virus. *Journal of Neuropsychiatry and Clinical Neuroscience*, **1**, 225–35.

Martinsson, T., Johannesson, T., Vujic, M., Sjöstedt, A., Steffenburg, S., Gillberg, C., Wahlström, J. (1994). Maternal origin of a supernumerary isodicentric chromosome 15–marker in infantile autism. *American Journal of Human Genetics*, Accepted for publication.

Mascari, M.J., Gottlieb, W., Rogan, P.K., Butler, M.G., Waller, D.A., Armour, J.A.L., Jeffreys, A.J., Ladda, R.L., Nicholls, R.D. (1992). The frequency of uniparental disomy in Prader–Willi syndrome. Implications for molecular diagnosis. *New England Journal of Medicine*, **326**, 1599–607.

Mazzocco, M.M.M., Pennington, B.F., Hagerman, R.J. (1994). Social cognition skills among females with fragile X. *Journal of Autism and Developmental Disorders*, **24**, 473–85.

Medalia, A., Isaacs-Glaberman, K., Scheinberg, H. (1988). Neuropsychological impairment in

Wilson's disease. *Archives of Neurology*, **45**, 502–4.

Meijer, A., Zakay-Rones, Z., Morag, A. (1988). Postinfluenzal psychiatric disorder in adolescents. *Acta Psychiatrica Scandinavica*, **78**, 176–81.

Menkes, J., Philippart, M., Clark, D.B. (1964). Hereditary partial agenesis of the corpus callosum. *Archives of Neurology*, **11**, 198–208.

Menkes, J.H., Kinsbourne, M. (1990). Workshop on neurologic complications of pertussis and pertussis vaccination. *Neuropediatrics*, **21**, 171–6.

Miller, C.A., Parker, W.D. (1985). Segmental neurofibromatosis. *Archives of Dermatology*, **113**, 837–8.

Miller, D.L., Ross, E.M., Alderslade, R., Bellman, M.H., Rawson, N.S. (1981). Pertussis immunisation and serious acute neurological illness in children. *British Medical Journal (Clin Res Ed)*, **282**, 1595–9.

Miller, H.G., Stanton, J.B., Gibbons, J.L. (1956). Para-infectious encephalomyelitis and related syndromes. *Quarterly Journal of Medicine*, **25**, 427–505.

Miyajima, I., Nakafuku, M., Nakayama, N., Brenner, C., Miyajima, A., Kaibuchi, K., Arai, K., Kaziro, Y., Matsumoto, K. (1987). GPA1, a haploid-specific essential gene, encodes a yeast homolog of mammalian G protein which may be involved in mating factor signal transduction. *Cell*, **50**, 1011–119.

Morrow, J.D., Whitman, B.Y., Accardo, P.J. (1990). Autistic disorder in Sotos syndrome: a case report. *European Journal of Pediatrics*, **149**, 567–9.

Moser, H. (1984). Duchenne muscular dystrophy: pathogenetic aspects and genetic prevention. *Human Genetics*, **66**, 17–40.

Murphy, M.B., Greenberg, F., Wilson, G., Hughes, M., DiLiberti, J. (1990). Williams syndrome in twins. *American Journal of Medical Genetics Suppl*, 97–9.

Musetti, L., Albizzati, A., Grioni, A., Rossetti, M., Saccani, M. & Musetti, C. (1993). Autistic disorder associated with congenital HIV infection. *European Child & Adolescent Psychiatry*, **2**, 221–5

Niedermeyer, E., Naidu, S. (1990). Further EEG observations in children with the Rett syndrome. *Brain and Development*, **12**, 53–4.

Nomura, Y., Segawa, M., Hasegawa, M. (1985). Rett syndrome – an early catecholamine and indolamine deficient disorder? *Brain and Development*, **7**, 334–41.

Noonan, J.A. (1968). Lexington hypertelorisma with Turner phenotype. A new syndrome with associated congenital heart disesase. *American Journal of Diseases of Children*, **116**, 373–80.

Nyhan, W.L., James, J.A., Teberg, A.J., Sweetman, L., Nelson, L.G. (1969). A new disorder of purine metabolism with behavioral manifestations. *Journal of Pediatrics*, **74**, 20–7.

Olegård, R., Sabel, K.G., Aronsson, M., Sanding, B., Johansson, P.R., Carlsson, C., Kyllerman, M., Iversen, K., Hrbek, A. (1979). Effects on the child of alcohol abuse during pregnancy – retrospective and prospective studies. *Acta Paediatrica Scandinavia Suppl*, **275**, 112–21.

Opitz, J.M., Westphal, J.M., Daniel, A. (1984). Discovery of a connective tissue dysplasia in the Martin-Bell syndrome. *American Journal of Medical Genetics*, **17**, 101–9.

Pascual-Castroviejo, I. (1987). Hypomelanosis of Ito. *In* Gomez, M. (Ed.) *Neurocutaneous Diseases: A Practical Approach*. London: Butterworths.

Peckham, C.S., Logan, G.S. (1988). Cytomegalovirus infection in pregnancy. Proceedings of the XIth European Congress of Perinatal Medicine.

Pearl, K.N., Preece, P.M., Ades, A., Peckham, C.S. (1986). Neurodevelopmental assessment after congenital cytomegalovirus infection. *Archives of Disease in Childhood*, **61**, 323–6.

Percy, A., Gillberg, C., Hagberg, B., Witt-Engerstrom, I. (1990). Rett syndrome and the autistic disorders. *Neurology Clinics*, **8**, 659–76.

Percy, A.K., Glaze, D.G., Schultz, R.J., Zoghbi, H.Y., *et al.* (1994). Rett syndrome: controlled study of an oral opiate antagonist, naltrexone. *Annals of Neurology*, **35**, 464–70.

Pietz, J., Lütcke, A., Sontheimer, D., Benninger, C., Pietz, B., Batzler, U., Heusser, A. (1990). EEG development in early treated PKU patients from birth to 6 months. *European Journal of Pediatrics*, **149 (Suppl.)**, S28–33.

Pollack, M.A., Golden, G.S., Schmidt, R., Davis, J.A., Leeds, N. (1978). Infantile spasms in Down syndrome: a report of 5 cases and review of the literature. *Annals of Neurology*, **3**, 406–8.

Price, D., Inglese, C., Jacobs, J. (1988). Pediatric AIDS: Neuroradiologic and neurodevelopmental findings. *Pediatric Radiology*, **18**, 445–48.

Randall, T. (1990). Marfan syndrome gene search intensifies following identification of basic defect. *Journal of the American Medical Association*, **264**, 1642–3.

Råstam, M., Gillberg, C., Wahlström, J. (1991). Chromosomes in anorexia nervosa. A case of 47 cases including a population-based group: a research note. *Journal of Child Psychology and*

Psychiatry, **32**, 695–701.

Ratcliffe, S.G., Butler, G.E., Jones, M. (1990). Edinburgh study of growth and development of children with sex chromosome abnormalities. IV. *Birth Defects*, **26**, 1–44.

Reiss, A.L., Freund, L. (1990). Fragile X syndrome. *Biological Psychiatry*, **27**, 223–40.

Reiss, A.L., Feinstein, C., Rosenbaum, K.N., Borengasser-Caruso, M.A., Goldsmith, B.M. (1985). Autism associated with Williams syndrome. *Journal of Paediatrics*, **106**, 247–9.

Riccardi, V.M. (1991a). Neurofibromatosis mimicry: editorial; comment: Comment on: *Arch Dermatol* 1991 Nov;127(11):1702–4. *Archives of Dermatology*, **127**, 1714–15.

Riccardi, V.M. (1991b). Neurofibromatosis: past, present, and future :editorial; comment: Comment on: *N Engl J Med* 1991 May 2;324(18):1264–6. *New England Journal of Medicne*, **324**, 1283–5.

Riccardi, V.M. (1991c). Neurogenetics and the neurosurgeon: editorial. *Neurosurgery*, **29**, 629–30.

Riccardi, V.M. (1993). Genotype, malleotype, phenotype, and randomness: lessons from neurofibromatosis-1 (NF-1). *American Journal of Human Genetics*, **53**, 301–4.

Riccardi, V.M., Eichner, J.E. (1986). *Neurofibromatosis: Phenotype, Natural History, and Pathogenesis*. Baltimore: Johns Hopkins University Press.

Robbins, T.O., Bernstein, J. (1988). Renal involvement. *In* Gomez, M. (Ed.) *Tuberous Sclerosis*. New York: Raven.

Rogers, P.T., Coleman, M. (1992). *Medical Care in Down Syndrome*. New York: Marcel Dekker.

Rolando, S. (1985). Rett syndrome: report of eight cases. *Brain & Development*, **7**, 290–6.

Rouleau, G.A., Wertelecki, W., Haines, J.L. (1987). Genetic linkage of bilateral acoustic neurofibromatosis to a DNA marker on chromosome 22. *Nature*, **329**, 246–8.

Rosemberg, S., Arita, F.N., Campos, C., Alonso, F. (1984). Hypomelanosis of Ito. Case report with involvement of the central nervous system and review of the literature. *Neuropediatrics*, **15**, 52–5.

Ross, D.L., Liwnicz, B.H., Gun, R.W.M., Gilbert, E. (1982). Hypomelanosis of Ito (incontinentia pigmenti achromians). A clinical study: macrocephaly and gray matter heterotopias. *Neurology*, **32**, 1013–16.

Ross, M.H., Galaburda, A.M., Kemper, T.L. (1984). Down's syndrome: is there a decreased population of neurons. *Neurology*, **34**, 909–16.

Rutter, M., Bartak, L. (1971). Causes of infantile autism: some considerations from recent research.

Journal of Autism and Childhood Schizophrenia, **1**, 20–32.

Rutter, S.C., Cole, T.R. (1991). Psychological characteristics of Sotos syndrome. *Developmental Medicine and Child Neurology*, **33**, 898–902.

Samuelsson, B. (1981). *Neurofibromatosis (von Recklinghausen's disease). A clinical-psychiatric and genetic study*. MD University of Göteborg.

Sanfield, J.A., Linares, O.A., Calahan, D.D., Forrester, J.M., Halter, J.B., Rosen, S.G. (1989). Altered norepinephrine metabolism in Shapiro's syndrome. *Archives of Neurology*, **46**, 53–7.

Schiavi, R.C., Theilgaard, A., Owen, D.R., White, D. (1988). Sex chromosome anomalies, hormones, and sexuality. *Archives of General Psychiatry*, **45**, 19–24.

Scriver, C.R. (1991). Phenylketonuria – genotypes and phenotypes: editorial; comment: Comment on: *N Engl J Med* 1991 May 2;324(18):1232–8. *New England Journal of Medicine*, **324**, 1280–1.

Seegmiller, J.E., Rosenbloom, F.M., Kelley, W.N. (1967). Enzyme defect associated with a sex-linked human neurological disorder and excessive purine synthesis. *Science*, **155**, 1682–4.

Selikowitz, M., Sunman, J., Pendergast, A., Wright, S. (1990). Fenfluramine in Prader–Willi syndrome: a double blind, placebo controlled trial. *Archives of Diseases in Childhood*, **65**, 112–14.

Semrud-Clikeman, M., Filipek, P.A., Biederman, J., Steingard, R., Kennedy, D., Renshaw, P., Bekken, K. (1994). Attention-deficit hyperactivity disorder: magnetic resonance imaging morphometric analysis of the corpus callosum. *Journal of the American Academy of Child and Adolescent Psychiatry*, **33**(6), 875–81.

Shannon, K.M., Ammann, A.J. (1985). Acquired immune deficiency syndrome in childhood. *Journal of Pediatrics*, **106**, 332–42.

Shapiro, W.R., Williams, G.H., Plum, F. (1969). Spontaneous recurrent hypothermia accompanying agenesis of the corpus callosum. *Brain*, **92**, 423–36.

Shepherd, C.W., Beard, C.M., Gomez, M.R., Kurland, L.T., Whisnant, J.P. (1991). Tuberous sclerosis complex in Olmsted County, Minnesota, 1950–1989. *Archives of Neurology*, **48**, 400–1.

Sherman, S.L. (1991). Genetic epidemiology of the fragile X syndrome with special reference to genetic counseling. *Progress in Clinical and Biological Research*, **368**, 79–99.

Shields, W.D., Nielsen, C., Buch, D., Jacobsen, V., Christenson, P., Zachau-Christenson, B., Cherry, J.D. (1988). Relationship of pertussis immunization to the onset of neurologic disorders: a retrospective epidemilogic study. *Journal of Pediatrics*, **113**, 801–5.

Silver, D.N., Lewis, R.A., Nussbaum, R.L. (1987). Mapping the Lowe oculocerebrorenal syndrome to Xq24–q26 by use of restriction fragment length polymorphisms. *Journal of Clinical Investigation*, **79**, 282–5.

Silverstein, F.S., Johnston, M.V., Hutchinson, R.J., Edwards, N.L. (1985). Lesch-Nyhan syndrome: CSF neurotransmitter abnormalities. *Neurology*, **35**, 907–11.

Smith, C., Sangster, G. (1972). Mucoplasma pneumoniae meningoencephalitis. *Scandinavian Journal of Infectious Diseases*, **4**, 69–71.

Smith, G.F., Berg, J.M. (1976). *Down's Anomaly*. 2nd edn. Edinburgh: Churchill Livingstone.

Smith, P.J., Hindmarsh, P.J., Kendall, B., Brook, G.G.D. (1986). Dysgenesis of the corpus callosum and hypopituitarism. *Acta Paediatrica Scandinavica*, **75**, 923–6.

Smith, I., Beasley, M.G., Wolff, O.H., Ades, A.E. (1988). Behavior disturbance in 8 year-old children with early treated phenylketonuria. *Journal of Pediatrics*, **112**, 403–8.

Smith, M., Smalley, S., Cantor, M., Pandolfo, M., Gomez, M.I., Baumann, R., Flodman, P., Yoshiyama, K., Nakamura, Y., Julier, C., et al. (1988). Mapping of a gene determining tuberous sclerosis to human chromosome 11. *Genomics*, **6**, 105–14.

Sollee, N.D., Latham, E.E., Kinden, D.J., et al. (1985). Neuropsychological impairment in Duchenne muscular dystrophy. *Journal of Experimental Neuropsychology*, **7**, 486.

Stafstrom, C.E., Patxot, O.F., Gilmore, H.E., Wisniewski, K.E. (1991). Seizures in children with Down syndrome: etiology, characteristics and outcome. *Developmental Medicine and Child Neurology*, **33**, 191–200.

Stagno, S., Whitley, R.J. (1985). Herpesvirus infection of pregnancy. Part I: Cytomegalovirus and Epstein–Barr virus infections. *New England Journal of Medicine*, **313**, 1270–4.

Steffanson, K., Wollman, R.L., Huttenlocher, P.R. (1988). Lineages of cells in the central nervous system. *In* Gomez, M. (Ed.) *Tuberous Sclerosis*. New York: Raven.

Steffenburg, S., Gillberg, C., Steffenburg, U. (1992, September 3–5). Psychiatric problems in children with mental retardation and seizure disorders. A population-based study. WHO 6th Invitational Child and Adolescent European Research Group Meeting. Göteborg, Sweden.

Steinbach, P., Adkins, W.N.J., Caspar, H.,

Dumars, K.W., Gebauer, J., Gilbert, E.F., Grimm, T., Habedank, M., Hansmann, I., Herrmann, J., Kaveggia, E.G., Langenbeck, U., Meisner, L.F., Najafzadeh, T.M., Opitz, M., Palmer, C.G., Peters, H.H., Scholz, W., Tavares, A.S., Wiedeking, C. (1981). The dup(3q) syndrome: report of eight cases and review of the literature. *American Journal of Medical Genetics*, **10**, 159–77.

Steinhausen, H.-C., Willms, J., Spohr, H.L. (1994). Correlates of psychopathology and intelligence in children with Fetal Alcohol Syndrome. *Journal of Child Psycholoy and Psychiatry*, **35**, 323–31.

Streissguth, A.P., Barr, H.M., Sampson, P.D. (1990). Moderate prenatal alcohol exposure: Effects on child IQ and learning problems at age 7 years. *Alcoholism, Clinical and Experimental Research*, **14**, 662.

Strömland, K., Nordin, V., Gillberg, C., Åkerström, B., Miller, M. (1994). Autism in thalidomide embryopathy. A population study. *Developmental Medicine and Child Neurology*, **36**, 351–6.

Tahernia, A.C. (1993). Cardiovascular anomalies in Marfan's syndrome: the role of echocardiography and beta-blockers. *Southern Medical Journal*, **86**, 305–10.

Takano, K., Kuroiwa, Y., Shimada, Y., Mannen, T., Toyokura, Y. (1983). CT manifestations of cerebral white matter lesion in Wilson disease. *Annals of Neurology*, **13**, 108–9.

Thase, M.E., Tigner, R., Smeltzer, D.J., Liss, L. (1984). Age-related neuropsychological deficits in Down's syndrome. *Biological Psychiatry*, **19**, 571–85.

Towfighi, J., Marks, K., Palmer, E., Vannucci, R. (1979). Moebius syndrome. Neuropathologic observations. *Acta Neuropathologica*, **48**, 11–17.

Trevathan, E., Moser, H.W., Opitz, J.M., Percy, A.K., Naidu, S., Holm, V.A., Boring, C.C., Janssen, R.S., Yeargin-Allsopp, M., Adams, M.J., Gillberg, C. (1988). Diagnostic criteria for Rett Syndrome. The Rett Syndrome Diagnostic Criteria Work Group. *Annals of Neurology*, **23**, 425–8.

Trombley, I.K., Mirra, S.S. (1981). Ultrastructure of tuberous sclerosis: cortical tuber and subependymal tumor. *Annals of Neurology*, **9**, 174–81.

Udwin, O. (1990). A survey of adults with Williams syndrome and idiopathic infantile hypercalcaemia. *Developmental Medicine and Child Neurology*, **32**, 129–41.

Udwin, O., Yule, W. (1990). Augmentative communication systems taught to cerebral palsied children – a longitudinal study. I. The acquisition of signs and symbols, and syntactic aspects of their use over time. *British Journal of Disorder in Communication*, **25**, 295–309.

Udwin, O., Yule, W., Martin, N. (1987). Cognitive abilities and behavioural characteristics of children with idiophathic hypercalcaemia. *Journal of Child Psychology and Psychiatry*, **2**, 297–309.

Uvebrant, P., Bjure, J., Sixt, R., Witt Engerström, I., Hagberg, B. (1993). Regional cerebral blood flow: SPECT as a tool for localization of brain dysfunction. *In* Hagberg, B. (Ed.) *Rett Syndrome – Clinical & Biological Aspects. Clinics in Developemental Medicine No. 127.* London: Mac Keith Press.

Verkerk, A.J., Pieretti, M., Sutcliffe, J.S., Fu, Y.H., Kuh, D.P., Pizzuti, A., Reiner, O., Richards, S., Victoria, M.F., Zhang, F.P., *et al.* (1991). Identification of a gene (FMR–1) containing a CGG repeat coincident with a breakpoint cluster region exhibiting length variation in fragile X syndrome. *Cell*, **65**, 905–14.

Volkmar, F.R., Poll, J., Lewis, M. (1984). Conversion reactions in childhood and adolescence. *Journal of the American Academy of Child Psychiatry*, **23**, 424–30.

Waldstein, G., Mierau, G., Ahmad, R., Thibodeay, S.N., Hagerman, R.J., Caldwell, S. (1987). Fragile X syndrome: skin elastin abnormalities. *Birth Defects*, **23**, 103–14.

Webb, D.W., Super, M., Normand, I.C., Osborne, J.P. (1993). Tuberous sclerosis and polycystic kidney disease. *British Medical Journal*, **306**, 1258–9.

Whitley, C.B., Ramsay, N.K., Kersey, J.H., Krivit, W. (1986). Bone marrow transplantation for Hurler syndrome: assessment of metabolic correction. *Birth Defects*, **22**, 7–24.

Williams, D.T., Pleak, R., Hanesian, H. (1987). Neuropsychiatric disorders of childhood and adolescence. *In* Hales, R.,Yudofsky, S. (Eds.). *The American Psychiatric Press Textbook of Neuropsychiatry*. Washington, DC: American Psychiatric Press.

Williamson, W.D., Desmond, M.M., LaFevers, N., Taber, L.H., Catlin, F.I., Weaver, T.G. (1982). Symptomatic congenital cytomegalovirus. Disorders of language, learning and hearing. *American Journal of Diseases of Children*, **136**, 902–5.

Wilson, P.M.Y., *et al.* (1989). Features of coxsackie B virus (CBV) infection in children with prolonged physical and psychological morbidity. *Journal of Psychosomatic Research*, **33**, 29–36.

Wilson, J.M., Young, A.B., Kelley, W.N. (1983).

Hypoxanthine-guanine phosphoribosyl transferase deficieny-the molecular basis of the clinical syndromes. *New England Journal of Medicine*, **309**, 900–10.

Wing, L. (1993). The definition and prevalence of autism: A review. *European Child & Adolescent Psychiatry*, **2**, 1–14.

Wisniewski, H.M. (1983). Neuritic (senile) and amyloid plaques. *In* Reisberg, B. (Ed.) *Alzheimer's Disease*. New York: Free Press.

Wisniewski, K., Dambska, M., Sher, J.H., Qasi, Q. (1983). A clinical neuropathological study of the fetal alcohol syndrome. *Neuropediatrics*, **14**, 197–201.

Witt-Engerström, I. (1993, October). Epidemiology and spectrum of disability in familial cases. Paper read at the World Congress on Rett Syndrome. Antwerp, Belgium.

Witt-Engerström, I., Gillberg, C. (1987). Rett Syndrome in Sweden. *Journal of Austism and Developmental Disorders*, **17**, 149–50.

Witte, R.A., (1985). The psychosocial impact of a progressive physical handicap and terminal illness (Duchenne muscular dystrophy) on adolescents and their families. *British Journal of Medical Psychology*, **58**, 179–87.

Woo, S.L., (1988). Collation of RFLP haplotypes at the human phenylalanine hydroxylase (PAH) locus: letter. *American Jouranl of Human Genetics*, **1988**, 5.

Woo, S.L., Lidsky, A.S., Güttler, F., Chandra, T., Robson, K.J.H. (1983). Cloned human phenylalanine hydroxylase gene allows prenatal diagnosis and carrier detection of classical phenylketonuria. *Nature*, **306**, 151–5.

Zappella, M. (1990*a*). A double blind trial of bromocriptine in the Rett syndrome. *Brain and Development*, **12**, 148–50.

Zappella, M. (1990*b*). Autistic features in children affected by cerebral gigantism. *Brain Dysfunction*, **3**, 241–4.

Zappella, M. (1992*a*). Hypomelanosis of Ito is common in autistic syndromes. *European Child & Adolescent Psychiatry*, **1**, 170–7.

Zappella, M. (1992*b*). The Rett girls with preserved speech. *Brain & Development*, **14**, 98–101.

Zappella, M. (1994). Rett syndrome. Like hand-washing developmental arrest and autistic symptoms in two Italian girls. *European Child and Adolescent Psychiatry*, **3**, 52–6.

Zori, R.T., Hendrickson, J., Woolven, S., Whidden, E.M., Gray, B., Williams, C.A. (1992). Angelman syndrome: clinical profile. *Journal of Child Neurology*, **7**, 270–80.

11 Psychotic disorders not elsewhere classified (including mania and depression with psychotic features)

Non-schizophrenic psychotic disorders constitute a relatively small proportion of all child and adolescent neuropsychiatric disorders (Steinberg, 1985). This group comprises mania, major depression with psychotic features, bipolar disorder, schizoaffective disorder and organic and toxic psychosis, including those that are precipitated by substance abuse (Gillberg *et al.*, 1986). Most of these conditions have reported onset at, or after, age 18 years and so fall outside the scope of this book. Nevertheless, premorbid emotional and behavioural abnormalities are common in the histories of people diagnosed in the categories mentioned (Hellgren, Gillberg & Enerskog, 1987; McClellan, Werry & Ham, 1993), and a number of investigators have reported on at least some individuals in the 6–17 year-old age range with any one of these diagnoses.

Mania

There is limited evidence for discrete episodes of adult type mania in prepubertal children, but some authorities believe that an atypical form of bipolar disorder characterized by periods of motor overactivity, inattention, behavioural disturbance, mood volatility and/or withdrawal occurs in genetically vulnerable children (Carlson, 1984). Clinical observations suggest that sleep problems may also be common in this group. There is anecdotal support for the notion that intermittent prostitution or promiscuous behaviour may signal underlying remitting mania. Uncontrolled studies suggest that

children showing such symptoms may be responsive to treatment with lithium (Weller *et al.*, 1986).

The existence of mania is considerably better validated in adolescents, and, according to one study, its prevalence in 13–19 year-olds is at least 3 in 10 000 (e.g. Gillberg *et al.*, 1986). Psychotic symptoms are prevalent in adolescent onset mania, with high rates of hallucinations, delusions and thought disorder (Carlson, 1990). Adolescents with mania more often have such 'schizophrenic-like' symptoms, and are more likely to be diagnosed as having schizophrenia or schizo-affective disorder than patients with adult onset bipolar disorder (Bashir, Russell & Johnson, 1987; McGlashan, 1988).

A whole host of medical conditions can produce the full-blown syndrome of mania. Thus, for instance encephalitis, severe influenza and AIDS infection have all been described to present with mania. Hyperthyroidism, Cushing syndrome and steroid medication can also produce the clinical picture. Large doses of sympathomimetics (such as if large quantities of some antitussis medications are ingested) are relatively common causes of manic episodes. Brain tumours (including meningiomas, gliomas and thalamic tumours), Wilson's disease, head trauma, multiple sclerosis and seizure disorders have all been described to produce mania in children and adolescents (Wise & Rundell, 1988).

The findings from open trials suggest that lithium may be useful in the treatment of mania in very young patients (Kelly, Koch & Buegel, 1976). There is also some data to suggest that prophylactic lithium may greatly reduce the risk of relapse in this group (Strober *et al.*, 1990), but further study is required before definite conclusions can be drawn in this respect. The problem of non-compliance should be recognized in this group. Lithium serum levels should be kept at 0.4–1.4 meq/l.

Major depression with psychotic features

Major depression with psychotic features may have a number of different etiologies, including genetic, brain damage and psychosocial trauma. For instance, in the study by Hellgren *et al.* (1987), a high rate of parental death was typical of adolescents with psychotic depression.

Depressive disorders in early and middle childhood are possibly often missed (Weller & Weller, 1991*a*), partly because the expressed symptom of depression may be less common in children and adolescents than in adults, and also because in many cases there have not been previous episodes of recognized depression (with complete recovery), which could have alerted the clinician (and family) to the possibility of depression.

The DSM-III-R diagnosis of depression requires the presence of at least five of the nine symptoms in Table 11.1. The diagnostic criteria of 'melancholic subtype' of major depression are also outlined in the table. The DSM-IV criteria for major depressive episode and dysthymia are virtually identical. However, for melancholia, there is no requirement of a specific response to treatment or of one or more prior episodes of depression. Personality disturbance does not exclude a melancholia diagnosis in the DSM-IV. Instead there are two new criteria, viz. 'distinct quality of depressed mood' and 'excessive or inappropriate guilt'. There may be a particular paucity of studies on children and adolescents with melancholic subtype depression because ECT, MAO inhibitors or lithium have rarely been used. It should be noted that major depression would not, according to the DSM-III-R, be an appropriate diagnosis, if there were associated major organic

Table 11.1. *The diagnosis of depressive disorders according to the DSM-III-R (see text for comparison with DSM-IV)*

At least five of the following nine symptoms have to be present in order to diagnose

Major depressive episode
1. Diminished interest or loss of pleasure in almost all activities
2. Sleep disturbance, either insomnia or hypersomnia
3. Observable psychomotor agitation or retardation
4. Weight change or appetite disturbance, either failure to gain weight as expected, weight loss or weight gain which is inappropriate for age
5. Recurrent thoughts of death
6. Difficulties concentrating or indecisveness
7. Feelings of worthlessness or inappropriate guilt
8. Fatigue or loss of energy
9. Depressed mood

Major depression, melancholic type
1. Loss of interest or pleasure in almost all activities
2. Sleep disturbance as manifested by waking up at least 2 hours earlier than usual
3. Observable psychomotor agitation or retardation
4. Weight change as manifested by loss of at least 5% body weight in a month
5. Depression worse in the morning
6. Lack of reactivity to usually pleasureable stimuli
7. No significant personality disturbance
8. One or more prior major depressive episodes followed by recovery
9. Previous good response to specific somatic treatment (e.g. ECT, MAO inhibitors, lithium)

In addition to depressed or irritable mood lasting for more than a year and not leaving the individual symptom free for more than 2 months, at least two of the following six symptoms have to be present in order to diagnose:

Dysthymia
1. Sleep change
2. Appetite change
3. Decreased energy
4. Low self-esteem
5. Difficulty making decisions/poor concentration
6. Feelings of hopelessness

conditions or the temporally associated loss of a loved one. However, even though this may be a reasonable approach in some types of research, in practice, it could be detrimental to the organically ill patient, who might be deprived of appropriate treatment for severe depressive symptoms.

In young children, somatic complaints, mood-congruent hallucinations (usually a single voice talking to the individual), avoidant behaviours and high levels of anxiety are common, and in later childhood and adolescence there is often considerable overlap with conduct disturbance and frank antisocial behaviour (Gillberg I.C. & Gillberg, 1983; APA, 1987; Weller & Weller 1991b; Werry, 1992a, b).

Clinically, depressive episodes in children and adolescents should be suspected whenever there is *change of behaviour lasting for more than a week* in combination with *hypothalamic symptoms* (such as loss of energy, frozenness, weight disturbance, appetite disturbance, constipation, sleep disturbance). Once this constellation of symptoms has been documented, a check on the more detailed list of depressive disorder criteria will help establish a diagnosis of true depressive disorder.

Early onset depressive disorders with psychotic features often have comorbid psychiatric conditions which may lead to misdiagnosis or negatively influence outcome (Carlson, 1990). There is a high rate of homotypic family psychiatric history, particularly if episodes of psychotic depression fluctuates with episodes of mania. According to the only population-based follow-up study published to date (Gillberg *et al.*, 1993), adolescents with depression (without manic episodes) with psychotic features may have considerably better outcomes than those with bipolar disorder, schizophrenia and other forms of psychosis.

Major depression without psychotic features is considerably more common than psychotic depression. Nevertheless, some studies have found that up to one in three (or more) of depressed adolescents have psychotic features (Carlson & Kashani 1988; Weller *et al.*, 1990).

Major depression without psychotic features may well respond to psychosocial and educational environmental measures alone. For instance, being the victim of scape-goating in school is a very serious stressor which may be alleviated by relatively simple intervention. Once such stress on the child is lifted, depressive symptoms may disappear quickly. In cases with depressed mood (and major depression) and co-morbid (pre-morbid) DAMP or other neurodevelopmental problems (dyslexia, Tourette syndrome), a proper diagnosis of the 'underlying' problems and appropriate information might well be the best way to deal with depression also. Psychotic depression may sometimes best be treated by hospitalization and a trial of antidepressant medication in daily doses ranging from 50–200 mg amitriptyline or imipramine. These are the two antidepressant drugs most widely used in child and adolescent psychiatry. They should be started in very small doses (5–10 mg/day) and then increased by 5–10 mg/day until side effects become too problematic or positive mood effects are noted. They should then be kept at this level for several months before discontinuation. They may well be useful in the treatment of moderately severe and severe cases of non-psychotic depression also. The tricyclic drugs have been used in millions of children (for enuresis, an indication which is not as valid today as it was ten years ago). This validates their low level of severe toxicity in young people. However, less than a handful of appropriate double-blind studies have been performed on the antidepressant effects of these drugs in children and adolescents (Puig-Antich, *et al.*, 1987; Preskorn *et al.*, 1987), and support for their efficacy has only been gained in some of these. Thus, antidepressant medication for the treatment of depression should be used with great caution in young people. Treatment with the new selective serotinin reuptake inhibitors cannot yet be recommended for clinical use with depressed children and adolescents. Their use in child and adolescence psychiatry must await proper clinical trials in the field.

Bipolar disorder

Unequivocal bipolar disorders with documented episodes of both mania and major depression are definitely rare conditions in childhood, but may increase in prevalence around the time of adolescence. There have been only a handful of reports in the literature documenting the occurrence of bipolar disorder in adolescence (Comings & Comings, 1987).

Lithium is the preferred pharmacological treatment both during manic episodes (see above) and for prophylaxis. Hospitalization may be required to ensure patient safety. Lithium should be given in doses of $300 + 300 + 300 - 600$ mg at 7–8 in the morning, 12 noon and 6 pm for children weighing 40–50 kg; $600 + 300 + 600$ mg for children and adolescents weighing 50–60 kg. Blood levels should be monitored 12 hours after last dose (in the morning before morning dose) once a week until two consecutive levels appear in the 0.4–1.2 meq/l. If no clinical improvement is seen, increase dose to reach no more than 1.4 meq/l (adapted from Weller et al., 1986).

Schizo-affective disorder

Schizo-affective disorder with psychotic features is uncommon. Nevertheless, two cases were found out of a total of 62 who almost met criteria both for schizophrenia and major affective disorder with psychotic features (Gillberg et al., 1986). In Eggers' follow-up study of 57 cases with 'schizophrenia', 15 (?) were reported to have schizoaffective psychosis, indicating that, although rare, it can be separated from schizophrenia (Eggers, 1982).

Although there have been no publications specifically addressing the topic of schizo-affective disorders in children and adolescents, a few prudent clinical conclusions may be warranted. In the author's experience, motility disturbance (closely imitating akathisia associated with neuroleptic medication) is often a hallmark of the disorder, particularly in connection with onset and before any kind of intervention has been tried. Religious and grandiose ideas are common as is confusion over time and place. Pregnancy may trigger episodes of schizo-affective disorder in some young women. Thus, whenever this diagnosis is suspected, a pregnancy test should be performed (not least in order to avoid medication that might harmfully affect the developing foetus). The author has personal clinical experience of two young women with schizo-affective disorder in association with the fragile-X syndrome. One of these women gave birth to a fragile-X positive son with classical autism. She later committed suicide.

Organic psychosis (including substance induced)

In the study by Gillberg et al. (1986), psychoses induced by known organic factors (such as viral infection of the brain) were more common than many of the aforementioned types of psychosis (only schizophrenia was more common) and accounted for 7 in 10 000 13–19 year-olds. About 20% of all psychosis cases with apparent teenage onset had a clear-cut organic origin/trigger.

Medication with large doses of stimulants (such as may occur with certain types of antitussive agents) may produce not only a full-blown manic episode (see above) but schizophreniform psychotic conditions as well.

Metabolic disorders and other systemic disorders, such as Wilson disease, porphyrias, and systemic lupus, can present (sometimes for long periods of time) with neuropsychiatric symptoms only. Such symptoms may cluster to suggest 'true' schizophrenia, mania or psychotic disorders which do not readily fit the criteria for any of the named syndromes.

Several individual case reports have shown certain infectious agents affecting brain functions to be particularly prone to triggering psychotic symptoms in young individuals. For instance, both mycoplasma pneumoniae and herpes encephalitis have been reported to cause psychotic disorders in childhood. Whether to diagnose such disorders as 'toxic psychosis', 'organic psychosis' or, depending on symptomatology, 'schizophrenic disorder' or 'mania' depends on whether or not one wants to accept the requirement of some of the diagnostic manuals that the existence of an underlying known organic disorder precludes the diagnosis of disorders which have, for reasons that are now either obscure or, depending on one's point of view, obsolete.

Psychosis not otherwise specified

Children and adolescents with emerging personality disorder may sometimes report psychotic symptoms, 'micropsychotic episodes' or 'psychotic-like' symptoms (Lewis, 1991; Nurcombe *et al.*, 1989; Nurcombe, 1991). The diagnosis of a personality disorder does not exclude the possibility of a primary psychotic disorder, and an association between borderline personality disorder and both adult and adolescent onset bipolar disorder has been reported (Kutcher, Marton & Korenblum, 1990; Brent *et al.*, 1990). The substance of this association of two purportedly separate disorder is in doubt, however, because of the overlap of diagnostic criteria. Some reviews of the literature (Gunderson & Phillips, 1991) suggest that borderline personality disorder is unrelated to either bipolar disorder or schizophrenia. Nevertheless, the confusion over labels in this field may well be due more to a lack of precision in defining the boundaries than to syndromes being discrete: there could be both overlap and discontinuity both of which may be obscured by the use of imprecise terminology. Thus, for instance, in the experience of the author, Asperger syndrome (for what that diagnosis is worth as a discrete entity) is a construct which is often 'missed' (= diagnosis not made) in children and adolescents, and labels of 'schizophreniform disorder', 'borderline' and 'paranoid psychosis' are instead applied by adult psychiatrists in early adult age. In missing out on the 'underlying' diagnosis, a whole host of other conditions are considered, which are probably conceptually inadequate, but which show some resemblance to the clinical picture exhibited by the patient.

Hallucinations that do not signal the onset of a chronic psychotic disorder occur in children and adolescents (Garralda, 1984*a*). In a follow-up study of 20 children with hallucinations, there was no increase in either schizophrenia, mood disorders or other psychiatric disorders when matched to psychiatric controls (Garralda, 1984*b*). However, hallucinations can, of course, be one of the most alarming presenting symptoms of psychosis in children (Garralda, 1984*c*).

References

American Psychiatric Association. (1987). *Diagnostic and Statistical Manual of Mental Disorders*. Third Edition – Revised. Washington, DC: APA.

Bashir, M., Russell, J., Johnson, G. (1987). Bipolar affective disorder in adolescence: a 10-year study. *Australian and New Zeeland Journal of Psychiatry*, **21**, 36–43.

Brent, D.A., Zelenak, J.P., Bukstein, O., Brown, R.V. (1990). Reliability and validity of the structured interview for personality disorders in adolescents. *Journal of the American Academy of Child and Adolescent Psychiatry*, **29**, 349–54.

Carlson, G.A. (1984). Classification issues of bipolar disorders in childhood. *Psychiatric Developments*, **4**, 273–85.

Carlson, G.A. (1990). Child and adolescent mania – diagnostic considerations. *Journal of Child Psychology and Psychiatry*, **31**, 331–41.

Carlson, G.A., Kashani, J.H. (1988). Manic symptoms in non-referred adolescent population. *Journal of Affective Disorders*, **15**, 219–26.

Comings, B.G., Comings, D.E. (1987). A controlled study of Tourette syndrome. V. Depression and mania. *American Journal of Human Genetics*, **41**, 804–21.

Eggers, C. (1982). Psychoses in childhood and adolescence. *Acta Paedopsychiatrica*, **48**, 81–98.

Garralda, M.E. (1984*a*). Hallucinations in children with conduct and emotional disorders: I. The clinical phenomena. *Psychological Medicine*, **14**, 589–96.

Garralda, M.E. (1984*b*). Hallucinations in children with conduct and emotional disorders: II. The follow-up study. *Psychological Medicine*, **14**, 597–604.

Garralda, M.E. (1984*c*). Psychotic children with hallucinations. *British Journal of Psychiatry*, **145**, 74–7.

Gillberg, C., Wahlström, J., Forsman, A., Hellgren, L., Gillberg, I.C. (1986). Teenage psychoses--epidemiology, classification and reduced optimality in the pre-, peri- and neonatal periods. *Journal of Child Psychology and*

Psychiatry, **27**, 87–98.

Gillberg, I.C., Gillberg, C. (1983). Three-year follow-up at age 10 of children with minor neurodevelopmental disorders. I: Behavioural problems. *Developmental Medicine and Child Neurology*, **25**, 438–49.

Gillberg, I.C., Hellgren, L., Gillberg, C. (1993). Psychotic disorders diagnosed in adolescence. Outcome at age 30 years. *Journal of Child Psychology and Psychiatry*, **34**, 1173–85.

Gunderson, J.G., Phillips, K.A. (1991). A current view of the interface between borderline personality disorder and depression. *The American Journal of Psychiatry*, **148**, 967–75.

Hellgren, L., Gillberg, C., Enerskog, I. (1987). Antecedents of adolescent psychoses: a population-based study of school health problems in children who develop psychosis in adolescence. *Journal of the American Academy of Child and Adolescent Psychiatry*, **26**, 351–5.

Kelly, J.T., Koch, M., Buegel, D. (1976). Lithium carbonate in juvenile manic-depressive illness. *Disorder of the Nervous System*, **37**, 90–219.

Kutcher, S.P., Marton, P., Korenblum, M. (1990). Adolescent bipolar illness and personality disorder. *Journal of the American Academy of Child and Adolescent Psychiatry*, **29**, 355–8.

Lewis, M. (Ed.) (1991). *Child and Adolescent Psychiatry. A Comprehensive Textbook*. Baltimore, Maryland: Williams & Wilkins.

McClellan, J.M., Werry, J.S., Ham, N. (1993). A follow-up study of early onset psychosis: comparison between outcome diagnoses of schizophrenia, mood disorders, and personality disorders. *Journal of Autism and Developmental Disorders*, **23**, 243–62.

McGlashan, T.H. (1988). Adolescent versus adult onset of mania. *American Journal of Psychiatry*, **145**, 221–3.

Nurcombe, B. (1991). The development of attention, perception, and memory. *In* Lewis, M. (Ed.) *Child and Adolescent Psychiatry. A Comprehensive Textbook*. Baltimore, MD: Williams & Wilkins.

Nurcombe, B., Seifer, R., Scioli, A., Tramontana, M.G., Grapentine, W.L., Beauchesne, H.C. (1989). Is major depressive in adolescence a distinct diagnostic entity? *Journal of the American Academy of Child and Adolescent Psychiatry*, **28**, 333–42.

Preskorn, S.H., Weller, E.B., Hughes, C.W., Weller, R.A., Bolte, K. (1987). Depression in prepubertal children: dexamethasone nonsuppression predicts differential response to imipramine vs. placebo. *Psychopharmacology Bulletin*, **23**, 128–33.

Puig-Antich, J., Perel, J.M., Lupatkin, W., Chambers, W.J., Tabrizi, M.A., King, J., Goetz, R., Davies, M., Stiller, R.L. (1987). Imipramine in prepubertal major depressive disorders. *Archives of General Psychiatry*, **44**, 81–9.

Steinberg, D. (1985). Psychotic and other severe disorders in adolescence. *In* Hersov, L., Rutter, M. (Eds.) *Child and Adolescent Psychiatry: Modern Approaches*. Oxford: Blackwell Scientific.

Strober, M., Morrell, W., Lampert, C., Burroughs, J. (1990). Relapse following discontinuation of lithium maintenance therapy in adolescents with bipolar I illness: a naturalistic study. *American Journal of Psychiatry*, **147**, 457–61.

Weller, E.B., Weller, R.A. (1991a). Grief. *In* Lewis, M. (Ed.) *Child and Adolescent Psychiatry. A Comprehensive Textbook*. Baltimore, Maryland: Williams & Wilkins.

Weller, E.B., Weller, R.A. (1991b). Mood Disorder. *In* Lewis, M. (Ed.) *Child and Adolescent Psychiatry. A Comprehensive Textbook*. Baltimore, Maryland: Williams & Wilkins.

Weller, E.B., Weller, R.A., Fristad, M.A., Bowes, J.M. (1990). Dexamethasone suppression test and depressive symptoms in bereaved children: a preliminary report. *Journal of Neuropsychiatry and Clinical Neuroscience*, **2**, 418–21.

Weller, R.A., Weller, E.B., Tucker, S.G., Fristad, M.A. (1986). Mania in prepubertal children: has it been underdiagnosed? *Journal of Affective Disorders*, **11**, 151–4.

Werry, J.S. (1992a). Child and adolescent (early onset) schizophrenia: a review in light of DSM-III-R. *Journal of Autism and Developmental Disorders*, **22**, 601–24.

Werry, J.S. (1992b). Child psychiatric disorders: are they classifiable? *British Journal of Psychiatry*, **161**, 472–80.

Wise, M.G., Rundell, J.R. (1988). *Concise Guide to Consultation Psychiatry*. Washington, DC: APA.

12 Traumatic brain injury and its neuropsychiatric sequelae

Traumatic brain injury occurs commonly. Yet it has attracted little study in childhood. It has been estimated that, in the US alone, each year about 75 000 people sustain 'new' brain injury and are left with significant disability (Kraus, Fife & Conroy, 1987). Many of these brain injuries pertain to children. In the late 1970s as many as 90% of closed head injury victims may have died. Nowadays 90% survive (Gualtieri, 1990). Traumatic brain injury to the brain is one of the most common causes of death in childhood and a common cause of chronic brain syndromes in children. Neurological damage can occur for a number of reasons. Acceleration and deceleration of the brain within the hard bone structure of the skull can produce contusion of the nervous system and subarachnoid haemorrhage. Shearing stress may develop during acceleration and deceleration because of the different densities of different parts of the brain. Cerebral oedema is a common complication, as are infection and haematoma. The repair process itself can contribute to further problems, for instance by unsuccessful rewiring. It is essential that the clinician responsible for the work-up and treatment of young people with traumatic brain injury regard each case individually: there are many causes and processes involved in brain injury and the cognitive and psychiatric sequelae will vary in severity and type from one child to another.

Epidemiology

Childhood accidents are the most common causes of acute brain injury. In several studies (Berfenstam et al., 1957; Sibert, Maddocks & Brown, 1981; Nathorst Westfelt, 1982), accidents have been reported to occur at an annual incidence of 10–20% of the child population (0–16 years). Of these, about one-third lead to injuries to the head and neck and less than 1% to fractures of the skull. In the study by Nathorst Westfelt (1982), from the city of Göteborg, 0.86% of all children under age 16 years sustained either a skull fracture or brain contusion during the course of one year. This incidence is similar to that found by Rune in Umeå (Rune, 1970): 1% of boys and 0.5% of girls aged 7–16 years suffered acute head injuries associated with primary cerebral symptoms of 'some degree of severity' during the course of one year.

Open head injuries are relatively uncommon, except in times of war. Closed head injuries represent the mainstay of traumatic head injuries incurred by young people today. The clinical problems of mild closed head injuries have been documented in several epidemiological studies, and although there is a literature maintaining that mild head injury is really of no, or at least very little, long-term consequence, the bulk of the evidence really suggests that it probably is (Gualtieri, 1990).

In closed head injury, damage to the central nervous system may occur anywhere in the cortex and in subcortical or brainstem structures. Diffuse degeneration of cerebral white matter (=axons) occurs after mechanical forces shear the nerve fibre at the moment of impact. Such diffuse degeneration has been described in humans as well as in subhuman primates (Blumbergs, Jones & North, 1989).

Perhaps the most unfortunate outcome for the survivor of closed head injury is that he/she will usually be confronted with a less than informed attitude on the part of psychiatrists and neurologists. Only conventional psychiatric diagnoses will be applied (in spite of generally being inadequate in this field), conventional neurological examination will show nothing or very little, and the victim of mild closed head injury may well be treated as if he/she were only imagining that something is wrong.

Neuropsychiatric outcome of traumatic brain injury

One of the very few students of traumatic brain injury, Thomas Gualtieri, recently summarized the neuropsychiatric outcome for people suffering traumatic brain injury in the following way: 'The neurobehavioral sequelae of TBI (traumatic brain injury) are effects on complex arrays of behavior, cognition, and emotional expression. They include psychiatric disorders such as depression, psychosis, disinhibition, abulia, dysregulation, hypochondriasis, insomnia, bulimia, and pathological drinking. They also include the traditional neurological sequelae, epilepsy, low arousal, hypersomnolence, post-traumatic headache, and migraine. They include, too, many of the higher cognitive functions that are usually the precinct of the neuropsychologist, like deficits in memory, attention, and executive function' (Gualtieri, 1990). Gualtieri was referring to traumatic brain injury generally, and not specifically to children or adolescents. Clinical experience suggests that the same type of problems that affect adults after closed head injuries may well pertain to adolescents also. Very little is known about preadolescent children in this respect.

In mild head injury, the post-concussion syndrome is said to be common, but data relating to children and adolescents are lacking. In adults, even after only transient unconsciousness or confusion and no anatomic evidence of brain damage there may be headache, dizziness, irritability, difficulty concentrating and alcohol intolerance. Fatigue, anergia, depression, insomnia and memory deficits are also commonly reported features.

The long-term neuropsychiatric sequelae of traumatic brain injury are only partly understood. There is a suggestion, inferred from the findings that adult patients suffering stroke have high rates of depression (Robinson, Starr & Price, 1984), that affective disorder may be one outcome. Indeed, one report by McKinlay et al. (1981) showed that more than 50% of patients with traumatic brain injury had depressive symptoms, and another one (Levin et al., 1987) showed that more than one-third of those with mild head injuries had such problems. However, none of these studies included adequate control measures, and they did not refer to children. Therefore, the possibility of a specific link with affective disorder remains tentative.

Delayed amnesia, occurring at about 2 years after injury, has also been reported (Gualtieri & Cox, 1991), but conclusions have to await further study in the field.

There is little doubt that post-traumatic epilepsy may occur even after closed head injuries, but that it is very much more common in the aftermath of open head injury (Annegers et al., 1980; Jennett, 1979; Salazar et al., 1985). Seizures may develop in the acute stage (up to 7 days after injury), but should not be taken as diagnostic of post-traumatic epilepsy. EEG abnormalities in the first few months do not necessarily predict later seizure activity, but the persistence of epileptogenic discharge on the EEG possibly does (Aicardi, 1986). True post-traumatic epilepsy usually takes more than several months, sometimes years, to develop.

Dementia of the Alzheimer type may develop as a long-term complication of traumatic brain injury. In patients with Alzheimer's disease, one of the few factors that are known to increase the risk is the record of traumatic brain injury earlier in life. It seems that the risk of developing dementia in a traumatic brain injury population is about four times that of the general population (French et al., 1985). There is also a considerable risk that symptoms of dementia may emerge at a younger age than in Alzheimer's disease without traumatic brain injury. Whether or not very young children sustaining traumatic brain injury have a considerably increased risk of developing dementia later in life is not known.

In severe traumatic brain injury, with prolonged unconsciousness, the range of outcomes is vast. Anything from mild sequelae to dementia and major motility problems may occur. For a fuller discussion of aspects of severe traumatic brain injury, the reader is referred to Gualtieri (1990).

In studies by Chadwick and colleagues (Chadwick *et al.*, 1981*a*, *b*, *c*), only children with injuries to the head severe enough to produce post-traumatic amnesia of at least 1 week developed behavioural and/or cognitive sequelae in the longer term. They also established that psychiatric disorder can arise *de novo* after severe head injury, even in the absence of any persistent neurological abnormalities. Socially disinhibited behaviour tended to be particularly common, but otherwise the same types of behaviour problems as shown by children in the general population were found. Cognitive impairment tends to be general rather than specific, even though speed of visuomotor information processing may be particularly affected. Furthermore, above a certain threshold (below which mild head injury will not lead to sequelae), there appears to be a dose-response relationship such that the degree of cognitive impairment can be predicted by the severity of the injury (Chadwick *et al.*, 1981*a*,*b*,*c*).

The locus of brain injury may be important in determining the type of symptoms: mania has developed in children with right hemisphere or limbic damage (Salle & Kindlon, 1987), whereas the symptom of depression has been noted more often when there have been injuries in the right frontal and left posterior regions (Shaffer *et al.*, 1985).

Children with the best recovery after severe brain trauma with unconsciousness lasting more than 90 days appear to be those who show minimal cerebral atrophy on CT 2 months after the injury (Kriel, Krach & Sheean, 1988).

There is a great need for intensified research on traumatic brain injuries in children. Pioneering studies were carried out already in the 1960s by Nylander and colleagues (Nylander &

Koersner, 1952;, Hjern & Nylander, 1962; Rune, 1970), but since then, except for occasional reports (Brown *et al.*, 1981), this clinically vitally important area of child neuropsychiatry, has been virtually abandoned by researchers. The crucial point to take into account when planning future studies in the field is the need to secure as close to a prospective approach as possible. Thus, in order to be able to study the emergence of psychiatric, behavioural and emotional problems after brain injury, one would have to ascertain the level of such problems immediately at first report that the injury has occurred. Retrospective studies in this field are likely to contribute little to our better understanding of brain–behaviour relationships.

Children at increased risk of sustaining traumatic brain injury

There appears to be a considerably increased risk for hyperactive children and children suffering from DAMP to be involved in accidents including the types that lead to fractures (Taylor, 1986; Gillberg & Gillberg, 1989; Taylor *et al.*, 1991; Hellgren *et al.*, 1993). Although, the type of injury involved is most often mild, some of these children and adolescents contract traumatic head injuries. Indirect data (Rune, 1970; Nathorst Westfelt, 1982) also support the view that children from disadvantaged psychosocial circumstances may have an increased risk of sustaining head injuries.

Children with autism and other forms of severe developmental disorders because of attention, motor control and planning deficits are liable to expose themselves to particularly dangerous situations (such as falling from rooftops and trees, being hit by buses, trains or cars, and drowning). They may well suffer traumatic brain injury as a result of this. Furthermore, a considerable proportion of the mentally retarded population (including those with autism) shows severe self-injury. It is not exceptional for a severely mentally retarded adolescent with autism to show frightening self-mutilating behaviours including smashing, knocking, banging and crashing of the skull. Such behaviour can lead to traumatic brain injury and contribute to a vicious circle in which the brain damage underlying the developmental disorder is aggravated, not only by the commonly occurring seizure activity, but also by the self-inflicted brain injury.

Children with epilepsy may also be at greatly increased risk of suffering traumatic brain injury. A very delicate interplay may occur in such cases. According to Gualtieri (1990), mesial temporal lobe sclerosis is a common result of brain injury. Such sclerosis, in turn, is commonly associated with epilepsy, and particularly with complex partial seizures. Such seizures are accompanied by severe psychiatric and adjustment problems in a majority of the cases (Lindsay, Ounsted & Richards, 1979, 1980). If the child is then exposed to further brain injury, such as might occur during a generalized seizure episode, both because of anoxia and trauma, a vicious circle may be perpetuated.

References

Aicardi, J. (1986). Consequences and prognosis of convulsive status epilepticus in infants and children. *Japan Journal of Psychiatry and Neurology*, **40**, 283–90.

Annegers, J.F., Grabow, J.D., Grover, R.D., Laws, E.R., Elverback, L.R., Kurland, L.T. (1980). Seizures after head trauma: a population study. *Neurology*, **30**, 683–9.

Berfenstam, R., Ehrenpreis, T., Ekström, G., Garsten, P., Myrin, S.O. (1957). Barnolycksfallen i Stockholm år 1955. *Svensk Läkartidning*, **54**, 1950 (In Swedish).

Blumbergs, P.C., Jones, N.R., North, J.B. (1989). Diffuse axonal injury in head trauma. *Journal of Neurology, Neurosurgery and Psychiatry*, **52**, 838–41.

Brown, G., Chadwick, O., Shaffer, D., Rutter, M., Traub, M. (1981). A prospective study of children with head injuries: III. Psychiatric sequelae. *Psychological Medicine*, **11**, 63–78.

Chadwick, O., Rutter, M., Brown, G., Shaffer, D., Traub, M.U. (1981a). A prospective study of children with head injuries: II. Cognitive sequelae. *Psychological Medicine*, **11**, 49–61.

Chadwick, O., Rutter, M., Shaffer, D., Shrou, P.E. (1981b). A prospective study of children with head injuries: IV. Specific cognitive deficits. *Journal of Clinical Neuropsychology*, **3**, 101–20.

Chadwick, O., Rutter, M., Thompson, J., Shaffer, D. (1981c). Intellectual performance and reading skills after localized head injury in childhood. *Journal of Child Psychology and Psychiatry*, **22**, 117–39.

French, L.R., Schuman, L.M., Mortimer, J.A., Hutton, J.T., Boatman, R.A., Christians, B. (1985). A case-control study of dementia of the Alzheimer type. *American Journal of Epidemiology*, **121**, 414–21.

Gillberg, I.C., Gillberg, C. (1989). Children with preschool minor neurodevelopmental disorders. IV: Behaviour and school achievement at age 13. *Developmental Medicine and Child Neurology*, **31**, 3–13.

Gualtieri, C.T. (1990). *Neuropsychiatry and Behavioral Pharmacology*. New York: Springer Verlag.

Gualtieri, T., Cox, D.R. (1991). The delayed neurobehavioural sequelae of traumatic brain injury. *Brain Injury*, **5**, 219–32.

Hellgren, L., Gillberg, C., Gillberg, I.C., Enerskog, I. (1993). Children with deficits in attention, motor control and perception (DAMP) almost grown up. General health at age 16 years. *Developmental Medicine and Child Neurology*, **35**, 881–92.

Hjern, B., Nylander, I. (1962). Late prognosis of severe head injuries in childhood. *Archives of Disease in Childhood*, **37**, 113–.

Jennett, B. (1979). Posttraumatic epilepsy. *Advances in Neurology*, **22**, 137–47.

Kraus, J.F., Fife, D., Conroy, C. (1987). Pediatric brain injuries: the nature, clinical course, and early outcomes in a defined United States' population. *Pediatrics*, **79**, 501–7.

Kriel, R.L., Krach, L.E., Sheean, M. (1988). Pediatric closed head injury: Outcome following prolonged unconsciousness. *Archives of Physical and Medical Rehabilitation*, **69**, 678–81.

Levin, H.S., Gary, H.E., High, W.M., et al. (1987). Minor head injury and the postconcussional syndrome: methodological issues in outcome studies. *In* Levin, H.S., Grafman, J.,Eisenberg, H.M. (Eds.) *Neurobehavioral recovery from head injury*. New York: Oxford University Press.

Lindsay, J., Ounsted, C., Richards, P. (1979). Long-term outcome in children with temporal lobe seizures. 3. Psychiatrics aspects in childhood and adult life. *Developmental Medicine and Child*

Neurology, **21**, 630–6.

Lindsay, J., Ounsted, C., Richards, P. (1980). Long-term outcome in children with temporal lobe seizures. IV: Genetic factors, febrile convulsions and the remission of seizures. *Developmental Medicine and Child Neurology*, **22**, 429–39.

McKinlay, W.W., Brooks, D.N., Martinage, D.P., Marschall, M.M. (1981). The short-term outcome of severe blunt head injury as reported by relatives of the injured person. *Journal of Neurology, Neurosurgery and Psychiatry*, **44**, 527–33.

Nathorst Westfelt, J. (1982). Evnironmental factors in childhood accidents. A prospective study in Göteborg, Sweden. *Acta Paediatrica Scandinavica*, **Suppl. 291**.

Nylander, I., Koersner, P.E. (1952). Electroencephalography and cerebral lesions. A clinical investigation on children. *Journal of Clinical and Experimental Psychopathology*, **13**, 164.

Robinson, R.G., Starr, L.B., Price, T.R. (1984). A two year longitudinal study of mood disorders following stroke: prevalance and duration at six months follow-up. *British Journal of Psychiatry*, **144**, 256–62.

Rune, V. (1970). *Acute Head Injuries in Children.*

An Epidemilogic, Child Psychiatric and Electroencephalographic Study on Primary School Children in Umeå. M.D. Thesis. University of Umeå.

Salazar, A.M., Jabbari, B., Vance, S.C., Grafman, J., Amin, D., Dillon, J.D. (1985). Epilepsy after penetrating head injury. I. Clinical correlates: a report of the Vietnam Head Injury Study. *Neurology*, **35**, 1406–14.

Salle, N.D., Kindlon, D.J. (1987). Lateralized brain injury and behavior problems in children. *Journal of Abnormal Child Psychology*, **15**, 479–91.

Shaffer, D., Schonfeld, I., O'Connor, P., Stokman, C., Trautman, P., Shafer, S., Ng, S. (1985). Neurological soft signs. Their relationship to psychiatric disorder and intelligence in childhood and adolescence. *Archives of General Psychiatry*, **42**, 342–51.

Sibert, J.R., Maddocks, G.B., Brown, B.M. (1981). Childhood accidents – an endemic of epidemic proportion. *Archives of Diseases in Childhood*, **56**, 225–7.

Taylor, E. (1986). Childhood hyperactivity. *British Journal of Psychiatry*, **149**, 562–73.

Taylor, E., Sandberg, S., Thorley, G., Giles, S. (1991). *The Epidemiology of Childhood Hyperactivity.* London: Institute of Psychiatry.

13 Epilepsy and psychiatric problems in childhood

Psychiatric, behavioural and emotional problems in children with various neurological disorders constitute a sadly neglected area from the point of view of systematic scientific study (Matthews, Barabas & Ferrari, 1982; Gillberg, 1991). In spite of the fact that behavioural and emotional problems are often extremely frustrating for families of children with neurological disorder (Taylor & Lochery, 1991), very little, in fact, is known about epidemiology or transactional chains of events in pathogenesis and intervention. The systematic study of behavioural effects (wanted and unwanted) of antiepileptic drugs in the treatment of children and adolescents has been extremely limited (Taylor, 1991).

Furthermore, neuropsychiatric disorders that are not epilepsy but that are akin to epilepsy also exist (Deonna, 1993). Regarding these disorders even less is known (Deonna et al., 1994). Surprisingly, there has been slightly more systematic study of anti-epileptic drug treatment in such disorders in children and adolescents.

Epilepsy is associated with a particularly high rate of psychiatric disorder. According to the Isle of Wight study, uncomplicated epilepsy carries a four-fold increase of the risk that the child will also have psychiatric problems. Almost 30% of 10–11 year-old children with uncomplicated epilepsy had psychiatric problems in that study (Rutter, Graham & Yule, 1970). Children with epilepsy accompanying other neurological disorders had psychiatric problems in 60% of cases. This latter figure represented a prevalence rate almost ten times that found in the general population on the Isle of Wight. Only children with deficits in attention, motor control and perception (DAMP) have severe psychiatric problems at an equally high rate (Gillberg, 1983).

The causes of psychiatric disorder in epilepsy are manifold and include (1) direct effects of the underlying aetiological factor, (2) specific effects of abnormal brain activity as such, (3) epilepsy itself, including its possible disruption of new learning, (4) neuropathic sequelae of fits, (5) the influence of various drugs and (6) experiential and social factors.

Direct effects of the underlying aetiologic factor can be seen, for instance, in tuberous sclerosis (Hunt & Shepherd, 1993), a neurocutaneous disorder which may present with behavioural problems long before the onset of seizure (Gillberg I.C., Gillberg & Ahlsén, 1994c). Similar associations may be seen in hypothyroidism (Gillberg I.C., Gillberg & Kopp, 1992) and Rett syndrome (Hagberg et al., 1983).

The type and location of the brain dysfunction causing epilepsy is important in determining the type and degree of problems encountered. Temporal lobe dysfunction (as in complex partial seizures which is often associated with mesial temporal sclerosis) tends to carry a particularly high risk for certain types of severe psychiatric problems, including hyperactivity, aggressiveness and psychosis (Taylor, 1969, 1975; Lindsay, Ounsted & Richards, 1979). Another example of the way the location of abnormal brain activity may affect the type of behavioural problems shown by the child is the so-called benign partial epilepsy of child-hood with Rolandic spikes. This is the most common type of partial motor epilepsy in child-hood, accounting for more than one in five of all school age epilepsies (Deonna, 1993). The seizure (often involving symptoms of the mouth and pharynx: drooling, dysarthria, dysphagia or speech loss (Deonna, 1993) and chewing and oral and vocal tics imitating Tourette syndrome (Gillberg & Törnblom, 1994)) is believed to be generated by (dominantly inherited) focal corti-cal (Rolandic–sylvian region in front of the sylvian fissure of the cerebral motor cortex which controls the movements of the mouth and pharynx) hyperexcitability, closely linked to brain maturation processes (such as those occurring around the time of puberty) and not associated with identifiable underlying circums-cribed brain lesions (Doose & Baier, 1989).

Psychotic behaviour can also be part of the ictal epileptic phenomena as such (Gillberg & Schaumann, 1983). It has been shown that temporary decrease in cognitive performance coincides with discharge activity on the EEG, even in cases where there are no other clinical manifestations of seizure activity (Aarts et al., 1984; Kasteleijn-Nolst Trénité et al., 1990).

Among the drugs that contribute to beha-vioural problems are, unfortunately, many of the substances used because of their anti-epilep-tic properties (Gillberg, 1991; Cueva et al., 1993).

Among the social factors that contribute most to the development of emotional problems in epilepsy (Hartlage & Green, 1972; Taylor & Lochery, 1991), stigmatization asso-ciated with prejudice and ignorance is clearly one of the most important (Taylor, 1969).

Type of psychiatric disorder associated with epilepsy

Any kind of psychiatric problem can co-exist with epilepsy and be either related (most likely) or unrelated to the epilepsy as such. In temporal lobe seizures, hyperkinetic syndromes, rage and 'psychosis' tend to be relatively common complications.

IQ is within the normal range in most child-ren and adolescents with epilepsy and it tends to remain at the same level over the years, unless there is clear associated brain *damage* (Ellen-berg, Hirtz & Nelson, 1986). School perfor-mance, however, is usually poorer than in the general population of children without epilepsy (Rodin, Schmaltz & Twitty, 1986). This is pro-bably a reflection both of subtle cognitive abnormalities (not necessarily picked up by the IQ-test), seizure activity interfering with learn-ing and a host of psychological and social factors.

It has been well documented that a minority of children with epilepsy show widely fluctuat-ing performance on IQ-tests over time and that some deteriorate in intellectual functioning or show associated language and social–commu-nication disorders (Chaudhry & Pond, 1961; Deonna, 1993).

Hyperkinetic syndrome (often associated with aggressiveness) was present in 30% of one relatively large British series of complex partial seizure patients followed through childhood to adult age (Lindsay, Ounsted & Richards, 1979). This was particularly common in males, if in the medical history there had been a clear insult to the brain, and if the onset of seizures was very early in life. Hyperkinetic syndromes tended to be associated with relatively low IQ (median 70 in the reported study) and the social outcome for adult life was relatively poor. Hyperkinetic syndromes may now be less common among children with complex partial seizures, partly because of the less widespread use of drugs that can lead to hyperkinetic behaviour (particularly phenobarbitone, primidone and some of the benzodiazepines).

Rage was also a common phenomenon in the British follow-up study (affecting about 40% of the whole group). A poor prognosis with regard to social adjustment and development of adult psychiatric disorder was common in this sub-group also. Girls with rage had very low IQ levels, whereas most boys functioned in the normal IQ range.

About 10% of the group with complex par-tial seizures had developed psychosis (often of a schizophreniform character) in early adult life.

Almost all of the patients were male, they had not shown early remission and were still on anticonvulsants. In no case did the EEG show a right-sided focus and there was a tendency for left-sided foci to be very common. Interestingly, on the basis of studies performed in adults with epilepsy, it has been suggested that left-sided foci may predispose to schizophreniform psychosis and right-sided foci to affective psychosis. In one study comparing individuals with epilepsy only with individuals with the combination of epilepsy and psychosis, PET-scan demonstrated a significant reduction of oxygen metabolism in the temporal and frontal lobes of the dominant hemisphere in the latter group (Gallhofer et al., 1985).

There might be two further psychiatric subgroups of people with temporal lobe seizures (most likely overlapping with some of the subgroups already described). Children with autism seem to show a very high risk of developing complex partial seizures (Gillberg, 1991). Whether or not there is also a high rate of autism or autism spectrum problems in complex partial seizures generally remains to be investigated. Obsessive–compulsive features in relation to such seizures have not been systematically examined, but clinical experience suggests that they may be relatively more common than in the general population (Taylor, D., 1991, personal communication).

Seizures that are particularly hard to treat are often strongly associated with psychiatric and behavioural deviance. Such seizures, i.e. convulsive disorders that require several different drugs and yet do not show good seizure control, are often of a mixed type and signal underlying widespread brain dysfunction. In a recent study, children with treatment-resistant epilepsy and mental retardation showed an extremely high rate of autistic symptoms, autistic disorder and hyperkinetic syndrome (Steffenburg et al., personal communication). Children with Lennox–Gastaut epilepsy (centrencephalic myoclonic–astatic petit mal), usually notoriously resistant to therapy, generally show stagnation and severe developmental regression (Doose & Völzke, 1979).

In other types of seizures, the evidence for a connection with specific emotional and behavioural problems is very limited. Autistic symptoms may accompany childhood absence epilepsy (Gillberg & Schaumann, 1983), juvenile myoclonic epilepsy and infantile spasms (Riikonen & Amnell, 1981; Coleman & Gillberg, 1985).

Paroxysmal multifocal discharges which tend to increase during sleep are characteristic of the Landau–Kleffner syndrome (see Chapter 8), also referred to as 'acquired epileptic aphasia'.

Childhood absence epilepsy is a rare, but important, underlying problem in certain cases of DAMP. Febrile seizures before age 5 years may be a sign of abnormal brain maturation which could present with DAMP symptoms in the school-age child without epilepsy or seizure activity (Hellgren et al., 1993).

The specific symptoms associated with benign epilepsy of childhood have already been mentioned. Because of the strong association of certain seizure types (e.g. myoclonic epilepsies) with mental retardation, there is also an especially strong correlation between such seizures and psychiatric disorder.

Anticonvulsant drugs

Behavioural side effects are very common, especially if drugs specifically targeted at influencing the brain are used. The anticonvulsants are such drugs. They constitute a major psychiatric risk for some children with epilepsy. Phenobarbitone and phenyotin both very often cause somnolence, irritability, restlessness, hyperactivity, rage and decreased learning. In the last 5 years, similar symptoms, sometimes even more dramatic, have been noted to concur with medication with the benzodiazepines. Drugs such as clonazepam appear to have a particularly deleterious effect in the treatment of early childhood epilepsies in which there are already at the time of commencing treatment some behaviour problems. It is not uncommon for major psychotic/autistic symptoms to develop (Gillberg, 1991). Withdrawal of the drug can occasionally lead to complete remission of such symptoms without increasing the seizure rate. Carbamazepine and valproic acid can also cause psychic reactions (Cueva *et al.*, 1993) (including increased compulsiveness, irritability and aggression, and, in exceptional cases, psychosis), but probably at much lower rates (Evans, Clay & Gaultieri, 1987). Also, both these drugs have been reported to have some genuinely positive effects on psychic functions.

These clinical observations of an occasionally deleterious effect on psychological and neuropsychiatric 'performance' of some antiepileptic drugs (Trimble & Cull, 1989) have to be tempered by the dearth of systematic study in the field. Most of the studies performed to date (and they are quite few) have severe methodological limitations (Taylor, 1991).

The teratogenicity of anticonvulsant drugs (Steinhausen, Rauss-Mason & Seidel, 1991) has been discussed in Chapter 3.

Psychosocial factors in epilepsy

Children with epilepsy, because of the nature of their ailment, may be more likely than other children with chronic illness to be dependent and experience control of events in their lives as external (Matthews *et al.*, 1982; Hoare, 1984*a*, *b*, *c*). Mothers of children with epilepsy tend to have less expectation of their achievement than they do for their siblings without epilepsy (Ferrari, 1984).

The dramatic psychological effects that seeing a child have a major seizure might have on parents, siblings, friends, peers, teachers and others can lead to transactional effects which may lead to stigmatization of the child. Most parents seeing their child have a first major convulsion feel convinced that the child is going to die. These almost inevitable psychological consequences need to be dealt with in tactful and neutral ways by the child's doctor. Lack of education about epilepsy may be one reason for the stigmatization so often associated with epilepsy and educative measures aimed at decreasing such ignorance are important in any treatment plan for childhood epilepsy, There may be all sorts of strange beliefs concerning epilepsy

which may lead to a generally prejudiced attitude to the child affected by seizures. One must not forget either that the child with seizures very often appears to have 'gone mad'. It is essential that the mechanisms underlying this 'madness' be explained to those involved in interactions with the child, so that in their eyes, the strange behaviour does not take on mystical implications.

Equally important is the implementation of a 'intervention strategy' in the case of seizures recurring in families of children who suffer from epilepsy. Parents and siblings need to be taught how to take care of the child once a seizure (perhaps producing lack of consciousness in the patient) has started. The strategy may have to differ considerably from one setting and situation to another. These matters will have to be dealt with in some detail, and, preferably, on several different occasions. Oral as well as written information should be provided. Some of the social and psychological handicaps of families with children and adolescents with epilepsy may be minimized if information of this kind is given early in the course of the seizure disorder.

Treatment of pscyhiatric problems in epilepsy

Before planning treatment of psychiatric problems in epilepsy it is necessary to analyse (1) the various factors which contribute to the psychiatric disorder (the epilepsy itself, the type of associated brain damage/dysfunction, the effects of drug treatment, constitutional factors related or unrelated to the epilepsy and various psychosocial factors) and (2) which type of problem (the epilepsy or the psychiatric disorder) is currently having the most negative impact on the child and family. The doctor will need to know the family's view and their need for specific help. Quite often the behavioural consequences of the seizure disorder, rather than the number of seizures *per se*, are perceived by brothers and sisters and mothers and fathers as considerably stronger contributors to negative effects on quality of life. In such cases, just monitoring the rate of seizures will not help improve family life. After an analysis of this kind, the doctor in charge will have to discuss the various treatment options at some length with the parents, and sometimes with the patient, depending on developmental level.

The management of psychiatric problems in epilepsy constitutes a very delicate balance between consideration of environmental measures, education, drugs, and, in treatment-resistant epilepsy, surgery. A neuropsychiatrist well acquainted with epilepsy must be an integral part of the team in charge of treatment of children with epilepsy. In the past, all too many children with epilepsy received drug treatment and diets and their seizure frequency was used as the only measure of outcome without due attention being paid to behaviour and emotion. Behavioural problems, once the seizure disorder has become less psychologically dramatic to people in the environment, are often considered by the parents and teachers as more difficult to cope with than the epilepsy as such. Alleviating some of the psychiatric problems in epilepsy often reduces the frequency and severity of fits.

Epilepsy brain surgery

Children with treatment resistant epilepsy who opt for surgical treatment, should receive a neuropsychiatric (and not only neuropsychological) assessment before, and a year after, surgery at the very least. In many centres at the present time, this need is sadly neglected. Outcome after surgical interventions can never be comprehensively evaluated unless there is a full appreciation of the neuropsychiatric problems associated with epilepsy. The fact that so many children with epilepsy are affected by severe psychiatric disorder (including DAMP, hyperactivity, autistic-like conditions and autism) before any intervention is undertaken should make the need for neuropsychiatric evaluation obvious. Taken with the evidence that anti-epileptic drug treatment may affect behaviour both positively and negatively, there should not be a need to discuss whether or not it is appro-

priate to include such evaluation in the follow-up of children who have been subjected to brain surgery in the treatment of seizure disorders.

There is already some data to indicate that behaviour and emotions can be positively affected by appropriate brain surgery in connection with treatment resistant epilepsy (Ounsted, Lindsay & Richards, 1987; Uvebrant et al., 1993). In the experience of the author, children with the combination of treatment-resistant epilepsy, autism or autistic features, explosive outbursts of rage and a tendency to generally disorganized negative behaviour (a common combination in treatment resistant epilepsy), may benefit greatly from epilepsy surgery. The few cases examined to date make generalized conclusions impossible, but it appears that, if the operation leads to dramatic reduction of seizure frequency, and if anti-epileptic drugs can be reduced or even withdrawn there is good hope that hyperactive, disorganized, negative and explosive behaviour problems will be considerably reduced, even in cases where there is little or no improvement in the basic deficits associated with the autistic symptoms.

References

Aarts, H.P., Binnie, C.D., Smit, A.M., Wilkins, A.J. (1984). Selective cognitive impairment during focal and generalized epileptiform EEG activity. *Brain*, **107**, 293–308.

Chaudhry, M.R., Pond, D.A. (1961). Mental deterioration in epileptic children. *Journal of Neurology, Neurosurgery and Psychiatry*, **24**, 213–19.

Coleman, M., Gillberg, C. (1985). *The Biology of the Autistic Syndromes*. New York: Praeger.

Cueva, J.E., Armenteros, J.L., Rosenberg, C.R., Campbell, M. (1993). Untoward effects of carbamazepine in hospitalized aggressive children with conduct disorder. Dept of Psychiatry, NYUMC.

Deonna, T. (1993). Annotation: cognitive and behavioural correlates of epileptic activity in children. *Journal of Child Psychology and Psychiatry*, **34**, 611–20.

Deonna, T., Davidoff, V., Despland, P.A., Roulet, E. (1994). Isolated disturbance of written language acquisition as an initial symptom of epileptic aphasia in a 7 year old child. A three years follow-up study. *Aphasiology*, In press.

Doose, H., Baier, W.K. (1989). Benign partial epilepsy and related conditions: multifactorial pathogenesis with hereditary impairment of brain maturation. *European Journal of Pediatrics*, **149**, 152–8.

Doose, H., Völzke, E. (1979). Petit mal status in early childhood and dementia. *Neuropediatrics*, **10**, 10–14.

Ellenberg, J.H., Hirtz, D.G., Nelson, K.B. (1986). Do seizures in children cause intellectual deterioration? *New England Journal of Medicine*, **314**, 1085–8.

Evans, R.W., Clay, T.H., Gualtieri, C.T. (1987). Carbamazepine in pediatric psychiatry. *Journal of the American Academy of Child and Adolescent Psychiatry*, **26**, 2–8.

Ferrari, M. (1984). Chronic illness: psychosocial effects on siblings. I. Chronically ill boys. *Journal of Child Psychology and Psychiatry*, **25**, 459–76.

Gallhofer, B., Trimble, M.R., Frackowiak, R., Gibbs, J., Jones, T. (1985). A study of cerebral blood flow and metabolism in epileptic psychosis using positron emission tomography and oxygen. *Journal of Neurology, Neurosurgery and Psychiatry*, **48**, 201–6.

Gillberg, C. (1983). Perceptual, motor and attentional deficits in Swedish primary school children. Some child psychiatric aspects. *Journal of Child Psychology and Psychiatry*, **24**, 377–403.

Gillberg, C. (1991). The treatment of epilepsy in autism. *Journal of Autism and Developmental Disorders*, **21**, 61–77.

Gillberg, C., Schaumann, H. (1983). Epilepsy presenting as infantile autism? Two case studies. *Neuropediatrics*, **14**, 206–12.

Gillberg, C., Törnblom, M. (1994). Tourette syndrome developing in a young woman with infantile autism, epilepsy, Rolandic spikes and neurofibromatosis. Submitted.

Gillberg, I.C., Gillberg, C., Ahlsén, G. (1994). Autistic behaviour and attention deficits in tuberous sclerosis. A population-based study. *Developmental Medicine and Child Neurology*, **36**, 50–6.

Gillberg, I.C., Gillberg, C., Kopp, S. (1992). Hypothyroidism and autism spectrum disorders. *Journal of Child Psychology and Psychiatry*, **33**, 531–42.

Hagberg, B., Aicardi, J., Dias, K., Ramos, O. (1983). A progressive syndrome of autism, dementia, ataxia and loss of purposeful hand use in girls: Rett's syndrome. Report of 35 cases.

Annals of Neurology, **14**, 471–9.

Hartlage, L.C., Green, J.B. (1972). The relation of parental attitudes to academic and social achievement in epileptic children. *Epilepsia*, **13**, 21–6.

Hellgren, L., Gillberg, C., Gillberg, I.C., Enerskog, I. (1993). Children with Deficits in Attention, Motor control and Perception (DAMP) almost grown up. General health at age 16 years. *Developmental Medicine and Child Neurology*, **35**, 881–92.

Hoare, P. (1984*a*). The development of psychiatric disorder among school children with epilepsy. *Developmental Medicine and Child Neurology*, **26**, 3–13.

Hoare, P. (1984*b*). Psychiatric disturbance in the families of epileptic children. *Developmental Medicine and Child Neurology*, **26**, 14–19.

Hoare, P. (1984*c*). Does illness foster dependency? A study of epileptic and diabetic children. *Developmental Medicine and Child Neurology*, **26**, 20–4.

Hunt, A., Shepherd, C. (1993). A prevalence study of autism in tuberous sclerosis. *Journal of Autism and Developmental Disorders*, **23**, 323–39.

Kasterleijn-Nolst Trénité, D.G.A., Smit, A.M., Velis, D.N., Villemse, J., van Emde, B.W. (1990). On-line detection of transient neuropsychological disturbances during EEG discharges in children with epilepsy. *Developmental Medicine and Child Neurology*, **32**, 46–50.

Lindsay, J., Ounsted, C., Richards, P. (1979). Long-term outcome in children with temporal lobe seizures. 3. Psychiatrics aspects in childhood and adult life. *Developmental Medicine and Child Neurology*, **21**, 630–6.

Matthews, W.S., Barabas, G., Ferrari, M. (1982). Emotional concomitants of childhood epilepsy. *Epilepsia*, **26**, 671–81.

Ounsted, C., Lindsay, J., Richards, P. (1987). *Temporal lobe epilepsy. A biographical study 1948–1986 (Clinics in Developmental Medicine No 103)*. Oxford: Mac Keith Press.

Riikonen, R., Amnell, G. (1981). Psychiatric disorders in children with earlier infantile spasms. *Developmental Medicine and Child Neurology*, **23**, 747–60.

Rodin, E.A., Schmaltz, S., Twitty, G. (1986). Intellectual functions of patients with childhood-onset epilepsy. *Developmental Medicine and Child Neurology*, **28**, 25–33.

Rutter, M., Graham, P., Yule, W. (1970). *A Neuropsychiatric Study in Childhood*. London: S.I.M.P./William Heinemann Medical Books Ltd.

Steinhausen, H.-C., Rauss-Mason, C., Seidel, R. (1991). Follow-up studies of anorexia nervosa: a review of four decades of outcome research. *Psychological Medicine*, **21**, 447–54.

Taylor, D. (1969). Some psychiatric aspects of epilepsy. *In* Herrington, C.R. (Ed.). *Current Problems in Neuropsychiatry. British Journal of Psychiatry, Special Publication No. 4.* Ashford, Kent: Hedley for the Royal Medico-Psychological Association.

Taylor, D. (1975). Factors influencing the occurrence of schizophrenia-like psychosis in patients with temporal lobe epilepsy. *Psychological Medicine*, **5**, 249–54.

Taylor, D.C., Lochery, M. (1991). Behavioral consequences of epilepsy in children. *Advances in Neurology*, **55**, 153–62.

Taylor, E. (1991). Developmental neuropsychiatry. *Journal of Child Psychology and Psychiatry*, **32**, 3–47.

Trimble, M.R., Cull, C.A. (1989). Antiepileptic drugs, cognitive function, and behavior in children. *Cleveland Clinical Journal of Medicine*, **56 Suppl**, S140–6; discussion S147–9.

Uvebrant, P., Bjure, J., Sixt, R., Witt Engerström, I., Hagberg, B. (1993). Regional cerebral blood flow: SPECT as a tool for localization of brain dysfunction. *In* Hagberg, B. (Ed.). *Rett Syndrome – Clinical & Biological Aspects. Clinics in Developemental Medicine No. 127.* London: Mac Keith Press.

14 Other neurological disorders/disabilities

Psychiatric aspects of other childhood neurological disorders have been dealt with even more summarily than behavioural and emotional problems in epilepsy. It is only in the last few years that interest in this clinically very important area has surfaced.

Infantile hydrocephalus

In the pre-surgical treatment days of infantile hydrocephalus, major neurological handicap was often so debilitating as to preclude the study of psychiatric problem.

In a recent Swedish study of a population-based group of surgically treated infantile hydrocephalus, behavioural problems and autistic symptoms were found to be very common. About one-fourth of all children with hydrocephalus had developed many autistic features by the time they reached school age. Hyperactivity problems and restlessness often associated with DAMP problems were also common. Autistic features and full-blown autism (which was present in 1 in 20 of all children with infantile hydrocephalus) were associated with severe mental retardation and severe brain damage. Other behavioural problems were associated with low IQ generally. Children with hydrocephalus who did not have a learning disorder did not appear to be at increased risk of psychiatric disorder (Fernell, Gillberg & von Wendt, 1991a, b). Self-esteem was somewhat lower than in children in general (Fernell, Gillberg & von Wendt, 1992).

In older studies (Hadenius et al., 1962), the so-called cocktail party syndrome was reported to be a common finding in children with hydrocephalus. This diagnosis was not made at all in the more recent Swedish study. The reason might be that surgical intervention (which was uncommon at the time when the older studies were performed) has changed the type of effects on the brain (and the behaviour) of the children. Another possibility is that some of the 'cocktail party symptoms' reported in the older studies may have been echolalia and lack of empathy. Such symptoms might now have been subsumed under the general heading of autistic features, so that, in fact, the difference between previous and recent findings, may be less pronounced than suggested by reported rates for cocktail party syndrome and autism. In a recent study, Dennis & Barnes (1993) found a high rate of deficits in the pragmatic use and understanding of language in discourse in a large group of shunt-operated 6–15 year-old children with hydrocephalus who had either, or both of, verbal or performance IQ above 70.

Cerebral palsy

Cerebral palsy is accompanied by an increased rate of psychiatric problems (at about the same level as or slightly higher than uncomplicated epilepsy) (Rutter, Graham & Yule, 1970). Nielsen (1966) reported that normally intelligent children with cerebral palsy exhibited three times higher rates of 'personality disorders' than age, sex-IQ and socioeconomic matched controls. However, to the author's knowledge, no systematic population-based study of psychiatric and behavioural problems in the whole spectrum of disorders diagnosed as cerebral palsy has ever been performed. Thus, very little is in fact known about the specifics of psychiatric and behavioural disorders in cerebral palsy.

Cognitive disability in CP is common, 50% to 70% are affected by mental retardation according to some surveys and a proportion suffers from milder learning disabilities (Scherzer & Tscharnuter, 1982). These cognitive impairments are likely to contribute to a high rate of psychiatric disorder. However, cognitive abilities are often very difficult to assess in a child with cerebral palsy who may, for instance, have quadriplegic motor disorder and be nonvocal due to neuromuscular involvement.

In severe cerebral palsy, such as spastic tetraplegia, indirect evidence suggests that the triad of autistic impairments may be very frequent (Wing & Gould, 1979; Edebol-Tysk, 1989a, b). This, if upheld in other systematic studies, could be taken to reflect the underlying severe widespread damage not only to high cortical brain areas, but to lower centres also.

In milder forms of cerebral palsy, clinical experience suggests that more common types of psychiatric problems may be prevalent. Emotional disorders, including anxiety states, are not uncommon in cerebral palsy, but since such problems are also common in the general population of children, it is quite difficult to decide whether such problems are more, or even less, common in cerebral palsy. In a study by Anderson, Clarke & Spain (1982) of physically handicapped 15 year-olds (comprising about 75% cases with cerebral palsy), depression, lack of self-confidence, worry and fearfulness were the most common problems. General irritability with tantrums or rages were also relatively common.

There are some case reports in the literature of Asperger syndrome (e.g. Gillberg, 1989) associated with mild cerebral palsy (hemiplegia, diplegia and ataxia). This association could represent clues to the underlying brain dysfunction in Asperger syndrome. Treatment in such cases should be along lines suggested both for the cerebral palsy problems and the Asperger-type problems.

Sibling relationships are affected in many cases of cerebral palsy (Dallas, Stevenson & McGurk, 1993a, b) with the disabled child being passive and lacking in assertiveness and the normal sibling being correspondingly more directive.

There are typical crisis points for the family with a child suffering from cerebral palsy. These have been described by Bax (1992) as follows: (1) the prediagnostic and diagnostic periods, (2) going to school and the realization that the child is not going to attend or function in an ordinary way in a normal school, (3) the attainment of puberty, and (4) the young adult's need to achieve independence. The family and child will need more (extra) counselling in connection with these crisis points. These general points could equally be made in relation to a whole host of other neuropsychiatric disorders, but they are definitely important to consider in cerebral palsy.

Even though the behavioural and emotional problems shown by many children with cerebral palsy may be similar to those encountered in normal children, this should not be taken to mean that the disability is not a factor in itself in causing the behaviour. This also holds in relation to the parents, who, in spite of not divorcing more often than other parents, if they divorce, often cite the child's disability as an important factor.

Brain tumours

Brain tumours, although rare, are among the most common forms of neoplasms in children, affecting as many as 5 in 100000 per year. Infratentorial tumours are the most common types. Increased intracranial pressure is common in such tumours, and onset of signs and symptoms may be insidious (Herskowitz & Rosman, 1982). Most tumours are of glial origin and metastases and meningiomas are rare.

Craniopharyngeomas and teratomas are

congenital tumours that arise from developmental malformations. The neurocutaneous syndromes (tuberous sclerosis, neurofibromatosis and ataxia-telangiectasia) often comprise intracranial tumours.

Infratentorial brain tumours

Tumours of the cerebellum, fourth ventricle and brainstem constitute the infratentorial brain tumours, all of which usually present with symptoms of increased intracranial pressure (mild, slowly progressing, morning headache; intermittent mild vomiting, slowly progressing; personality changes including irritability and restlessness, sometimes memory loss and academic impairment; double vision and strabismus; papilloedema; bulging fontanelle and delayed fontanelle closure and widened sutures in infants; increased blood pressure and *in*creased or decreased pulse, irregular respirations; diffuse slowing on EEG; generalized seizures). Other symptoms may be caused by brainstem compression and include progressive cranial nerve dysfunction (usually involving ocular and facial muscles), head tilt, cervical pain, nystagmus, ataxia and spasticity.

Astrocytomas (usually relatively benign) and medulloblastomas (rapid growing and highly malignant) are the two tumour types localized to the cerebellum. Onset in the former is usually insidious, in the latter dramatic. Medulloblastomas often affect the reticular activating system and may, in addition to vomiting, headache and ataxia, cause akinetic mutism (Daly & Love, 1958). Astrocytomas should be resected, shunting of CSF achieved if required, and radiation therapy given depending on degree of malignancy and extent of resection. Outcome is relatively good. In contrast, outcome in medulloblastomas, even if treated with resection, radiation therapy and chemotherapy, is often poor, and the five-year survival rate is only about 40% (Laurent & Cheek, 1986).

Ependymomas and choroid plexus papillomas are the two most common types of tumours in the fourth ventricle. Treatment is by resection and radiation therapy. The choroid plexus papillomas produce CSF and hence raise the intracranial pressure. Separation anxiety, school refusal and fearfulness for more than a year in addition to various somatic complaints have been reported in a 12 year-old boy with choroid plexus papilloma (Blackman & Wheeler, 1987). He had had macrocephaly, mild ataxia and motor incoordination from about age 2 years. Tumour resection resulted in amelioration of the psychiatric symptoms.

Brainstem tumours are usually gliomas of the pons and there is often a classic triad of progressive cranial nerve dysfunctions, hemiparesis (caused by compression of the pyramidal tracts) and ataxia/nystagmus (caused by compression of the cerebellar tracts). Radiation therapy and chemotherapy are treatments of first choice, as surgery does not alter outcome (Laurent & Cheek, 1986). Outcome is usually very poor.

Supratentorial brain tumours

The cerebral hemispheres are sometimes affected by brain tumours and include astrocytomas and glioblastomas together with a whole host of other tumour types which are very much rarer. Raised intracranial pressure is uncommon, except in very late stages. Personality changes are often the presenting symptoms, but may be very difficult to ascertain in young children. Intermittent irritability, depressions and decrements in school achievements, memory skills, social awareness and personal hygiene are common. Papilloedema and, particularly, localizing neurological signs usually occur considerably later and, unfortunately, are often the only problems which will lead the treating physician to consider a diagnosis of brain tumour (at a time when successful therapy may no longer be possible).

Parasellar tumours (arising in the proximity of the sella) usually cause endocrine and psychiatric symptoms. Cranipharyngiomas are much the most common of these (Richmond & Wilson, 1982), followed by optic nerve chiasm gliomas and astrocytomas and pinealomas. Craniopharyngiomas probably arise from remnants of the pharyngeal duct (the embryonic

Rathke pouch) in the proximity of the pituitary stalk. Growth retardation and delayed sexual maturation are common symptoms, but may be ascertained only in retrospect, once the diagnosis has already been made. Obesity, visual and olfactory hallucinations and alterations in body temperature may ensue. Somnolence, apathy, irritability, mood swings, sulkiness and social dysfunction (non-autistic, but with reduced empathy skills in group settings) are common neuropsychiatric symptoms. Focal neurological signs are uncommon. Diabetes insipidus is a common sign.

Work-up

If there is suspicion that a child may be suffering from a brain tumour, a full neurological examination is indicated, even though, sometimes, this will not provide firm evidence for or against the diagnosis. .A CT-scan and an MRI-scan should be performed. A skull X-ray may be indicated if there is a suspicion of craniopharyngioma. This examination may demonstrate midline calcification, erosion of the dorsum sellae or enlargement of the sella turcica or all three of these. If all these examinations are negative, the individual may nevertheless need further follow-up and examinations. Repeated EEGs may show changes (including diffuse slowing) over time. A SPECT may also help in diagnosis. A full neuropsychological work-up, including appropriate IQ-tests repeated at 2–6 month intervals may also aid in diagnosis in difficult cases with slow-growing tumours.

Once a diagnosis of brain tumour has been made, the child should always receive a full neuropsychiatric assessment, including in-depth examination by a trained child neuropsychiatrist and a trained child neuropsychologist. This evaluation should be undertaken as soon as possible after diagnosis to secure 'baseline' assessments for follow-up of outcome and intervention results. Since it is now clear that both the tumours themselves and the interventions used (radiation therapy in particular) cause psychiatric problems, and many young individuals survive for many years after a diagnosis of brain tumour, it is essential to monitor the neuropsychiatric development. This will help in identifying the causes of the child's psychological and psychiatric problems and aid in opting for the best type of intervention.

Psychiatric sequelae of brain tumours and treatments for brain tumours

It is clear that brain tumours, depending on type, location and size, may in themselves, cause a plethora of psychiatric symptoms. The long-term neuropsychiatric outcome of infratentorial brain tumours is variable with 30–60% of patients suffering severe neuropsychiatric problems or behaviour problems and are in need of special education (Mulhern, Crisco & Kun, 1983). Supratentorial tumours possibly have a poorer outcome, with 50–85% of patients showing these types of impairment at follow-up (Kun, Mulhern & Crisco, 1983). It seems that children with temporal lobe tumours may have a particularly poor long-term neuropsychiatric outcome with universal impulse control problems and need for special education (Mulhern et al., 1983). However, most studies to date in this field have included very small numbers of individuals with specific types of brain tumours, which means that generalized conclusions cannot be drawn.

So far, it has not been possible definitely to single out the negative effects of brain irradiation from those associated with the brain tumour itself. However, the comparison of children who receive CNS irradiation for acute lymphocytic leukemia (ALL) and children with brain tumours treated with various doses of brain irradiation and/or neurosurgery, is helpful when trying to evaluate the contribution of brain irradiation to neuropsychiatric problems in children. Thus, it appears that (1) an immediate post-irradiation syndrome occurring 4–8 weeks after treatment and comprising somnolence, anorexia and lethargy, (2) a longer term post-irradiation syndrome comprising increased distractibility, poor attention span, declining IQ and (3) cerebral atrophy may be specific effects of the radiation therapy. These effects tend to be more pronounced in younger children and to become more pronounced after

2–5 years even when initial improvement has occurred (Duffner *et al.*, 1985; Mulhern & Kun, 1985; Packer *et al.*, 1989). Also, long-term growth hormone suppression with resulting growth stunting, hypothyroidism, hearing deficits and oncogenesis, may occur.

Clearly, any family faced with the diagnosis of brain tumour in a child, will be devastated. There is usually very little time to adjust to the awful news before treatment and operations have to be started. Neuropsychiatric teams must be educated to meet the psychological and educational as well as the assessment needs of such families. National and local children's brain tumour or children's malignancies support groups will help in providing much-needed support for the family (and child).

References

Anderson, E.M., Clarke, L., Spain, B. (1982). *Disability in Adolescence*. London: Methuen.

Bax, M. (1992). Integration/mainstreaming. *Developmental Medicine and Child Neurology*, **34**, 659–60. (Editorial).

Blackman, M., Wheeler, G.H.T. (1987). A case of mistaken identity: A fourth ventricle tumour presenting as school phobia in a 12 year old boy. *Canadian Journal of Psychiatry*, **32**, 584.

Dallas, E., Stevenson, J., McGurk, H. (1993a). Cerebral-palsied children's interactions with siblings-I. Influence of severity of disability, age and birth order. *Journal of Child Psychology and Psychiatry*, **34**, 621–47.

Dallas, E., Stevenson, J., McGurk, H. (1993b). Cerebral-palsied children's interactions with siblings-II. Interactional structure. *Journal of Child Psychology and Psychiatry*, **34**, 649–71.

Daly, D.D., Love, J.G. (1958). Akinetic mutism. *Neurology*, **8**, 238.

Dennis, M., Barnes, M.A. (1993). Oral discourse after early-onset hydrocephalus linguistic ambiguity, figurative language, speech acts, and script-based inferences. *Journal of Pediatric Psychology*, **18**, 639–52.

Duffner, P.K., Cohen, M.E., Thomas, P.R.M. *et al.* (1985). The long-term effects of cranial irradiation on the central nervous system. *Cancer*, **56**, 1841.

Edebol-Tysk, K. (1989a). Evaluation of care-load for individuals with spastic tetraplegia. *Developmental Medicine and Child Neurology*, **31**,

737–45.

Edebol-Tysk, K. (1989b). *Spastic Tetraplegic Cerebral Palsy*. MD Göteborg: University of Göteborg.

Fernell, E., Gillberg, C., von Wendt, L. (1991a). Autistic symptoms in children with infantile hydrocephalus. *Acta Paediatrica Scandinavica*, **80**, 451–7.

Fernell, E., Gillberg, C., von Wendt, L. (1991b). Behavioural problems in children with infantile hydrocephalus. *Developmental Medicine and Child Neurology*, **33**, 388–95.

Fernell, E., Gillberg, C., von Wendt, L. (1992). Self-esteem in children with infantile hydrocephalus and their siblings. Use of the Piers-Harris self-concept scale. *European Child & Adolescent Psychiatry*, **1**, 227–32.

Gillberg, C. (1989). Asperger syndrome in 23 Swedish children. *Developmental Medicine and Child Neurology*, **31**, 520–31.

Hadenius, A.-M., Hagberg, B., Hyttnäs-Bensch, K., Sjögren, I. (1962). The natural prognosis of infantile hydrocephalus. *Acta Paediatrica Scandinavica*, **51**, 117–18.

Herskowitz, J., Rosman, N. (1982). *Neurology and Psychiatry – Common Ground*. New York: MacMillian.

Kun, L.E., Mulhern, R.K., Crisco, J.J. (1983). Quality in life in children treated for brain tumors: Intellectual, emotional, and academic function. *Journal of Neurosurgery*, **58**, 1.

Laurent, J.P., Cheek, W.R. (1986). Brain tumors in children. *In* Fishman, M.A. (Ed.) *Pediatric Neurology*. New York: Grune & Stratton.

Mulhern, R.K., Crisco, J.J., Kun, L.E. (1983). Neuropsychological sequelae of childhood brain tumors. *Journal of Clinical Child Psychology*, **12**, 66.

Mulhern, R.K., Kun, L.E. (1985). Neuropsychologic function in children with brain tumors. III: Interval changes in the six months following treatment. *Medical Pediatric Oncology*, **13**, 318.

Nielsen, H.H. (1966). *A Psychological Study of Cerebral Palsied Children*. Copenhagen: Munksgaard.

Packer, R.J., Sutton, L.N., Atkins, T.E. *et al.* (1989). A prospective study of cognitive function in children receiving whole-brain radiotherapy and chemotherapy. *Journal of Neurosurgery*, **70**, 707.

Richmond, I.L., Wilson, C.B. (1982). Parasellar tumors in children. I. Clinical presentation, preoperative assessment, and differential diagnosis. *Child's Brain*, **7**, 73–84.

Rutter, M., Graham, P., Yule, W. (1970). *A Neuropsychiatric Study in Childhood*. London: S.I.M.P./William Heinemann Medical Books Ltd.

Scherzer, A.L., Tscharnuter, I. (1982). *Early Diagnosis and Therapy in Cerebral Palsy: A Primer on Infant Developmental Problems*. New York: Marcel Dekker.

Wing, L., Gould, J. (1979). Severe impairments of social interaction and associated abnormalities in children: epidemiology and classification. *Journal of Autism and Developmental Disorders*, **9**, 11–29.

Part III:
Assessment

15 Neuorodevelopmental examination of the child with neuropsychiatric problems

First of all, it is important to realize that the neuropsychiatric diagnosis of a child with neuropsychiatric problems is often (although by no means always) a long and sometimes complicated task without short cuts. The child and adolescent presenting with neuropsychiatric symptoms *always needs a neuropsychiatric work-up comprising a psychiatric examination and a neurodevelopmental evaluation. Laboratory work-up of some kind is often required also as is a neuropsychological assessment.* It is always difficult to draw the clinical line in deciding what is (and what is not) a 'neuropsychiatric symptom'. Whenever there is a suspicion of a named disorder reflecting brain problems, a genetic disorder or when there are symptoms such as social withdrawal, empathy deficits, psychotic symptoms (hallucinations, delusions, confusion), pervasive attention deficits, learning problems, motor control problems, tics (motor or vocal), grossly disturbed eating behaviour, or significant weight loss in children or adolescents, a full neuropsychiatric work-up is always required. The neurodevelopmental work-up includes a detailed family history, review of the pregnancy and early developmental history, evaluation of social and academic settings and a developmental and neuromotor evaluation.

Psychiatric examination

The psychiatric history-taking will depend on the type of problem investigated and is suggested in this book in connection with all the named disorders under the heading of 'Behavioural and Physical Phenotype'. There is also a neuropsychiatric symptom checklist at the back of the book (Appendix II) which is intended to be used for differential diagnostic purposes, but which also suggests the symptom areas which need to be covered in any in-depth neuropsychiatric evaluation.

The psychiatric examination of the individual should be made at direct interview and examination. The neurodevelopmental examination often provides a good starting point for talking to, and psychiatrically examining, the pre-adolescent child. In adolescents, the need to establish as trusting a relationship as possible in order to properly understand the psychological problems may be precluded by vigorous somatic examination. It is often best to perform the neurodevelopmental and physical examination in connection with the first meeting, when it is usually expected by the teenager and the interpersonal rapport between him/her and the examiner is not yet firmly established.

If the evaluation concerns an adolescent rather than a young child, it may well be appropriate to provide the parent with oral and written information about certain types of problems and their early childhood presentation (such as DAMP, ADHD, Tourette syndrome, Asperger syndrome) if the clinical suspicion is raised that the individual might suffer from one of these disorders. Sometimes it is only after carefully studying a pamphlet on one or several of these that the parent begins to put the adolescent's problems in a more coherent frame and starts to provide an in-depth

Table 15.1. *Neurodevelopmental examination of child with neuropsychiatric disorder*

Area	Item	Specifics to note
Neuropsychiatric	Cognition	Level of consciousness, awareness, power of concentration, orientation (room, time), general level of information, curiosity
	Speech/language	Vocal tics, stuttering, articulation deficits, muffled speech, abnormal pitch, speed or volume of voice, failure to adjust volume and language communication to demands of situation, semantic problems
	Social reciprocity	Stand-offish manner, withdrawal, negativism, talking without noting comments from parent or examiner, 'autistic aloneness/isolation'
	Gaze	Staring gaze, stiff gaze, gaze avoidance, failure to reciprocate
	Attention	Short attention span, overfocused attention
	Motor activity	Hyperactivity, inability to sit still, motor restlessness, fidgets, squirms, hypoactivity
	Repetitive movements	Motor stereotypies (hand flapping, finger flicking, knocking, toe-walking, body rocking, head rolling etc.), motor tics
	Emotional aspects	On the verge of tears, depressed, psychomotor retardation, shyness, irritability, anger
	Thought content	Delusional thinking, hallucinations. extreme phobias
Paediatric general	Height	At every consultation
	Weight	At every consultation
	OFC	Always measure on first consultation, thereafter depending on clinical findings
Neurodevelopment	Minor physical anomalies	See Table 15.3
	Overall movements	Clumsiness, ataxia, poor balance
	Soft neurological signs	See Table 15.4
	Hard neurological signs	Reflex abnormalities, asymmetries

account of the symptoms that do, and do not, fit the clinical stereotypes of the disorders. However, it is also necessary to consider the risk that providing all the diagnostic information even before taking an unbiased history may well skew the results of the subsequent diagnostic evaluation.

The areas that need to be covered at direct examination are briefly listed in Table 15.1 together with the neurodevelopmental items that should be included depending on the age and developmental level of the individual being examined.

Neurodevelopmental assessment

Family history

Every child with a neuropsychiatric disorder needs to be assessed from the point of view of familial and genetic loading. The parents (often the mother only) should be interviewed concerning social interaction problems, eccentric and odd personality styles, learning disorders (including mental subnormality, dyslexia and need for special education), hyperactivity, motor clumsiness, tics, Tourette syndrome, epilepsy, eating disorders and psychosis in the first- and second-degree relatives. It is often prudent to start by asking about grandparents, uncles and aunts and then to proceed to siblings, father and mother. Every one of these needs special attention/asking. It will never do simply to ask: 'Is there anyone in your family (or your husband's family) who suffers from . . .' Instead this could be the opening question serving only to furnish the basis for further probing along the lines of 'And what about your brother? Did any of the problems I just mentioned ever pertain to him? For instance, did he require special schooling or special help in reading or writing or other subjects? . . . And what about your sister? . . .'

In addition to this highly structured systematic inquiry into the general neuropsychiatric family history, there may be other needs in some families: if, for instance, there is suspicion that the child might be suffering from tuberous sclerosis or neurofibromatosis, the screen for family genetic problems should include questions tapping specific skin lesions, renal lesions, etc.

A comprehensive family history often cannot be obtained at first contact with the family but will need probing into at intervals during the course of the further work-up of the child. It is common for families to negate a positive family history of any type of disorder on first consultation, but then gradually to open up and provide a more reasonable account of the family background. It is always untrue to say: 'No relevant hereditary factors'! All families have positive history for something!

Gestational and early developmental history

Mothers often only remember major events in pregnancy when asked to recollect several years later. Thus, the best approach in trying to recapitulate a comprehensive picture of the gestational period may be to get the mother's permission to obtain copies of the maternity care and medical reports. It is often useful to check a list of pregnancy, intrapartal and neonatal factors (Table 15.2) in order to compile a measure of reduced optimality in the pre- and perinatal periods (see Chapter 3 on 'Back-

Table 15.2 *Pre, peri-, and neonatal conditions studied*

Pre-, peri-, and neonatal factors	Optimal
Prenatal factors	
Maternal age	20–30
Parity	1–2
Abortions in history	0–2
Bleedings in pregnancy	absent
Severe infections in pregnancy	absent
Generalized oedema	absent
Albuminuria	absent
Blood pressure	< 140/95
Psychiatric specialist care	no
Maternal diabetes or epilepsia	absent
Medication	< 1 week[a]
Gestational age (weeks)	36–41
Smallness for gestational age	no[b]
Intrapartal factors	
Twins or multiple birth	no
Breech, foot, or other abnormal presentation	no
Vacuum extraction	no
Epidural anaesthesia	no
Apgar score	9–10
Cord prolapse/around neck/knot	no
Amniotic fluid	clear
Child severely traumatized (fractures, lots of petechiae)	no
Neonatal factors	
Respiratory distress	absent
Septicaemia/meningitis	absent
Hyperbilirubinaemia	absent[c]
Anaemia requiring transfusion	absent
Irritable infant, floppy infant/convulsions	no
Difficulties regulating temperature	no
Clinical dysmaturity	no[d]
Oxygen treatment > 30%	no

Notes:
[a] Only medication with well-known or suspected negative effect on the foetus (barbiturates, sulphonamides, chlorotalidon, furosemide, and hydrochlorothiazide in the present study).
[b] Weight below the $-2\,SD$ limit for gestational age.
[c] > 15 mg % in children with birthweight ≤ 2500 g; > 20 mg % in children with birthweight ≥ 2500 g.
[d] Scaling skin that appears to be too large for the body – included only if diagnosed by experienced paediatricians.

ground factors'). From the list of 29 conditions/ factors detailed in the Table, most normal pregnancies, intrapartal and neonatal periods would lead to an accumulation of reduced optimality corresponding to 0–3 'events'. Reductions by 4–5 points are also fairly common in normal circumstances, but are more prevalent in populations of children who are later diagnosed with psychosis and DAMP (Gillberg *et al.*, 1986; Gillberg & Rasmussen, 1982). Reductions by 6–8 points are common in cerebral palsy and autism (Kyllerman, 1981; Kyllerman & Hagberg, 1983; Gillberg & Gillberg, 1983) and are quite uncommon in children later evaluated and found to be normal.

For some conditions and in certain cases, the record data is considerably less reliable than the information obtained from the mother, even when this latter data is collected with several years hindsight. This may be true with mothers who abused alcohol or drugs in pregnancy, and who have later recovered from the substance abuse disorder. Eating disorders are more likely to be tapped at personal interview than by reviewing medical records. However, as in the case with substance abuse disorder, if recovery from the disorder is not complete at the time of evaluation, neither the medical record review, nor the personal clinical interview with the mother is likely to reveal the problem.

If the mother has a notebook in which she has recorded her child's development (sometimes including even the gestational period), or if there are home videos available containing reliable dates, information from such sources is likely to be reliable and useful.

Concerning the early psychomotor development (including speech and language) of the child, it is noteworthy that specific dates for developmental milestones provided by the parent several months to years after they actually occurred tend to be very unreliable (unless a notebook is consulted) (Hart, Bax & Jenkins, 1978). However, asking about development in more general terms ('Was his/her development normal, somewhat slow, delayed?'), may well prompt reliable answers. Parents, at least most mothers, are generally much better at this sort of overall judgement about their child's development than doctors give them credit for.

Social background

It is essential never to exclude the possibility that psychosocial factors may have contributed to the symptoms and type of presentation in a child or adolescent with a neuropsychiatric disorder.

Early deprivation, nutritional as well as psychosocial, is a common background factor in children who have been adopted from faraway cultures. Traumatic repeated separations in the first few years of life (and later) can contribute to emotional and behavioural problems (Provence, 1991). All types of psychopathology may be associated with such separations. Anxiety disorders and depression may be most common, but severe hyperactivity is also a possibility (Garralda, 1988). It is not clear how possible effects of repeated separations are mediated, and at present, all that can be concluded is that they may be regarded as covarying factors in some cases of child and adolescent psychopathology.

Loss, such as occurs if one or both parents die, is generally followed by grief in the child (Weller & Weller, 1991). Sometimes major depression ensues. This may be very severe and include psychotic features (Hellgren, Gillberg & Enerskog, 1987). A history of loss of first-degree relatives appears to be more common both in adolescent psychosis and anorexia nervosa than in sex- and age-matched controls (Hellgren *et al.*, 1987; Råstam, 1992). Preliminary data indicate that the risk of developing more severe depressive symptoms is much increased in those bereaved children who have a positive dexamethasone suppression test (Weller *et al.*, 1990). The whole developmental period, and perhaps particularly the pre-adolescent years, should be seen as a time of vulnerability to the stress of experiencing the death of close relatives. A positive history in this field always needs to be weighed in with the rest of the data in the formulation of a plausible hypothesis of the pathogenetic chain of events in the individual child with the neuropsychiatric disorder. Even if, in disorders like autism, parental death was not in any way responsible for the development of the child's autistic disorder, it is unlikely that the event had no effects whatsoever on the child's general psychosocial situation. In hyperactivity disorders, parental death may well in itself have contributed significantly to the development of some of the symptoms.

There is a plethora of other psychosocial factors that may contribute to the development, shaping or maintenance of symptoms in child neuropsychiatric disorders. This is not the place to review such factors in depth. The reader is referred to specific texts on this subject (e.g. Rutter & Garmezy, 1983). However, the clinical conclusion that social factors need to be equally well covered in the work-up of a child with a neuropsychiatric disorder as in the work-up of any child with emotional or behavioural problems, is reiterated here to emphasize their major importance.

Academic functioning screen

Often missed in the work-up of children and adolescents with psychiatric disorders is the mandatory evaluation of the individual's academic progress. Parents (and the individual him/herself after about the age of 6–7 years) should be asked about their child's progress in day-nursery, pre-school, school, home and peer group settings. Specific questions should be asked about reading, writing and maths skills. It is often useful to obtain (if possible) a copy of a recent school report including the child's grades.

Neurodevelopmental examination

The neurodevelopmental work-up (see Table 15.1) comprises general paediatric status (weight, height, and head circumference, skin, eyes, ears and mouth inspection at the very least, evaluation of pubertal development in children over age 8 years) and a neuromotor examination tailored to the individual's sex and age. The latter examination should include an assessment of physical stigmata (including 'minor physical anomalies', see Table 15.3) which might suggest a chromosomal or other congenital disorder (including corpus callosum dysgenesis in hypertelorism), overall agility (in naturalistic gross and fine motor movements),

Table 15.3. *List of anomalies and scoring weights*

Anomaly	Weight
Head	
Two or more hair worls	0
Circumference out of normal range:	
For each age level, $> 1.0\,SD \leq 1.5\,SD$	1
$> 1.5\,SD$	2
Eyes	
Epicanthus:	
Where upper and lower lids join the nose, point of union is:	
Partly covered	1
Deeply covered	2
Hypertelorism:	
Approximate distance between tear ducts:	
For 6 and 7 year-olds, $= 3.2$ cm	1
≥ 3.3 cm	2
For 8 and 9 year-olds, ≥ 3.4 cm	1
For 10, and 11, and 12 year-olds,	
$= 3.4$ cm	1
≥ 3.5 cm	2
Ears	
Low seated:	
Top juncture of ear is below line extended from nose bridge through outer corner of eye by $\leq .5$ cm	1
$> .5$ cm	2
Adherent lobes:	
Straight back toward rear of neck	1
Lower edges of ears extended:	
Upward and back toward crown of head	2
Malformed ears	1
Asymmetrical ears	1
Soft and pliable ears	0
Mouth	
High palate:	
Roof of mouth:	
Definitely steepled	2
Flat and narrow at the top	1
Furrowed tongue (one with deep ridges)	
Smooth–rough spots on tongue	0
Hands	
Fifth finger:	
Slightly curved inward toward other fingers	1
Markedly curved inward toward other fingers	2
Single transverse palmar crease	1

Table 15.3. (*cont.*)

Anomaly	Weight
Feet	
Third toe:	
Appears equal in length to second toe	1
Definitely longer than second toe	2
Partial syndactylia of two middle toes	1
Gap between first and second toe	
(approximately $\geq 1/4$ inch)	1

balance (in unprovoked and provoked states, such as during standing on one leg) and tonus (evaluated both by passive movements of limbs and clinical judgement of the child's movements and posture, pronounced lordosis of the lumbar back, flat feet and drooling sometimes signalling underlying generalized moderate degrees of hypotonus) plus a brief examination for 'hard' and 'soft' neurological signs.

Some of the neurological soft signs have been shown to have at least face validity (in that they tend to be associated with neuropsychiatric disorders such as DAMP, Rasmussen *et al.*, 1983) and predictive validity (in that persistence of dysfunction over time tends to remain associated with neuropsychiatric disorder, Shaffer *et al.*, 1985; Hellgren *et al.*, 1993). These include dysdiadochokinesis, tracing in a mace, difficulties jumping up and down on one foot, standing on one foot, cutting out a paper circle and walking on the lateral sides of the feet (Gillberg, I.C., 1987). How to score these items and assign ratings of 'normality'/'abnormality' depend on the age (chronological and developmental) and sex of the individual (Touwen, 1979; Gillberg I.C., 1987). No precise limits for cut-off can be presented here, but a general description and rough guidelines are provided in Table 15.4.

A general rating of overall gross motor skills/clumsiness made by a trained observer is often informative. Teenagers who are clumsy have usually been clumsy from a very young age and the clumsiness is associated with many different kinds of neuropsychiatric abnormality, including DAMP, dyslexia and Asperger syndrome (Hellgren *et al.*, 1993).

Children with neuropsychiatric disorders are often referred to neurologists for evaluation of 'neurological status'. Both the psychiatrist and neurologist often assume that what is expected at this evaluation is an assessment of all the various types of 'classic' neurological reflexes, such as deep tendon reflexes and ocular/conjunctival reflexes to mention but a few. In practice, the yield of such examination is often very limited, unless there is a strong suspicion of disorder presenting with focal signs (such as may be the case with multiple sclerosis, brain tumours, etc.).

A detailed neurological examination, similar to that performed in adult neurology may well be required in some cases, but it can never substitute for a functional neuromotor evaluation. The absence of focal neurological signs certainly should not be taken to mean that the child does not suffer from brain dysfunction, brain damage or even specific neurological disorder (Rutter, 1982). Unfortunately, even though few doctors would dispute this conclusion, in clinical practice it is very common for the psychiatrist to consider the 'negative' neurological examination as a '*carte blanche*' sign of non-organicity. Psychological factors are often taken to be the cause of a psychiatric disorder for which no neurological focal signs can be found.

Clinical interviews, rating scales and self-report questionnaires

A large number of clinical interviews, rating scales and self-report questionnaires are now available for use in research and clinical practice. Since this is a clinically oriented book, only a few of the most widely used of these will be reviewed here. Psychometric properties of these instruments (reliability, validity and standardization, see Chapter 17) are generally good or excellent unless specifically discussed.

It is necessary to emphasize the fact that questionnaires and structured interviews cannot substitute for good clinical judgement and comprehensive clinical diagnosis in which all the information provided about the individual

Table 15.4. *The examination for soft neurological signs*

Item	Comment
Standing on one leg	Normal children aged 6–7 years manage more than 10 s wihtout putting down other foot for support; over age 7 years 20 s
Hopping on one leg	Normal children aged 6 years and over manage 20 hops up and down without putting down other foot for support; time taken less than 11 s; the whole foot has to leave the floor for result to be scored normal
Walking on lateral aspects of feet (Fog & Fog, 1963)	Normal children aged 7 years and older manage this test without major associated movements or major asymmetries; abduction of shoulder or flexion of elbow less than 60 degrees
Walking on heels	Normal children aged 6 years and older manage this without major associated movements or asymmetries (see previous item)
Diadochokinesis	Performed separately for right and left hand; other hand hanging down; alternating pro-supination; children aged 6–7 years manage more than 15 complete pro-supinations with only minor interruptions in switching from pro- to supination; over age 8–9 years more than 20 with no interruption; non-preferred hand 2–3 pro-supinations less
Handedness	Prompt child to draw, comb hair, brush teeth, eat with spoon and throw small ball (pretend if objects not available). Complete righthandedness = right hand preferred in 5/5, complete lefthandedness = left hand preferred in 5/5, varying degrees of ambidexterity in other cases. Handedness normally established in children over age 5 years
Maze-tracing task (Bishop, 1980)	After age 7 years, performance with non-preferred hand not more than 5 errors poorer than with preferred hand
Cutting out paper circle with diameter of about 4 inches	After age 6 years, less than 20% of circle area cut 'away' or 'included extra', time taken less than 90 s
Prechtl test for elicitation of tremor and choreoathetoid movements	No clear age-norms available; pronounced tremor or choreoathetoid movements are always abnormal

Note: The above list is just a suggestion of easy-to-perform tests that may be used to elicit possible soft neurological signs and atypical handedness. Most of the instructions and norms have been modified from Touwen (1979) and Gillberg IC (1987).

is comprehensively reviewed. In research, there is now sometimes a tendency to rely almost solely on structured interviews, rating scales and questionnaires. Although originally reflecting a healthy move away from the merely subjective, there is a risk that this tendency might eventually impinge on the need continuously to evaluate the information available using the gestalt acumen of the experienced clinician. Nevertheless, even experienced clinicians can be completely mistaken, and the use of structured instruments like those briefly reviewed in the following, when sensibly applied, is definitely a major step forward in clinical child neuropsychiatry.

Clinical interviews

For adolescents in the late teens, many of the interviews used for adults, are appropriate, either in their original format, or in slightly modified versions that have been particularly adapted for use with teenagers. Thus, for instance, the structured clinical interview for DSM-III-R diagnosis (SCID), is available in two parts, one for diagnosis on axis I and one for diagnosis on axis II (SCID-I and SCID-II, Spitzer *et al.*, 1992), and can be used with confidence in 17–22 year-olds (Råstam, Gillberg & Gillberg, 1994; Gillberg, Råstam & Gillberg, 1994). The diagnostic interview for children and adolescents (DICA, Herjanic & Campbell, 1977; Welner *et al.*, 1987) and the diagnostic interview schedule for children (DISC, Costello *et al.*, 1984) also cover axis I and axis II disorders, but they have been designed specifically for use with younger individuals. This is both a great asset and a problem. The advantage is that they cover disorders beginning in childhood. The disadvantage is the discontinuity *vis-à-vis* adult structured interviews. The DICA is particularly useful in the area of attention deficit and conduct disorder. The Kiddie-schedule for affective disorders and schizophrenia (K-SADS) (Chambers *et al.* 1985) covers a more limited field of disorders. Even narrower in scope are the autism diagnostic interview (ADI, Le Couteur *et al.*, 1989) and the Asperger syndrome diagnostic interview (ASDI, Ehlers & Gillberg, 1993). Some of these interviews (the SCID-I and II, K-SADS, ADI and ASDI) are investigator-based, i.e. they provide structured questions to cover all the diagnostic criteria for the disorders outlined in the DSM-III-R or ICD-10, but the scoring decision rests with the clinician performing the interview. Others are purportedly structured interviews which require no clinical judgement on the part of the interviewer (DICA), although some degree of common sense will be necessary. Others still (DISC) are extremely structured and contain an explicit skip formula so that when a primary symptom is negative, no probes are asked.

Rating scales

The rating scales are similar in that the subjective rating is performed by somebody other than the patient. For instance, the childhood behaviour checklist (CBCL, Achenbach & Edelbrock, 1983) exists in a parent and teacher rating version (and there is also a self-report questionnaire for adolescents, see below) containing about 120 items. It takes 25–60 minutes to complete and yields 'factor diagnoses' which are not equivalent to clinical DSM-III-R diagnoses but which have been used to equate these. The Rutter scales (Rutter, Graham & Yule, 1970), containing about 20–30 questions and requiring 3–10 minutes to complete yield valid estimates of overall 'marked psychiatric abnormality' with subgroups of 'antisocial' and 'neurotic' problems. In addition, a hyperactivity factor consisting of three items has been construed. The Conners teacher and parent scales (Conners, 1969) are probably the most widely used of all children's rating scales. In their various versions (containing 10–39 questions) they all tap attention deficits and conduct disorder and are often used to make a preliminary decision whether or not pervasive ADHD is present (when both parent and teacher ratings agree that the child is a high-scorer). For rarer problems, the Autism behavior checklist (ABC, Krug, Arick & Almond, 1980), the Asperger syndrome screening questionnaire (ASSQ, Ehlers & Gillberg, 1993), Yale global tic severity scale (Leckman *et al.*, 1989) and the eating attitudes test (EAT, Garner & Garfinkel, 1979) may all be useful in quantifying the amount of symptoms or alerting the investigator to the possibility of a specific diagnosis. However, none of these instruments should be considered diagnostic instruments in themselves.

Self-report questionnaires

The diagnostic self-report questionnaires developed specifically for use with children and adolescents include the Birleson depression inventory (Birleson, 1981), the Millon clinical multiaxial inventory for personality features and problems (MCMI, Millon, 1982) and the CBCL adolescent version (Rey, Schrader & Morris-Yates, 1992). What is rarely appreciated in the use of these instruments is the possibility that the individual may be suffering from dyslexia and other learning disorders, and that, in such cases, responses to various questions may not correspond to the individual's actual evaluation of himself/herself.

Observation scales

Some scales should be completed by the clinician only after observation of the child. These include the childhood autism rating scale (CARS, Schopler, Reichler & Renner, 1988) and the autism diagnostic observation schedule (ADOS, Lord *et al.*, 1989).

Summary and clinical conclusions

No one of the instruments reviewed is appropriate for use with all children and adolescents with neuropsychiatric disorder (or suspected neuropsychiatric disorder). Not reviewed here, but generally useful is a DSM-III-R or DSM-IV checklist in which all the childhood diagnoses are listed (and the criteria items included with brief descriptors). No formal checklist of this kind exists, and would have to be compiled by the individual clinician to suit his/her needs. The structured and semistructured interviews are very useful (indeed necessary) in clinical research, and may be very helpful in clinics catering for children and adolescents with more circumscribed problems (movement disorders, autism and autisticlike conditions, obsessive–compulsive disorders, eating disorders, etc.). However, in the clinic serving a broader neuropsychiatric clientele, the clinical examination and screening will have to be left with the experienced clinician who does not rely on any one particular instrument. Only after initial screening out of a great number of disorders in this way will it be meaningful to focus on a narrower set of diagnoses, and only then will the interview schedules reviewed (both the

slightly broader, like the DICA, and the very narrow, like the ADI) enter the picture.

The self-report questionnaires and parent and teacher rating scales are particularly helpful in the work-up of young individuals with depression (the Birleson), eating disorders (EAT), attention disorders (Conners) and personality disorders (MCMI). However, none of them should be used other than as aids to clinical diagnosis and as measures of amount of symptomatology. For general psychiatric problems, the CBCL is exceptional in that it covers broad areas of psychopathology and has been subjected to more systematic epidemiological study than any other similar instrument.

For children suspected of suffering from one of the behavioural phenotype syndromes (Chapter 10), a whole host of more or less specific interview and screening questionnaires exists (O'Brien, 1992), but the *diagnosis* of these syndromes usually is not aided by these instruments. Rather, at the present stage, they should be seen as research instruments established as tools for examining intra- and intersyndrome comparability of neuropsychiatric symptoms.

References

Achenbach, T.M., Edelbrock, C.S. (1983). *Manual for the Child Behavior Checklist and Revised Child Behavior Profile*. Burlington, VT: University of Vermont.

Bax, M., Dennis, J., O'Brien, G., Gillberg, C., Yule, W., Udwin, O. (1993). The Behavioural Phenotype Study Questionnaire. *Unpublished manuscript*.

Birleson, P. (1981). The validity of depressive disorder in childhood and the development of a self-rating scale: a research report. *Journal of Child Psychology and Psychiatry*, **22**, 73–88.

Bishop, D.V.M. (1980). Handedness, clumsiness and cognitive ability. *Develpmental Medicine and Child Neurology*, **22**, 569–79.

Chambers, W.J., Puig-Antich, J., Hirsch, M., Paez, P., Ambrosini, P.J., Tabrizi, M.A., Davies, M. (1985). The assessment of affective disorders in children and adolescents by semistructured interview. Test-retest reliability of the schedule for affective disorders and schizophrenia for school-age children, present episode version. *Archives of*

General Psychiatry, **42**, 696–702.

Conners, C.K. (1969). A teacher rating scale for use in drug studies with children. *American Journal of Psychiatry*, **126**, 884–8.

Costello, A.J., Edelbrock, C.S., Dulcan, M.K. *et al.* (1984). Development and testing of the NIMH Diagnostic Interview Schedule for Children in a Clinic Population. Final Report. Rockville, MD, Center for Epidemilogic Studies, National Institute of Mental Health.

Ehlers, S., Gillberg, C. (1993). The epidemiology of Asperger syndrome. A total population study. *Journal of Child Psychology and Psychiatry*, **34**, 1327–50.

Fog, E., Fog, M. (1963). Cerebral inhibition examined by associated movements. In Bax, M., Mackeith, R. (Eds.). *Minimal Cerebral Dysfunction. Clinics in Developmental Medicine No. 10*. London: S.S.M.E.I.U./William Heinemann Medical Books Ltd.

Garner, D.M., Garfinkel, P.E. (1979). The Eating Attitudes Test: an index of the symptoms of anorexia nervosa. *Psychological Medicine*, **9**, 273–9.

Garralda, M.E., Bailey, D. (1988). Child and family factors associated with referral to child psychiatrists. *British Journal of Psychiatry*, **153**, 81–9.

Gillberg, C., Rasmussen, P. (1982). Perceptual, motor and attentional deficits in seven-year-old children: background factors. *Developmental Medicine and Child Neurology*, **24**, 752–70.

Gillberg, C., Wahlström, J., Forsman, A., Hellgren, L., Gillberg, I.C. (1986). Teenage psychoses – epidemiology, classification and reduced optimality in the pre-, peri- and neonatal periods. *Journal of Child Psychology and Psychiatry*, **27**, 87–98.

Gillberg, I.C. (1987). *Deficits in Attention, Motor Control and Perception: Follow-up from Pre-School to Early Teens*. M.D. Thesis. University of Uppsala.

Gillberg, I.C., Gillberg, C. (1983). Three-year follow-up at age 10 of children with minor neurodevelopmental disorders. I: Behavioural problems. *Developmental Medicine and Child Neurology*, **25**, 438–49.

Gillberg, I.C., Råstam, M., Gillberg, C. (1994). Anorexia nervosa 6 years after onset. Part I. Personality disorders. *Comprehensive Psychiatry*, in press.

Hart, H., Bax, M., Jenkins, S. (1978). The value of a developmental history. *Developmental Medicine and Child Neurology*, **20**, 442–52.

Hellgren, L., Gillberg, C., Enerskog, I. (1987). Antecedents of adolescent psychoses: a population-based study of school health problems in children who develop psychosis in adolescence. *Journal of the American Academy of Child and Adolescent Psychiatry*, **26**, 351–5.

Hellgren, L., Gillberg, C., Gillberg, I.C., Enerskog, I. (1993). Children with Deficits in Attention, Motor control and Perception (DAMP) almost grown up. General health at age 16 years. *Developmental Medicine and Child Neurology*, **35**, 881–92.

Herjanic, B., Campbell, W. (1977). Differentiating psychiatrically disturbed children on the basis of a structured interview. *Journal of Abnormal Child Psychology*, **5**, 127–34.

Krug, D.A., Arick, J., Almond, P. (1980). Behavior checklist for identifying severely handicapped individuals with high levels of autistic behavior. *Journal of Child Psychology and Psychiatry*, **21**, 221–9.

Kyllerman, H. (1981). Dyskinetic cerebral palsy: II. *Acta Paediatrica Scandinavica*, **71**, 551–8.

Kyllerman, M., Hagberg, B. (1983). Reduced optimality in pre and perinatal conditions in a Swedish newborn population. *Neuropediatrics*, **14**, 37–42.

Le Couteur, A., Rutter, M., Lord, C., Rios, P., Robertson, S., Holdgrafer, M., McLennan, J. (1989). Autism diagnostic interview: a standardized investigator-based instrument. *Journal of Autism and Developmental Disorders*, **19**, 363–87.

Leckman, J.F., Riddle, M.A., Hardin, M.T., Ort, S.I., Swartz, K.L., Stevenson, J., Cohen, D.J. (1989). The Yale Global Tic Severity Scale: initial testing of a clinician-rated scale of tic severity. *Journal of the American Academy of Child and Adolescent Psychiatry*, **28**, 566–73.

Lord, C., Rutter, M., Goode, S., Heemsbergen, J., Jordan, J., Mawhood, L., Schopler, E. (1989). Autism diagnostic observation schedule: a standardized observation of communicative and social behavior. *Journal of Autism and Developmental Disorders*, **19**, 185–212.

Millon, T. (1982). *Millon Clinical Multiaxial Inventory (MCMI)*. Minneapolis, Minnesota: National Computer Systems.

O'Brien, G. (1992). Behavioural phenotypes and their measurement. *Developmental Medicine and Child Neurology*, **34**, 365–7.

Provence, S. (1991). Separation and deprivation. *In* Lewis, M. (Ed.) *Child and Adolescent Psychiatry. A Comprehensive Textbook*. Baltimore, Maryland:

Williams & Wilkins.

Rasmussen, P., Gillberg, C., Waldenström, E., Svenson, B. (1983). Perceptual, motor and attentional deficits in seven-year-old children: neurological and neurodevelopmental aspects. *Developmental Medicine and Child Neurology*, **25**, 315–33.

Råstam, M. (1992). Anorexia nervosa in 51 Swedish adolescents. Premorbid problems and comorbidity. *Journal of the American Academy of Child and Adolescent Psychiatry*, **31**, 819–29.

Råstam, M., Gillberg, C., Gillberg, I.C. (1994). Anorexia nervosa 6 years after onset. Part II. Comorbid psychiatric problems. *Comprehensive Psychiatry*, in press.

Rey, J.M., Schrader, E., Morris-Yates, A. (1992). Parent–child on children's behaviours reported by the Child Behaviour Checklist (CBCL). *Journal of Adolescence*, **15**, 219–30.

Rutter, M. (1982). Syndromes attributed to minimal brain dysfunction in childhood. *American Journal of Psychiatry*, **139**, 21–33.

Rutter, M., Garmezy, N. (1983). Developmental psychopathology. *In* Hetherington, E.M. (Ed.) *Socialization, Personality, and Social Development.* New York: Wiley.

Rutter, M., Graham, P., Yule, W. (1970). *A Neuropsychiatric Study in Childhood.* London: S.I.M.P./William Heinemann Medical Books Ltd.

Ryan, N.D., Puig-Antich, J., Cooper, T., Rabinovich, H., Ambrosini, P., Davies, M., King, J., Torres, D., Fried, J. (1986). Imipramine in adolescent major depression: plasma level and clinical response. *Acta Psychiatrica Scandinavica*, **73**, 275–88.

Schopler, E., Reichler, R.J., Renner, B.R. (1988). *The Childhood Autism Rating Scale (CARS).* Revised. Los Angeles: Western Psychological Services, Inc.

Shaffer, D., Schonfeld, I., O'Connor, P., Stokman, C., Trautman, P., Shafer, S., Ng, S. (1985). Neurological soft signs. Their relationship to psychiatric disorder and intelligence in childhood and adolescence. *Archives of General Psychiatry*, **42**, 342–51.

Spitzer, R.L., Williams, J.B., Gibbon, M., First, M.B. (1992). The Structured Clinical Interview for DSM-III-R (SCID). I: History, rationale, and description. *Archives of General Psychiatry*, **49**, 624–9.

Touwen, B.C.L. (1979). *Examination of the Child with Minor Neurological Dysfunction.* 2nd Edition. London: S.I.M.P./William Heinemann Medical Books Ltd.

Weller, E.B., Weller, R.A. (1991). Grief. *In* Lewis, M. (Ed.) *Child and Adolescent Psychiatry. A Comprehensive Textbook.* Baltimore, Maryland: Williams & Wilkins.

Weller, E.B., Weller, R.A., Fristad, M.A., Bowes, J.M. (1990). Dexamethasone suppression test and depressive symptoms in bereaved children: a preliminary report. *Journal of Neuropsychiatry and Clinical Neuroscience*, **2**, 418–21.

Welner, W., Reich, W., Herjanic, B., *et al.* (1987). Reliability, validity and parent-child agreement studies of the Diagnostic Interview for Children and Adolescents. *Journal of the American Academy of Child and Adolescent Psychiatry*, **26**, 649–53.

16 Laboratory work-up

It is impossible comprehensively to review the growing literature on the 'laboratory neuro-work-up' of individuals with child neuropsychiatric disorders in a brief chapter. The following presentation instead includes some clinical guidelines in respect of why and how to use the available laboratory examinations in the work-up of individuals with neuropsychiatric disorders with childhood or adolescent onset.

Neurochemistry, molecular genetics and cytogenetics

Only a few years ago, it was still possible to treat neurochemistry, cytogenetics and molecular genetics as separate. Today, such subdivision is no longer possible. Neurotransmitters, neuro-modulators, enzymes, other proteins, ions, vitamins and co-factors are all part of 'neurochemistry' and the intricate interplay of neural and glial structures in the central nervous system. Most of them (and their sites of action) are ruled by specific genes. Abnormalities of these genes can now often be detected at the molecular level. Sometimes the gene abnormalities engage portions of the genome large enough to allow visualization in the light microscope and the deviation then becomes classifiable as 'cytogenetic'.

There is no way in which a laboratory work-up of the individual patient with neuropsychiatric disorder could be performed without the guidance of the differential diagnostic considerations. In other words, there is no neurochemical, blood, urine or CSF test that should be performed in all patients presenting with neuropsychiatric symptoms. The clinician will have to consult the chapters on specific disorders for detailed instructions.

Nevertheless, a few basic guidelines can be provided here. *A cytogenetic examination* should be undertaken in all cases presenting with autistic symptoms. A chromosomal culture in a folic acid deficient medium is still to be preferred since molecular genetic diagnosis of the fragile X syndrome will not provide information about other chromosomal disorders that may (more rarely) be associated with autistic symptomatology. Equally, all children and adolescents presenting with dysmorphic features and neuropsychiatric disorders should have a chromosomal culture analysed. Females with severe dyslexia should be evaluated to rule out the fragile X syndrome. In mental retardation generally, the comprehensive work-up should include a chromosomal culture.

For many disorders, such as Angelman syndrome, Huntington chorea, Prader–Willi syndrome and von Recklinghausen disease, *specific molecular genetic diagnosis* is now possible. The clinician working in child and adolescent neuropsychiatry will need the assistance of a good neurogenetic laboratory. A working relationship should be established, and the clinical neuropsychiatrist should never hesitate to consult the clinical geneticist to enquire about whether or not a particular syndrome can now be genetically diagnosed at the molecular level. Development in this field is so rapid that it is difficult, if not impossible, for the clinician to keep pace with it.

Blood screens for thyroid disorder should always be high on any list of priorities in the field of laboratory work-up in neuropsychiatrically disordered children and adolescents. Even though in many industrialized countries, newborn screening for thyroid disorder is performed, there is a risk that mistakes may be made in this procedure. Also, thyroid disease, not present at birth, may develop several years later.

PKU is usually not missed at newborn screening, but there is no guarantee and it is advisable to include *a screen (urine or blood) for aminoacidopathies* in all cases with neuropsychiatric disorder with early childhood onset.

Infections should be considered as possible pathogenic agents in child neuropsychiatric disorder. Borrelia infection (Lyme disease) is known to masquerade as known syndromes as well as hitherto unknown, strange combinations of syndromes. HIV-infection is gradually becoming a more important aetiology of child neuropsychiatric disorder (Musetti *et al.*, 1993), and the need to rule out HIV, as well as other infectious agents, by blood tests needs highlighting here.

In the future, it is possible that simple blood tests of, for example serotonin, might be used as a screen for particular variants of child neuropsychiatric disorder (high serotonin autism and hypothyroidism, low serotonin conduct disorder associated with high levels of aggression and suicide risk). However, we are presently nowhere near such a position. The clinician working in child and adolescent neuropsychiatry needs to be aware of the lack of evidence for any blood, urine or CSF screening tests that will help focus the diagnostic process, unless such testing is guided by specific differential diagnostic speculation.

Neurophysiology

An ordinary resting *EEG* should be performed in all cases presenting with autism, Asperger syndrome, childhood schizophrenia, Tourette disorder, DAMP and in many of the behavioural phenotype syndromes (such as the fragile X syndrome, Bourneville disease, Rett syndrome and Angelman syndrome to mention but a few). The reason for this statement is the fact that, in many of these disorders, epilepsy occurs at a very much increased rate as compared with the general population, and even in cases in which it does not, the distinction between attentional dysfunction and absences may be very difficult, particularly if the child is generally uncooperative.

It is desirable (but often impossible) to obtain additional EEG recordings after hyperventilation, during exposure to flickering light, sleep deprivation and drowsiness. Many EEG changes (including spike and wave activity typical of epileptic phenomena) only occur under these specific circumstances.

In DAMP, and other disorders involving delayed development of motor and attentional functions, there is often a significant increase in low frequency activity in the resting EEG, described as 'moderate increase of low frequency activity' (Gillberg *et al.*, 1981). 'Paroxysmal activity on activation' is a common finding in the severely disturbed DAMP group with autistic features, according to one study (Gillberg *et al.*, 1981).

The argument is often raised whether EEG changes commonly occur in normal people and, if so, what their diagnostic significance might be. There can be little doubt that EEG changes (such as slight increase of low frequency activity) often occur in control populations, not meeting criteria for psychiatric disorder (Eeg-Olofson, 1970). However, blind child psychiatric assessment of children selected from the normal population because they have been exposed to a minimum of risk factors which might cause brain dysfunction, reveals that, in those with EEG changes (including the commonly reported 14/6 Hz positive spikes activity), there are problems and personality traits that, although not qualifying for diagnosis of major disorder, do not occur in those without the EEG changes (Bosaeus, 1978).

An EEG should, of course, also be performed in all children and adolescents clinically suspected of suffering from a seizure disorder.

Telemetric EEG recordings (for hours to

several days) performed in the home of the patient (or on the ward) could potentially be very informative, but, unfortunately, such examinations are not clinically available in most clinical settings.

Various kinds of *evoked response/potential examinations* are available. For instance, in autism, the use of auditory brainstem response (ABR) examinations, has helped elucidate both the role of brainstem dysfunction and hearing impairment in this disorder. ABR is now a standard examination in autism in many centres.

At the present stage, the use of evoked potentials, including P300-examinations and visual and somatosensory evoked response examinations, is often a matter for active researchers rather than clinicians. It is quite possible that such examinations will eventually become a more integral part of clinical laboratory work-up in young people with neuropsychiatric disorders.

Neuroradiology

X-ray examinations of the skull and central nervous system can be conceptually divided into those that demonstrate (a) the structure of the skull, (b) the structure of the brain, and (c) the function of the brain.

(a) is represented by the ordinary skull X-ray, the indications of which are relatively few in child psychiatry. However, in the case of hypothalamic and hypophyseal tumours (which might be suspected on the basis of symptoms of hormonal change in the child), it is still often the best screening method.

(b) is represented by computerized axial tomography (CAT or CT) and magnetic resonance imaging (MRI) techniques. The latter type of examination is also referred to as nuclear magnetic resonance (NMR) imaging.

(c) comprises single photon emission computed tomography (SPECT), positron emission tomography (PET) and magnetoencephalography (MEG). MEG is not yet in clinical use and will not be covered in this presentation.

CT (computerized axial tomography) of the brain

CT is currently the most widely available imaging method and can be applied at moderate costs. CT relies on multiple measurements of X-ray transmissions at different angles in a slice through the brain and the fact that there will be variation in the amount of X-ray attenuation according to the properties of the tissue through which the X-rays pass. Computer methods are then used to analyse the resulting vast amounts of data.

CT is very useful for the detection of focal lesions (particularly those that are calcified, haemorrhagic or space-occupying). A contrast can be injected intravenously to allow the separation of lesions associated with vascular abnormalities.

The general use of CT in the evaluation of neuropsychiatrically disordered child patients is still controversial. However, in the work-up of patients with severely autistic behaviour it should be standard, because of its excellent ability to pick out calcified lesions (such as may occur in tuberous sclerosis and intrauterine infection syndromes). In all neuropsychiatrically disordered individuals for which no reasonable, plausible clinical diagnosis can be made, it should also be included in the work-up. Whenever there is clinical suspicion (such as when the neurological, and neurofunctional, examination produces clearly asymmetrical findings) of a space-occupying lesion, both CT and MRI scans may be called for.

MRI (magnetic resonance imaging of the brain)

MRI is generally viewed as a better imaging technique, but is more expensive and less available than CT. CT uses ionizing radiation whereas MRI instead utilizes manipulation and measurement of the electromagnetic properties of biological tissues. The use of MRI is limited by conditions adversely affected by the magnetic field used (including pacemakers, aneurysm clips, ferromagnetic foreign bodies and calcified lesions).

Some of the atomic nuclei found in the brain behave as magnetic dipoles that can be aligned in one plane by placing the head within a strong magnetic field. The magnetic field induces the dipoles to perform complex periodic movement. The frequency of this movement is characteristic of each nuclear species at given field strengths. The field strength is measured in tessla. A radio signal tuned to the frequency of the nuclear species is applied, and nuclear magnetic resonance results. A radio frequency signal is emitted which can be measured by the MRI apparatus. Hydrogen nuclei (protons) are generally utilized for the creation of magnetic resonance imaging because they are abundant and have a high signal amplitude. Certain properties of the decay of the resonant frequency signal are used to generate images based upon three different types of relevant information (Andreasen, 1989):

T1 images that portray normal cerebral anatomy are constructed from that aspect of resonance decay which is useful for depicting high contrast between white and grey matter and CSF;

T2 images that portray many forms of cerebral pathology are constructed from that aspect of resonance decay which is useful for depicting regions of high free-water content (typical of such conditions as infection, inflammation, infarction, edema and demyelination);

Proton density images that portray the quantity of hydrogen nuclei in a particular sample.

MRI provides excellent differentiation between white and grey matter. It has heightened sensitivity for most pathological lesions as compared with CT. Furthermore, it visualizes structures that in CT are partly obscured by bone artifact interference (such as the posterior fossa contents). Its applicability in clinical child neuropsychiatry is fast expanding at the time of going to press with this book. Posterior

fossa and subcortical abnormalities have been reported in autism by several different groups (Gaffney et al., 1988; Courchesne et al., 1988; Piven et al., 1990). MRI often provides an almost pathognomonic diagnostic picture in tuberous sclerosis (Gomez, 1988).

SPECT (single photon emission computed tomography) of the brain

Single photon emission computed tomography or SPECT is currently expanding its territory as a diagnostic tool in clinical child neuropsychiatry, particularly in the fields of autism and epilepsy (Gillberg I.C. et al., 1993). It is possibly the most rapidly developing technique for three-dimensional clinical imaging of brain functions.

The recent introduction of Seretec has led to the relatively non-invasive technique of intravenous injection of a radioactive substance whose circulation in the brain allows the determination and imaging of regional cerebral blood flow (rCBF), and hence, albeit indirectly, neural activity, through single photon emission computed tomography. The scan generated depicts rCBF at the moment of tracer binding (which is usually not equivalent to the moment of scanning).

SPECT monitors brain metabolism and regional variations in brain activity at relatively low costs and minimal radiation exposure. It shows good temporal and spatial resolution. However, as yet, no exact measurements of blood flow are possible (for instance, the procedure cannot yet measure glucose metabolic rates), and other than the comparison of 'regions of interests' on one side with the corresponding area on the other, no numerical results can be presented. SPECT remains a visually impressive, but subjective instrument (Fig. 16.1, 16.2, 16.3). White matter lesions are often missed. The main disadvantage, however, is the relatively limited clinical experience so far, making conclusions about specificity of findings difficult. For instance, the recent demonstration of temporal lobe hypoperfusions in all of a considerable number of high-functioning young individuals with autism (Gillberg et al.,

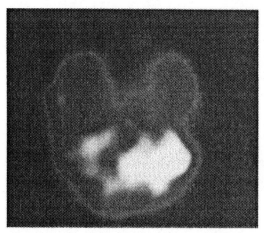

Fig. 16.1. 22-year-old man with autism without epilepsy. The transaxial slice shows left temporal lobe hypoperfusion (right side in photograph) with a normally perfused right temporal lobe (left side in photograph). (The occipital lobes appear yellowish-white).

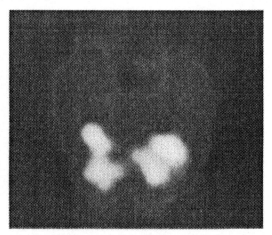

Fig. 16.3. Six-year-old boy with autism without epilepsy. The transaxial slice shows hypoperfusion in the left temporal lobe (right side in photograph) with some hypoperfusion with the right temporal lobe. (The occipital lobes appear yellowish-white.)

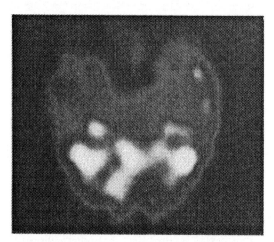

Fig. 16.2. 11-year-old boy with autism without epilepsy. The transaxial slice shows right temporal lobe hypoperfusion (left side in photograph) with some medical hypoperfusion within the right temporal lobe. (The occipital lobes appear yellowish-white).

1993) remains to be put in perspective with SPECT findings from other neuropsychiatrically disordered patients.

The SPECT findings in autism, speech–language disorders and dyslexia all signal the possibility that SPECT may soon become clinically indicated in the work-up of these disorders. In the diagnosis of patients evaluated for epilepsy surgery (many of whom are behaviourally disturbed and have hyperkinetic symptoms and autistic behaviour), SPECT is already part of the routine clinical work-up in many centres.

PET (Positron emission tomography)

Positron emission tomography (PET) has many advantages including the breadth of specific biochemical processes that can be monitored. However, the relatively enormous costs and high doses of radiation exposure currently incurred with PET precludes its applicability for clinical purposes at the present stage. It remains a research instrument. As such, it has already produced thought-provoking findings in depression (Buchsbaum et al., 1982), Tourette syndrome (Chase *et al.*, 1986) and Huntington chorea (Clark *et al.*, 1986). There are currently no clinical indications for this procedure.

Neuropathology

Brain biopsies are not indicated in child and adolescent neuropsychiatric disorders. Thus, the degree to which neurohistopathology can contribute to clinical child neuropsychiatry is very limited. However, brain autopsies should be undertaken in children and adolescents with neuropsychiatric disorders who die (whether expectedly or not). There may be more than theoretical interest in this area: tuberous sclerosis is sometimes only diagnosed at autopsy, and the diagnosis of this disorder in a family may prompt the need for intensive genetic counselling. Furthermore, for many families who have been living with a neuropsychiatrically disordered child for many years, brain autopsy may contribute to a better understanding of the nature of the child's problems, help alleviate feelings of guilt and promote better psychological functioning in the family.

In order to accomplish a meaningful analysis of the implications of the results of a thorough clinical report and a detailed brain autopsy, the interested clinician should establish a working relationship with the neuropathologist, who, in turn, will need to keep abreast of recent developments in the field in order to provide the best possible examination of the brain.

References

Andreasen, N.C. (1989). Nuclear magnetic resonance imaging. *In* Andreasen, N.C. (Ed.) *Brain Imaging: Applications in Psychiatry.* Washington, DC: American Psychiatric Press.

Bosaeus, E. (1978). *Psychiatric assessment of healthy children with various EEG-patterns.* MD Thesis. University of Göteborg.

Buchsbaum, M.S., Ingvar, D.H., Kessler, R., Waters, R.N., Cappelletti, J., van Kammen, D.P.,

King, A.C., Johnson, J.L., Manning, R.G., Flynn, R.W., Mann, L.S., Bunney, W.E.J., Sokoloff, L. (1982). Cerebral glucography with positron tomography. Use in normal subjects and in patients with schizophrenia. *Archives of General Psychiatry*, **39**, 251–9.

Chase, T.N., Geoffrey, V., Gillespie, M., Burrows, G.H. (1986). Structural and functional studies of Gilles de la Tourette syndrome. *,Revue Neurologique*, **142**, 851–5.

Clark, C., Hayden, M., Hollenberg, S., Li, D., Stoessl, A.J. (1987). Controlling for cerebral atrophy in positron emission tomography data. *Journal of Cerebral Blood Flow Metabolism*, **7**, 510–2.

Courchesne, E., Yeung-Courchesne, R., Press, G.A., Hesselink, J.R., Jernigan, T.L. (1988). Hypoplasia of cerebellar vermal lobules VI and VII in autism. *New England Journal of Medicine*, **318**, 1349–54.

Eeg-Olofsson, O. (1970). The development of the electroencephalogram in normal children and adolescents from the age of 1 through 21 years. *Acta Paediatrica Scandinavica, suppl 208.*

Gaffney, G.R., Kuperman, S., Tsai, L.Y., Minchin, S. (1988). Morphological evidence for brainstem involvement in infantile autism. *Biological Psychiatry*, **24**, 578–86.

Gillberg, C., Matousek, M., Petersén, I., Rasmussen, P. (1984). Perceptual motor and attentional deficits in seven-year-old children. Electroencephalographic aspects. *Acta Paedopsychiatrica*, **50**, 243–53.

Gillberg, I.C., Bjure, J., Uvebrant, P., Gillberg, C. (1993). SPECT (Single Photon Emission Computed Tomography) in 31 children and adolescents with autism and autistic-like conditions. *European Child & Adolescent Psychiatry*, **2**, 50–9.

Gomez, M.R. (1988). *Tuberous Sclerosis.* New York: Raven Press.

Musetti, L., Albizzati, A., Grioni, A., Rossetti, M., Saccani, M., Musetti, C. (1993). Autistic disorder associated with congenital HIV infection. *European Child & Adolescent Psychiatry*, **2**, 221–5.

Piven, J., Berthier, M.L., Starkstein, S.E., Nehme, E., Pearlson, G., Folstein, S. (1990). Magnetic resonance imaging evidence for a defect of cerebral cortical development in autism. *American Journal of Psychiatry*, **147**, 734–9.

17 Neuropsychological work-up

General review

The neuropsychological work-up, its extent and contents, varies from one case to another, and there is no one formula for work-up which will suffice as a general model. Some neuropsychiatric patients need little in the way of neuropsychological assessment, and others will require an exhaustive battery of tests. In the 'average' case, there will be a need to include one of the commonly used intelligence/developmental tests (like the WISC, the Griffiths or the Leiter to mention but a few). Occasionally this needs to be complemented by using specific language tests, attentional tests, or batteries purporting to tap specific problems relating to dysfunction of particular brain areas.

In this chapter, some of the most commonly used tests will be briefly surveyed. There is no assumption that this represents a comprehensive review, or that it could be used to substitute for a text of neuropsychology. Rather, it should be seen as a short introduction to the area of neuropsychological work-up as it relates particularly to the examination of neuropsychiatrically disordered children and adolescents.

Before we go on to examine these tests, a few basic concepts need to be familiar to the reader. These are: (a) content validity, (b) criterion-related validity, (c) construct-related validity, (d) test-retest reliability, (e) inter-rater reliability and (f) inter-item consistency.

Content validity refers to the degree to which the item content of a test covers a representative sample of the measured domain. For instance, in order to have good content validity, a speech–language test needs to include a variety of items providing information on many different aspects of both speech and language.

Criterion-related validity refers to the degree to which an instrument is effective in predicting an individual's performance in a specified activity. For instance, in order to have good criterion-related validity, a reading test should be able to predict a pupil's reading performance in the class-room.

Construct-related validity refers to the degree to which a particular test measures a theoretical construct on which the test is based. For instance, in order to have good construct-related validity, a test like the Sally-Anne test (Chapter 6), purportedly specific to theory of mind functions, should correlate strongly with other tests purporting to tap this theoretical construct.

Test-retest reliability refers to the degree to which a score on a particular test can be reproduced over time.

Inter-rater reliability refers to the degree to which two independent assessors will agree concerning the scoring of a result obtained at simultaneous examination of an individual.

Inter-item (or internal) consistency refers to the degree of homogeneity of the domain that the test is purported to sample, i.e. how the various items correlate with each other and with the overall score of 'abnormality'.

Finally, in order to be well standardized, an instrument has to be pretested on a large, demographically representative sample of subjects. Only standardization of this kind will provide a sound background for making reasonable assumptions about the meaning of the test result in any given individual.

For research purposes, in well-controlled studies, standardization norms may be less important, but in every-day clinical practice, no controls exist for comparison, and so reliance has to be placed on a standardized sample.

The Wechsler scales

The Wechsler scales, i.e. the WPPSI (Wechsler pre-school and primary scale of intelligence) (Wechsler, 1967), the WISC-R (Wechsler intelligence scale for children–revised) (Wechsler 1974), the WISC-III (third version, Wechsler, 1992) and the WAIS-R (Wechsler adult intelligence scale–revised) (Wechsler, 1981) are the most widely used scales for assessing intelligence. Among these, the WISC-R has, by far, the most extensive documentation in the field of neuropsychiatric disorders with childhood onset, and will be reviewed in some detail in the present context. However, in the last few years it has been widely replaced by the WISC-III, broadly similar (indeed, in many aspects almost identical) to the WISC-R. However, the clinical validation of the WISC-III is not nearly as extensive as it is for the WISC-R. It has been more recently standardized than the WISC-R and norms are available that correspond to a population mean of 100. The WISC-R, for reasons which are still somewhat unclear, gradually yielded higher and higher mean IQ, so that the population mean in the late 1980s was 112–114 rather than 100. For this reason in particular, but also because in some instances the language is more modern, the WISC-III is to be preferred over the WISC-R.

The Wechsler childhood scales represent downward extensions of the adult scale (the WAIS-R). The scales were constructed on the inherent notion that intelligence may be construed as the individual's overall capacity to understand and cope with the world (Wechsler, 1974). The author emphasized that, in assessing intelligence, it is essential not to put undue emphasis on any one ability, and that there have to be many subtests in order to try to attempt to

challenge an individual's abilities in a broad variety of ways so as to provide a fuller estimate of capacity. The tasks require children to answer verbal queries and solve various types of visual and visuo-motor puzzles.

The Wechsler scales have long been considered 'merely' intelligence tests, but, in recent years a reappraisal of their usefulness in clinical practice has led to the realization that they can also, to a considerable extent, be used as differential diagnostic tools in child neuropsychiatry.

As with any other neuropsychological instrument, a result on the WISC needs to be viewed in relation to available normative data, clinical assessment setting, 'profile of subscores' and the experience of the psychologist performing the testing.

For instance, mean IQ on the WISC-R (for which normative studies were performed in Sweden in the early 1970s), is no longer 100, at least not in Sweden. Rather, it is close to 112 (Hagberg & Hagberg, 1989). The reasons for this upward shift are unclear, but could be associated with early stimulation programmes (such as are provided in some day nurseries and pre-schools) (Hagberg et al., 1981) and gradually less stringent adherence to instructions in the test manual with decreasing clinical experience on the part of the examining psychologists (Gillberg et al., 1983). In any case, there is, of course, the need to adjust levels for 'normal intelligence' even in a clinic sample. Thus, an IQ of 85 on the WISC-R is clearly indicative of cognitive functioning close to the cut-off for 'mental retardation' (defined as an IQ of 70 or less if mean IQ in the population is 100).

On the other hand, it would not be appropriate to say that a child with specific language impairment examined in a clinic had mental retardation just because his full scale (FS) IQ was 68. His verbal IQ (VIQ) was only 40, but his performance IQ (PIQ) was 100. Looking at some of the subscores even within the verbal scale revealed that this was a case with normal abstract and logical reasoning but with severe verbal expressive deficits. The clinical diagnosis of specific language impairment would have to be qualified by the information that the child 'functioned in the mentally retarded range but had normal non-verbal intelligence' rather than by an additional diagnosis of 'global' mental retardation.

The experience of the testing psychologist is essential in assuring optimal cooperation on the part of the child and optimal performance and interpretation of the test results.

The individual profile of subscores, is usually considerably more informative than the full scale intelligence quotient (FS IQ) obtained.

The WISC-R is divided into a verbal and a performance part, each of which comprises six subsets of tests (Table 17.1).

Just recently, the WISC-III (1992) was introduced in Sweden, containing some changes as compared with the WISC-R and yielding new norms. With the appearance of this new instrument, it seems likely that the idea of a substantial reduction in the rate of mental retardation in the young Swedish population cannot survive.

The WISC scales (the WISC-R in particular) have outstanding reliability properties (Sattler, 1988) and internal consistency is excellent (Wechsler, 1974). Satisfactory – excellent concurrent, criterion and construct validity have also been reported in a plethora of studies (Sattler, 1988).

In the author's experience, and supported by findings by Frith (1989), specifically poor results on the comprehension and picture arrangement subtests on the WISC are indicative of theory of mind dysfunction or 'empathy disorder' (Gillberg, 1992).

The WAIS-R and the WISC-R (and WISC-III) overlap between the ages of 16 and 16 years 11 months. According to Sattler (1988), a more thorough sampling of ability is obtained with the WISC-R with children of low normal or below normal intelligence in the overlapping age range.

The WPPSI (Wechsler, 1967) is a downward extension of the WISC. It has excellent reliability and validity and has recently been re-standardized in many countries. It is possible that this more detailed test of young children's intellectual abilities will eventually replace other tests currently more commonly used (including

the Griffiths). Eight of the subtests are also found on the WISC. In addition, there are three more scales (sentences, animal house and geometric design). The test is intended for children aged 4 years to 6 years 6 months. The major objection to the WPPSI in clinical practice in the 1970s and 1980s has been that it has been considered relatively lengthy to administer. However, this may have reflected the overall negative attitude to 'intelligence testing' in the 1970s and 1980s rather than any inherent aspects of the test itself.

Often mentioned as supporting right-hemisphere dysfunction is a particular pattern of low results on the ACID subtests (arithmetic, coding, information and digit span) of the WISC-R. However, even though theoretically interesting, and certainly supported by some clinical data, the empirical evidence for this notion is weak.

The Griffiths scales

The Griffiths Developmental Scale (Griffiths, 1970) is in widespread use in some countries (like Sweden), but is used only occasionally in other parts of the world (like the UK). In yet other countries, it is not used at all (such as in some states of the USA).

The Griffiths has the advantage of providing one version for infants (0–2 years) and an another one for slightly older children (3–8 years), making it possible to follow children at risk in a longitudinal fashion using a similar instrument at several different points in time from early infancy through the early school years. However, the infant version shows relatively poor predictive values (DQs = developmental quotients, grossly equivalent to IQ-scores), other than in cases with severe and profound mental retardation. Also, one scale (the Practical reasoning scale, see below) is only included in the Griffiths II scale.

There are additional disadvantages with the Griffiths scale. First, it only contain six rather broad subscales (A. Motor, B. Personal–social, C. Hearing and speech, D. Eye–hand coordination, E. Performance and F. Practical reason-

Table 17.1. *Subscales and characteristics of the WISC-III*

Subscale	Contents	Taps impairments in	Comments
Verbal			
Information	Recall of names, dates, geographical, literary, anatomical and other information	Storage and retrieval of old data	Sensitive to stimulation; often poor result in dyslexia and other disorders associated with distractibility
Comprehension	Questions about which action should be pursued in a number of social settings	Judgement, 'common sense', abstract and propositional thinking, social awareness	Often very poor result in autism and occasionally Asperger syndrome
Similarities	Questions such as 'What is the similarity between an apple and a pear?'	Concept formation, associative and abstract thinking	Often very poor result in mental retardation, specific language impairment and high-level autism, especially after age 10 yrs
Digit span	Repeat series (of varying length) of digits forwards and backwards	Recent memory, concept formation and retrieval (backwards) and ability to attend and concentrate	Often poor result in ADHD and memory deficits; in autism often superior forwards, poor backwards
Vocabulary	Meaning of words	Comprehension and expression of word meaning	Sensitive to stimulation; Often poor result in DAMP, dyslexia and specific language impairment, usually excellent in Asperger syndrome after early school years
Arithmetic	Verbal (oral or written) instructions to mathematical problems requiring verbal/written (motor) activity	Attention, reading, concept formation, specific mathematical problems	Often poor in dyslexia Tourette, ADHD, DAMP and developmental arithmetic disorder, sometimes poor result in Asperger syndrome
Performance			
Picture completion	Oral–verbal response to questions about details missing in pictures	Ability to differentiate parts from whole, naming and word finding	
Block design	Construction of pattern according to visual instruction	Visuospatial skills, concrete logic	Often superior results in autism, often good result in dyslexia; often poor result in visuo-motor problems
Picture arrangement	Arranging pictures according to logic underlying theme	Logical progress and social awareness, 'theory of mind'	Very poor result in autism and Asperger syndrome

Table 17.1. (*cont.*)

Subscale	Contents	Taps impairments in	Comments
Object assembly	Construction of well-known forms such as car or hand without external visual instruction	Visuo-spatial skills and mental concepts, conceptualization of 'wholes' rather than detail	Poor results in visuo-motor problems, sometimes poor in Asperger syndrome and anorexia nervosa
Digit symbol (Coding)	Matching digit and symbol	Concrete symbol processing, attention, learning, memory, sequencing and precision	Poor results in ADHD, DAMP and dyslexia, very poor results in hypothyroidism, sometimes good results in autism often poor results in Asperger syndrome
Mazes	Tracing with a pen through mazes	Visuo-motor skills, attention, precision	Poor results in DAMP
Symbol search	Matching one symbol with one in a set of symbols	Attention, speed	–

ing), none of which is detailed enough to allow a finer discrimination between various levels of functioning. Secondly, it is a mixture of experimental testing and interview (many items are accepted as scorable on the basis of interview alone, whereas other items require experimental observation for scoring). Finally, like the WISC-R, it tends to overrate IQ, and the mean DQ in the child population is probably currently close to 110 on this scale.

The Griffiths is useful for diagnosing clumsiness (on the A. Motor scale), severe and profound mental retardation and for approximating the level of intellectual functioning in young children with autism. In the latter condition there is usually a very typical profile with peaks in the A. Motor, B. Personal–social and E. Performance scales and troughs in the C. Hearing and speech and F. Practical reasoning scale. If the Griffiths scale has been used in the work-up of a young child, a WISC-III-test should always (whenever possible; very severely mentally retarded children may not score at all on this test and some non-verbal children will only be able to do (parts of) the performance scale) be performed in the school-age period to corro-

borate or refute previous findings. A definitive diagnosis of mental retardation should never be made on the basis of testing with the Griffiths alone.

The Leiter international performance scales

The Leiter international performance scales are excellent instruments for estimating IQ in non-verbal children aged 3–7 years (or with a mental age roughly corresponding to this range). It consists of a number of subtests and makes use only of cubes (that the children are requested to organize according to specific principles that are presented in non-verbal ways). It has been shown to yield good agreement with other measures of IQ and social quotients (such as derived from the Vineland social maturity scale) in certain non-communicative children (Shah & Holmes, 1985). However, one must keep in mind the typical peaks in visual performance skills shown by some children with autism, which infer that superior results on the Leiter scales need not necessarily reflect overall superior IQ.

The Vineland social maturity scales

The Vineland social maturity scale (Doll, 1965) was recently revised to produce the Vineland adaptive behaviour scale (Sparrow, Balla & Cicchetti, 1984). This scale assesses an individual's personal and social functioning/self-support. A semi-structured interview is conducted by the examiner with a respondent (the parent/carer) familiar with the subject. Communication, daily living skills, socialization and motor skills (the latter scale only under age 5 years) are the domains surveyed. These are then combined to generate an adaptive behaviour composite. There is also an additional checklist tapping maladaptive behaviours.

There are three forms of the Vineland adaptive behaviour scale: survey form, expanded form and classroom edition. The survey form, which requires about 1 hour to administer is the most widely used. The expanded form proves more details on the skills included in the survey form and is often used with severely handicapped individuals in order to design an appropriate intervention programme. The classroom edition is intended for completion by the child's teacher and takes about 20 minutes to fill out.

The Vineland scale is very useful, particularly when trying to obtain overall estimates of functioning in children who are difficult to test in a formalized test setting. However, the means and range of scores tend to vary considerably across age groups, suggesting that the scales may not be appropriate for longitudinal follow-up comparisons.

The NEPSY

The NEPSY (Neuropsychological Investigation for Children) (Korkman & Peltomaa, 1991) is a comprehensive neuropsychological assessment of cognitive and psychomotor development. The target group is children aged 4–8 years who suffer from learning disorders and various types of brain dysfunction.

The NEPSY comprises five parts: (1) tests of attention, orientation and executive functions, (2) language tests, (3) sensory–motor tests, (4) visuo-spatial tests and (5) tests of motor and learning. Each part includes several separate tests which are designed to represent the main components of the broader areas of mental functioning.

The assessment provides information of the nature and mechanism of learning disorders by assessing separately the subcomponents of a disturbed function. If, for example, the child presents with a language problem, this disorder may be analysed by assessing oral motor series, sensory–motor differentiation, auditory and phonological analysis of speech, recognition with meaning, comprehension of complex speech, short-term memory, conception of syntax and logical–verbal relations, naming, and word fluency.

The NEPSY tests are standardized and psychometrically elaborated. The inter-rater reliabilities and the internal consistency of the tests are adequate, and the validity has been analysed in a number of studies (Korkman, 1988a, b, c). In a recent validation study one type of test profile was shown to predict attention disorders at school (Korkman & Peltomaa, 1991). Another study demonstrated that children with ADHD performed poorly on a test measuring impulse control, whereas children with reading and spelling problems performed poorly on a number of language tests (Korkman & Pesonen, 1993).

An extended American version for children aged 3–12 years will be published shortly (Korkman, Kirk & Kemp. 1993)

Other tests

A number of other tests are available for use with children. These include the Peabody picture vocabulary test, the Illinois test of psycholinguistic abilities, the British abilities scales, the Benton and Bender visual and visual motor tests and the neuropsychological test batteries of Halstead-Reitan and Luria (see Table 17.2).

The Peabody picture vocabulary test–revised (PPVT-R) has been very well standardized, and

Table 17.2. *Commonly utilized child and adolescent neruopsychological assessment instruments*

Test	Age (years)	Comments
IQ/Overall development		
WPPSI	4–6.5	Similar to WISC, 8 of 11 scales have same title
WISC-R	6–16.9	Most widely used IQ-test available. Twelve subscales yielding verbal, performance, and full scale IQ
WISC-III	6–16.9	Recently standardized. Same as WISC-R but containing additional subtest (symbol search) (see Table 17.1)
Griffiths I	0–2	Mixture of observation and interview. Useful for distinguishing cases with severe mental retardation. Five subscales
Griffiths II	2–8	Mixture of observation and interview. Useful for distinguishing cases with mental retardation from normality. Six subscales (motor, personal/social, hearing–speech, eye-hand coordination, performance and practical reasoning). Characteristic autism profile in mildly retarded range: low hearing–speech and practical reasoning and intermediate eye–hand coordination, relatively better results on remaining three subscales
Stanford–Binet	2–adult	General IQ test
Raven Coloured Matrices	5.5–11.5	Non-verbal test of IQ for children with different cultural background
Leiter international performance scales language (including autism)	3–7	Non-verbal test of IQ, consisting of various types of block design and block arrangement tests. Very useful in language-disordered and non-native-speaking populations
Language/vocabulary		
Peabody picture vocabulary test	4–adult	Measures receptive vocabulary acquisition. Requires reasonably good visuo-spatial receptive skills. Provides standard scores, percentiles and age-equivalents. Employed by some as an overall screen measure of intelligence (because of its overall score's moderate correlation with WISC-R IQ)
Illinois test of psycholinguistic abilities (ITPA)	4–9.9	A wide range of subtests given titles which suggest the measurement of specific language functions, although most studies suggest that it may be better used as an overall IQ-test
Adaptive behaviour		
Vineland adaptive behaviour scales	0–19 retarded: all ages	Standard scores for adaptive behaviour composite, communication, daily living skills, socialization and motor; percentiles, developmental age score and age equivalents. Separately standardized (and scores available) for normal, visually impaired, hearing impaired, emotionally disturbed and mentally retarded

it is reliable and valid (Sparrow, Fletcher & Cicchetti, 1985). The test consists of 175 plates that are displayed consecutively to the subject on a small easel. Each plate contains four pictures, and the subject is instructed to point to (or announce) the number of the picture that depicts the vocabulary word read by the examiner. The limited demands for responsiveness made placed upon the child make this test particularly appealing for children who, for various reasons, are less than co-operative. The overall score correlates well with that of the overall WISC-R IQ.

The Illinois Test of Psycholinguistic Abilities (ITPA) (Kirk, McCarthy & Kirk, 1968) has been developed in order to diagnose disorders of speech and language. However, it is doubtful whether it validly measures language functions rather than overall IQ, and, except for some of its subtests (modifications of which appear in the NEPSY), it has been used less in recent years.

The British Abilities Scales (BAS) () were developed in order to measure more aspects of abilities than are included in most other tests. It has been standardized in UK child populations, and is a reliable test. Its construct validity and applicability remain to be established.

The Bender-Gestalt test (Bender, 1938; Koppitz, 1968) and the Benton visual retention test (Benton, 1974) are commonly used visual–motor tests which purportedly tap 'brain damage'. The child is shown cards on which are reproduced geometric designs and is asked to copy each design directly from the original (Bender) or memory (Bender, Benton). There is some (relatively old) normative data, but by and large these tests have little validity in terms of the 'brain damage' construct.

The Halstead-Reitan (Reitan & Wolfson, 1985) and Luria-Nebraska (Golden, 1987) neuropsychological test batteries are flexible and permit putting different degrees of emphasis on various aspects of the child's functioning. However, both tests are time-consuming (3–6 hours are required for completion), and it is still unclear what underlying constructs they tap.

Furthermore, the Luria childhood battery is a downward extension of an adult battery, which has led to criticism (Sattler, 1988), because of the implicit assumption that developmental changes in brain function are not important. Thus, considerable caution is warranted in the clinical interpretation of results obtained using this battery.

The Wisconsin card sorting test (WCST) is a test purportedly measuring such frontal lobe functions as planning, strategy, flexibility and persistence.

Summary including clinical recommendations

The WISC is the best researched of all children's IQ-tests and should be regarded as the 'method of choice' when evaluating children with neuropsychiatric disorder. It is useful not only for providing a reliable measure of the child's overall IQ, but also for suggesting fairly typical clinical profiles in certain conditions, such as autism. The WISC-III, providing the most recently updated version of this test, should be used in most cases. However, in many situations, the WISC is not appropriate. For instance, in non-verbal children, only the performance scale can be employed, and even this may be too demanding since some of the subscales are difficult to administer without any verbal prompts. The Leiter and the Raven may be excellent alternatives in such cases. The Vineland adaptive behaviour scale is often a useful tool for making an overall judgement with regard to the child's functional level. Achievements tests, such as in respect of reading and writing, are required in cases of dyslexia and other types of scholastic failure. More in-depth neuropsychological evaluation (such as with the NEPSY) may be necessary in some cases. However, before a decision is taken to extend the neuropsychological work-up beyond that of an IQ-test and an achievement test, the rationale for this should be made clear. For instance, in patients planned for/undergoing epilepsy surgery, other kinds of brain surgery and brain irradiation/chemotherapy work-up and follow-up, a comprehensive neuropsychological work-up is always required. In combination with a careful neuropsychiatric assessment, it provides the best basis for evaluating change over time (Table 17.2).

References

Bender, L. (1938). *Visual Motor Gestalt and Its Clinical Use*. New York: American Orthopsychiatry Association.

Benton, A.L. (1974). *Revised Visual Retention Test: Manual*. San Antonio, TX: The Psychological Corporation.

Doll, E. (1965). *Vineland Social Maturity Scale*. Revised. Minnesota: American Guidance Service, Inc.

Frith, U. (1989). Autism and 'theory of mind'. *In* Gillberg, C. (Ed.) *Diagnosis and Treatment of Autism*. New York: Plenum Press.

Gillberg, C. (1992). The Emanuel Miller Memorial Lecture 1991: Autism and autistic-like conditions: subclasses among disorders of empathy. *Journal of Child Psychology and Psychiatry*, **33**, 813–42.

Gillberg, C., Svenson, B., Carlström, G., Waldenström, E., Rasmussen, P. (1983). Mental retardation in Swedish urban children: some epidemiological considerations. *Applied Research in Mental Retardation*, **4**, 207–18.

Golden, C.J. (1987). *Luria-Nebraska Neuropsychological Battery: Children's Revision*. Los Angeles: Western Psychological Services.

Griffiths, R. (1970). *The Abilities of Young Children*. London: Child Research Centre.

Hagberg, B., Hagberg, G. (1989). Neuropediatric aspects of prevalence, etiology, prevention, and diagnosis. *In* Clarke, A.M., Clarke, A.D.B.,Berg, J.M. (Eds.) *Mental Deficiency: The Changing Outlook*. 4th. London: Methuen & Co. Ltd.

Hagberg, B., Hagberg, G., Lewerth, A., Lindberg, U. (1981). Mild mental retardation in Swedish school children. I. Prevalence. *Acta Paediatrica Scandinavia*, **70**, 441–4.

Kirk, S., McCarthy, J., Kirk, W. (1968). *The Illinois Test of psycholinguistic Abilities*. Rev. Ed. Urbana: University of Illinois Press.

Koppitz, E. (1968). *Psychological Evaluation of Children's Human Figure Drawings*. New York: Grune & Stratton.

Korkman, M. (1988a). *NEPSY. A neuropsychological test battery for young developmentally disabled children*. Helsinki University.

Korkman, M. (1988b). NEPSY. An adaptation of Luria's investigation for young children. *The Clinical Neuropsychologist*, **2**, 375–92.

Korkman, M. (1988c). *NEPSY. A proposed neuropsychological investigation for children – Revised version*. Helsinki: Psykoligien kustannus.

Korkman, M., Kirk, U., Kemp, S.L. (1993). NEPSY. Developmental assessment of neuropsychological function. Accepted for publication.

Korkman, M., Peltomaa, K. (1991). A pattern of test findings predicting attention problems at school. *Journal of Abnormal Child Psychology*, **19**, 451–67.

Korkman, M., Pesonen, A.-E. (1993). Comparison of neuropsychological test profiles of children with attention disorder and/or reading and spelling disorder. *Journal of Learning Disabilities*, In press.

Reitan, R.M., Wolfson, D. (1985). *The Halstead–Reitan Neuropsychological Test Battery*. Tucson, AZ: Neuropsychology Press.

Sattler, J.M. (1988). *Assessment of Children*. San Diego: J.M. Sattler.

Shah, A., Holmes, N. (1985). The use of the Leiter International Performance Scale with autistic children. *Journal of Autism and Developmental Disorders*, **15**, 195–203.

Sparrow, S.S., Balla, D.A., Cicchetti, D.V. (1984). *The Vineland Adaptive Behavior Schales*. Circle Pines, MN: American Guidance Service.

Sparrow, S.S., Cicchetti, D.V. (1984). The behavior inventory for rating development (BIRD): assessments of reliability and factorial validity. *Applied Research into Mental Retardation*, **5**, 219–31.

Sparrow, S.S., Fletcher, J.M., Cicchetti, D.V. (1985). Psychological Assessment of Children. *In* Michels, R., Cavenar, J.O., Brodie, H.K.H., *et al.* (Eds.) *Psychiatry*. Philadelphia: JB Lippincott.

Wechsler, D. (1967). *Manual of the Wechsler Pre-School and Primary Scale of Intelligence for Children*. New York: Psychological Corporation.

Wechsler, D. (1974). *Manual of the Wechsler Intelligence Scale for Children – Revised*. New York: Psychological Corporation.

Wechsler, D. (1981). *Manual for the Wechsler Adult Intelligence Scale – Revised*. San Antonio, TX: The Psychological Corporation.

Wechsler, D. (1992). *Manual of the Wechsler Intelligence Scale for Children. Third Edition – Revised*. New York: Psychological Corporation.

Part IV:
Intervention

18 The impact of childhood neuropsychiatric disorders on the family

The effect of neuropsychiatric disorders on the children

The reactions of children with various types of neuropsychiatric disorder to their own ailment have already been briefly reviewed in Chapter 3. The purpose of highlightling these reactions here is to suggest that intervention cannot be properly planned without taking them into account. The child with DAMP/ADHD/ clumsy child syndrome who has judged himself to be 'different from the rest', 'abnormal' or 'not good enough/not wanted' is likely to behave very differently from the child with the same type of neuropsychiatric disorder who has, instead, developed an aggressive stance, blaming parents, peers and teachers for all his/her problems. Only a proper analysis of the interactions between underlying neuropsychiatric disorder and the coping style of the child (Rutter & Garmezy, 1983) can guide the intervention/ treatment in directions that are likely to be helpful to the affected individual and his/her environment (Williams, Pleak & Hanesian, 1991).

Sibling reactions

There is a considerable literature on the interactions of siblings (Dunn & McGuire, 1992), but the number of studies that directly address the issue of the effects on siblings of having a neuropsychiatrically disordered brother or sister is limited. It is generally concluded that siblings of neuropsychiatrically disordered brothers and sisters have more emotional and behavioural problems than children with non-handicapped siblings. The problems are partly correlated with factors characterizing the handicapped child (severity and type of illness), the non-handicapped sibling him/herself (birth order and gender) and of parental relations (Senapati & Hayes, 1988).

Recent research has drawn more attention to the finding that most siblings of neuropsychiatrically disordered children fall within the normal range of functioning (McHale & Gamble, 1989), and, even though a minority may be severely distraught by having a handicapped brother or sister, there are also those who will attest to the experience of having a handicapped sibling as 'rewarding' (e.g. Bågenholm & Gillberg, 1991).

The possible importance of siblings in intervention/treatment should not be underestimated. In families containing a child with anorexia or bulimia nervosa, it appears that siblings may actually be highly effective therapists (Vandereycken & van Vreckem, 1990).

Parental reactions

There is a considerable literature on the reactions of parents to the birth of a handicapped child (with cleft palate, spina bifida and Down syndrome to mention but a few conditions) (Oberfield & Gabriel, 1991). The psychological effects of giving birth to a child who is immediately perceived as or diagnosed deviant at birth (such as in the case of Down syndrome) and of slowly having to adapt to the fact that the seemingly normal child is abnormal (such as in autism) are likely to be very different. In the first instance, 'ordinary' principles for crisis intervention (Drotar *et al.*, 1975), such as early information and short-term psychotherapy, will probably be helpful. In the case of neuropsychiatric disorders which are only diagnosed when the child is several years of age, a crisis may not even occur or be so atypical that it would be highly inappropriate to expect short term psychotherapy to be effective.

A number of factors interact in the shaping of a parent's reaction to having a neuropsychiatrically disordered child: societal attitudes, parental age, gender and marital status, previous experiences, whether the child is first- or later-born, the nature of the child's disorder, and the presence or absence of networks of social and emotional support to mention but a few. Economic factors should not be ignored, and, if problematic to the family, should be alleviated, if at all possible.

Genetic stoppage (i.e. the conscious decision on the part of the parents not to have more children because they have already given birth to a handicapped individual) is probably in operation in many families containing neuropsychiatrically disordered children. For instance, there is evidence that parents of children with autism more often than parents of other children decide they will not 'take the risk associated with having more children' (Szatmari & Jones, 1978; Gillberg, Gillberg & Steffenburg, 1992). This, in turn, implies that, at least theoretically, genetic counselling could contribute to less distress on the part of the parents in making decisions of this kind: knowing more about the genetic risk may help parents feel more secure (whether the risk is low or high).

Many parents have felt rejected by teachers, psychologists and doctors before. They may be either suspicious, reticent or hostile. They may expect the neuropsychiatrist to be 'just another one of those specialists who will put the blame on the parents'. It is essential not to contribute to the vicious circle of child disorder–parental distress–specialist failure to make appropriate diagnosis–parental perplexity–specialist reassurance–parental guilt–aggravation of child's symptoms–parental distress, etc. Neutral information about the nature of the child's disorder and reassurance that it has not been *caused* by parental failure will usually help break a circle of this kind.

Most parents feel bereaved (Caplan, Mason & Kaplan, 1965) and their reactions can be understood in terms of grief. Any doctor working with children suffering from neuropsychiatric disorders will need to be well informed about the emotional processes associated with grief, his/her own attitudes and ways to cope with a spectrum of different patterns of reactions. Parents whose infants are born with severe and obvious abnormalities, as well as those who bear children who are only gradually recognized as deviant may have to face a lifetime of adjustment to a situation they had not expected and to a child who will continue to place special demands on them. One of the most important tasks of the clinical neuropsychiatrist is to support such parents throughout the years so that they may feel that they will not need to go searching for better support elsewhere. This is not to say that parents' seeking advice from other specialists would signal a failure on the part of the neuropsychiatrist. To the contrary, if the parents feel such 'second opinions' would be helpful, the neuropsychiatrist should aid them in finding appropriate consultation, rather than warn them of the risks of seeing 'one more doctor'.

Transactional effects

Sameroff proposed a transactional model for development (Sameroff, 1975; Sameroff & Chandler, 1975) which is, at least in parts, equally applicable to the understanding of development of normal as well as abnormal children. The child's characteristics (sex, age, temperament, disorders) affect how the child behaves, how parents treat the child (differently, for instance, when the child has ADHD treated or not treated with stimulants, Barkley *et al.*, 1982) and how the parents' behaviour affects the child. The parent's characteristics may have the same principal effects. This view of transactional effects renders simplistic cause and effect relationships naive.

How individual families cope with their particular child, and how the child affects and reacts to their specific family situation, should be the focus of exploration before any in-depth intervention plan is offered. Again, it is important to stress that parents need to be taken seriously. The biological origin of the child's disorder should be stressed. It is usually only after detailed diagnostic information of this kind that it will be possible to start other types of exploration and intervention that may, with time, foster positive effects on the bilateral forces involved in the transactional chain of events.

References

Bågenholm, A., Gillberg, C. (1991). Psychosocial effects on siblings of children with autism and mental retardation: a population-based study. *Journal of Mental Deficiency Research*, **35**, 291–307.

Barkley, R.A., McMurray, M.B., Edelbrock, C.S., Robbins, K. (1989). The response of aggressive and nonaggressive ADHD children to two doses of methylphenidate. *Journal of the American Academy of Child and Adolescent Psychiatry*, **28**, 873–81.

Caplan, G., Mason, E., Kaplan, D. (1965). Four studies of crisis in parents of prematures. *Community Menthal Health Journal*, **1**, 149–61.

Drotar, D., Baskiewicz, A., Irvin, N. *et al.* (1975). The adaptation of parents to the birth of an infant with a congenital malformation: A hypothetical model. *Pediactrics*, **56**, 710–17.

Dunn, J., McGuire, S. (1992). Sibling and peer relationships in childhood. *Journal of Child Psychology and Psychiatry*, **33**, 67–105.

Gillberg, C., Gillberg, I.C., Steffenburg, S. (1992). Siblings and parents of children with autism. A controlled population based study. *Developmental Medicine and Child Neurology*, **34**, 389–98.

McHale, S.M., Gamble, W.C. (1989). Siblings relationships of children with disabled and nondisabled brothers and sisters. *Developmental Psychology*, **25**, 421–9.

Oberfield, R., Gabriel, H.P. (1991). Prematurity, birth defects, and early death: Impact on the family. *In* Lewis, M. (Ed.) *Child and Adolescent Psychiatry. A Comprehensive Textbook*. Baltimore, Maryland: Williams & Wilkins.

Rutter, M., Garmezy, N. (1983). Developmental psychopathology. *In* Hetherington, E.M. (Ed.) *Socialization, Personality, and Social Development*. New York: Wiley.

Sameroff, A.J. (1975). Early influences on development: fact or fantasy? *Merrill-Palmer*, **21**, 267–94.

Sameroff, A., Chandler, M. (1975). Reproductive risk and the continuum of caretaker causality. *In* Horowitz, F. (Ed.) *Review of Child Development Research*. Chicago: University of Chicago Press.

Senapati, R., Hayes, A. (1988). Sibling relationships of handicapped children: a review of conceptual and methodological issues. *International Journal of Behavioral Development*, **11**, 89–115.

Szatmari and Jones 1978 Szatmari, P., Jones, M.B. (1991). IQ and the genetics of autism. *Journal of Child Psychology and Psychiatry*, **32**, 897–908.

Vandereycken, W., van Vreckem, E. (1990). Siblings as co-patients and co-therapists in eating disorders. Paper presented at the First International Symposium on Brothers and Sisters. Leiden, December.

Williams, D.T., Pleak, R.R., Hanesian, H. (1991). Neurological disorders. *In* Lewis, M. (Ed.) *Child and Adolescent Psychiatry. A Comprehensive Textbook*. Baltimore, Maryland: Williams & Wilkins.

19 Interventions and treatments

The impact of diagnosis and information; the psychoeducational approach

The word intervention is sometimes taken to mean 'treatment'. This is often not appropriate. Treatment should be aimed at a specific problem/dysfunction/pathology which can be positively affected by the treatment; a cure is intended. The typical example is antibiotic treatment of a bacterial infection; cures are often achieved. Treatment in this sense, more often than not, does not apply in child and adolescent psychiatry. Child and adolescent psychiatry is certainly not unique in this respect. Contrary to popular belief, treatment in this sense, is not available in the vast majority of problems in any branch of medicine.

Almost all the neuropsychiatric disorders of childhood are severely handicapping subchronic or chronic conditions. In the majority of cases no cures are available to date, and any intervention should be performed in order to improve the situation of the individual and family rather than to cure the underlying disorder.

Diagnosis and information are often major components of good treatment. They always constitute essential elements of intervention.

In general, information about the diagnosis, work-up and implications should be as open and detailed as possible, taking into account the specifics and needs of the individual and his/her family. Optimally, often both parents should be present when the information is shared. Written information to supplement the oral communication is usually helpful. A written summary of the diagnostic evaluation should be provided in most cases. Excellent leaflets, booklets and books are available in several different languages on many topics ranging from autism and attention deficit syndromes through Prader–Willi and Williams syndromes.

Prognosis should be discussed after a diagnosis has been made. This issue should *never* be treated lightly or in terms of definitive statements. Outcome is *always* unknown, whether one is dealing with a post-viral chronic fatigue syndrome or autism. The information should always be based on the most up-to-date review of the outcome literature relating to the particular disorder. In most disorders there is huge variation in respect of outcome, and this range should be acknowledged. It is essential to take a realistic view. Striking over-optimistic or over-pessimistic attitudes is inappropriate and usually serves to prolong the phase in which a family is trying unsuccessfully to reorientate after a period of shock and confusion.

Models for crisis development and intervention are very often hopelessly off key in child neuropsychiatry. Shock is rarely a matter of a one-time-thing in disorders such as autism, DAMP and Asperger syndrome. Rather, a slow re-learning process (cognitive and affective), trying to adjust to the situation of having an abnormal or unusual child, is set in motion before, at, or years after, initial diagnosis. There is no simple solution to the various problems faced by a family with a handicapped child, and no two crises are the same. Thus, it is often grossly inappropriate to speak of the need for crisis psychotherapy. What most parents need in connection with a diagnosis of a childhood onset neuropsychiatric disorder is information, empathic support and practical help in arranging financial matters, daycare and respite care, for example.

Parent associations

Parent associations, when knowledgeable and effectively organized, can be exceptionally helpful to families of individuals suffering from child or adolescent neuropsychiatric disorders and also to the professionals catering for them within the health care system. There has been a tradition that parents and professionals work separated from each other, both with the goal of providing the best available help to affected children. Slowly, this tradition is breaking down, and we are beginning to see the coming together of parents and professionals, both in organizing conferences, writing books and in everyday clinical practice.

In tailoring services to meet the needs of neuropsychiatrically disordered children, adolescents and their families, it is essential to find out just what families need, and not impose interventions that are felt by those closest to the patient to be irrelevant. Thus, whenever considering major changes, improvements, or the implementation of new services, relevant parent associations should be consulted.

Support groups of other kinds

Apart from parent associations, there are other support groups, including 'handicap' institutions of various kinds, siblings associations, and associations of individuals with a particular disorder without the 'admixture' of parents or siblings.

Changing societal attitudes

One of the most important intervention aspects in child neuropsychiatry is the changing of societal attitudes to specific disorders and handicapping conditions. This has to be a continuous process that has to be informed by updated knowledge accumulated in research, clinical practice and results obtained in investigations of attitudes on the part of those affected, their families and carers, and people in the community not affected by a particular disorder.

Diets

For a few child and adolescent neuropsychiatric disorders, diets are important. This applies both in preventive and clinical child neuropsychiatry. In prevention, a phenylalanine-free diet to those individuals who have been screened positive for PKU in the first week of life, will interrupt the destruction of nerve tissue and hinder the evolution of autistic symptoms and intellectual deterioration in some cases. In rare cases of lactic acidosis with autism and cognitive problems, identifying the correct metabolic enzyme error may lead to a specific dietary treatment which will then lead to amelioration of autistic symptoms (Coleman & Blass, 1985).

It is quite possible that a number of those (very few) young children with severe autistic symptoms who grew up to become normally functioning adults may have metabolic disorders which may be, inadvertently, 'treated' by a change of diet (a change which was not informed by knowledge about the metabolic disorder, but rather occurred by chance in relation to the underlying problem).

Psychopharmacology

The field of neuropsychopharmacology is currently growing at a fast rate. After decades of being relegated to the position of 'second best' interventions in child psychiatry, the emergence of safe and effective psychopharmacological treatments for disorders such as Tourette syndrome and obsessive–compulsive disorder has finally opened the door to a more reasonable, scientifically validated stance on the part of clinicians in relation to the question of neuropsychopharmacology. What was once by some regarded as an almost shameful suggestion, the option to treat a child with a severe neuropsychiatric disorder with an appropriate pharmacological agent, is now considered in the management of many cases.

Table 19.1 outlines some of the most important diagnostic categories and problem types for which drug treatment should be considered, and the types of pharmacological agents which might merit appraisal in the individual case. This table draws on data and clinical experience from Green (1991); Gualtieri (1990) and Gadow (1992), as well as on the author's own experience and limited empirical study in the field. As is obvious already on surveying the table, a relatively limited group of drugs have been properly evaluated in psychopharmacological studies. In addition to those drugs shown in the table, an even smaller number has been tried in double-blind, placebo-controlled studies and found to be ineffective in most instances. Fenfluramine (Gadow, 1992) belongs in this group. The fact that it has been omitted from the table does not mean that it is never useful in the treatment of any of the disorders listed. However, in autism, the disorder for which it was purported to be particularly useful in the early 1980s, it has been shown to be ineffective in most instances. In preliminary studies it has shown some promising effects in the treatment of bulimia nervosa, but the evidence is not yet such that it warrants special mention in the table. On the other hand, haloperidol is cited as being useful in autism. However, any conclusion to this effect is in need of qualification. While clearly effective in reducing some autism symptoms (Green, 1991), haloperidol has such potentially severe side effects (Campbell, 1989) that it is very much in doubt whether it can be considered a safe enough treatment, even in a disorder as severe as autism. Thus, the table should be seen only as a suggestion as to what type of medication might be useful in the individual case with a particular disorder. In order for a reasonable decision to be made in each case, the section on each disorder and the brief section on each class of drugs should be consulted first.

The rest of this section on psychopharmacological interventions will be devoted to a brief overview of the various classes of drugs used in the management of child and adolescent neuropsychiatric disorders.

Neuroleptics and other so-called antipsychotic drugs

The two classes of psychopharmacological drugs that appear to have been scientifically examined the most, are the neuroleptics and the tricyclic antidepressants. However, this statement applies primarily to adults, and the empirical study of such drugs in children and adolescents has been relatively limited. Overall, the use of neuroleptics in children has been (and continues to be) limited, at least in Europe. Their effectiveness seem to be less striking in children than in adults. However, the main reason for their restricted use is possibly the awareness of the potentially very negative side effects and the risk that irreparable nerve damage may be incurred.

The neuroleptics have been subjected mainly to empirical study in three types of childhood/adolescent onset disorders, viz. autism, Tourette syndrome and psychosis.

Campbell and her group in New York have published excellent work on the wanted and unwanted effects of neuroleptics (particularly haloperidol) in the treatment of autism (Campbell, 1989). The results of these studies, showing a number of beneficial effects of haloperidol on several symptoms (such as hyperactivity, stereotypies and social withdrawal) in autism as well as a high risk of concomitant extrapyramidal and other side effects, are not automatically generalizable to other children and adolescents with autism. First of all, almost all the studies, pertain to young children who have been hospitalized and closely monitored in a less than lifelike setting. Gains demonstrated in a setting of this kind cannot be projected on to children with autism living in the community and facing the interaction of families, a normal (or abnormal) peer group, teachers in a sometimes less than well-structured environment. Because of the relatively high risk of extrapyramidal side

Table 19.1 *Child neuropsychiatric problems for which psychopharmacotherapy may be therapeutically indicated and types of appropriate, scientifically validated, medication*

Diagnosis/problem	Medication	Reference
Aggression regardless of other diagnosis	Neuroleptics	Gadow, 1992
	Stimulants	Gadow et al., 1990
	Lithium	Campbell et al., 1984
	Carbamazepine	Evans, Clay & Gualtieri, 1987
	Propranolol	Gadow, 1992
Mental retardation with severe psychiatric problem including self-injury	Lithium	Campbell et al., 1984
	Naltrexone	Gadow, 1992
Autism and autistic-like conditions	Vitamin B6	Gillberg & Coleman 1992
	Haloperidol	Campbell et al., 1983
		Perry et al., 1989
	Lithium	Campbell, 1989
DAMP/ADHD/Hyperactivity	Stimulants	Gadow, 1992
	Tricyclics	Gadow, 1992
	Carbamazepine	Cueva et al., 1993
Dyslexia	Piracetam	Wilsher, Atkins & Manfield, 1985
Tourette syndrome	Pimozide	Green, 1991
	Haloperidol	Green, 1991
	Clonidine	Leckman et al., 1991
Obsessive–compulsive disorder	Clomipramine	Flament et al., 1985
	Fluoxetine	Riddle et al., 1990
	Fluvoxamine?	
Bulimia nervosa	Tricyclics	Goldbloom et al., 1989
Schizophrenia	Neuroleptics	Gadow, 1992
Epilepsy (particularly if associated with neuropsychiatric disorder of other type)	Carbamazepine	Evans, Clay & Gualtieri, 1991
	Valproic acid	Evans, Clay & Gualtieri, 1991
	Other antiepileptics	Gillberg, 1992
Enuresis	Oxytocin	Hjälmås, Passerini-Glazel & Chiozza, 1992
Fragile X syndrome	Folic acid	Hagerman et al., 1992
Sleep disorders		
Insomnia[a]	Diphenylhydramine	Gadow, 1992
Sleep-wake schedule disorder[a]	Diazepam	Green, 1991
Pavor nocturnus[b]	Diazepam	Green, 1991
Somnabulism[a]	Diazepam	Green, 1991
Narcolepsy	Stimulants	Kotagal, Hartse & Walsh, 1990
Kleine–Levin syndrome	Stimulants	Lishman, 1978
	Lithium	referens

Notes:

[a] sleep disorders should not be treated with drugs other than during exceptional circumstances, see text!

[b] pavor nocturnus is probably best treated with abrasio of nasal adenoid; drug treatment indicated only in a limited number of cases.

effects (tardive dyskinesias) of haloperidol in the treatment of autism (almost 20–30% according to some of the New York studies (Perry *et al.*, 1985)), many clinicians refrain from using them in very young children. However, in the US, the neuroleptics are considered drugs of first choice even in the treatment of very young children with autism (Green, 1991). Also, according to Green (1991), the tardive dyskinesias seen so often in the treatment of children with autism, are always reversible. In Scandinavia the neuroleptics are mostly used in adolescence in order to control hyperactivity, negativism and angry and labile affect in autism, symptoms which are known to be ameliorated by treatment with haloperidol (and other drugs from the butyrophenone group). The two most commonly used drugs are haloperidol and pimozide. Haloperidol is used in doses of 0.25 mg–1 mg (occasionally 2–3 mg in severe cases) twice daily for children and 0.5–5 mg twice daily for adolescents. Pimozide is usually given only to adolescents at a dose of 1–4 mg twice daily or 2–8 mg in one daily dose. Experience with this drug in the very young age group is limited.

In Tourette syndrome, a drug trial is often indicated, and haloperidol is, without doubt the best researched drug in this disorder. Since Tourette syndrome is not generally as severely a handicapping disorder as autism, the pros and cons of medication have to be weighed even more carefully. When drug treatment is used, doses should be kept as low as possible, usually in the range of 1–3 mg twice daily (starting out with 0.5 mg twice daily). Pimozide may be given at similar doses to control extreme tics.

In psychotic disorders, doses may have to be higher than those recommended for autism and Tourette syndrome. In the case of pimozide, recent studies suggest that a daily dose exceeding 10 mg is not indicated. Haloperidol is often preferred to low-potency drugs (such as chlorpromazine and thioridazien) because they are less likely to cause severe sedation and adrenolytic reactions such as hypotension. However, the risk of producing extrapyramidal side effects is possibly greater, and perhaps particularly so in young children, who appear to be prone to developing dystonic reactions on haloperidol. Some clinicians prefer thirodiazin because of its relatively low risk of producing severe extrapyramidal symptoms. On the negative side, excessive sedation and gradual weight gain (in turn leading to less mobility and more inactivity, which may both set the patient moving in a negative spiral) are common side effects of thioridazin.

In psychotic depression, there is often a need to combine neuroleptics (for one to two weeks) and antidepressants. In a study using chlorpromazine (50–100 mg/day) and nortriptyline (20–35 mg/day) in psychotic depressed adolescents, the combined drug treatment was very effective, and even though the addition of nortriptyline after a couple of weeks reduced the chlorpromazine blood level (possibly through induction of liver enzymes), the reduction was not significant and had no obvious clinical effect.

Dosage

In addition to what has already been said in the foregoing, only a few general statements are appropriate here. Dosage should usually be proportionate to adult doses on a weight basis, but can sometimes be higher without any obvious negative side effects and considerable positive gains. Nevertheless, it is also clear that a clinically positive response can often be achieved at doses considerably lower than those recommended in the literature. This observation appears to hold true regardless of the type of problem treated. Perhaps these observations should be interpreted to mean that the range of responses in children and adolescents is even greater than that observed in adults, and that one should retain an open mind as to optimal dosage whenever one embarks on treatment with any of the neuroleptics in child disorders.

Side effects

The extrapyramidal side effects (*acute dystonia*, which can occur after single doses, and *tardive dyskinesias*, including akathisia, and *rabbit syndrome* (characterized by rapid movements of perioral muscles), which usually develop only after long-term administration of antipsychotic drugs and believed to represent up-regulation of dopamine receptors after chronic blockade) have already been mentioned, and are probably the best known of all the side effects that can occur with neuroleptic treatment. Only the acute dystonias and rabbit syndrome are amenable to treatment with anti-Parkinsonian drugs. Campbell *et al.* (1988) reported that 30% of children with autism who participated in a long-term haloperidol-treatment study developed dyskinesia. Of these 30%, 80% developed withdrawal dyskinesias, which emerged approximately 2 weeks following the discontinuation of medication. The dyskinesias lasted from several days to several months, but they were all reversible. Persistent tardive dyskinesias have also been reported in 30–40% of individuals with mental retardation who are treated with neuroleptics (and withdrawal dyskinesias in an additional 29%) (Gadow, 1992). These figures are so high as to warrant extreme caution in the prescription of this class of drugs in mentally retarded populations (including those with the combination of autism and mental retardation). However, it should be emphasized that dyskinesias can sometimes be very difficult to distinguish from the stereotyped movements and tics often seen in mentally retarded individuals. Not all the published studies have taken this into account. This means that a proportion of cases reported to have tardive dyskinesias may actually have unwanted symptoms of their underlying disorder rather than side effects of the drug treatment (Campbell, personal communication, 1993).

Behavioural toxicity is not as well known and is often misinterpreted as being due to too low dosage of the medication. Irritability, depressive feelings, hyperactivity or hypoactivity increasing to apathy may all be unwanted symptoms of neuroleptic medication. School phobia, dysthymia and aggression has been reported in children with Tourette syndrome in connection with haloperidol treatment (Mikkelson, Detlor & Cohen, 1981; Bruun, 1988).

After long periods (several months) of treatment with antipsychotic drugs, one must expect rebound symptoms on withdrawal. The fact that most antipsychotic medication leads to blocking of neurotransmitter receptors of several types is probably one reason for increased receptor sensitivity, and this, in turn, accounts for rebound symptoms, mostly of the cholinergic type. Nausea, loss of appetite, vomiting, profuse sweating, insomnia, agitation, aggressiveness, destructiveness and irritability may appear in any combination. These symptoms usually take 8–12 weeks to subside. When withdrawing antipsychotic medication, parents, staff and children (whenever appropriate) should be warned of these possible developments. Weight change has been observed on withdrawal of neuroleptic medication in children with autism (Green *et al.*, 1984).

Clozapine is an atypical antipsychotic drug. Pharmacologically it is a dibensodiazepine. It has strong affinity for dopamine$_1$ and low affinity for dopamine$_2$ receptor and thus causes few, if any, extrapyramidal side effects. It resembles chlorpromazine and thioridazine in being (even more) strongly anticholinergic, antihistaminic, serotoninolytic and adrenolytic. Its use, so far, has been restricted to the treatment of schizophrenia and other severe psychotic disorders not responding to other treatments. As such, it seems to be exceptionally helpful in some severely dysfunctional cases (Kane *et al.*, 1988*a*, *b*, 1993). Studies on young people are only just beginning to be reported. Siefen and Remschmidt (1986) administered 225–800 mg per day of clozapine for an average of 4 months to 12 adolescents with psychosis and reported that a majority did very well on this medication. Further investigations in child and adolescent populations will be necessary to determine the efficacy of clozapine in this age group. The reason why clozapine, which has been used for more than 15 years, has been unsuccessful in emerging as a first choice drug is the high rate of agranulocytosis associated with its use. At least 1% of all treated patients develop agranulocytosis. However, with weekly blood cell monitoring and discontinuation at significant white cell count drop, all, or almost all agranulocytosis cases are reversible and fatalities have not been reported for several years in cases that have been carefully monitored on a regular basis. Other side effects are relatively minor and include sedation (mostly early in treatment), sleepiness, dizziness and orthostatic hypotension with tachycardia.

In summary, antipsychotic drugs should be used with great caution and surveillance. They should never be considered the treatment of first choice except in psychosis. In autism and Tourette syndrome, their use might be indicated in certain cases, but they should be considered substitutes for other kinds of intervention. They are not recommended in other disorders in child psychiatry, because of the short- and long-term side effects, which, although rarely life-threatening can cause much discomfort and/or linger for long periods of time. The appearance of negative behavioural effects, cognitive dulling and extrapyramidal side effects should be anticipated and explained to the parents and child as appropriate. Lowering the dosage may often effectively deal with problems of this kind. Cautious prescription, periodic discontinuation and careful monitoring will maximize the number of cases benefiting from treatment with these drugs.

Antidepressants

Controlled studies of the use of tricyclic antidepressants in children and adolescents pertain mainly to three patient groups: those with (1) enuresis, (2) DAMP/ADHD and (3) obsessive–compulsive disorder. Limited study has also been done in the field of eating disorders, notably bulimia (in which imipramine, desipramine and fluoxetine have all been shown to effectively reduce bingeing and vomiting). Comparatively few studies have been performed in these fields, but the number of controlled studies examining the effects of tricyclic antidepressant in depressive disorders is, surprisingly, even smaller (Green, 1991). Furthermore, no controlled studies of antidepressants, have documented the superiority of tricyclics (imipramine, nortiptyline) to placebo in depression in young patients.

Antidepressants should be used with great care, if at all, in the treatment of depression of children under age 13 years. In the treatment of

depression in adolescence, guidelines similar to those pertaining to adults should be followed.

Antidepressants have been used for many years in the treatment of enuresis. However, in the author's opinion, because of potentially very severe side effects and because of the very high rate of enuresis in the population, antidepressants should no longer be on the list of treatment options in enuresis (diagnosis, information, enuresis alarms or oxytocin should be used instead, see section on enuresis).

Antidepressants have been used in the treatment of children and adolescents with DAMP/ADHD, but since almost all comparative studies show stimulants (see below) to be both superior from the point of view of treatment success and to have considerably fewer and less severe side effects, there is little to advocate their use in the treatment of attention disorders. Nevertheless, occasionally, if a child has failed to respond to stimulants, a trial of a tricyclic (like imipramine or clomipramine) might well be indicated, and, although rarely, effective.

The current optimism regarding clomipramine's effectiveness in the treatment of obsessive–compulsive disorder in childhood and adolescence might not survive once many more empirical studies have been performed (Flament et al., 1985). Although clearly clinically effective in controlling some obsessions and compulsions in some young people, the side effects can be such that treatment has to be discontinued, even when starting treatment has been initiated in a very slow and careful way. Also, it seems clinically clear to the author that, quite often clomipramine is not effective at all in the treatment of childhood obsessive–compulsive disorder.

The pharmacological action of the tricyclic antidepressants is partly known, but it is still much less completely understood why they are sometimes effective clinically. They all have some monoamine reuptake blocking properties, and it has been hypothesized that they exercise their clinical effects through enhancing the effect of the endogenous monoamines in the central nervous system. However, most of the tricyclics have a number of additional, including anticholinergic and neuroendocrine, effects, and its is unclear how much of their clinical effectiveness can be attributed to these, or yet other, properties.

Dosage

All the side effects tend to be of less clinical importance if dosage is started at a very low level (such as 5–10 mg imipramine or clomipramine in the evening) with gradual increases of 5–10 mg every two or three days. If treatment is managed in this way, it is usually possible to keep to a once a day dosage formula, which makes compliance much better than if the doses are divided into two or three.

Side effects

The side effects of the tricyclic antidepressants range from mild–moderate to severe. In general, one must admit that they have been well tolerated, given that tricyclics have been used in general medical practice for more than 30 years without falling into disrepute. Nevertheless, it is uncommon, if not unheard of, for any given individual not to experience any of the mild–moderate side effects. These include dryness of the mouth, double vision, constipation, low blood pressure (particular when changing from the supine to the prone position), micturation problems and weight gain. All of these are clearly dose dependent, and will subside with lowering of dosage or withdrawal of the drug.

The severe side effects mainly comprise those that involve central nervous system unwanted effects. On starting medication, it is quite common for mood to become more negative. After a few weeks of treatment, mood may swing well into a manic state (although this is rare in children and adolescents). Concentration, attention and vigilance all often go down during the initial 10 to 20 days of treatment. Lethargy and social withdrawal may be seen. All these effects may be enhanced by the simultaneous intake or use of alcohol. Mild tremor is common as is paresthesias of the arms and legs. Occasionally ataxia and even seizures can occur, although usually only in cases of self-inflicted suicidal ideation intoxication. Other central nervous system symptoms which may

occur are thought disorder, hallucinations, delusions, disorientation, memory defects, agitation and confusion. These symptoms may be common only in certain individuals who tend to metabolize the tricyclics slowly (Preskorn et al., 1987). Therefore, close monitoring of blood levels should be performed in all adolescents who are put on tricyclics for any length of time.

Cardiovascular side effects are of concern in all age groups, perhaps particularly so in children and young adolescents. Tachycardia, cardiac arrhythmias, increases in PR and QRS intervals and even heart block have been reported. An ECG PR interval < 200 ms and QRS duration < 120 ms appear to be more important clinical dosing parameters than accepting a rather arbitrary absolute dosage limit in optimizing responses and avoiding cardiovascular toxicity (Gadow, 1992). At least four case reports of sudden death in children on treatment with imipramine and desipramine have been published (Saraf et al, 1974; Biederman, 1991; Riddle et al., 1991; Abramowicz, 1990; Campbell, Perry & Green, 1984). These reports signal the need to retain a very cautious attitude when prescribing tricyclics to young children.

So far, the only tricyclics that can be said to have at least some validation in child and adolescent psychiatry are imipramine and clomipramine, and, except in controlled drug trials, these are the ones that should be used, at least until there have been more validating studies on young people with the newer drugs, such as the selective serotonin reuptake blockers (fluvoxamine, fluoxetine etc.). Fluoxetine has been used increasingly in children and adolescents in recent years, but, so far, almost exclusively in open trials or anecdotal cases (Cook et al., 1992). A double-blind, placebo-controlled study in children and adolescents showed some positive results of fluoxetine treatment in OCD (Riddle et al., 1992).

Lithium

Lithium should be considered as a possible drug treatment (usually in combination with other treatments) in children and adolescents showing severe aggression (Campbell *et al.*, 1984), autism with mood swings (Gillberg & Coleman, 1992), mental retardation with uncharacteristic relapsing behaviour problems or bipolar disorder (Glue, 1989) and in bipolar disorder in adolescents (Gadow, 1992).

For most indications, lithium treatment should be given according to guidelines provided in the literature on young adult patients.

Dosage

The dosage should be kept at a level which keeps the serum level in the range of 0.4–1.1 meq/l. Clinical experience suggests that effectiveness is usually (if at all) achieved at a serum level in the 0.4–0.7 range (although occasionally, at least in the case of treatment of aggression, blood levels of up to 1.5 meq/l may be needed, Campbell *et al.*, 1984). Lithium has to be given at least twice, usually three to four times a day (both because of its toxicity, see below, and its pharmacokinetics).

Side effects

It appears that the risk of kidney damage, thyroid hypofunction and cardiac abnormalities is low when serum levels are kept at the low level of 0.4–0.7 meq/l, in spite of the fact that none (or little) of the positive behavioural effect is lost. Lithium has a low therapeutic index, and toxicity may occur at doses close to therapeutic levels. Diarrhoea, vomiting, ataxia (including mild symptoms), *coarse* tremor (not mild, high-frequency tremor which is usually benign), sedation, slurred speech and impaired coordination may occur. Patients and carers need to be carefully instructed (orally and in writing) to immediately discontinue medication and contact their physician if such signs and symptoms should occur. Life-threatening toxic effects (cardiac arrhythmias, confusion, seizures and coma followed by death) may occur if serum levels continue to go up.

Stimulants

The stimulants are the best researched of any class of drugs prescribed for the treatment of childhood disorder. The literature on this one class of drugs is enormous. The stimulants are widely used, but prescription practice varies enormously. In the US, several per cent of all school-age children are currently treated with stimulants on a daily basis, usually under the diagnosis of ADHD. In some parts of New York City in 1993, 25% of all school-age boys received treatment under the alleged diagnosis of ADHD (Kowallis 1993, personal communication). In the whole of the US in the late 1980s, at least 10% of all children were treated with stimulants for attention deficit problems (Ciaranello, 1993). In Sweden about 0.01% of this population group are treated with stimulants, and only after special prescription that has to be approved by the Swedish FDA in each individual case. Psychiatrists in most western countries have adopted a 'middle of the road' strategy between these two extremes.

There can be little question that the stimulants are effective in the short-term treatment of childhood attention deficit problems. Stimulants increase not only the attention span and the amount of on-task behaviour in the educational setting, they also improve the quality of social interactions within the family and the peer group (Barkley *et al.*, 1990). They reduce hyperactive behaviour and possibly some conduct problems. It appears that they may also contribute to better academic performance, even though in this domain results are less strikingly clear-cut than with regard to behaviour. Furthermore, stimulants are generally much less sedative than most of the other classes of drugs used in the treatment of behaviour disorders in childhood and adolescence. While it has been shown beyond any reasonable doubt that a majority of children with severe attention deficit improve their attentional functioning while on short-term treatment with stimulant drugs, it is less clear whether such treatment alters the outcome of such disorders in the longer-term perspective (Jacobvitz *et al.*, 1990).

ADHD is a diagnosis which is used widely in the US, but probably less frequently in Europe. It is a diagnosis which shows great diagnostic overlap with other conditions including conduct disorder, learning problems (including dyslexia), speech-and language disorders, motor control problems and autism spectrum disorders (Gillberg, 1992). It is also quite possible that major depression in young children may present with or show co-morbid attention deficit problems. Sometimes the co-morbid problem is a better indication of the type of treatment needed than ADHD as such. This is probably true both of conduct disorder (although some data (Taylor *et al.*, 1991) indicate that stimulants may be effective in the treatment of conduct symptoms also, at least if co-morbid with ADHD) and autism spectrum disorder. Perhaps one of the reasons why stimulant treatment is so widely used in the US is the fact that once a diagnosis of ADHD is made, regardless of the co-morbidity, stimulants will be tried, whereas in Europe, the co-morbid problems are likely to be the focus instead.

Apart from ADHD, stimulant treatment may be indicated in narcolepsy and Kleine–Levin syndrome.

Narcolepsy is a poorly defined condition in childhood, and the literature on the syndrome is scant. General guidelines cannot be provided here because of the lack of any supportive data.

Kleine–Levin syndrome, on the other hand, is receiving increasing attention. Both stimulant treatment (during episodes of hypersomnia) and lithium (for long-term prevention of new attacks) have been advocated (Lemire, 1993). It seems reasonable to try short-term stimulant treatment in connections with episodes first. Lithium may be useful if stimulant treatment fails, and the disorder tends towards a subchronic course.

Dosage

The dosage of amphetamine (D-amphetamine) for school-age children (usually the only age group in which stimulant treatment may be indicated) should be 5–15 mg two to four times a day depending on clinical response, sleep patterns, etc. Stimulants have a tendency to increase (usually already existing) problems of calming down and going off to sleep in the evening if the last dose of the day is given too close to bedtime.

The dosage of methylphenidate (the drug most often used in the US) needs to be about twice that of amphetamine. However, individual variation in this respect is considerable, and, as always in childhood psychopharmacology, titration of the individually most effective dose is necessary.

Methylphenidate is often the preferred initial drug. If it fails to produce significant improvement, dextroamphetamine should be tried instead (Shaywitz & Shaywitz, 1991). Ward, Wender & Reimherr (1993) recently suggested that methamphetamine might be more useful in clinical practice than any of the other two stimulants. His reasons for doing this was methamphetamine's allegedly more specific central (and less peripheral) effects and the fact that it can be given in a more long-acting formulation.

Side effects

Side effects are comparatively few and benign in stimulant treatment. In fact, stimulants seem to be one of the least problematic classes of drug when it comes to psychopharmacological treatment of childhood disorders. This statement contrasts sharply with the general belief that stimulants are probably the drugs that have the potentially most severe side effects of all. Anorexia, nausea, weight loss (usually in the range of 1–3 kg), depressed motor performance (including limited facial expression) and mild symptoms of depressed mood are the most common negative effects. Final height and weight is usually not affected, even when treatment has been going on for many years in childhood and adolescence (Klein & Mannuzza, 1988). It seems likely, however, that a small subgroup of children may be at greater risk of growth suppression, and careful serial heights and weights of any child receiving stimulant medication should be plotted and monitored on a growth chart (Hamill *et al.*, 1976). Some parents are, understandably, concerned that stimulant treatment will predispose the child to later drug addiction. All the available data indicates that this is not the case (Weiss & Hechtman, 1986; Green, 1991). It is generally believed that as many as 60–80% of all school-age children with ADHD or attention deficit problems not meeting full ADHD criteria benefit greatly from stimulant medication. However, Jacobvitz *et al.* (1990) recently challenged this view, pointing out the need for careful evaluation in the long term and the use of alternative or additional interventions (educational, psychotherapeutical, psychopharmacological, etc.). Also, it should be remembered that stimulants do not work well in at least 30% of cases (Barkley, 1990), disruptive effects on appetite and sleep may occur (Hunt *et al.*, 1985), the short half-life of the drugs may contribute to roller coaster effects on mood and self-control throughout the day (Hunt *et al.*, 1985), irritability, anxiety and depression (often co-morbid with ADHD) will usually not be controlled and irritability and dysphoria may occasionally be induced by stimulant treatment (Barkley, 1990)

Antiepileptic drugs: carbamazepine

The antiepileptics, other than the benzodiazepines, are used in children and adolescents first and foremost in the treatment of epilepsies of various kinds. Recently, they have also been tried in the treatment of some behaviour disorders with or without epilepsy. Carbamazepine has received more attention in this respect than any of the other anti-epileptic drugs.

Carbamazepine is a compound sharing structural features both with the tricyclic antidepressants, chlorpromazine and maprotiline (Rodin, 1983). It also shares structural features with the anticonvulsants phenytoin, phenobarbital and clonazepam (Dalby, 1975). Clinically, it has both psychotropic and anticonvulsant properties. It has special affinity for limbic structures, an antikindling (anti-epileptic) effect in addition to a generally depressant effect on neurotransmission and a possibly stabilizing neuronal effect, similar to that of lithium.

In conduct disorder, recent research suggests that carbamazepine may be useful in some cases (Jeanette Cueva, personal communication, 1993). This may be true particularly when there are explosive behaviours, including aggressiveness and destructiveness, and there appear to be no or minimal triggers. 'Episodic dyscontrol syndrome' (or intermittent explosive syndrome) may sometimes be successfully controlled with carbamazepine treatment, although the literature on this point is largely anecdotal (Gualtieri, 1990).

In DAMP and other ADHD syndromes, carbamazepine may be helpful in controlling explosive and otherwise aggressive behaviour. Remschmidt (1976) reviewed the data from 7 double-blind and 21 open studies, together comprising more than 800 children and adolescents with behaviour disorders without epilepsy who were treated with carbamazepine. He found positive mood change, increased initiative, decreased anxiety and positive clinical results on target symptoms such as poor activity control (hyper- and hypoactivity), impaired attention/concentration, aggressiveness and dysphoric mood.

There has been considerable debate over the usefulness of some antiepileptic drugs, carbamazepine in particular, in the treatment of various kinds of behaviour problems associated with paroxysmal EEG abnormalities. While no empirical studies can be called upon to decide this issue either way, it seems that a trial of carbamazepine may be indicated in episodic or explosive behaviours associated with EEG abnormalities (Kuhn-Gebhart, 1976). In the author's experience, particular attention has to be paid to the risk of behavioural and neurological toxicity of antiepileptic drug treatment in such cases.

The positive effects of carbamazepine in the treatment of behaviour disorders in children and adolescents are supported mostly by clinical experience. Empirical validation through double-blind, placebo-controlled studies is only just emerging. Therefore, even though the weight of clinical experience is substantial, and carbamazepine has become one of the favourite drugs of neuropsychiatrists, caution is warranted in its prescription.

Dosage

In children over age 10 years and adolescents, dosage can often be started at a level of 5 mg/kg/day divided into two doses. Increments can usually be made every three days. Blood levels are not clearly related to clinical response and should only be monitored when toxic levels are suspected or when there is a suspicion of non-compliance.

Side effects

Carbamazepine is usually well tolerated. However, about 3% develop allergies with skin rashes and medication; in such cases, it usually has to be discontinued. Considerable sedation is common during the first few days of treatment. This usually subsides, but if it does not, may be the cause for discontinuation. Slight ataxia is also common in the early days of treatment. Behavioural toxicity is much more common than generally believed and includes irritability, disorganization and agitation. Rarely, hallucinations and frank psychosis develop. Carbamazepine also shows proclivity to induce or aggravate the occurrence of centrencephalic seizures. Dyskinetic movements may be triggered, and children already suffering from dyskinesia and akathisia may have symptom aggravation during treatment with carbamazepine. It is not helpful in the treatment of Tourette syndrome (Gualtieri, 1990).

Antiepileptic drugs: valproic acid

In recent years, the possible psychotropic effects of valproic acid, another drug originally introduced for the treatment of generalized seizures, have become the focus of considerable attention, even though empirical study of such effects in children and adolescents is lacking (Gualtieri, 1990).The anticonvulsant effects of valproic acid appear to be related to its effect on GABA-ergic nerve transmission (it potentiates GABA-mediated inhibition in the brain), but it is also effective in reducing non GABA-ergic spike generation. The reason for the possible psychotropic effects is not known, but may also be related to GABA-ergic effects. The positive effects in psychiatric disorders, if any, are probably similar to those seen with carbamazepine.

Dosage

Dosage should be in the range of 5–30 mg/kg/day depending on clinical response. The author has seen young children (2–6 years of age) who

have responded very favourably, both with regard to a seizure disorder and concomitant autistic symptoms, on even smaller doses of valproic acid, administered in one daily dose. It is not clear that blood levels (usually reported to be therapeutically effective in the range of 300–700 μmol/l are a good guide to monitor clinical response and so, just as in the cases of carbamzepine, should be used to monitor compliance and suspected 'overdosage' rather than to meticulously follow for control of efficacy.

Side effects

The very serious hepatic side effects, including fatal hepatotoxicity, are extremely uncommon. They usually occur in the first 6 months of treatment and tend to be confined to the youngest age group of treated patients (Gualtieri, 1990). Although rare, they remain the reason why valproic acid is mostly used only in the treatment of severe epilepsy. Trombocytopenia may occur at any time during treatment, even after several years of medication. Gastrointestinal problems including anorexia, indigestion, nausea and even vomiting are relatively common side effects. Behavioural toxicity is similar in type to that seen with carbamazepine, but possible rare. Valproic acid is probably particularly beneficial in the treatment of epilepsy in autism and autism spectrum disorders, given that it does not seem negatively to affect autistic symptoms (and sometimes may even ameliorate withdrawal and other autism symptoms).

Benzodiazepines

The benzodiazepines have little room in child and adolescent psychopharmacology other than in the treatment of epilepsy and, occasionally, in the short-term treatment of sleep disorders.

The benzodiazepines may, in fact, be more useful in the treatment of child and adolescent psychiatric disorders than hitherto acknowledged. However, there is a dearth of studies in the field, and no clear recommendations can be afforded at the present time.

Dosage

Until better evidence is available from systematic research, the bensodiazepines should be given in doses that are proportionate to adult doses on a weight basis or according to observed clinical effects.

Side effects

The long half-life and the possible teratogenic effects (Laegreid, Hagberg & Lundberg, 1992) of the bensodiazepines have contributed to their relatively negative standing in the field of child and adolescent psychopharmacology today.

Clinical experience and open clinical trials of clonazepam and nitrazepam (and other anti-epileptics) in the treatment of epilepsy in autism (Gillberg, 1991) indicate that, in some cases, side effects of these particular drugs may clearly outweigh any benefits. In individual cases, clonazepam can actually increase autistic symptomatology with, or without, associated reduction of seizure activity. Drooling, dulling, hyperactivity and increased withdrawal often result from treatment of epilepsy in autism with bensodiazepines. The author has even seen one case with full-blown autistic disorder and epilepsy in which the autistic symptoms completely subsided after discontinuation of clonazepam.

If the bensodiazepines are to be used at all in child and adolescent psychopharmacology, a drug with a relatively short half-life should be chosen over those with more than a ten-hour half-life (e.g. oxazepam may be more adequate than diazepam).

Vitamin B6

Vitamin B6, usually in combination with magnesium, has been shown, by several different groups, to be effective in the treatment of severe behaviour problems in autism in a small subgroup of cases (Gillberg & Coleman, 1992). Vitamin B6 acts a cofactor in the metabolism of the monoamines. The monoamines have all been implicated in the pathogenesis of autism.

Dosage

Vitamin B6 has been given in doses ranging from 300–900 mg/day divided into two or three doses in most of the studies performed to date. Magnesium supplementation has usually been with magnesium sulphate in doses of?.

Side effects

Vitamin B6 in large doses is not necessarily a harmless drug. In animals it may cause peripheral neuropathy (Yamamoto, 1991). When given in large quantities, it uses magnesium as a co-factor. Therefore, only a month or so after the start of vitamin B6 treatment, magnesium may be depleted from the body, and supplementation will become necessary lest permanent neuropathy should occur.

Folic acid

Folic acid has been reported to have some positive effects in the treatment of attention problems and hyperactivity in the fragile X syndrome (Gillberg & Coleman, 1992). Originally, this positive effect was believed to be a result of some direct effect on the chromosomal abnormality, but in recent years it has been suggested that, whatever positive effects occur are likely to be due to the mild stimulant action of folic acid.

Dosage

In the treatment of behaviour problems associated with the fragile X syndrome, folic acid has been administered in doses of 0.5–2.0 mg/kg/day divided in two to three doses. The average dose that has been used in the studies that demonstrated some effectiveness of the drug has been 1.0 mg/kg/day.

Side effects

The reported side effects have been minimal in the studies performed to date. Some increase of appetite and minimal to moderate weight gain has been reported in a few cases. According to one study (Gillberg, Persson & Wahlström, 1986), and clinical experience with a group of ten young males with the fragile X syndrome, those who are reported to be helped by folic acid in the prepubertal period may develop aggressive outbursts in adolescence, and these may subside with the discontinuation of drug treatment.

Piracetam

Piracetam has been shown to be moderately effective in increasing reading speed and reading comprehension in dyslexia in a considerable number of, double-blind placebo-controlled studies (Wilsher, 1987). The fact that the drug company has sponsored several of these investigations has led to a critical attitude (Gadow, 1992) and a general reluctance on the part of the scientific community to accept the results *prima facei*. Nevertheless, the data is such that piracetam should definitely be considered an interesting investigational drug, and there is still good reason to retain a hopeful attitude that it may actually hold promise for the treatment of specific reading retardation.

Dosage

For dyslexia, piracetam has been recommended in doses of 3.3–9.9 g/day divided in two to three daily doses depending on age and body weight of the child.

Side effects

The reported side effects of piracetam in the treatment of dyslexia have been few and generally benign. The most commonly reported unwanted effect has been that of a certain kind of increased nervousness, defined by some individuals as a feeling of overalertness and by others as restlessness. Minor gastrointestinal problems have also been reported.

Other drugs

Other drugs that may occasionally be useful in child and adolescent neuropsychiatry include:

(a) beta-blockers,
(b) alpha-blockers (clonidine),
(c) bromocriptine,
(d) paraldehyde,
(e) fenfluramine, and
(f) naltrexone.

The beta-blockers, commonly employed in the treatment of hypertensive states in adults, in preliminary open studies, have been demonstrated to have some potential in the treatment of severe behaviour problems in autism (Smith & Perry, 1992). Unfortunately, no corroborating evidence exists in the field, and so there is no rationale for suggesting a reasonable clinical practice. More research is required in this area before any conclusions can be drawn.

Clonidine has been used in the treatment of tic disorders. It has even been proclaimed as the second drug of choice in the treatment of Tourette syndrome, in spite of the fact that very little empirical data actually exists (Cohen *et al.*, 1980; Leckman *et al.*, 1985). It is also sometimes used in the treatment of severe ADHD (Hunt, Minderra & Cohen, 1985), but only one double-blind (cross-over) placebo-controlled study of 12 children (10 of whom completed the study) has been performed to date to the author's knowledge. Thus, even though positive results were reported, clonidine can only be regarded as an investigational treatment for ADHD at the present stage. There is a risk that clonidine treatment may trigger or aggravate covert or co-morbid affective disorders (including depression) (Green, 1991).

Bromocriptine, a dopamine agonist, has been advocated as a useful adjunct in the treatment of withdrawal and apraxia in Rett syndrome and similar behavioural syndrome (Zappella, 1990; Zappella *et al.*, 1990).

Paraldehyde has been used as a hypnotic sedative for more than a century. As with digitalis, its continued use for more than 100 years in medicine, appears to be ample proof of its efficacy. Nevertheless, it is used less and less. In particularly severe sleep disorders, such as in autism, it can sometimes be very effective in inducing sleep. However, its tendency to recirculate and cause episodic drowsiness over the next couple of days, detracts from its overall usefulness in child and adolescent psychopharmacology.

Fenfluramine was launched in the early 1980s as somewhat of a miracle cure in autism. Although this view has since been challenged (Campbell, 1989), and fenfluramine is no longer considered a drug that may be helpful in anything but a small minority of individuals affected by autism, the first report led to the growth of a considerable literature on fenfluramine for the treatment of childhood neuropsychiatric disorder. It may be helpful in controlling hyperactivity in children with mental retardation and autism. Perhaps the most interesting outcome of research in this area so far is the finding that fenfluramine may be helpful in controlling some of the most severe symptoms of bulimia nervosa (Campbell et al., 1989).

Naltrexone, a blocker of endogenous and exogenous opioids, is currently under investigation by a number of different research groups (e.g. Campbell et al., 1993). Mostly it is being tried in the treatment of autism, after mid-1980 reports (Gillberg, Terenius & Lönnerholm, 1985) of endorphin hyperfunction in autism, particularly in those individuals with autism who also showed self-injurious behaviours. Naltrexone appears to be relatively harmless with regard to toxicity. Perhaps it is also relatively inefficient in controlling negative behaviours and promoting socialization in autism, even though mildly-moderately positive effects on ratings of hyperactivity seem to be consistent. More research is needed before conclusions can be drawn in this field. Self-injury has been reported to respond favourably to opiate antagonists (Campbell et al., 1989), but, here too, more investigations are necessary before conclusions can be drawn.

General guidelines before starting drug treatment in child neuropsychiatric disorders

Before starting any drug treatment in child and adolescent neuropsychiatric disorders it is essential to monitor a number of things. The following need to be systematically recorded:

(a) weight,
(b) height,
(c) neurological examination including for tics, stereotypies, extrapyramidal symptoms (including signs of tardive dyskinesias).

The AIMS (abnormal involuntary movements scale) (Campbell, 1985) or some such similar scale should be used in the rating of involuntary movements. This is essential because of the difficulty encountered in trying to tease apart motor symptoms associated with the underlying disorder and side effects of drug treatment,

(d) complete blood count, and blood tests of liver and kidney function. These tests need to be repeated at least once every six months. After a six-month period it is usually wise to discontinue medication for 4–12 weeks, and make a decision as to the need for continued medication on the combined evidence from evaluation of the clinical disorder, side effects of drug treatment and the overall benefits and hazards of continued/discontinued medication.

References

Abramowicz, M. (1990). Sudden death in children treated with a tricyclic antidepressant. *The Medical Letter on Drugs and Therapeutics*, **32**, 53.

Barkley, R.A. (1990). *Attention Deficit Hyperactivity Disorder*. New York: Guilford Press.

Barkley, R.A., Fischer, M., Edelbrock, C.S., Smallish, L. (1990). The adolescent outcome of hyperactive children diagnosed by research criteria: I. An 8-year prospective follow-up study. *Journal of the American Academy of Child and Adolescent Psychiatry*, **29**, 546–57.

Biederman, J. (1991). Sudden death in children treated with a tricyclic antidepressant. *Journal of the American Academy of Child and Adolescent Psychiatry*, **30**, 495–8.

Bruun, R.D. (1988). The natural history of Tourette's syndrome. *In* Cohen, D.J., Bruun, R.D.,Leckman, J.F. (Ed.) *Tourette's Syndrome and Tic Disorders*. New York: John Wiley & Sons.

Campbell, M. (1985). Timed stereotypies rating scale. Special feature: Rating scales and assessment instruments for use in pediatric psychopharmacology research. *Psychopharmacology Bulletin*, **21**, 102.

Campbell, M. (1989). Pharmacotherapy in autism: An overview. *In* Gillberg, C. (Ed.) *Diagnosis and treatment of autism.* New York: Plenum.

Campbell, M., Small, A.M., Sokol, M.S., *et al.* (1987). Naltrexone in autistic children: An acute dose range tolerance trial. Stallone Foundation. San Diego, CA.

Campbell, M., Adams, P., Perry, R., Spencer, E.K., Overall, J.E. (1988). Tardive and withdrawal dyskinesia in autistic children: A prospective study. *Psychopharmacology Bulletin*, **24**, 251–5.

Campbell, M., Overall, J.E., Small, A.M., Sokol, M.S., Spencer, E.K., Adams, P., Foltz, R.L., Monti, K.M. Perry, R., Nobler, M., Roberts, E. (1989). Naltrexone/autistic children: an acute open dose range tolerance trial. *Journal of the American Academy of Child Adolescent Psychiatry*, **28**, 200–6.

Campbell, M., Anderson, L.T., Small, A.M., Adams, P., Gonzalez, N.M., Ernst, M. (1993). Naltrexone in autistic children: behavioral symptoms and attentional learning. in press.

Campbell, M., Perry, R., Bennett, W.G., Small, A.M., Green, W.H., Grega, D., Schwartz, V., Anderson, L. (1983). Long-term therapeutic efficacy and drug-related abnormal movements: a prospective study of haloperidol in autistic children. *Psychopharmacology Bulletin*, **19**, 80–3.

Campbell, M., Perry, R., Green, W.H. (1984). The use of lithium in children and adolescents. *Psychosomatics*, **25**, 95–106.

Ciaranello, R. (1993). Editorial. *New England Journal of Medicine*, **328**, 1038–9.

Cohen, D.J., Detlor, J., Young, J.G., Shaywitz, B.A. (1980). Clonidine ameliorates Gilles de la Tourette syndrome. *Archives of General Psychiatry*, **37**, 1350–7.

Coleman, M., Blass, J.P. (1985). Autism and lactic acidosis. *Journal of Autism and Developmental Disorders*, **15**, 1–8.

Cook, E.H.J., Rowlett, R., Jaselskis, C., Leventhal, B.L. (1992). Fluoxetine treatment of children and adults with autistic disorder and mental retardation. *Journal of the American Academy of Child and Adolescent Psychiatry*, **31**, 739–45.

Cueva, J.E., Armenteros, J.L., Rosenberg, C.R., Campbell, M. (1993). Untoward effects of carbamazepine in hospitalized aggressive children with conduct disorder. Dept of Psychiatry, NYUMC.

Dalby, M.A. (1975). Behavioural effects of carbamazepine. *Advances in Neurology*, **11**, 331–44.

Evans, R.W., Clay, T.H., Gualtieri, C.T. (1987). Carbamazepine in pediatric psychiatry. *Journal of the American Academy of Child and Adolescent Psychiatry*, **26**, 2–8.

Flament, M., Rapoport, J.L., Berg, C.J., Sceery, W., Kilts, C., Mellstrom, B., Linnoila, M. (1985). Clomipramine treatment of childhood obsessive compulstive disorder; a double blind controlled study. *Archives of General Psychiatry*, **42**, 977–83.

Gadow, K.G. (1992). Pediatric psychopharmacotherapy: a review of recent research. *Journal of Child Psychology and Psychiatry*, **33**, 153–95.

Gadow, K.D., Nolan, E.E., K., S., Sprafkin, J., Paolicelli, L. (1990). Methylphenidate in aggressive-hyperactive boys. I. Effects on peer aggression in public school settings. *Journal of the American Academy of Child and Adolescent Psychiatry*, **29**, 710–18.

Gillberg, C. (1991). The treatment of epilepsy in autism. *Journal of Autism and Developmental Disorders*, **21**, 61–77.

Gillberg, C. (1992). The Emanuel Miller Memorial Lecture 1991: Autism and autistic-like conditions: subclasses among disorders of empathy. *Journal of Child Psychology and Psychiatry*, **33**, 813–42.

Gillberg, C. (1992). Psychiatric and behavioural problems in epilepsy, hydrocephalus and cerebral palsy. *In* Aicardi, J. (Ed.) *Diseases of the Nervous System in Childhood.* London: Mac Keith Press.

Gillberg, C., Coleman, M. (1992). *The Biology of the Autistic Syndromes.* 2nd edition. London, New York: Mac Keith Press, Cambridge University Press.

Gillberg, C., Terenius, L., Lönnerholm, G. (1985). Endorphin activity in childhood psychosis. Spinal fluid levels in 24 cases. *Archives of General Psychiatry*, **42**, 780–3.

Gillberg, C., Persson, E., Wahlström, J. (1986). The autism-fragile-X syndrome (AFRAX). A population-based study of ten boys. *Journal of Mental Deficiency Research*, **30**, 27–39.

Glue, P. (1989). Rapid cycling affective disorders in the mentally retarded. *Biological Psychiatry*, **26**, 250–6.

Goldbloom, D.S., Kennedy, S.H., Kaplan, A.S., Woodside, D.B. (1989). Anorexia nervosa and bulimia nervosa. *Canadian Medical Association Journal*, **140**, 1149–54.

Green, W.H. (1991). *Child and Adolescent Clinical Psychopharmacology.* Baltimore: Williams and Wilkins.

Green, W.H., Campbell, M., Hardesty, A.S.,
Grega, D.M., Padron-Gayol, M., Shell, J.,
Erlenmeyer-Kimling, L. (1984). A comparison of
schizophrenic and autistic children. *Journal of the
American Academy of Child Psychiatry*, **23**,
399–409.

Gualtieri, C.T. (1990). *Neuropsychiatry and
Behavioral Pharmacology*. New York: Springer
Verlag.

Gualtieri, C.T. (1993). The problem of tardive
akathisia. *Brain Cognition*, **23**, 102–9.

Hagerman, R.J., Jackson, C., Amiri, K.,
Silverman, A.C., O'Connor, R., Sobesky, W.
(1992). Girls with fragile X syndrome: physical
and neurocognitive status and outcome.
Pediatrics, **89**, 395–400.

Hamil, P.V.V., Drizd, T.A., Johnson, C.L., Reed,
R.B., Roche, A.F. (1976). NCHS growth charts,
1976. Monthly vital statistics report, health
examination survey data. *National Center for
Health Statistics Publication (HRA)*, **25**, suppl 3,
1.22.

Hjalmas, K., Passerini-Glazel, G., Chiozza, M.L.
(1992). Functional daytime incontinence:
pharmacological treatment. *Scandinavian Journal
of Urology and Nephrology Suppl*, 108–14;
discussion 115–16.

Hunt, R.D., Minderra, R., Cohen, D.J. (1985).
Clonidine benefits children with attention deficit
and hyperactivity. *Journal of the American
Academy of Child and Adolescent Psychiatry*, **24**,
617–29.

Jacobvitz, D., Sroufe, L.A., Stewart, M., Leffert,
N. (1990). Treatment of additional and
hyperactivity problems in children with
sympathomimetric drugs: a comprehensive
review. *Journal of the American Academy of Child
and Adolescent Psychiatry*, **29**, 677–88.

Kane, J.M. (1993). Newer antipsychotic drugs. A
review of their pharmacology and therapeutic
potential. *Drugs*, **46**, 585–93.

Kane, J.M., Honigfeld, G., Singer, J., Meltzer, H.
(1988*a*). Clozapine in treatment-resistant
schizophrenics. *Psychopharmacology Bulletin*, **24**,
62–7.

Kane, J.M., Honigfield, G., Singer, J., Meltzer, H.,
Group, and the Clozaril Collaborative Study
Group. (1988*b*). Clozapine for the treatment-
resistant schizophrenic. *Archives of General
Psychiatry*, **45**, 789–96.

Klein, R.G., Mannuzza, S. (1988). Hyperactive
boys almost grown up. III. Methylphenidate
effects on ultimate height. *Archives of General
Psychiatry*, **45**, 1131–4.

Kotagal, S., Hartse, K.M., Walsh, J.K. (1990).
Characteristics of narcolepsy in preteenaged
children. *Pediatrics*, **85**, 205–9.

Kuhn-Gebhart, V. (1976). Behavioral disorders in
non-epileptic children and their treatment with
carbamazepine. *In* Birkmayer, W. (Eds.) *Epileptic
Seizures – Behaviour – Pain*. Bern: Hans Huber.

Laegreid, L., Hagberg, G., Lundberg, A. (1992).
The effect of benzodiazepines on the fetus and the
newborn. *Neuropediatrics*, **23**, 18–23.

Leckman, J.F., Hardin, M.T., Riddle, M.A.,
Stevenson, J., Ort, S.I., Cohen, D.J. (1991).
Clonidine treatment of Gilles de la Tourette's
Syndrome. *Archives of General Psychiatry*, **48**,
324–8.

Leckman, J.F., Detlor, J., Harcherik, D.F., Ort, S.,
Shaywitz, B.A., Cohen, D.J. (1985). Short- and
long-term treatment of Tourette's syndrome with
clonidine: A clinical perspective. *Neurology*, **35**,
343–51.

Lemire, I. (1993). Revue de syndrome de Kleine–
Levin: vers une aproche intégrée. Review of
Kleine–Levin syndrome: toward an integrated
approach. *Canadian Journal of Psychiatry*, **38**,
277–84.

Lishman, W.A. (1978). *Organic Psychiatry. The
Psychological Consequenses of Cerebral Disorder*.
Oxford: Blackwell Scientific Publications.

Mikkelsen, E.J., Detlor, J., Cohen, D.J. (1981).
School avoidance and social phobia triggered by
haloperidol in patients with Tourette's disorder.
American Journal of Psychiatry, **138**, 1572–6.

Perry, R., Campbell, M., Green, W.H., Small,
A.M., Die Trill, M.L., Meiselas, K., Golden,
R.R., Deutsch, S.I. (1985). Neuroleptic-related
dyskinesias in autistic children. A prospective
study. *Psychopharmacology Bulletin*, **21**, 140–3.

Perry, R., Campbell, M., Adams, P., Lynch, N.,
Spencer, E.K., Curren, E.L., Overall, J.E. (1989).
Long-term efficacy of haloperidol in autistic
children: Continuous vs. discontinuous drug
administration. *Journal of the American Academy
of Child and Adolescent Psychiatry*, **28**, 93–6.

Preskorn, S.H., Weller, E.B., Hughes, C.W.,
Weller, R.A., Bolte, K. (1987). Depression in
prepubertal children: dexamethasone
nonsuppression predicts differential response to
imipramine vs. placebo. *Psychopharmacology
Bulletin*, **23**, 128–33.

Remschmidt, H.S. (1976). The psychotropic effect
of carbamazepine in non-epileptic patients with
particular reference to problems post by clinical
studies in children with behavioral disorders. *In*
Birkmeyer, W. (Ed.) *Epileptic Seizures –*

Behaviour – Pain. Bern: Hans Huber.

Riddle, M.A., Scahill, L., King, R., Hardin, M.R., Towbin, K.E., Ort, S.I., Leckman, J.F., Cohen, D.J. (1990). Obsessive compulsive disorder in children and adolescents: phenomenology and family history. *Journal of the American Academy of Child and Adolescent Psychiatry*, **29**, 766–72.

Riddle, M.A., Nelson, J.C., Kleinman, C.S., Rasmusson, A., Leckman, J.F., King, R.A., Cohen, D.J. (1991). Sudden death in children receiving Norpramin: a review of three reported cases and commentary. *Journal of the American Academy of Child and Adolescent Psychiatry*, **30**, 104–8.

Riddle, M.A., Scahill, M., King, R.A., Hardin, M.T., Anderson, G.M., Ort, S.I., Smith, J.C., Leckman, J.F., Cohen, D.J. (1992). Double-blind, crossover trial of fluoxetine and placebo in children and adolescents with obsessive-compulsive disorder. *Journal of the American Academy of Child and Adolescent Psychiatry*, **31**, 1062–9.

Rodin, E.A. (1983). Carbamazepine (tegretol). *In* Brown, T.R., Feldman, R.G. (Eds.) *Epilepsy Diagnosis and Management.* Boston: Little Brown.

Saraf, K.R., Klein, D.F., Gittelman-Klein, R., Groff, S. (1974). Imipramine side effects in children. *Psychopharmacologia*, **37**, 265–74.

Shaywitz, B.A., Shaywitz, S.E. (1991). Co-morbidity – a critical issue in attention deficit disorder. *Journal of Child Neurology*, 6 (Suppl.), S13-S22.

Siefen, G., Remschmidt, H. (1986). Behandlungsergebnisse mit Clozapin bei schizophrenen Jugendlichen: Results of treatment with clozapine in schizophrenic adolescents. *Zeitschrift f«F0»G«01»«F0»r Kinder Jugendpsychiatrie*, **14**, 245–57.

Smith, D.A., Perry, P.J. (1992). Nonneuroleptic treatment of disruptive behavior in organic mental syndromes. *Annals of Pharmacotherapy*, **26**, 1400–8.

Taylor, E., Sandberg, S., Thorley, G., Giles, S. (1991). *The Epidemiology of Childhood Hyperactivity.* London: Institute of Psychiatry.

Ward, M.F., Wender, P.H., Reimherr, F.W. (1993). The Wender Utah Rating Scale: an aid in the retrospective diagnosis of childhood attention deficit hyperactivity disorder. *American Journal of Psychiatry*, **150**, 885–90.

Weiss, G., Hechtman, L.T. (1986). *Hyperactive Children Grown Up.* New York: Guilford Press.

Wilsher, C.R. (1987). A brief review of studies of piracetam in dyslexia. *Journal of Psychopharmacology*, **2**, 95–100.

Wilsher, C.R., Atkins, G., Manfield, P. (1985). Effect of piracetam on dyslexic's reading ability. *Journal of Learning Disabilities*, **18**, 19–25.

Yamamoto, T. (1991). Pathologic processes of lumbar primary sensory neurons produced by high doses of pyridoxine in rats – morphometric and electron microscopic studies. *Sangyo Ika Daigaku Zasshi*, **13**, 109–23.

Zappella, M. (1990). A double blind trial of bromocriptine in the Rett syndrome. *Brain and Development*, **12**, 148–50.

Zappella, M., Genazzani, A., Facchinetti, F., Hayek, G. (1990). Bromocriptine in the Rett syndrome. *Brain & Development*, **12**, 221–5.

Appendix I
Some important terms: Glossary

Cognitive and social cognitive terms

Central coherence: The cognitive process by which high-level meaning is derived from the weaving together of otherwise piecemeal information.

Empathy: The ability to (fully) understand the perspectives of other people.

Executive functions: Cognitive processes, such as planning, orienting towards goal, ability to postpone, etc., believed to reflect frontal (or prefrontal) neural activiy.

Eye direction detector: Hypothetical construct. Refers to the ability within the visual modality to build representations of self-other-object relations, which, in turn, enables joint attention.

Joint attention: A behaviour shown already by infants prior to one year of age signifying that the child shows that s/he is attending to the same thing or event that also attract the attention of another person.

Theory of mind: The ability to impute mental states to others and to oneself.

Genetic terms

Autosomes: Chromosome pairs numbers 1 to 22, in contrast to the gonosomes (see below).

Centromere: Constricted portion of the chromosome which divides it into long and short arms.

Deletion: Part of a chromosome arm broken off. Usually abbreviated 'del' or symbolized by p- if occurring on the short 'p-arm' (from the French word 'petit', meaning small) and by q- if occurring on the long arm of the chromosome.

DNA: Deoxyribonucleic acid, a sequence of so-called nucleotides (bases), usually double stranded.

Dominant trait: A trait which is expressed in the phenotype in the heterozygous condition.

Duplication: Presence of a segment of a chromosome in a double dose on the same chromosome.

Exons: Coding parts of genes for structural proteins (non-coding parts are called introns).

Genes: Unit of genetic information consisting of DNA.

Genetic mutation: Error in the exact sequence of constituent DNA. (It is like a misspelling of the DNA sequence.)

Genome: All the chromosomal DNA (in humans, about 3×10^9 base pairs of DNA).

Genomic imprinting: Gene expression is modified by whether it is the mother or the father who passes on the chromosomal material to the child.

Genosomes: The sex chromosomes X and Y.

Haplotypes: Sets of RFLPs (see below).

Histones: Basic proteins with 50 to 200 amino acids, notably arginine, lysine and histidine.

Chromosomes are composed of DNA on a framework of histones.

Inversion: A fragment of a chromosome may break off, become inverted, and fuse again with the same chromosome so that a distorted sequence of genes results.

Isochromosome: Chromosome with two identical halves (sometimes two identical short arms, sometimes two identical long arms).

Isodicentric: Chromosome complexes with two centromeres.

Karyotyping: The analysis of the chromosomes in a cell arranged according to size and banding patterns.

Marker chromosome: Chromosome material (from the regular chromosomal set-up) which appears as a separate chromosome not part of the normal karyotype.

Mosaicism (mixoploidy): Two or more cell populations (clones), each with a different karyotype, in the same individual.

Recessive trait: A trait which is expressed in the phenotype in the homozygous condition.

RFLPs: Restriction fragment length polymorphisms, or suite of DNA markers; they are inherited.

Ring chromosome: A chromosome in the form of a ring. There is deletion of the long and short arms and fusion of the two break-points, leading to the formation of a ring.

RNA: Ribonucleic acid: a sequence of nucleotides (bases), usually single-stranded.

Tetrasomy: Two haploid sets of 23 chromosomes plus two extra chromosomes. Partial tetrasomy refers to the condition when only a part of one chromosome occurs in two extra copies.

Translocation: Transfer of a piece of one chromosome to another chromosome. If two non-homologous chromosomes exchange pieces, the translocation is balanced.

Trisomy: Two haploid sets of 23 chromosomes plus one extra chromosome.

Uniparental (maternal or paternal) disomy: An individual carries two copies of a chromosome (or part of a chromosome) which are inherited from the same parent.

Some technical abbreviations

ADD: Attention deficit disorder.

ADHD: Attention deficit hyperactivity disorder.

C(A)T-scan: Computed (axial) tomography (often used for neuroimaging).

CP: Cerebral palsy.

CSF: Cerebro-spinal fluid.

DAMP: Deficits in attention, motor control and perception.

DSM: Diagnosis and Statistical Manual of Mental Disorders.

ICD: International Statistical Classification of Diseases and Related Health Problems.

MR(I)-scan: Magnetic resonance imaging (often used for neuroimaging). No radioactivity involved.

MR: Mental retardation.

OCD: Obsessive–compulsive disorder.

OCPD: Obsessive–compulsive personality disorder.

PET-scan: Positron emission tomography (often used for evaluating cerebral metabolism).

SPECT: Single proton emission computed tomography (often used for evaluating cerebral blood flow).

Appendix II
Some brief differential diagnostic considerations

In this section a brief listing of symptoms and syndromal diagnoses is made with indications of which clinical differential diagnoses should be considered. The list is alphabetical. It should not be assumed that the list is exhaustive, neither as regards presenting symptom/syndrome, nor in respect of possible differential diagnoses.

ADHD

Attention deficits are common in almost all psychiatric disorders and in many neurodevelopmental disorders, including autism, Asperger syndrome, Tourette syndrome, dyslexia, OCD, depression, anxiety disorders and schizophrenia. In addition, many children with mental retardation have attentional dysfunction inappropriate to their overall level of intellectual functioning. Attention deficits are often, but not necessarily associated with hyperactivity of varying degrees. It is possible that attention deficits in Tourette syndrome and OCD (and perhaps also in schizophrenia) may be of a different kind than usually associated with the diagnosis of ADHD and be characterized more by intrusion of obsessive ideas and compulsions to do things (or psychotic thinking) than of primary attention deficits. It is useful to diagnose attention deficits even in the presence of the other diagnoses mentioned. Treatment options could vary depending on the degree of associated attention deficits.

Anxiety

Anxiety states in children are, as yet, poorly understood. Specific study of anxiety has been scant. Panic attacks, similar to panic attacks in adulthood, but sometimes presenting in even more dramatic forms, occur in school age children and may be part of a panic disorder syndrome. Panic amounting to confusional states may be seen in disorders on the autism spectrum (including autistic disorder) and can often be linked to (auditory) overstimulation or verbal misunderstanding. Separation anxiety disorder definitely occurs even in preschool children and may signal as kindergarten or school refusal. Simple phobias are almost universal in young children and, if not severely socially or academically handicapping, should not prompt specific intervention measures. Excessive worrying is common in some shy, but well-adjusted children who have long been referred to as children with emotional disorders. Outcome in such conditions is probably fair or good in most cases. The long-term follow-up of clumsy children indicates that anxiety (and mood) disorders may be one of the most common type of outcome in such cases.

Asperger syndrome

This diagnosis should prompt a consideration of the same type of medical disorders that are associated with autism, even though the yield of medical work-up is likely to be fairly low, with probably less than 10% having an associated medical disorder. From the symptomatic differential diagnostic point of view OCD and schizophrenic disorder are clinically most important, because they may imply different treatment approaches. Autistic disorder is conceptualized as being on a spectrum with Asperger syndrome. Diagnostic boundaries are blurred *vis-à-vis* autistic disorder, on the one hand, and personality disorder/personality traits, on the other.

Autistic disorder/autistic symptomatology

Autistic symptoms should be regarded as a warning that an underlying medical condition might be present. The most common medical disorders associated with autistic symptomatology are some neurocutaneous disorders (tuberous sclerosis neurofibromatosis, Ito's hypomelanosis), fragile X syndrome and, in females, Rett syndrome. A whole host of other conditions should be considered (see Table 6 in Chapter 6) before a diagnosis of idiopathic autistic disorder/childhood autism is made. If onset of autistic symptoms is in the first two years of life, and such symptoms are accompanied (or preceded) by epileptic seizures then a diagnosis of tuberous sclerosis is highly suspect. The presence of skin symptoms and a combination of CAT-scan, MRI-scan and ophthalmological examination will aid in diagnosis. Any girl with very early onset autistic symptoms should raise suspicion of suffering from Rett syndrome. The most salient feature of this diagnosis is the deterioration or complete loss of acquired purposeful hand movements. All individuals with pronounced autistic symptoms (regardless of whether full criteria for autistic disorder/childhood autism are met or not) should be screened for chromosomal abnormality, including fragile X.

Delusions

Delusions are very difficult to diagnose in children with a mental age under 6 years. Further-more, if the parent (or another close person) has delusions, it may be impossible to tease out the extent to which the child is kept in a *folie-à-deux* relationship with the other person or has 'primary' delusions. In Asperger syndrome and high-functioning autism (and perhaps also some cases of Tourette syndrome and borderline intellectual functioning without associated severe psychiatric disorder), concrete thinking and autism-type communication dysfunction may well lead to misinterpretation of events and this may be perceived as 'delusional thinking', even when there is no indication that the delusions are part of, or predisposing to, schizophrenic disorder.

Depression

Depressed mood is a common concomitant of DAMP-syndromes and other neurodevelopmental disorders, particularly in the 9–11 year-old age range. Asperger syndrome, panic disorder and OCD are also commonly superseded by depression in early adolescence. It is also an almost universal symptom in adolescent onset anorexia nervosa. Chronic fatigue syndrome may present with overwhelming depression. Major depression with familial roots may have its onset in childhood. If none of the disorders referred to can account for depression and there is no family history of major depression/bipolar disorder, then there is a need to exclude (at least) thyroid and parathyroid disorder and brain tumours before a diagnosis of major depression is made in a child or adolescent. This holds even if a major psychosocial trigger can be identified. 'Psychological triggers' can often be found in children who do not suffer from depression.

Dyslexia

Dyslexia is a common concomitant of a large number of neuropsychiatric disorders including ADHD, DAMP, Tourette syndrome and Asperger syndrome. These should not be considered alternative, but rather overlapping diagnoses. If there is no family history of dyslexia, a reasonable cause for the reading and spelling problems needs to be identified. Dyslexia is relatively uncommon in females. All girls with dyslexia should be worked up with a view to diagnosing chromosmal abnormality (including fragile X). Some boys also need a work-up of this kind.

Eating disorders/disturbed eating behaviour

Disturbed eating behaviours are very common in young children. Food fads and food refusal are probably the most common types of abnormal eating behaviours in preschool children. Children with autistic disorder, Asperger syndrome, OCD and teenagers who develop anorexia nervosa are particularly likely to have (had) food fads and pica. Other reasons for food refusal and failure to thrive in the first years of life include severe physical disorders (e.g. kidney and heart disease), psychosocial dwarfism, Williams syndrome and Prader-Willi syndrome. Prader–Willi syndrome should always be considered in a young child who is overeating. Abnormal eating behaviours that cannot be reasonable accounted for in young children should prompt a search for an underlying hypothalamic and other endocrine disorders (including tumours such as craniopharyngioma, hypothyroidism, etc.). Anorexia and bulimia nervosa are usually readily diagnosable on the basis of typical behavioural symptoms, but the threshold should be low for in-depth physical work-up, including CAT- and MRI-scans if there is anything atypical in the clinical picture.

Elective mutism

Many normal children refuse to speak for a little while in new surroundings. This is not to be confused with elective mutism. An IQ-test, hearing test and neurodevelopmental examination should always be performed in elective mutism because of its frequent association with low IQ, hearing deficit and specific develop-

mental disorders. Elective mutism sometimes develops in children with high-functioning autism or Asperger syndrome. When occurring without prior warning (i.e. when there has been no clear indication of abnormal development or personality dysfunction), both major psychosocial and biological trauma/change need to be considered in detail.

Explosive behaviour

Explosive behaviours (aggression, attack-behaviours, rage, self-injury) should always lead to EEG examination, which need to be repeated if not informative at first evaluation. Epilepsies of various kinds (complex partial in particular) and intermittent explosive disorder may be the most common diagnoses. Other diagnoses that need to be considered are Prader–Wiili syndrome, tuberous sclerosis, de Lange syndrome, Lesch–Nyhan syndrome, Rett syndrome variant with preserved speech, thyroid disorder, hypoglycaemia (including in diabetes mellitus), cryptogenic autistic disorder, cryptogenic conduct disorder, antisocial and borderline personality disorders.

Hallucinations

Hallucinations occur in children and adolescents, not only in schizophrenic disorder, but for a variety of reasons. Hallucinations are difficult to diagnose in children with a mental age under 6 years. Diagnoses of hallucinations, particularly auditory hallucinations, should be made with extreme restriction in pre-school children. Migraine, epilepsy, side effects of medication and brain tumours (e.g. craniopharyngioma and other tumours in the vicinity of the optic tract) should be considered in all cases of (particularly visual) hallucinations in very young children. In certain cultures (e.g. parts of the West Indies) hallucinations are considered normal phenomena and a child with hallucinations might be considered 'special' in a positive way. Alternatively, there may even be concern that the child is not developing normally if he/

she has never admitted to hallucinations. Some children with severe conduct disorder claim that they are hallucinating and yet do not show other symptoms indicating major psychotic disorders. Grief reactions may be accompanied by hallucinatory experiences, which may be perceived as positive by the affected individual. Hallucinations should always be clearly separated from illusional phenomena. Hallucinations occur in mood disorders, particularly major depression with mood-congruent hallucinations (e.g. hearing a voice telling the child to kill him/herself). Hallucinations in schizophrenic disorder are often less readily admitted to, and may be consciously concealed from, the psychiatrist. Some children with DAMP and Asperger syndrome report strange, 'concrete' hallucination-like experiences. It is unclear to what extent such experiences represent 'true' hallucinations.

Hyperactivity

See ADHD, minor physical anomalies and motor clumsiness. Hyperactivity (hyperkinetic disorder) is a common feature of many neuropsychiatric and physical disorders. Extremes of motor over-activity are often encountered in autism, childhood disintegrative disorder, severe mental retardation without autism, foetal alcohol syndrome, thyroid disorder and, intermittently, in connection with constipation and anal pruritus in young children. Hyperkinetic disorders unassociated with these disorders are usually associated with motor coordination problems, speech–language disorders and/or dyslexia. There is a high rate of minor physical anomalies in groups of children with pervasive hyperkinesis.

Left-handedness

Handedness should be assessed by using a battery of tests (such as the one suggested by Annett, 1970). The preferred hand in at least five different situations should be examined or enquired about. Handedness in children with a mental age of less than 3–5 years is not as informative as in older children. However, most normal children have a clear preference for one hand over the other in many activities already around age 1–4 years. Mixed handedness is a common finding in developmental disorders. A larger proportion of left-handers than right-handers have brain disorder, including epilepsy and autism. Also, unilateral brain damage is more common. If the non-preferred hand has *very* poor motor skills (such as might be demonstrated in the maze-tracing task suggested by Bishop (1980)), this could be an indication that contralateral brain damage has occurred which led to poor motor skills in that hand. The evidence from examination of handedness and motor skills should be combined with family history data regarding the possibility of familial sinistrality before a clinical conclusion regarding the meaning of the child's handedness is made.

Minor physical anomalies

Minor physical anomalies are often found in child neuropsychiatric disorders, including ADHD, DAMP, autism and schizophrenia. Sometimes they may themselves suggest underlying disorder such as in the case of many of the so called 'behavioural phenotype syndromes' (e.g. de Lange syndrome, Down syndrome, Prader–Willi syndrome or Williams syndrome). In most cases, however, they are more unspecific and do not combine to suggest a particular disorder. Nevertheless, they are usefully monitored by rating on a structured scale (such as suggested by Waldrop & Halverson, 1971), and when present at a higher rate than in normal children, may suggest the need for further, including chromosomal, work-up.

Mood disorder

Mood disorders are often misclassified or missed altogether in child psychiatric diagnostic practice. They have not received as comprehensive coverage in the research literature as the other disorders covered in this book, and hence have not been the focus of attention in many pages of this book.

Motor clumsiness/motor coordination problems/soft neurological signs

Motor clumsiness and motor coordination problems are part and parcel of many neuropsychiatric disorders, including DAMP, Asperger syndrome, autistic-like conditions and the fragile X syndrome. Soft neurological signs (dysdiadochokinesis, abnormal associated movements, choreiform movements, etc.) may be the neurological examination equivalent of such clinical symptoms. Soft neurological signs are common not only in the disorders mentioned but also in anorexia nervosa. Prospective studies of children with soft neurological signs in childhood often develop anxiety and mood disorders in adolescence.

OCD/OCPD/obsessive-compulsive symptomatology

Obsessive and compulsive symptoms are common in the general population. It is only when the severity of such problems is sufficient to prompt referral or when there is personal suffering that a diagnosis of OCD should be considered. Obsessions and compulsions are common not only in OCD, but also in Tourette disorder, DAMP, Asperger syndrome, high-functioning autism and anorexia nervosa. OCPD may and may not be associated with severe OCD symptoms. Obsessions and compulsions are often reported to be egodystonic, but this is very often not the case in children and adolescents.

Regression in skills

Whenever a child loses a skill that was previously unequivocally present, this should be taken very seriously and lead to a full neuropsychiatric evaluation as soon as possible. How-

ever, in very young children (under age 2 years), it is sometimes impossible to determine with any degree of accuracy whether a particular skill was present or not, and so the report that one skill, and one skill only, has deteriorated, should always be regarded with slightly more caution, and a full work-up might not be indicated. Nevertheless, even in this young age group, the report of developmental arrest or loss of skills may well signal onset of symptoms in very serious disorders including Rett syndrome and mucopolysaccharidoses. It is often wise to repeat IQ-tests at 3–6 month intervals if there are unsubstantiated claims of deterioration. Parents are often very good at picking up early signs of regression of skills even when the neuropsychiatrist or neurologist cannot make a positive diagnosis or document deterioration (or even plateauing), and should always be 'trusted' until proven wrong. Regression of skills (particularly in the field of fine manipulation) in a female around age 6 months–2 years is highly suspect of Rett syndrome. Regression of skills (particularly in the fields of language and social interaction) around age 3–5 years in children of both sexes suggests the possibility of encephalopathy, encephalitis, childhood disintegrative disorder or Landau–Kleffner syndrome. Regression of academic skills, or plateauing, is seen in many chromosomal disorders, including Down syndrome and the fragile X syndrome. Schizophrenia and major depression with psychotic features may also present with academic deterioration. Anorexia nervosa is often preceded by plateauing of academic achievement, but probably not by intellectual decline. Loss of skills at any age may suggest the presence of a progressive neurometabolic disorder. The reader will need to consult a textbook of child neurology in order to be able to cover all of the possibilities in this field (e.g. Aicardi, 1992).

Schizophrenic disorder

Schizophrenic disorder is extremely uncommon in preadolescent children. A definite diagnosis should not be made in any child until at least two years of intensive clinical follow-up has been achieved. Children with a preliminary diagnosis of schizophrenia during the early school years often have a multitude of neurodevelopmental/neuropsychiatric problems on follow-up a few years later. Neurological and metabolic disorder may well lead to schizophrenic symptoms. A full medical work-up should be performed, similar to that recommended for autistic disorders (see Chapter 6). Encephalitis from viral or bacterial infection is a definite aetiological possibility.

School refusal

School refusal is usually unassociated with specific neuropsychiatric problems. However, occasionally it may be the first 'clinical' sign of severe separation anxiety disorder, panic disorder, elective mutism, Asperger syndrome or neurodevelopmental disorders involving learning problems. Thus, school refusal should not be treated as a purely psychological problem until such disorders have been ruled out.

Self-injurious behaviour

Severe self-injury with a high risk of body injury is the hallmark of Lesch–Nyhan syndrome. Lip-biting and cheek-chewing is particularly common. Ocular self-mutilation may occur specifically in certain metabolic disorders, some of which may be associated with hypocalcinuria and be alleviated by calcium supplementation. Severe self-injury is also common in all variants of autistic disorder/autistic-like conditions. The risk of such behaviour is very high (about 50%) if there is associated mental retardation. Individuals with the fragile X syndrome are prone to mild–moderate wrist/knuckle-biting. Individuals with Tourette syndrome and DAMP often have a history of head-banging/crashing in infancy and early childhood. Such behaviours may be followed by milder self-injury (often involving nails and fingers) at a later age. The type of self-injury inflicted by adolescent girls (wristcutting and -slashing) can be a symp-

tom of underlying borderline personality disorder.

Sleep disorders

Sleep and its disorders should be closely monitored in all children presenting with neuropsychiatric problems or for neuropsychiatric evaluation. Sleep is disturbed in autism, autistic-like conditions, certain forms of epilepsy, some cases of ADHD and DAMP, Tourette disorder, major depression, mania, Kleine–Levin syndrome, narcolepsy and other disorders specifically labelled 'sleep disorders'. Decreased need for sleep is common in autism, autistic-like conditions and mania. Increased need for sleep is common in some cases of DAMP, Kleine–Levin syndrome and narcolepsy. Disruption of the normal diurnal sleep cycle is common in major depression and Tourette disorder. In addition to other abnormal sleep patterns, such disruption also often occurs in mania and certain variants of epilepsy.

Speech–language disorders

Speech–language delay is one of the most universal early signs that a child might be suffering from a neuropsychiatric disorder. It may also be the first symptom of an underlying neurodevelopmental disorder which will later be diagnosed as mental retardation or dyslexia. Thus, any child with clear speech–language delay should be followed closely at least for a few years to determine whether or not clinically relevant neuropsychiatric symptoms (mental retardation, autistic symptoms, semantic pragmatic disorder with social deficits, ADHD, DAMP, dyslexia) will follow in its footsteps. Speech–language delay in girls is almost always a sign of a severe underlying neuropsychiatric/neurodevelopmental disorder, whereas in boys it is sometimes part of a less severe maturational delay. However, even relatively mild speech problems (such as considerable articulation problems at age 5 years) at follow-up are often shown to be precursors of more widespread language dysfuncton. Complete and pervasive speech–language arrest and regression raises the possibility that the child may have Landau–Kleffner syndrome or childhood disintegrative disorder or other major neurological disorder.

Thought disorder

The definition of thought disorder remains a problem in child psychiatry. Thought disorder defies simple operationalization, and diagnostic criteria are difficult to apply reliably. Children with mental retardation, autism and autistic-like conditions all have immature or abnormal thought processes, and many young individuals with Tourette syndrome and OCD have compulsive disruption of 'normal' thinking. However, thought disorder usually infers another type of disturbed thinking, *viz.* that encountered in adults with schizophrenic disorder. In the author's opinion, thought disorder should not be diagnosed in children with a mental age under about 6 years, and, until research provides different guidelines, should be diagnosed very sparingly, if at all, in prepubertal children.

Tics

Tics need to be distinguished from other motor phenomena, including extrapyramidal side effects of neuroleptic medication and motor stereotypies encountered in autism. Sometimes all three groups of phenomena coincide in the same individual. Simple motor tics are extre-

mely common, occurring in more than 10% of all children, and can be difficult to distinguish from normal repetitive movements that children in the first school years can engage in. The more elaborate the tics and the more muscle groups they involve, the more likely that one is dealing with a true tic disorder. It is often difficult (sometimes clinically impossible) to distinguish tics from non-tic-compulsions. If there are vocal tics in combination with multiple motor tics, Tourette disorder is probably the correct diagnosis. Tics and Tourette disorder are common co-morbid problems in Asperger syndrome, high-functioning autism, OCD, DAMP and other attention deficits and should not be considered an 'either-or-diagnosis' if such problems/disorders are present. It is essential to consider the possibility that abnormal muscle twitching seen in severe and progressive neurological disorder may masquerade as 'tics' in the early stages of the disorder.

References

Aicardi, J. (Ed.) (1992). *Disease of the Nervous System in Childhood. Clinics in Development Medicine, N. 115/118.* London: MacKeith Press.

Annett, M. (1970). A classification of hand preference by association analysis. *British Journal of Psychology,* **16**, 303–21.

Bishop, D.V.M. (1980). Handedness, clumsiness and cognitive ability. *Developmental Medicine and Child Neurology,* **22**, 569–79.

Waldrop, M., Halverson, C. (1971). Minor physical anomalies hyperactive behaviour in young children. *In* Helmuth, J. (Eds.) *The Exceptional Infant.* New York: Brunner-Mazel.

INDEX

354